ESSENTIAL PSYCHOTHERAPIES

ESSENTIAL PSYCHOTHERAPIES

Second Edition

Theory and Practice

Edited by

ALAN S. GURMAN
STANLEY B. MESSER

THE GUILFORD PRESS
New York   London

© 2003 The Guilford Press
A Division of Guilford Publications, Inc.
72 Spring Street, New York, NY 10012
www.guilford.com

Printed in the United States of America

This book is printed on acid-free paper.

Last digit is print number: 9 8 7 6 5 4 3 2 1

Library of Congress Cataloging-in-Publication Data

Essential psychotherapies : theory and practice / edited by Alan S.
Gurman, Stanley B. Messer.—2nd ed.
        p. cm.
Includes bibliographical references and index.
     ISBN 1-57230-766-8
  1. Psychotherapy.   I. Gurman, Alan S.   II. Messer, Stanley B.
     RC480.E69 2003
     616.89′14—dc21   2003003983

To our children—
Jesse and Ted Gurman
Elana, Leora, and Tova Messer

About the Editors

Alan S. Gurman, PhD, is Professor of Psychiatry and Director of Family Therapy Training at the University of Wisconsin Medical School. He has authored and edited a number of highly acclaimed books, including *Clinical Handbook of Couple Therapy, Handbook of Family Therapy,* and *Theory and Practice of Brief Therapy.* A past editor of the *Journal of Marital and Family Therapy* and past president of the Society for Psychotherapy Research, Dr. Gurman is a pioneer in the development of integrative approaches to marital therapy and has received numerous awards for his contributions to the family therapy field. He also practices psychotherapy in Madison, Wisconsin.

Stanley B. Messer, PhD, is Professor and Dean of the Graduate School of Applied and Professional Psychology at Rutgers University. He is coauthor of *Models of Brief Psychodynamic Therapy: A Comparative Approach* and coeditor of several volumes, including *Theories of Psychotherapy: Origins and Evolution, History of Psychotherapy: A Century of Change, Hermeneutics and Psychological Theory,* and *Psychoanalytic Therapy and Behavior Therapy: Is Integration Possible?*. Dr. Messer has also written many articles on psychotherapy integration, brief psychodynamic therapy, and case formulation, among other topics, and has conducted empirical research on the process of psychotherapy. He was Associate Editor of *American Psychologist* and is on the editorial board of several journals. Dr. Messer also practices psychotherapy in Highland Park, New Jersey.

Contributors

Martin M. Antony, PhD, Anxiety Treatment and Research Center, St. Joseph's Healthcare, and Department of Psychiatry and Behavioral Neurosciences, McMaster University, Hamilton, Ontario, Canada

Arthur C. Bohart, PhD, Department of Psychology, California State University–Dominguez Hills, Carson, California, and Saybrook Graduate School and Research Center, San Francisco, California

Sara K. Bridges, PhD, Counseling Psychology Program, Department of Counseling, Educational Psychology, and Research, University of Memphis, Memphis, Tennessee

Marianne Celano, PhD, Department of Psychiatry and Behavioral Sciences, Emory University School of Medicine, Atlanta, Georgia

Rebecca C. Curtis, PhD, Derner Institute of Advanced Psychological Studies, Adelphi University, Garden City, New York, and William Alanson White Institute for Psychoanalysis, New York, New York

Barbara M. Dausch, PhD, Veterans Administration Health Care System, Palo Alto, California

Robert R. Dies, PhD, private practice, New Port Richey, Florida

Arthur Freeman, EdD, Department of Clinical Psychology, Philadelphia College of Osteopathic Medicine, Philadelphia, Pennsylvania

Jerry Gold, PhD, Derner Institute of Advanced Psychological Studies, Adelphi University, Garden City, New York

Alan S. Gurman, PhD, Department of Psychiatry, University of Wisconsin–Madison, Madison, Wisconsin

Irwin Hirsch, PhD, William Alanson White Institute for Psychoanalysis, New York, New York, and Derner Institute of Advanced Psychological Studies, Adelphi University, Garden City, New York

Michael F. Hoyt, PhD, Kaiser Permanente Medical Center, San Rafael, California, and University of California School of Medicine, San Francisco, California

Nadine J. Kaslow, PhD, Department of Psychiatry and Behavioral Sciences, Emory University School of Medicine, Atlanta, Georgia

Stanley B. Messer, PhD, Graduate School of Applied and Professional Psychology, Rutgers University, and Robert Wood Johnson Medical School, Piscataway, New Jersey

Robert A. Neimeyer, PhD, Department of Psychiatry, University of Memphis, Memphis, Tennessee

Mark A. Reinecke, PhD, Department of Psychology and Behavioral Science, Northwestern University, Chicago, Illinois

Lizabeth Roemer, PhD, Department of Psychology, University of Massachusetts at Boston, Boston, Massachusetts

Kirk J. Schneider, PhD, Existential–Humanistic Institute and Saybrook Graduate School and Research Center, San Francisco, California

George Stricker, PhD, Department of Psychology, Adelphi University, Garden City, New York

David L. Wolitzky, PhD, Department of Psychology, New York University, New York, New York

Contents

1. **Contemporary Issues in the Theory and Practice of Psychotherapy: A Framework for Comparative Study**   1
   Alan S. Gurman and Stanley B. Messer

2. **The Theory and Practice of Traditional Psychoanalytic Treatment**   24
   David L. Wolitzky

3. **Relational Approaches to Psychoanalytic Psychotherapy**   69
   Rebecca C. Curtis and Irwin Hirsch

4. **Person-Centered Psychotherapy and Related Experiential Approaches**   107
   Arthur C. Bohart

5. **Existential–Humanistic Psychotherapies**   149
   Kirk J. Schneider

6. **Behavior Therapy**   182
   Martin M. Antony and Lizabeth Roemer

7. **Cognitive Therapy**   224
   Mark A. Reinecke and Arthur Freeman

8. **Postmodern Approaches to Psychotherapy**   272
   Robert A. Neimeyer and Sara K. Bridges

9. **Integrative Approaches to Psychotherapy**   317
   George Stricker and Jerry Gold

10. **Brief Psychotherapies**   350
    Michael F. Hoyt

11. **Family Therapies**   400
    Nadine J. Kaslow, Barbara M. Dausch, and Marianne Celano

12. **Marital Therapies**   463
     Alan S. Gurman

13. **Group Psychotherapies**   515
     Robert R. Dies

     Author Index   551

     Subject Index   565

1

Contemporary Issues in the Theory and Practice of Psychotherapy

A Framework for Comparative Study

ALAN S. GURMAN
STANLEY B. MESSER

This book presents the core theoretical and applied aspects of essential psychotherapies in contemporary clinical practice. For us, "essential" approaches do not include those that appear to be generating momentary enthusiasm but are likely to soon vanish from the therapeutic scene. In our view, essential psychotherapies are those that form the conceptual and clinical bedrock of psychotherapeutic training, practice, and research. We believe there are two quite distinct categories of essential psychotherapies. First, there are those approaches whose origins are found in the earliest phases of the history of psychotherapy. Although the foundational and defining attributes of these methods have largely endured across several generations of psychotherapists, they have been revised and refined considerably over time. Examples of such time-honored approaches are traditional and relational approaches to psychoanalytic psychotherapy; existential–humanistic, person-centered, and experiential approaches; behavior therapy; and group therapy. Second, the essential psychotherapies presented here include several

that have been developed relatively recently; have had undeniably strong effects on practice, training, and research; and are likely to endure long into the future. Examples are the cognitive, postmodern, brief, family, marital, and integrative approaches.

INTRODUCING *ESSENTIAL PSYCHOTHERAPIES*

As intended in its first edition, *Essential Psychotherapies* has become a primary reference source for comprehensive presentations of the most prominent contemporary influences in the field of psychotherapy. Although there are literally hundreds of differently labeled "psychotherapies" (the great majority of which are really only partial methods, single techniques, or minor variations on existing techniques or approaches) (Bergin & Garfield, 1994), we continue to believe that those can be subsumed by about a dozen quite distinguishable types. As editors, we have challenged our contributing authors to convey not only what

1

is basic and core to their ways of thinking and working but also what is new and forward-looking in theory, practice, and research. Our contributors, all eminent clinical scholars (and all practicing clinicians, as well), have aggregately helped to forge a volume that is well suited to exposing advanced undergraduates, beginning graduate students, and trainees in all the mental health professions to the major schools and methods of modern psychotherapy. Because all the chapters were written by cutting-edge representatives of their therapeutic approaches, there is something genuinely new to these presentations that will be of value to more experienced therapists as well.

As in the first edition, each chapter offers a clear sense of the history, current status, assessment approach, and methods of the therapy being discussed, along with its foundational ideas about personality and psychological health and dysfunction. As both academicians and practicing psychotherapists, we endorse the adage that there is nothing so practical as a good theory. Each chapter balances the discussion of theory and practice and emphasizes the interplay between them.

Before detailing our organizing framework for the chapters in this book, three comments about its contents are in order. First, while *Essential Psychotherapies* provides substantive presentations of the major "schools" of psychotherapeutic thought and general guidelines for practice, it does not emphasize treatment prescriptions for specific disorders or "special populations." Although forces in the contemporary world of psychotherapy support a rather broad movement to specify particular techniques for particular problems and types of persons, we continue to believe that the majority of practitioners approach their work from the standpoint of theory as it informs general strategies and techniques of practice. Moreover, we believe that such an emphasis on the interplay between theory and practice is consistent with an emerging, balanced approach to psychotherapy training,

which attends not only to exposure to empirically supported treatments and techniques but also to those aspects of the psychotherapy relationship that have a marked effect on our work (Gurman & Razin, 1977; Norcross, 2002).

Second, there is today a great deal of energy being devoted to the development and refinement of integrative approaches to psychotherapy (see Stricker & Gold, Chapter 9, for a comprehensive view of integrative approaches). While we value the search for integrative principles and common factors that transcend particular therapies (Gurman, 2001, 2002; Messer, 2001), we support the continuing practice of teaching about relatively distinct schools or systems of psychotherapy. For therapists to become integrative effectively, they must master the foundational theories from which such integrations evolve. Moreover, theoretical integration itself cannot evolve without these basic theories remaining intact (Liddle, 1982).

Relatedly, an aspect of therapeutic integration that is rarely discussed (cf. Lebow, 1987) is how the method or methods to which a therapist primarily adheres and the therapist's personality interact to increase his or her attraction to such methods (and probably his or her disinterest in, or even distaste for, other approaches). As Gurman (1983) has emphasized, "The choice of a favorite method of psychotherapy . . . is always very personal." The field of psychotherapy provides enough variety of styles and ideas to match the personal predilections of any aspiring clinician.

THE EVOLUTION OF PSYCHOTHERAPY AND OF *ESSENTIAL PSYCHOTHERAPIES*

The essential psychotherapies of the new millennium are not the same essential psychotherapies of the era in which the editors of this book were graduate students. Though the essential approaches are largely the same as when this volume first appeared in 1995, there have been some important changes in the landscape of psychotherapy since then. First, Gestalt therapy and transactional analysis, popular and prominent approaches in earlier times, seem largely to have evaporated from view, as psychotherapy generally has become increasingly pragmatic, short term, and problem focused. As a result, the separate chapters on these approaches that appeared in the first edition of this volume do not appear in the present edition (although Gestalt therapy is discussed in Bohart, Chapter 4, on person-centered and related experiential approaches).

Conversely, two approaches to psychotherapy that did not appear in the first edition appear here for the first time. Postmodern approaches to psychotherapy, which have their origins in both midcentury academic psychology (e.g., the Personal Construct Therapy of George Kelly, 1955/1991) and the social constructionist movement in psychotherapy during the last decade or so (e.g., Michael White's [White & Epston, 1990] influential "Narrative" therapy), have widely influenced the practice of both individual and more family- and couple-oriented clinical work. Marital (or couple) therapy, most often considered to be a subspecialty of family therapy, is probably the most widely practiced form of family therapy. In the last decade, marital therapy has evolved in some directions so independently of the broader family field, however, that it now has a conceptual, clinical, and empirical identity quite its own (Gurman & Fraenkel, 2002). For these reasons, marital therapy is included here in a separate chapter from the one dealing with family therapy.

The various models of psychotherapy appearing here stem from different views of human nature, about which there is no universal agreement. These schools of therapy embrace fundamentally different ways of getting to know clients, which stem from different epistemological outlooks (e.g., introspective vs. extraspective; Messer & Winokur, 1980). In addition, these therapies encompass distinct visions of reality (e.g., tragic, comic, romantic, and ironic views of life; Messer & Winokur, 1984). They also vary in the extent to which they incorporate the belief that fundamental change is possible, or even what constitutes that change.

We believe that it is important for the field, and for a volume such as this one, to respect the search for common principles in theory and practice while continuing to appreciate and highlight the different perspectives each model or school of therapy exemplifies.

A FRAMEWORK FOR COMPARING THE PSYCHOTHERAPIES

It is not the answer that enlightens, but the questions.
—Eugene Ionesco

Our theories are our inventions; but they may be merely ill-reasoned guesses, bold conjectures, hypotheses. Out of these we create a world, not the real world, but our own nets in which we try to catch the real world.
—Karl Popper

As in the first edition of *Essential Psychotherapies*, we provided the authors a comprehensive set of guidelines. These guidelines have proven useful in facilitating readers' comparative study of the major models of contemporary psychotherapy and may also be used by the student as a template for studying therapeutic approaches not included here. We believe that these guidelines include the basic and requisite elements of an adequate description of any approach to psychotherapy.

In presenting these guidelines to our authors, we aimed to steer a midcourse between constraining the authors' expository creativity and providing the reader with sufficient anchor points for comparative study. We believe that our contributors succeeded in following these guidelines while describing their respective approaches in an engaging way. We encouraged authors to sequence their material within chapter sections according to their own preferences. They were also advised that they need not limit their presentations to the matters raised in the guidelines, and certainly need not address every point identified in the guidelines, but that they should address these matters if they were relevant to the treatment approach being described. Authors were also allowed to merge sections of the guidelines, if doing so helped them communicate their perspectives more meaningfully.

We believe that the authors' flexible adherence to the guidelines helped to make clear how theory helps to organize clinical work and facilitates case conceptualization. The inclusion of clinical case material in each chapter serves to illustrate the constructs and methods described previously.

Although most of our author guidelines remained unchanged from the first edition, we did make some significant additions to and modifications of those original guidelines. We added two new sections— "Research Support" and "Current and Future Trends" in the therapeutic approach. Moreover, we instructed our authors to pay more attention than in the first edition to the role of the therapeutic relationship, the relevance of cultural diversity, the place of psychiatric diagnosis and the use of medications, and method-specific ethical considerations.

We now present these author guidelines, along with our rationale and commentaries on each area. In this fashion, we hope to bring the reader up to date on continuing issues and controversies in the field.

HISTORICAL BACKGROUND

History is the version of past events that people have decided to agree on.
                                    —NAPOLEON BONAPARTE

Purpose: To place the approach in historical perspective within the field of psychotherapy.

Points to consider:

1. Cite the major influences that contributed to the development of the approach (e.g., people, books, research, theories, conferences). What were the sociohistorical forces or *Zeitgeist* that shaped the emergence and development of this approach (Victorian era, American pragmatism, modernism, postmodernism, etc.)?
2. The therapeutic forms, if any, that were forerunners of the approach (psychoanalysis, learning theory, organismic theory, etc.).
3. Types of patients with whom the approach was initially developed, and speculations as to why.
4. Early theoretical speculations and/or therapy techniques.

People's lives can be significantly influenced for the better in a wide range of ways—for example, a parent adopts a new approach toward his defiant adolescent, a member of the clergy facilitates a congregant's self-forgiveness, an athletic coach serves as a life-altering "role model" for a student, and so on. Yet none of these, or other commonly occurring, healing, or behavior-changing experiences, qualifies as psychotherapeutic. That is, *psychotherapy is not defined as any experience that leads to desirable psychological outcomes. Rather, it refers to a particular process.* Although written over three decades ago, Meltzoff and Kornreich's (1970) definition of psychotherapy seems to us not to have yet been improved upon:

> Psychotherapy is . . . the informed and planful application of techniques derived from established psychological principles, by persons qualified through training and experience to understand these principles and to apply these techniques with the intention of assisting individuals to modify such personal characteristics as feelings, values, attitudes and behaviors which are judged by the therapist to be maladaptive or maladjustive. (p. 4)

Given such a definition of (any) psychotherapy, we believe that developing an understanding and appreciation of the professional roots and historical context of psychotherapeutic models is an essential aspect of one's education as a therapist. Lacking such awareness, the student of psychotherapy is likely to find therapy theories rather disembodied abstractions that seem to evolve from nowhere, and for no known reason. We noted earlier that each therapist's choice of a theoretical orientation (including any variation of an eclectic or integrative mélange) ultimately reflects a personal process. In addition, an important aspect of a therapist's ability to help people change lies not only in his or her belief in the more technical aspects of the chosen orientation but also in the worldview implicit in it (Frank & Frank, 1991; Messer & Winokur, 1984). Having some exposure to the historical origins of a therapeutic approach helps clinicians comprehend such an implicit worldview. The reader interested in detailed analyses of the historical backdrops against which most major systems of therapy were developed is referred to Freedheim and colleagues (1992).

In addition to appreciating the professional roots of therapeutic methods, it is enlightening to understand why particular methods, or sometimes clusters of related methods, appear on the scene in particular historical periods. The intellectual, economic, and political contexts in which therapeutic approaches arise often provide meaningful clues about the emerging social, scientific, and philosophical values that frame clinical encounters. Such values may have a subtle but salient impact on whether newer treatment approaches endure. For example, until quite recently, virtually all the influential and dominant models of psychotherapy (cf. Bergin & Garfield, 1994; Bongar & Bentler, 1995; Corsini & Wedding, 1995; Lynn & Garske, 1985) have derived from three philosophic traditions: psychoanalysis, humanism, and behaviorism. In the last two decades in particular,

however, two newer conceptual forces have shaped the landscape of psychotherapy in visible ways. The systems-oriented methods of family and couple therapy have grown out of an increasing awareness of the contextual embeddedness of all human behavior. Relatedly, even more traditional therapeutic approaches, such as those grounded in psychoanalytic thinking, have become more relational in recent times. And postmodernism, a modern multinational intellectual movement that extends well beyond the realm of psychotherapy into the worlds of art, drama, literature, political science, and so on, questions the time-honored notion of a fully knowable and objective external reality, arguing that all "knowledge" is local, relative, and socially constructed.

Likewise, emerging integrative and brief psychotherapeutic approaches have gained increased recognition and stature in the last two decades, in part in response to increased societal (as well as professional) expectations that psychotherapy demonstrate both its efficacy and its efficiency.

THE CONCEPT OF PERSONALITY

Children are natural mimics—they act like their parents in spite of every attempt to teach them good manners.
—ANONYMOUS

Purpose: To describe within the therapeutic framework the conceptualization of personality.

Points to consider:

1. Is the concept of "personality" meaningful within your approach, or is there some other psychological or physical unit that is more meaningful?
2. What are the basic psychological concepts used to understand patients?
3. What is the theory of personality development in this approach?

PSYCHOLOGICAL HEALTH AND PATHOLOGY

Utopias will come to pass when we grow wings and all people are converted into angels.
—FYODOR DOSTOYEVSKI

Purpose: To describe the way in which psychological health and pathology are conceptualized within the approach.

Points to consider:

1. Describe any formal or informal system for diagnosing or typing patients.
2. How do symptoms or problems develop? How are they maintained?
3. What determines the type of symptoms or problems to appear?
4. Are there other dimensions that need to be considered in describing psychological dysfunction?
5. Is there a concept of the ideal or healthy personality within this approach?

All approaches to psychotherapy are attempts to change or improve some aspect of personality or problematic behavior. Yet *not all theories of therapy include a concept of personality, nor do all theories of personality necessarily have a companion theory of change.* For example, one form of personality theory is known as trait theory, the most prominent current form of which is the "five-factor model" (Hofstee, 2003). The five factors or dimensions said to describe personality as derived from factor-analytic studies are Neuroticism, Extroversion, Openness to Experience, Agreeableness, and Conscientiousness. There is no therapy or change process corresponding to this theory. On the flip side of the coin, and more pertinent to this volume, is that there are some theories of therapy that are not linked to a specific theory of personality. A good example is behavior therapy, which accounts for consistency in people's behavior with concepts such as conditioned and operant learning, stimulus generalization, and modeling.

Although there are different definitions of what constitutes personality, three elements are usually included:

1. Personality is not merely a collection of individual traits or disconnected behaviors, but is structured, organized and integrated.
2. This structural criterion implies a degree of consistency and stability in personality functioning. Behavioral manifestations of that structure may vary, however, according to the situational context. This is due to behavior being a function of the interaction of personality and situational factors.
3. There is a developmental aspect to personality, which takes into account childhood and adolescent experience. That is, personality emerges over time out of a matrix of biological and social influences.

There exists an intimate connection between personality theory and the mechanisms posited to bring about change by any theory of psychotherapy. Psychoanalysis, for example, emphasizes unconscious aspects of human functioning, including disguised motives, ambivalence in all human relations, and intricate interactions among the structures of mind, namely, id, ego, and superego. Thus, it is not surprising that an essential curative factor in this theory is interpretation of motives, defenses, conflicts, and other hidden features of personality. A cognitive theory of personality, by contrast, is based on the assumption that there are mental structures that determine how an individual comes to evaluate and interpret information related to the self and others. In particular, this theory posits "scripts" (Abelson, 1981) or "schemas" (Neisser, 1967) that organize and determine individuals' behavior, affect and experience. Psychotherapy, within this approach, involves cognitive reeducation, in the course of which old, irrational, or maladaptive cognitions are unlearned and replaced by new, more adaptive ones. As well, areas of deficiency are remedied by the learning of new cognitive skills (Messer & Warren, 1990).

Much can go awry in the developing personality due to biological or psychosocial factors. Symptoms can result from contemporaneous stresses and strains or, more typically, from the interaction of a personality disposition with a current event that triggers emotional disturbance or maladaptive interpersonal behavior. Although some theories avoid the use of language and labels that pathologize human experience, they still speak clearly about what constitutes maladaptive behavior. Thus, even schools of therapy that do not formally judge the health of a person based on external criteria such as symptoms or interpersonal difficulties do attend to the consequences of behavior in terms of that person's welfare and interest.

It should be noted that psychological disorders possess no natural boundaries but only loose categorical coherence. This is not an instance in which nature is carved at its joints. All efforts to date have failed to identify objective features that underlie the various mental disorders as characterized by *Diagnostic and Statistical Manual of Mental Disorders* (DSM), the manual of psychiatric disorders. What people seem to agree on is their undesirability, which is more a moral than a scientific valuation (Woolfolk, 1998). In fact, *a therapy may reveal its esthetic and moral values by how it conceptualizes mental health and psychological well-being.* For example, "Psychoanalysis puts forth the ideal of the genital personality, humanistic psychology the self-actualized person, and cognitive-behavior therapy, the objective problem-solving human being" (Messer & Woolfolk, 1998, p. 257).

In other words, the terms of personality theory, psychopathology, and the goals of psychotherapy are not neutral (cf. London, 1986). They are embedded in a value structure that determines what is most important to know about and change in an individual, couple, family or group. Even schools of

psychotherapy that attempt to be neutral with regard to what constitutes healthy (and, therefore, desirable) behavior and unhealthy (and, therefore, undesirable) behavior inevitably, if unwittingly, reinforce the acceptability of some kinds of client strivings more so than others.

Modes of assessing personality and pathology are closely linked to the underlying theory. If the latter focuses on unconscious factors, for example, collecting dreams and early memories may be considered a more fertile model of assessment than self-report questionnaires (Messer & Warren, 1990). In the following chapters, the reader is encouraged to look for the links among personality theory, mode of describing psychopathology, manner of assessing these dimensions, and the kind of change that is sought after.

THE PROCESS OF CLINICAL ASSESSMENT

If you are sure you understand everything that is going on, you are hopelessly confused.
—WALTER MONDALE

Purpose: To describe the methods used to gain understanding of an individual's style or pattern of interaction, symptomatology, and adaptive resources.

Points to consider:

1. At what unit level(s) is assessment made (e.g., individual, dyadic, system)?
2. At what psychological levels is assessment made (e.g., intrapsychic, behavioral, systemic)?
3. To what extent and in what ways are cultural factors (e.g., ethnicity, race, religion, social class, gender) considered in your assessment?
4. Are any tests, devices, questionnaires, or structured observations typically used?
5. Is assessment separate from treatment or integrated with it; for example, what is

the temporal relation between assessment and treatment?

6. Are the patient's strengths/resources a focus of your assessment? If so, in what way?

7. What other dimensions or factors are typically involved in assessing dysfunction?

8. What, if any, is the role of standard psychiatric diagnosis in your assessment?

The practicality of a good theory of psychotherapy, including ideas about personality development and psychological dysfunction, becomes evident as the therapist tries to make sense of both problem stability (how problems persist) and problem change (how problems can be modified). As indicated earlier in Meltzoff and Kornreich's (1970) definition of psychotherapy, the therapist is obligated to take some purposeful action in regard to his or her understanding of the nature and parameters of whatever problems, symptoms, complaints, or dilemmas are presented. Therapists typically will be interested in understanding what previous steps patients have taken to resolve or improve their difficulties, and what adaptive resources the patient, and possibly other people in the patient's world, has for doing so. Moreover, the therapist will pay attention to the cultural (ethnic, racial, religious, social class, gender) context in which clinically relevant concerns arise. Such contextualizing factors can play an important role in how the therapist collaboratively both defines the problem at hand and selects a general strategy for addressing the problem therapeutically. As Hayes and Toarmino (1995) have emphasized, understanding the cultural context in which problems are embedded can serve as an important source of hypotheses about what maintains problems and what types of interventions may be helpful.

How therapists actually engage in clinical assessment will vary from one approach to another, but all include face-to-face clinical interviews. Probably the majority of therapists emphasize the immediate therapist–patient conversation as the source of such understanding. A smaller number of therapists will also opt to complement such conversations with direct observations of the problem as it occurs (e.g., in family and couple conflict situations, or in cases involving anxiety-based avoidance of specific stimuli). In addition, some therapists regularly include in the assessment process a variety of patient self-report questionnaires or inventories and may also use structured interview guides, which are usually research-based instruments. Generally, therapists who use such devices have specialized clinical practices (e.g., focusing on a particular set of clinical disorders for which such measures have been specifically designed).

The place of standard psychiatric diagnosis in the clinical assessment phase of psychotherapy likewise varies widely. The overwhelming majority of psychotherapists of different theoretical orientations routinely consider the traditional diagnostic psychiatric status of patients according to the criteria of the fourth edition of DSM (American Psychiatric Association, 1994), at least to meet requirements for financial reimbursement, maintenance of legally required treatment records, and other such institutional contingencies. Although engaging in such formal diagnostic procedures may provide a useful orientation to the general area of a patient's concerns, every method of psychotherapy has developed and refined its own, more fine-grained, idiosyncratic ways of understanding each individual patient's problem. Moreover, some newer approaches to psychotherapy argue that "diagnoses" do not exist "out there" in nature but merely represent the consensual labels attached to certain patterns of behavior in particular cultural and historical contexts. Such therapy approaches see the use of diagnostic labeling as an unfortunate and unwarranted assumption of the role of "expert" by therapists, which may inhibit genuine collaborative exploration between therapists and "patients" (or "clients"). For such therapists, what matters more are the more fluid issues that people struggle with, not the diagnoses they are given.

All things considered, the primary dimension along which clinical assessments vary is the intrapersonal–interpersonal. Some therapy models emphasize "intrapsychic" processes, whereas others emphasize social interaction. In fact, there is a constant interplay between people's "inner" and "outer" lives. Emphasis on one domain "versus" another reflects an arbitrary punctuation of human experience that probably says as much about the theory of the perceiver as it does about the client who is perceived.

THE PRACTICE OF THERAPY

All knowledge is sterile which does not lead to action and end in charity.
—CARDINAL MERCIER

Purpose: To describe the typical structure, goals, techniques, strategies, and process of a particular approach to therapy and their tactical purposes.

Points to consider:

A. *Basic Structure of Therapy*
   1. How often are sessions typically held?
   2. Is therapy time-limited or unlimited? Why? How long does therapy typically last? How long are typical sessions?
   3. Who is typically included in therapy? Are combined formats (e.g., individual plus family or group sessions) ever used?
   4. How structured are therapy sessions?
B. *Goal Setting*
   1. Are there treatment goals that apply to all or most cases for which the treatment is appropriate (see "Treatment Applicability") regardless of presenting problem or symptom?
   2. Of the number of possible goals for a given patient group, how are the cen-

tral goals selected? How are they prioritized?
   3. Do cultural factors (e.g., race, religion, social class, ethnicity, gender) typically influence the setting of treatment goals?
   4. Do you distinguish between intermediate or mediating goals and ultimate goals?
   5. Who determines the goals of treatment? Therapist, individual, both, or other? How are differences in goals resolved? To what extent and in what ways are therapist values involved in goal setting?
   6. Is it important that treatment goals be discussed with patients explicitly? If yes, why? If not, why not?
   7. At what level of psychological experience are goals established (are they described in overt, behavioral terms, in affective-cognitive terms, etc.)?
C. *Process Aspects of Treatment*
   1. Identify, describe, and illustrate with brief case vignettes major commonly used techniques and strategies.
   2. How is the decision made to use a particular technique or strategy at a particular time? Typically, are different techniques used in different phases of therapy?
   3. Are "homework" or other out-of-session tasks used?
   4. What are the most commonly encountered forms of resistance to change? How are these dealt with?
   5. What are both the most common and the most serious technical errors a therapist can make operating within your therapeutic approach?
   6. Are psychotropic medications ever used (either by the primary psychotherapist or in collaboration with a medical colleague) within your approach? What are the indications/contraindications for their use?
   7. On what basis is termination decided and how is termination effected?

Psychotherapy is not only a scientific and value-laden enterprise but also part and parcel of its surrounding culture. It is a significant source of our current customs and worldviews and thus possesses significance well beyond the interactions between clients and therapists. For example, when laypeople refer to Freudian slips, defenses, guilt complexes, conditioned responses, existential angst, identity crises, co-dependency, enabling partner, or discovering their true self, they are demonstrating the impact of psychological and psychotherapeutic categories on their vocabulary and cultural conversations. Similarly, when they explain their problems in terms of childhood occurrences such as parental neglect, repressed memories, conditioned emotional reactions, or lack of unconditional positive regard, they are affirming that the institution of psychotherapy is much more than a technical, medical, or scientific endeavor. It helps to shape the very terms in which people think, and even constitutes the belief system they use to explain and make sense out of their lives (Messer & Woolfolk, 1998).

At the same time, psychotherapy is a sensitive barometer of those customs and outlooks, which the different modes of practice are responsive to and incorporate within their purview. The relation between psychotherapy and culture, then, is one of reciprocal influence (Messer & Wachtel, 1997). For example, two currently important cultural phenomena affecting the practice of psychotherapy are the corporatization of the mental health service delivery system and the medicalization of how psychological disorder is treated. Regarding the former, *the advent of managed health care* has had a strong impact on the practice of psychotherapy. Managed care itself was a response to rapidly rising health care costs and the efforts of large businesses to curtail them. Managed care organizations (MCOs) were created to handle health care for such large corporations and did so by charging a dollar amount per month for each person they contracted to cover. The MCOs,

which were assuming the health care financial risks, could only make a profit if costs were held down, thus producing a strong incentive to keep payments to health service providers to a minimum.

What this typically meant was that MCOs would cover only a certain number of psychotherapy sessions, or a certain dollar amount per year. This, in turn, brought about the flourishing of brief or time–limited therapy and, simultaneously, decreased the affordability and attractiveness of longer-term therapies. As it happens, the more behavioral, cognitive, family, and marital therapies tend to be short term in outlook (e.g., Gurman, 2001), whereas the psychoanalytic (both traditional and relational), existential, and experiential therapies are more open ended. The former group of therapies is briefer because they are typically problem focused and goal oriented, whereas the latter are typically more exploratory and depth oriented in their modus operandi. In this way, an economic issue reverberated through the health care culture, supporting certain kinds of practice and diminishing others. We wish to emphasize that this effect is not due primarily to scientific findings, clinical judgment, or popular demand but, rather, to the economic needs of American business and the nation at large. Although we value the practice of brief therapy (e.g., Messer, Sanderson, & Gurman, 2003), we also believe that both short- and long-term therapy should be available as possible choices for patients according to professionally judged and documented need. To illustrate that the provision of long-term therapy in the United States is a possible option, we note that psychoanalysis is included in government health care coverage in Germany.

Regarding the medicalization of mental health treatment, the language of medicine has long been prominent in the field of psychotherapy. We talk of "symptoms," "diseases," "disorders," "psychopathology," and "treatment." As Messer and Wachtel (1997) remarked, "it is a kind of new narrative that reframes people's conflicts over value and moral questions as sequelae of 'disease' or 'disorder,' thereby bringing into play the prestige (and hence curative potential) accruing to medicine and technology in our society" (p. 3). Modern psychotherapy started with Freud, who was a physician. As the major practitioners of therapy were physicians for at least the first half of the last century, the language of medicine came naturally to them. In addition, they wished to see psychotherapy as an integral part of the medical profession. Quite aside from these historical influences, in the latter half of the 20th century there has been good reason to consider treatment of mental disorders as medical. There are now medications that have been at least moderately successful in treating various mental conditions such as bipolar disorder, schizophrenia, depression, and anxiety. The popular success and research backing of some medications has even led some psychologists to lobby for attainment of prescription privileges. Were this to occur, it would have a huge impact on the practice of psychotherapy.

Medication for conditions such as anxiety, social phobia, and depression are now promoted on TV directly to the consumer, with the promise of the pill removing a person's worries and blues. Thus, the drug companies have played their part in promoting a biological approach to mental disorder. Many such symptoms, however, are closely related to interpersonal conflicts and other problems in living which are not so readily dispatched. Regarding the symptoms of depression, at least among outpatients, psychotherapy and medication are usually equivalent in the short run, with psychotherapy (usually cognitive-behavioral therapy) reducing the risk of relapse. In the case of depression, research has shown that about three-quarters of the effect of medication is placebo or suggestion (Kirsch & Sapirstein, 1999). Brief forms of cognitive therapy, behavior therapy, and interpersonal therapy have all been shown to do as well as medication in alleviating depression, with-

out side effects or the loss of empowerment that the former may entail (Hollon, Thase, & Markowitz, 2002). Recent research indicates, however, that there is some advantage in combining psychotherapy with medication in the treatment of depression, which may lead to more integrative modes of practice (de Jonghe, Kool, van Aalst, Dekker, & Peen, 2001).

The point we wish to make is that the spread of the biological way of understanding psychopathology and personality traits, as well as the biological mode of treating emotional disorders, has had its effects on the practice of psychotherapy. Clients and therapists are more likely to consider having medication prescribed. Psychologists and other nonmedical therapists are collaborating more frequently with physicians in treating their patients. Courses in psychopharmacology are now routinely offered or even required in counseling, clinical, and psychiatric social work training programs. This trend has also been supported by MCOs, which consider medication a less expensive alternative to psychotherapy. Thus, there are two powerful challenges to traditional psychotherapy that threaten to diminish its status and cloud its future. From our standpoint, it would be unfortunate if the range of essential therapies that are herein described were not taught and practiced, if the psychological outlook these essential therapies convey were not respected, and if the important kind of psychological help these therapies offer were less available.

THE THERAPEUTIC RELATIONSHIP AND THE STANCE OF THE THERAPIST

It is only an auctioneer who can equally and impartially admire all schools of art.

—OSCAR WILDE

Purpose: To describe the stance the therapist takes with patients, and the role of the therapist–patient relationship in fostering change.

Points to consider:

1. How does the therapeutic relationship influence the outcome of therapy?
2. What techniques or strategies are used to create a treatment alliance? Describe and illustrate.
3. To what degree does the therapist overtly control sessions? How active/directive is the therapist?
4. Does the therapist assume responsibility for bringing about the changes desired? Is responsibility left to the patient? Is responsibility shared?
5. Does the therapist use self-disclosure? What limits are imposed on therapist self-disclosure? In general, what role does the "person" of the therapist play in this approach?
6. Does the therapist's role change as therapy progresses? Does it change as termination approaches?
7. Is countertransference recognized or employed in any fashion?
8. What are the clinical skills or other therapist attributes most essential to successful therapy in your approach?

In recent years, a great deal of effort has been expended to identify empirically supported treatments (ESTs) among the many existing forms of psychotherapy (e.g., Nathan & Gorman, 1998). Although such efforts can be useful for important public policymaking decisions, they tend to focus heavily on one particular domain of the therapy experience—the role and power of therapeutic techniques. Increasingly, but only quite recently, EST-oriented efforts have been counterbalanced by efforts to investigate and understand the essential characteristics of empirically supported relationships (ESRs) (Norcross, 2002). Such undertakings rest on a solid empirical basis for arguing that *the therapist as a person exerts large effects on the outcome of psychotherapy, and that these effects often outweigh the effects that are attributable to treatment techniques per se. In addition, the relationship established between therapist and patient may be more powerful than particular interventions* (Wampold, 2001). Even symptom-focused therapy encounters, which rely substantially on the use of clearly defined change-inducing techniques, occur in the context of human relationships characterized by support and reassurance, persuasion, and the modeling of active coping.

The kind of therapeutic relationship required by each approach to psychotherapy includes the overall "stance" the therapist takes to the experience (e.g., how the working alliance is fostered, how active and self-disclosing the therapist is, etc.). Thus, different therapeutic orientations appear to call forth and call for somewhat different therapist attributes and interpersonal inclinations. Therapists with a more or less "take charge" personal style may be better suited to practicing therapy approaches that require a good deal of therapist activity and structuring than those requiring a more reflective style, and so on.

Given the presumed equivalence of effectiveness of the major methods of psychotherapy (Garfield & Bergin, 1994; Wampold, 2001), it is not surprising that idiosyncratic personal factors would influence therapists' preferred ways of practicing. Thus, Norcross and Prochaska (1983) found that therapists generally do not advocate different approaches on the basis of their relative scientific status but are more influenced by their own direct clinical experience, personal values and philosophy, and life experiences. As British psychiatrist Robin Skynner (personal communication, March 1982) once quipped, we need "different thinks for different shrinks."

Finally, it is worthwhile to remember that therapeutic techniques themselves may significantly alter the nature of the therapist–patient relationship (Messer, cited in Lazarus & Messer, 1991). Although all techniques are born within an originating "home theory," they are often "exported" for use within other frameworks. Messer (2001) has referred to this process as "assimilative integration." Although helpful techniques may not lose their effectiveness when they are imported, their introductions are also communications within a given therapist–patient contextual pairing.

CURATIVE FACTORS OR MECHANISMS OF CHANGE

You can do very little with faith, but you can do nothing without it.

—SAMUEL BUTLER

Purpose: To describe the factors (or mechanisms of change) that lead to change and to assess their relative importance. Include research findings if possible.

Points to consider:

1. What are the proposed curative factors or mechanisms of change in this approach?
2. Do patients need insight or understanding in order to change? (Differentiate between historical–genetic insight and interactional insight.)
3. Are interpretations of any sort important and, if so, do they take history into account? If interpretations of any kind are used, are they seen as reflecting a psychological "reality" or are they viewed rather as a pragmatic tool for effecting change?
4. Is the learning of new interpersonal skills seen as an important element of change? If so, are these skills taught in didactic fashion, or are they shaped as approximations that occur naturalistically in treatment?
5. Does the therapist's personality or psychological health play an important part in bringing about change?
6. How important are techniques as opposed to just "being with" the patient?
7. What factors or variables enhance or limit the probability of successful treatment in your approach?
8. To what extent does the management of termination of therapy determine outcome?
9. What aspects of your therapy are *not* unique to your approach, i.e., characterize all therapy?

A current controversy in the psychotherapy research literature is whether change is brought about largely by specific ingredients of therapy or factors common to all therapies. The former usually refers to specific technical interventions such as biofeedback, systematic desensitization, *in vivo* exposure, cognitive reframing, interpretations, or empathic responding, which are said to be the ingredient(s) responsible for client change. Quite frequently, these techniques are set out in detail in manuals to which the practitioner is expected to adhere in order to achieve the desired result. The specific ingredient approach is in keeping with the medical model insofar as one treats a particular disorder with a psychological technique (akin to administering a pill), producing the psychological equivalent of a biological effect. Its proponents tend to fall in the cognitive and behavioral camps, but at least in theory could hail from any of the psychotherapy schools. Followers of the "empirically supported treatment" movement are typically adherents of this approach, advocating specific modes of intervention for different forms of psychopathology.

Common factors refer to features of therapy that are not specific to any one approach. Because outcome studies comparing different therapies have found few differences among the therapies (see commentary in "Research Support" section), it has been conjectured that this finding is due to the importance of therapeutic factors held in common by the various therapies. Thus, instead of running horserace research to discern differences among the therapies, proponents argue that effort should be redirected to their commonalities. These include *client factors* such as positive motivation and expectation for change; *therapist qualities* such as warmth, ability to form a good alliance, and empathic attunement; *strategic processes* such as providing feedback, exposing clients to the elements of the problem in thought or behavior, and helping them to acquire mastery; and *structural features* of the treatment, such as the provision of a rationale for the person's disorder, and having a coherent theoretical framework for interventions (Grencavage & Norcross, 1990; Weinberger, 1995).

Drawing on the common factors approach, Wampold (2001) developed what he refers to as a "contextual" model. In it, "the purpose of specific ingredients is to construct a coherent treatment that therapists believe in, and this provides a convincing rationale to clients. Furthermore, these ingredients cannot be studied independently of the healing context and atmosphere in which they occur" (Messer & Wampold, 2002, p. 22). In a sense, this is a common factors model which also takes account of the context in which those factors occur—namely, a healing atmosphere, and the employment of a specific theoretical model. In his important recent book, *The Great Psychotherapy Debate,* Wampold has made the case for the centrality of common factors such as the therapy alliance, the therapist's allegiance to his or her theory or rationale for treatment, and the personality qualities and skill of the therapist. He reviews the evidence for the specific ingredients model and finds it wanting. Nevertheless, proponents have also presented convincing evidence in favor of the specific ingredients model (e.g., Chambless & Ollendick, 2001).

An appealing way of thinking about curative factors that defuses the tension in this debate is provided by Beutler (2002). He and his colleagues "inspected the separate contributions to outcome of initial patient qualities, types of intervention, strength of the therapeutic relationship, and the overall fit of four patient and treatment variables" (p. 33). They found that patient qualities, specific interventions, and quality of the therapeutic relationship each added something to the prediction of treatment outcome. In addition, the fit of the treatment to the patient was important. Thus, support was found for both the specific ingredients and common factors models.

TREATMENT APPLICABILITY AND ETHICAL CONSIDERATIONS

All who drink this remedy recover in a short time, except those whom it does not help, who all die and have no relief from any other medicine. Therefore, it is obvious that it fails only in incurable cases.

—GALEN

Purpose: To describe those patients for whom your approach is especially relevant and any ethical issues that are particular to your approach.

Points to consider:

1. For what kinds of patients is your approach particularly relevant?
2. For whom is your approach either not appropriate or of uncertain relevance?
3. What is the applicability of your approach to people of diverse cultural backgrounds (e.g., as a function of ethnicity, race, religion, social class, and gender)?
4. When, if ever, would a referral be made for another (i.e., different) type of therapy?
5. When would no treatment (of any sort) be recommended?
6. Are there aspects of your approach that raise particular ethical issues that are different from those raised by psychotherapy in general?

In the end, questions about the applicability, relevance, and helpfulness of particular psychotherapy approaches to particular kinds of symptoms, problems, and issues are best answered through painstaking research on *treatment efficacy* (as determined through randomly controlled trials) and *effectiveness* (field studies). Testimonials, appeals to established authority and tradition, and similar unsystematic methods are insufficient to the task. Psychotherapy is too complex to track the interaction among, and impact of, the most relevant factors in therapeutic outcomes on the basis of only participants' perceptions. Moreover, the contributions to therapeutic outcomes of therapist, patient, and technique factors probably vary from one method to another.

When Galen's observations about presumptively curative medicines are applied to psychotherapy nowadays, they are certainly met with a knowing chuckle and implicit recognition of the inherent limits of all our treatment approaches. Still, *new therapy approaches rarely, if ever, make only modest and restrained claims of effectiveness, issue "warning labels" for "customers" for whom their ways of working are either not likely to be helpful or may possibly be harmful, or suggest that alternative approaches may be more appropriate under certain conditions.*

If therapy methods continue to grow in number (and we see no reason to predict otherwise), the ethical complexities of the psychotherapy field may grow commensurately. There are generic kinds of ethical matters that therapists of all orientations must deal with, for example, confidentiality, adequacy of recordkeeping, duty to warn, respecting personal boundaries regarding sexual contact and dual relationships, and so forth. And yet, more recently influential approaches, especially those involving multiperson clientele (e.g., marital and family therapy) raise practical ethical matters that just do not emerge in more traditional modes of practice—for example, balancing the interests and needs of more than one person against the interests and needs of another person, all the while also trying to help maintain the very viability of the patient system (e.g., marriage) itself.

Such potential influences of new perspectives on ethical concerns in psychother-

apy are perhaps nowhere more readily and saliently seen than when matters involving cultural diversity are considered. Certainly, all psychotherapists must be sensitive in their work to matters of race, ethnicity, social class, gender, sexual orientation, and religion, adapting and modifying both their assessment and treatment-planning activities and perspectives and active intervention styles as is deemed functionally appropriate to the situation at hand (Hayes & Toarmino, 1995). To do otherwise would risk the imposition, wittingly or unwittingly, of the therapist's own values onto the patient, for example, in terms of the important area of setting goals for their work together.

A culture-sensitive/multicultural theoretical orientation has been predicted by experts in the field of psychotherapy (Norcross, Hedges, & Prochaska, 2002) to be one of the most widely employed points of view in the next decade. And feminism, which shares many philosophical assumptions with multiculturalism (Gurman & Fraenkel, 2002), is also predicted to show an increasing impact on psychotherapy (Norcross et al., 2002). Together, these modern perspectives have usefully challenged many normative assumptions and practices in the general field of psychotherapy, forcing the field to recognize the diversity of social and psychological experience and the impact of relevant broader social beliefs that often confuse clinical description with social prescription. Critiques of various psychotherapies from these contemporary perspectives have sensitized therapists to the potential constraining and even damaging effects of a failure to recognize the reality of one's own necessarily limited perspective.

It must be recognized, nonetheless, that such critiques of established therapeutic worldviews do not necessarily provide clear guidelines about the ways in which culture-sensitive and gender-sensitive therapists should actually practice psychotherapy. As Hardy and Laszloffy (2002) make clear, a multicultural perspective "is not a set of codified techniques or strategies . . . but rather a philosophical stance that significantly informs how one sees the world in and outside of therapy (p. 569). Relatedly, Rampage (2002) has stated that "How to *do* feminist therapy is much less well understood than is the critique of traditional . . . therapy" (p. 535).

Like other attitudes, perspectives, and worldviews, multiculturalism and feminism, then, are not clinical methodologies to be taught and refined. As psychotherapists of all theoretical orientations strive to enhance their awareness of and sensitivity to the kinds of societal concerns brought to their attention by such modern perspectives, it is ethically incumbent upon therapists that they focus on the larger lesson of these perspectives. This larger lesson is that the responsibility and primary loyalty of therapists are to their clients, not their theories, strategies, or techniques.

RESEARCH SUPPORT

If all the evidence as you receive it leads to but one conclusion, don't believe it.
                                        —MOLIÈRE

The process of being scientific does not consist of finding objective truths. It consists of negotiating a shared perception of truths in respectful dialogue.
                                    —ROBERT BEAVERS

Purpose: To summarize existing research that supports the efficacy and/or effectiveness of your approach.

Points to consider:

1. Describe the nature and extent of empirical research that supports the efficacy and/or effectiveness of your approach.
2. If supportive research is not abundant, on what other bases can the effectiveness of your approach be argued?

Each chapter in this volume provides a snapshot of the *outcome research* backing its particular model of therapy. *There have been hundreds, if not thousands, of studies on the outcome of psychotherapy,* which is a testament to investigators' efforts to place the field on a firmer scientific footing. In recent times, a statistical process known as *meta-analysis* has been applied across large numbers of these studies. This procedure compares the efficacy of a particular therapy either to a waiting-list control group, to another therapy, or to other treatment modalities such as medication. Two major findings have emerged from these meta-analyses. The first is that being treated in psychotherapy is considerably more effective than not being treated. In fact, to be more precise, four out of five people will be better off because of therapy.

Here is the conclusion offered by the editors of the recent *Handbook of Psychological Change* (Snyder & Ingram, 2000) on the value of psychotherapy, based on comprehensive empirical reviews:

> Across a wide variety of approaches differing in their foci, operations, and temporal (short- to long-term) perspectives for engendering change; as applied by practitioners of varying age, gender, ethnicity, and amounts of experience; as delivered to a wide range of clientele varying in age, ethnicity, diagnostic label, and chronicity of problems, psychotherapy enables people to increase their personal satisfaction, interpersonal effectiveness, job and school performance, adaptive physiological responding to aversive circumstances, and a myriad of other behaviors in the human repertoire. Furthermore, the effects for psychotherapy appear to be as robust as those for educational interventions or medical procedures. . . . (p. 716)

Nevertheless, in the same volume, Karoly and Anderson (2000) present a more skeptical view of the findings, pointing to their shortcomings. In effect, they say, there is insufficient evidence to declare that psychotherapy works. Specifically, they point out that the meta-analytic findings are probably due to nonspecific effects, such as optimism, expectancies, and cognitive dissonance ("if I spent time, energy, and money on this, it must be worthwhile"), rather than to any process unique to therapy or to the theories of therapeutic change. Second, the findings are based on short-term outcomes, typically less than a year. There is some reason to believe that there is a deterioration of treatment gains that takes place over time, producing a less rosy picture of outcome. For example, Westen and Morrison (2001) found that most patients with depression and generalized anxiety disorder do not remain improved after 1 to 2 years and that many seek further treatment. Finally, Karoly and Anderson point out that too many studies use symptom alleviation as the criterion of improvement rather than the broader kinds of changes in personality that psychotherapy theories attempt to bring about.

The second major finding is that there is little difference in the effectiveness of the therapies that have been extensively practiced and researched. Time and again the results of comparative studies have shown that when pitted against one another, each therapy is more effective than sitting on a wait list, but not better than any other standard therapy (e.g., Lipsey & Wilson, 1993; Luborsky et al., 2002; Smith, Glass, & Miller, 1980; Wampold et al., 1997).

The other major kind of therapy research is known as *process research*. Rather than focusing on the question of whether therapy works, it studies the processes that attempt to answer the question of how it works. The effects of client factors (e.g., race, age, defensiveness, motivation), therapist factors (e.g., warmth, attunement, experience), different kinds of interventions (reflection, giving advice, interpretations), and the interaction among these and other variables are all part of process research. There is often an attempt to relate such process variables to change within a session or to therapy outcome. For example, one may study whether the therapist's providing interventions in keeping with the formulation of the case results in therapy progress (Messer,

Tishby, & Spillman, 1992). There are thousands of such studies, which cannot be as neatly summarized as the outcome results. The reader will find further examples in the research sections or elsewhere in the body of the individual chapters.

CASE ILLUSTRATION

A good example is the best sermon.
—YANKEE PROVERB

Purpose: To illustrate the clinical application of this model by detailing the major assessment, structural, technical and relational elements of the process of treating a person/couple/group viewed as typical, or representative, of the kinds of patients for whom this approach is appropriate.

Points to consider:

1. Relevant case background (e.g., presenting problem, referral source, previous treatment history).
2. Description of relevant aspects of your clinical assessment: functioning, structure, dysfunctional interaction, resources, individual dynamics/characteristics, including how this description was arrived at.
3. Description of the process and content of goal setting.
4. Highlight the major themes, patterns, etc., of the therapy over the whole course of treatment. Describe the structure of therapy, the techniques used, the role and activity of the therapist, and so on.
   Note: Do not describe the treatment of a "star case," in which therapy progresses perfectly. Select a case which, while successful, also illustrates the typical course of events in your therapy.

The first psychotherapist to use case illustrations was none other than the founder of modern psychotherapy, Sigmund Freud.

Here is what he wrote about the case history approach:

It still strikes me as strange that the case histories I write read like short stories and that, as one might say, they lack the serious stamp of science. I must console myself with the reflection that the nature of the subject is evidently responsible for this, rather than any preference of my own. . . . A detailed description of mental processes such as we are accustomed to find in the works of imaginative writers enables me, with the use of a few psychological formulas, to obtain at least some kind of insight into the course of that affliction [i.e., hysteria]. [The case histories provide] an intimate connection between the story of the patient's suffering and the symptoms of his illness. (Breuer & Freud, 1893–1895/1955, p. 160)

There are several advantages to the case report as a method for presenting the process of therapy. The therapist is in a privileged position to know what has happened over the course of therapy. A *case study* summarizes large quantities of case material in a richly textured, narrative fashion. Well-written cases bring material alive in a compelling way and bring us in on the unfolding sequence of events, major emergent theses, and the results of the therapy. The treating therapist permits readers to participate in his or her sense of discovery and excitement in elaborating new ideas and techniques (Messer & McCann, in press).

There are disadvantages to the case report as well, particularly from a scientific standpoint. First, it is one person's view only, albeit that of a trained observer. What is not recorded may be technical mistakes that are not remembered or are simply omitted to avoid guilt or shame (Spence, 1998). We cannot assume that accounts prepared for publication are veridical because we know that memory is affected by wishes and confirmatory bias. The summary report, therefore, is not a substitute for the recording of actual dialogue between client and therapist because the data are selected in terms of both what is reported and the inferences that are drawn by the reporting therapist.

There are new research endeavors in the area of single case study that vitiate at least some of these concerns. One is the "hermeneutic single case efficacy design" (Elliott, 2001). It uses a "mixture of quantitative and qualitative information to create a rich case record that provides both positive and negative evidence for the causal influence of therapy and client outcome" (p. 317). It searches for negative evidence to rule out competing explanations as to how events external to therapy might have caused client improvement. Another new approach is known as "multiple case depth research" (Schneider, 1999) which combines both case-study methodology and depth-experiential therapeutic principles. In its effort to achieve validity, it poses three questions: Are the data plausibly linked to theory? Is the theory generalizable? Is the conclusion plausibly disconfirmable? Despite the value of these efforts, there will probably continue to be a trade-off between the advantages of a more free-flowing, narrative presentation of the case report and the efforts to bring it within normative science.

CURRENT AND FUTURE TRENDS

None of us understand psychotherapy well enough to stop from learning from all of us.
—FRANK PITTMAN

Progress always looks like destruction.
—JOHN STEINBECK

Purpose: To outline the major challenges, opportunities and obstacles to the further growth and development of your approach.

Points to consider:

1. What are the major positive emerging trends within the theory and practice of your approach?

2. What stands in the way of the further development of your approach from cultural, economic or research perspectives?

There are two major areas of psychotherapy in which important trends can be identified, and which readers of the chapters that follow might usefully keep in mind as they study the therapeutic approaches discussed in this volume.

The Science and Practice of Psychotherapy

There is a long history of disconnection between psychotherapy practitioners and psychotherapy researchers. Researchers typically criticize clinicians for engaging in practices that lack empirical justification, and clinicians typically criticize researchers as being out of touch with the complex realities of doing psychotherapy. Though reflecting caricatured positions, such characterizations on both sides are unfortunately not entirely unwarranted.

As already noted, the world of psychotherapy has seen an increased pressure placed on the advocates of particular therapeutic methods to document both the efficacy of their approaches through carefully controlled clinical research trials and the effectiveness of these methods via patients' evaluations in uncontrolled, naturalistic clinical practice contexts (Nathan & Gorman, 1998). This movement to favor ESTs has even more recently been challenged by a complementary movement of psychotherapy researchers who assert the often overlooked importance of ESRs (Norcross, 2002).

At the risk of oversimplification, those who advocate an EST perspective tend to be associated with certain theoretical orientations (behavioral, cognitive, cognitive-behavioral) and styles of practice (brief), whereas those who adopt an ESR perspective tend to be associated with other theoretical orientations (psychoanalytic and psychodynamic, person-centered, experiential,

existential–humanistic, and postmodern), with other dominant approaches (integrative, family and marital, group) standing somewhere in the middle.

The questions raised by such unfortunately competing points of view are not at all insignificant—for example:

1. Will ESTs, which tend to emphasize technical refinement, symptomatic change and changes in presenting problems, not only survive, but thrive?
2. Will ESR-oriented approaches, which tend to emphasize enhancing client resources and resilience and self-exploration and personal discovery, fade from view?
3. Will the influence of brief approaches expand, while the influence of long-term approaches contracts?
4. Can research better inform us not only how to disseminate effective psychotherapy methods but also how to better identify effective psychotherapists?
5. Can both qualitative and quantitative research methods be brought to bear on theoretically and clinically important questions, or will they, like researchers and clinicians, tend to operate quite independently?

In the end, and in various possible manifestations, a collaboratively oriented way of framing questions such as these may be, (how) can the field of psychotherapy foster more evidence-based practice, without unduly constraining the kinds of evidence that are allowed to inform practice? In other words, *can we create a truly scientific practice while also creating a truly practical science?*

Integration and Specialization in Psychotherapy

The modern trend toward integration in psychotherapy goes back at least to Dollard and Miller's (1950) classic, *Personality and Psychotherapy,* which sought to bring together the psychoanalytic and behavioral orientations. Almost exactly midway through the period from Dollard and Miller's book until today, appeared Wachtel's (1977) highly influential *Psychoanalysis and Behavior Therapy.* This domain of psychotherapy has progressed over the years from a rather singular emphasis on the integration of particular therapeutic approaches, to a parallel emphasis on the actual process and principles of integrating apparently disparate points of view and clinical methods (see, e.g., Messer, 2001). Certainly, one of the main forces behind the "integration movement" has been empirical—that is, the repeated finding of rough equivalence of treatment outcomes among different approaches, leading to an increased interest in identifying the common factors involved in psychotherapeutic change, as discussed earlier. But empirical foundations notwithstanding, many integrative efforts have grown more out of conceptual and clinical concerns and questioning than out of research findings per se. This is an important attribute of the integration movement. Without it, there may evolve merely a series of rather arid integrations of formerly unconnected approaches, which, as the latest "products" of integration, take on lives of their own and merely add to the already very long list of identifiable psychotherapies. Moreover, the integrative movement necessarily always relies on the continued existence of original theories of therapy to serve as its own launching pad. *Perhaps seemingly ironically, integrative development cannot continue without original theories remaining vital.*

At the same time that the integration movement is likely to persist, there will certainly be a continuing parallel movement in the world of psychotherapy toward increased specialization. This specialization, a logical outgrowth of the EST movement, will emphasize a model of therapy practice (and training) which places a premium on the application of highly specific treatment interventions to the remediation of highly specif-

ic disorders and problems. Already, it appears that significant numbers of recently trained psychotherapists are opting to specialize in their clinical work, often by limiting their clinical activities to the treatment of a narrow range of patient problems or diagnoses. Ironically and dialectically, the field's push toward specialization may help to fuel the movement toward integration. In the end, competition between these two movements may strengthen the growth of each.

SUGGESTIONS FOR FURTHER READING

The most impressive of all kinds of Professors is the Full Professor. It is not apparent at first glance what it is full of, but there is an obvious fullness.
—RICHARD ARMOUR

Purpose: To aid the instructor in assigning relevant readings as a supplement to the text.

Points to include:

1. Two articles or accessible book chapters that provide detailed, extensive clinical case studies.
2. Two research-oriented articles or chapters, preferably one of which includes an overview of research finding or issues pertinent to your approach.
3. Two books that could serve as reference volumes for the student.

CONCLUSION

Start at the beginning, proceed through the middle, and stop when you get to the end.
—LEWIS CARROLL, *Alice in Wonderland*

REFERENCES

Abelson, R. P. (1981). Psychological status of the script concept. *American Psychologist, 36,* 715–729.

American Psychiatric Association. (1994). *Diagnostic and statistical manual of mental disorders* (4th ed.). Washington, DC: Author.

Bergin, A. E., & Garfield, S. L. (Eds.). (1994). *Handbook of psychotherapy and behavior change* (4th ed.). New York: Wiley.

Beutler, L. E. (2002). The Dodo bird is extinct. *Clinical Psychology: Science and Practice, 9,* 30–34.

Bongar, B., & Beutler, L. E. (Eds.). (1995). *Comprehensive textbook of psychotherapy: Theory and practice.* New York: Oxford University Press.

Breuer, J., & Freud, S. (1955). Studies on hysteria. In J. Strachey (Ed. & Trans.), *Standard edition of the complete psychological works of Sigmund Freud* (Vol. 2, pp. 1–305). London: Hogarth Press. (Original work published 1893–1895)

Chambless, D. L., & Ollendick, T. H. (2001). Empirically supported psychological interventions: Controversies and evidence. *Annual Review of Psychology, 52,* 685–716.

Corsini, R. J., & Wedding, D. (Eds.). (1995). *Current psychotherapies* (5th ed.). Itasca, IL: Peacock.

de Jonghe, F., Kool, S., van Aalst, G., Dekker, J., & Peen, J. (2001). Combining psychotherapy and antidepressants in the treatment of depression. *Journal of Affective Disorders, 64,* 217–229.

Dollard, J., & Miller, N. E. (1950). *Personality and psychotherapy.* New York: McGraw-Hill.

Elliott, R. (2001). Hermeneutic single-case efficacy design: An overview. In K. J. Schneider, J. F. T. Bugental, & J. F. Pierson (Eds.), *The handbook of humanistic psychology* (pp. 315–326). Thousand Oaks, CA: Sage.

Frank, J. D., & Frank, J. B. (1991). *Persuasion and healing.* Baltimore: Johns Hopkins University Press.

Freedheim, D. K., Freudenberger, H., Kessler, J., Messer, S., Peterson, D., Strupp, H., & Wachtel, P. (Eds.). (1992). *History of psychotherapy: A century of change.* Washington, DC: American Psychological Association.

Garfield, S. L., & Bergin, A. E. (1994). *Handbook of psychotherapy and behavior change* (4th ed.). New York: Wiley.

Grencavage, L. M., & Norcross, J. C. (1990). Where are the commonalities among the therapeutic common factors? *Professional Psychology: Research and Practice, 21,* 372–378.

Gurman, A. S. (1983). *Psychotherapy research and the practice of psychotherapy.* Presidential address, Society for Psychotherapy Research, Sheffield, England.

Gurman, A. S. (2001). Brief therapy and family/couple therapy: An essential redundancy. *Clinical Psychology: Science and Practice, 8,* 51–65.

Gurman, A. S. (2002). Brief integrative marital therapy: A depth-behavioral approach. In A. S. Gurman & N. S. Jacobson (Eds.), *Clinical handbook of couple therapy* (3rd ed., pp. 180–220). New York: Guilford Press.

Gurman, A. S., & Fraenkel, P. (2002). The history of couple therapy: A millennial review. *Family Process, 41,* 199–160.

Gurman, A. S., & Razin, A. M. (Eds.). (1977). *Effective psychotherapy: A handbook of research.* New York: Pergamon Press.

Hardy, K. V., & Laszloffy, T. A. (2002). Couple therapy using a multicultural perspective. In A. S. Gurman & N. S. Jacobson (Eds.), *Clinical handbook of couple therapy* (3rd ed., pp. 569–593). New York: Guilford Press.

Hayes, S. C., & Toarmino, D. (1995, February). If behavioral principles are generally applicable, why is it necessary to understand cultural diversity? *The Behavior Therapist,* pp. 21–23.

Hofstee, W. K. B. (2003). Structures of personality traits. In T. Millon & M. J. Lerner (Eds.), *Handbook of psychology: Vol. 5. Personality and social psychology* (pp. 231–254). New York: Wiley.

Hollon, S. D., Thase, M. E., & Markowitz, J. C. (2002). Treatment and prevention of depression. *Psychological Science in the Public Interest, 3,* 39–77.

Karoly, P., & Anderson, C. W. (2000). The long and short of psychological change: Toward a goal-centered understanding of treatment durability and adaptive success. In C. R. Snyder & R. E. Ingram (Eds.), *Handbook of psychological change* (pp. 154–176). New York: Wiley.

Kelly, G. A. (1991). *The psychology of personal constructs.* New York: Routledge. (Original work published 1955)

Kirsch, I., & Sapirstein, G. (1999). Listening to Prozac but hearing placebo: A meta-analysis of antidepressant medication. In I. Kirsch (Ed.), *How expectancies shape experience* (pp. 303–320). Washington, DC: American Psychological Association.

Lazarus, A. A., & Messer, S. B. (1991). Does chaos prevail? An exchange on technical eclecticism and assimilative integration. *Journal of Psychotherapy Integration, 1,* 143–158.

Lebow, J. L. (1987). Developing a personal integration in family therapy: Principles for model construction and practice. *Journal of Marital and Family Therapy, 13,* 1–14.

Liddle, H. A. (1982). On the problems of eclecticism: A call for epistemologic clarification and human scale theories. *Family Process, 21,* 81–97.

Lipsey, M. W., & Wilson, D. B. (1993). The efficacy of psychological, educational and behavioral treatment: Confirmation from meta-analysis. *American Psychologist, 48,* 1181–1209.

London, P. (1986). *The modes and morals of psychotherapy* (2nd ed.). Washington, DC: Hemisphere.

Luborsky, L., Rosenthal, R., Diguer, L., Andrusyna, T. P., Berman, J. S., Levitt, J. T., Seligman, D. A., & Krause, E. (2002). The Dodo bird verdict is alive and well—mostly. *Clinical Psychology: Science and Practice, 9,* 2–12.

Lynn, S. J., & Garske, J. P. (Eds.). (1985). *Contemporary psychotherapies: Models and methods.* Columbus, OH: Charles E. Merrill.

Meltzoff, J., & Kornreich, M. (1970). *Research in psychotherapy.* New York: Atherton.

Messer, S. B. (2001). Assimilative integration [Special issue]. *Journal of Psychotherapy Integration, 11,* 1–154.

Messer, S. B., & McCann, L. (in press). Research perspectives on the case study: Single-case method. In J. S. Auerbach, K. N. Levy, & C. E. Schaffer (Eds.), *Relatedness, self-definition, and mental representation: Essays in honor of Sidney J. Blatt.* London: Routledge.

Messer, S. B., Sanderson, W. C., & Gurman, A. S. (2003). Brief psychotherapies. In G. Stricker & T. A. Widiger (Eds.), *Handbook of psychology: Vol. 8. Clinical psychology* (pp. 407–430). New York: Wiley.

Messer, S. B., Tishby, O., & Spillman, A. (1992). Taking context seriously in psychotherapy research: Relating therapist interventions to patient progress in brief psychodynamic therapy. *Journal of Consulting and Clinical Psychology, 60,* 678–688.

Messer, S. B., & Wachtel, P. L. (1997). The contemporary psychotherapeutic landscape: Issues and prospects. In P. L. Wachtel & S. B. Messer (Eds.), *Theories of psychotherapy: Origins and evolution* (pp. 1–38). Washington, DC: American Psychological Association.

Messer, S. B., & Wampold, B. E. (2002). Let's face facts: Common factors are more potent than specific ingredients. *Clinical Psychology: Science and Practice, 9,* 21–25.

Messer, S. B., & Warren, C. S. (1990). Personality change and psychotherapy. In L. A. Pervin (Ed.), *Handbook of personality: Theory and research* (pp. 371–398). New York: Guilford Press.

Messer, S. B., & Winokur, M. (1980). Some limits to the integration of psychoanalytic and behavior therapy. *American Psychologist, 35,* 818–827.

Messer, S. B., & Winokur, M. (1984). Ways of knowing and visions of reality in psychoanalytic and behavior therapy. In H. Arkowitz & S. B. Messer (Eds.), *Psychoanalytic therapy and behavior therapy: Is integration possible?* (pp. 53–100). New York: Plenum Press.

Messer, S. B., & Woolfolk, R. L. (1998). Philosophical issues in psychotherapy. *Clinical Psychology: Science and Practice, 5,* 251–263.

Nathan, P. E., & Gorman, J. M. (Eds.). (1998). *A guide to treatments that work.* New York: Oxford University Press.

Neisser, U. (1967). *Cognitive psychology.* New York: Appleton-Century-Crofts.

Norcross, J. C. (Ed.). (2002). *Psychotherapy relationships that work: Therapist contributions and responsiveness to patients.* New York: Oxford University Press.

Norcross, J. C., Hedges, M., & Prochaska, J. O. (2002). The face of 2010: A Delphi poll on the future of psychotherapy. *Professional Psychology, 33,* 316–322.

Norcross, J. C., & Prochaska, J. O. (1983). Clinicians' theoretical orientations: Selection, utilization and efficacy. *Professional Psychology, 14,* 197–208.

Rampage, C. (2002). Working with gender in couple therapy. In A. S. Gurman & N. S. Jacobson (Eds.), *Clinical handbook of couple therapy* (3rd ed., pp. 533–545). New York: Guilford Press.

Schneider, K. J. (1999). Multiple-case research: Bringing experience-near closer. *Journal of Clinical Psychology, 55,* 1531–1540.

Smith, M. L., Glass, G. V., & Miller, T. I. (1980). *The benefits of psychotherapy.* Baltimore: Johns Hopkins University Press.

Snyder, C. R., & Ingram, R. E. (2000). Psychotherapy: Questions for an evolving field. In C. R. Snyder & R. E. Ingram (Eds.), *Handbook of psychological change* (pp. 707–726). New York: Wiley.

Spence, D. P. (1998). Rain forest or mud field: Guest editorial. *International Journal of Psychoanalysis, 79,* 643–647.

Wachtel, P. L. (1977). *Psychoanalysis and behavior therapy.* New York: Basic Books.

Wampold, B. E. (2001). *The great psychotherapy debate: Models, methods and findings.* Mahwah, NJ: Erlbaum.

Wampold, B. E., Mondin, G. W., Moody, M., Stich, F., Benson, K., & Ahn, H. (1997). A meta-analysis of outcome studies comparing bona fide psychotherapies: Empirically "All must have prizes." *Psychological Bulletin, 122,* 203–215.

Weinberger, J. (1995). Common factors aren't so common: The common factors dilemma. *Clinical Psychology: Science and Practice, 2,* 45–69.

Westen, D., & Morrison, K. (2001). A multidimensional meta-analysis of treatments for depression, panic and generalized anxiety disorder: An empirical examination of the status of empirically supported therapies. *Journal of Consulting and Clinical Psychology, 69,* 875–899.

White, M., & Epston, P. (1990). *Narrative means to therapeutic ends.* New York: Norton.

Woolfolk, R. L. (1998). *The cure of souls: Science, values and psychotherapy.* San Francisco: Jossey-Bass.

2

The Theory and Practice of Traditional Psychoanalytic Treatment

David L. Wolitzky

The aim of this chapter is to introduce the theory and practice of Freudian psychoanalysis and the psychoanalytic psychotherapy that derived from it. The term "psychoanalysis" refers to (1) a theory of personality and psychopathology, (2) a method of investigating the mind, and (3) a theory of treatment. I shall be concerned primarily with the theory of treatment but will need to present some of the basic theoretical and methodological concepts as the context for understanding the theoretical rationale for therapeutic intervention.

Sigmund Freud (1856–1939) was the founder of psychoanalysis and the father of modern psychotherapy. Although he was confronted with the exigencies of the clinical situation, Freud's primary aspiration was to develop psychoanalysis as a theory of the human mind and secondarily to develop it as a therapeutic modality. Accordingly, his theoretical writings consume the bulk of the 23 volumes of his collected works, published as the definitive *Standard Edition*.

As a comprehensive theory of personality and psychopathology, psychoanalysis has had a profound impact on 20th-century thought and culture, an impact that is unrivaled by any other conception of personality. Psychoanalytic theorizing not only has aimed at understanding and explaining the nature of adult psychopathology but also has addressed the broader domain of normal personality functioning and the development of personality. In this sense it can be regarded as a general psychology. As such, it ranges from biological and protobiological explanations of key aspects of mental life (e.g., cognition, affect, and motivation) to sociocultural, historical theorizing about the origins of society and the family. Attempts to understand art, literature, music, religion, and virtually all other aspects of human experience according to psychoanalytic principles (so-called applied psychoanalysis) have filled innumerable journals and books for nearly a full century.

The origins of psychoanalysis can be traced back to the last two decades of the 19th century in the cultural context of turn–of–the–century Vienna. It has evolved throughout the past century and spread throughout the world, particularly to the rest of Europe, the United States, and South America. Freud's life and the psychoanalytic movement he inspired and led have been the subject of a multitude of books and articles through the years.

In the past century, we have seen many developments of psychoanalytic theory and practice. All of them have taken their point of departure from Freud, either by extending or by modifying a line of thought implicit or undeveloped in Freud's work or by rejecting essential Freudian assumptions yet referring to their alternate conceptions by the term "psychoanalytic." Indeed, there have been many heated professional squabbles through the years about whether one should call certain "deviations" from the original theory and practice of psychoanalysis by that name. For instance, the so-called neo-Freudians (e.g., Adler, Jung, and Horney) have been called deviant in that each departs from Freud's emphasis on the importance of childhood sexuality. Whether a new school of psychoanalytic thought evolves and becomes assimilated into the mainstream of the prevailing psychoanalytic paradigms or whether it becomes a "deviant" school often has more to do with the existing sociohistorical *Zeitgeist* than with the extent to which the theory advanced departs from Freud's views. A most recent case in point is Kohut's (1971, 1977) self psychology which departs in fundamental ways from basic Freudian tenets yet did not create the kinds of schisms that characterized earlier theoretical differences (Eagle, 1987).

There is by now significant diversity within what has been termed "the common ground of psychoanalysis" (Wallerstein, 1990). Therefore, it is no longer accurate to refer to *the* psychoanalytic theory of personality or of treatment. Rather, we need to specify the particular theoretical perspective from which we are approaching the topic. In this chapter, I focus primarily on traditional Freudian theory and its ego-psychological extensions. That is, I provide an ac-

count of Freud's core concepts and their implications for treatment as well as a brief reference to the contributions of later theorists who sought to extend Freud's thinking. Together, this body of thought constitutes what has been called traditional Freudian theory and forms the basis for the so-called classical psychoanalytic approach to treatment.

For present purposes, we may follow Pine (1990) and divide theoretical changes in psychoanalytic thinking into four main eras. First, of course, was Freud's theory of unconscious motivation with its ultimate postulation *of libidinal and aggressive drives* as the prime movers of mental life and behavior. The second wave of theorizing was the development of *ego psychology* with its focus on the defensive and coping devices used to deal with conflicted wishes. Third, we saw the evolution of versions of *object relations theory* with its focus on the mental representation of objects, the relationship of the self to one's world of inner objects (mostly people), and the repetitive reenactment of this internal world in the context of ongoing interpersonal relationships and fantasies of such relationships. The fourth, and most recent change in psychoanalytic thinking is the advent of *self psychology,* as created by Heinz Kohut (1971, 1977), in which the cohesion and fulfillment of the self came to be regarded as the individual's primary aim. Writing in 1990, Pine could not have foreseen the next wave of psychoanalytic theorizing that has shown enormous popularity in the last decade. I am referring to the widespread influence of what broadly can be termed "American relational theory." Developed mainly by Mitchell (1988), this approach is an amalgam of Sullivan's (1953) interpersonal theory and British object relations theories, primarily Fairbairn (1941) and Winnicott (1965).

This chapter focuses on the first and second eras of psychoanalytic theorizing and on the contemporary extensions, revisions, and understandings of those views. In what follows, I use the terms "traditional," "modern," and "contemporary" interchangeably, and, at times, in seemingly oxymoronic combinations (e.g., "contemporary classical") to mean "the current Freudian theory and practice of psychoanalysis and psychoanalytic psychotherapy," an approach that continues to adhere to most of the core propositions of Freud's theories in the context of subsequent modifications and extensions of those theories. Freud's changing views did not result in a comprehensive statement of a theory of treatment. His followers have rarely presented a formal, systematic exposition of a theory of the therapeutic action of psychoanalysis. Having created an orienting context with this brief introduction, I proceed to focus on the origins and the current application of traditional psychoanalytic theory to the treatment of psychopathology.

HISTORICAL BACKGROUND

The kinds of patients first treated by Freud were usually late adolescent women who presented with hysterical symptoms. The kinds of hysterical symptoms prevalent in the Victorian society in which Freud worked were disturbances in the senses and/or the musculature—for example, blindness, paralyses, mutism, convulsive-like motor actions (e.g., trembling), and anesthesia (i.e., loss of or diminished sensation in one or more parts of the body). These symptoms came to be regarded as psychological when no organic basis for them could be found. It is quite likely that some organic conditions were mistaken for neurotic ones and vice versa.

Prior to the development of any form of psychoanalytic therapy, the main methods of treating emotional and mental disturbances were rest, massage, hydrotherapy (warm baths), faradic therapy (the application of low-voltage electrical stimulation to areas of the body that were symptomatic), and hypnosis. As we shall see later, psychoanalysis evolved from attempts to treat

symptoms via hypnosis (Bernheim, 1886; Charcot, 1882; Janet, 1907).

Dissatisfied with the existing methods of treating these "nervous conditions," Freud, impressed by Charcot's demonstrations of hypnotic effects, became particularly interested in the potential of hypnotic suggestion as a therapeutic tool. He began to employ hypnosis in his practice, at first using the direct suggestion that the symptom(s) disappear. This approach generally met with limited success. Some patients could not readily be hypnotized; in others, symptoms would dissipate but return. These early clinical experiences led Freud to become more curious about the causes and mechanisms of symptom formation and to search for more effective therapeutic methods. With regard to the latter, Freud sometimes used the so-called "pressure technique" in which he placed his hand on the patient's forehead and gave the strong suggestion that the patient would remember the original experience associated with the onset of the symptoms. These early variations in technique evolved into the method of *free association* in which the patient is asked to say whatever comes to mind without the usual editing and inhibition characteristic of typical social interactions.

The patient known as Anna O provided a critical turning point for Freud and for the development of psychoanalysis. Anna O was suffering from a variety of hysterical symptoms for which she was being treated by Josef Breuer, an eminent Viennese physician. Breuer attempted to hypnotize her and to suggest away her symptoms. However, she wanted to talk (to have a "catharsis") and as he allowed her to do so, she began to recall the memories and affective states that turned out to be the context in which the symptoms originated. This was the birth of the "talking cure."

In the intimate setting of recounting emotionally vivid and meaningful experiences, patients developed an attachment to the doctor. At one point in the course of her treatment with Breuer, Anna O developed a pseudocyesis (a fantasy of being pregnant) which featured the fantasy that Breuer was the father. Breuer, unsettled by this development, left for vacation with his wife. These kinds of emotional reactions by the patient and the therapist led to the development of the central concepts of transference and countertransference (discussed later).

Breuer and Freud (1895) published their ideas about their early cases in *Studies in Hysteria,* the key idea contained in this work being that "hysterics suffer from reminiscences." That is, a painful memory is dissociated from the mass of conscious experience and the "quota of affect" associated with that memory is converted to a bodily symptom. The release of the dammed-up affect via talking about the memory allows for the "associative reabsorption" of the blocked idea and causes the symptom to disappear. Breuer and Freud (1895) offered a two-factor theory as to why the memory and its affect were not in consciousness in the first place. The first factor was that the experience in question occurred in an altered state of consciousness (a so-called hypnoid state) so that it failed to connect with the dominant mass of conscious ideas. The second factor was a motivational one, namely, the person did not *want* to remember the experience.

Here we have the beginnings of a *dynamic* point of view. In this view, the patient is seen as being motivated to keep an idea and its associated affect out of awareness. This defensive effort arises because the idea and its associated affect are considered by the person to be incompatible with the dominant mass of ideas and attitudes making up the ego. *Repression* (i.e., the motivated forgetting of the disagreeable idea or conflicted wish) is a way of repudiating or disavowing impulses that are anxiety arousing or repugnant to one's sense of morality. A key accomplishment of successful defense is self-deception. But, such efforts always weaken the personality by impairing its integrated functioning.

THE CONCEPT OF PERSONALITY

In this early phase of Freud's work, the focus was on the symptom. Symptoms were regarded as circumscribed, disembodied foreign objects to be excised, not unlike an impacted wisdom tooth. The nature of the person in whom the symptoms resided was not considered important. However, Freud soon realized that patients' symptoms were meaningful expressions of their character and overall personality functioning. Over the next several decades Freud evolved his theory of personality development and psychopathology. His followers have extended and modified his ideas, sometimes within the spirit of Freud's core concepts, at other times with significant rejection of those core concepts. Freud himself changed central aspects of his theory many times in the course of his long career. Clearly, I cannot present a complete account of all these theoretical developments, but I do offer a brief statement of the essential concepts. The interested reader should consult Brenner (1982).

For Freud, the basic unit of study was the intrapsychic life of the individual, that is, the basic motives, wishes, anxieties, defenses, and regulatory capacities of the developing child, as seen primarily from the perspective of conflicts within the person. The formation of the psychic structures in which these dynamic conflicts were expressed was dependent on the interaction of genetic and experiential factors. Freud postulated an initial state of "primary narcissism" in which interest in objects was not inherently present from birth but forced on the infant by the realization that not relating to anybody in the outside world was an untenable strategy for survival. The biological helplessness of the infant requires, as a matter of survival, that the mother serve as the supplier and homeostatic regulator of the infant's basic needs. Thus, from the start the infant had to relate to the social world. The formation of psychic structures thus inevitably takes place in the context of social interactions that the developing infant internalizes as its "representational world."

Freud believed that there were two basic tendencies governing mental life, the *pleasure principle* and the *reality principle*. According to the pleasure principle, the basic tendency of the organism is to maximize pleasure and to minimize pain and to do so in as rapid and automatic a way as possible. Increases in endogenous excitation were regarded as unpleasant, whereas decreases were associated with pleasure. Hence, the aim of the organism was to rid itself of excitation as soon as possible. Reality forces the organism to give up sole reliance on the pleasure principle. For example, if the hungry infant hallucinates the mother's breast, it learns that it can achieve a partial, temporary satisfaction. But, it also learns that this gratification is short-lived and turns to pain if its hunger pangs continue for any length of time. Thus, "finding" the breast (i.e., turning to reality) is essential for satisfaction and survival. In other words, the infant has to adopt the reality principle, if only as an expedient, if it is to find pleasure and survive.

As the infant perceives, thinks, and lays down memories, we have the beginnings of what is called *psychic structure*. In his paper *Formulations on the Two Principles of Mental Functioning,* Freud (1911) distinguished between two kinds of thinking, primary-process thinking and secondary-process thinking. *Primary-process thinking* is governed by the pleasure principle. It is not governed by the rules of logic but is primitive and directed by the desire for immediate drive discharge. *Secondary-process thinking* is reality oriented and based on a conceptual organization of memories.

The memory of previous experiences of satisfaction forms the basis for wishes. A *wish,* according to Freud, is a desire to reinstate a condition of "perceptual identity"; that is, to have a current experience that matches the memory of a prior experience of satisfaction. To the extent that the wish is

pursued without regard to reality considerations, the cognitive elaboration of it should show hallmarks of primary-process thinking. The symbolization, condensation, and displacement seen in dreams and/or in hallucinatory wish fulfillment are instances of primary-process thinking. Even in dreams, however, we see the residual operation of secondary-process thinking. For example, the choice of a symbol is not arbitrary but is based on the structural and functional similarity of the symbol and the thing symbolized.

What are the basic tensions one must reduce to avoid unpleasure? This question brings us to Freud's basic theory of motivation. Freud always postulated two major classes of instinctual drives. At first, the two drives were the sexual or *libidinal* and the self-preservative or *ego instincts.* Later, Freud theorized that the two major drives were the *libidinal* (or sexual) drive and the *aggressive* drive. According to the theory, a drive is the psychical representative of the instinct. It is a demand made on the mind for work. It impels the organism to mental and physical activity the aim of which is to discharge the nervous system excitation produced by the drive. According to Freud, sexuality (broadly conceived as sensual) and aggression were the two basic human motivational sources of behavior.

There are four main characteristics of an instinctual drive; it has a source (a bodily tension), an impetus (a degree of intensity), an aim (to lessen the drive tension), and an object (the means whereby the drive tension is reduced, e.g., sucking one's thumb, milk from mother's breast). The object is the most variable aspect of the drive (i.e., the drive can be more or less satisfied in a number of ways). We do not directly observe drives but infer them on the basis of "drive derivatives" (i.e., wishes). The energy that derives from the instinctual drives is *psychic energy.* The term "cathexis" refers to the amount of sexual or aggressive drive or psychic energy invested in a particular idea, wish, or unconscious fantasy. These energic concepts, which were a key aspect of Freud's "metapsychology," have been cogently criticized in the past two decades as pseudoscientific explanations that are at best descriptive metaphors designed to capture the force and quantitative aspects of behavior and experience (Holt, 1989).

At first Freud believed that accumulated drive pressure that was not discharged was transformed into anxiety. For example, the practice of coitus interruptus was believed to lead to anxiety. In this connection, he made a distinction between the *actual neuroses* and the *psychoneuroses*. Neurasthenia, anxiety neurosis, and hypochondria were classified as actual neuroses. These syndromes, each of which has clear somatic aspects, were distinguished from the psychoneuroses on the grounds that the latter have a primarily psychological etiology.

Although Freud never quite abandoned the idea of actual neuroses, the concept of *intrapsychic conflict* became the core notion of Freudian theory. If the person believes that the satisfaction of a wish, or even the desire to satisfy it, is dangerous, an approach–avoidance situation is created. This formulation assumed certain typical danger situations in childhood. In developmental order, they are loss of the object, loss of the object's love, castration anxiety, and guilt (the latter two presume the loss of the object's love). Although the term "object" sounds quite impersonal and strange when applied to a person, it is used in psychoanalytic theory as a general term to indicate that wishes can be directed to inanimate objects and, especially, to so-called internalized objects (mental representations of the other).

The anticipation of each of these dangers gives rise to signal anxiety and leads to a *defense* against a potentially traumatic anxiety. For example, suppose a young boy has incestuous wishes toward his mother but believes and fears that such wishes are wrong and will lead to castration by the father. The boy, who loves the father as well as fears him and resents him as an unwanted rival,

now needs to defend against his sexual wishes toward his mother. This, of course, is the classic *Oedipal conflict* so central to Freudian theory.

Freud's theory has a strong developmental emphasis. The nature of the child's wishes and preoccupations, and therefore of the corresponding anxieties, differs at different ages. There is an invariant sequence of phases or *stages of psychosexual development*. These stages are the oral, anal, phallic, and genital. Each stage is influenced by the preceding ones and in turn influences subsequent stages. As the name implies, the *oral* stage centers on concerns with hunger, with the mouth as the chief bodily zone involved, but is conceived of more broadly as including maternal care and comfort. At this stage the primary fear is loss of the object—that is, of the mother as the supplier and regulator of the infant's needs. In the *anal* phase, the focus is on toilet training and the major anxiety is loss of the parent's love. In the *phallic* phase, the boy is subject to *castration anxiety* (and the girl to *penis envy*), and in the *genital* stage, guilt is the major danger. Erikson (1950) presented a psychosocial elaboration of Freud's psychosexual stages in which he emphasized the psychological experiences central to each Freudian stage (e.g., describing the oral stage as the time when the infant first establishes a "basic trust" or "mistrust" of the social world).

Two other key Freudian concepts need to be noted here: *fixation* and *regression*. According to Freud, excessive frustration or satisfaction could lead to a rigid clinging to a particular mode of satisfaction characteristic of that stage. For example, excessive oral satisfaction (or frustration) could lead to the persistence of thumb-sucking long after it is age appropriate. Regression refers to the reinstatement of a mode of seeking satisfaction that is no longer age appropriate. If, for example, the birth of a sibling leaves the older sibling feeling terribly unloved he or she might revert to thumb-sucking. Freud believed that the major modes of adaptation to the environment and to the regulation of tension states are well developed by the time a child is 6 years old and change relatively little after that.

Given this sketch of personality functioning, we may say that the mind is always in a state of dynamic equilibrium as it tries to secure for itself maximum satisfaction with a minimum of pain. Another way of stating this point is that there is always a balance between the attempt to express and satisfy wishes and the attempt to defend and disguise those wishes that are considered likely to arouse more anxiety than pleasure. If we listen to someone free associate in therapy, we can expect to see indications of the expression of and the defense against wishes. That is, we expect to observe the ways in which a person deals with conflict.

Following are some of the core, interrelated propositions of traditional Freudian theory:

1. The principle of psychic determinism states that there is a lawful regularity to mental life; that is, even seemingly random or "accidental" mental phenomena have causes.

2. A substantial part of mental life takes place outside conscious awareness. Unconscious wishes and motives exert a powerful influence on conscious thought and behavior and can explain seemingly random or "accidental behaviors" (e.g., slips of the tongue and many other kinds of parapraxes described by Freud, 1901, in *The Psychopathology of Everyday Life*).

3. All behavior is motivated by a desire (a) to avoid being rendered helpless by excessive stimulation, and (b) to maximize pleasure and minimize pain (the pleasure principle).

4. Inner conflict is inevitable and ubiquitous; all behavior reflects efforts at effecting a compromise among the various components of the personality, principally one's desires for instinctual drive gratification (sexual and aggressive) and the constraints against such gratification (physical reality,

social constraints, and superego prohibitions). This proposition takes its fullest form in Freud's (1923, 1926) structural theory of id, ego, and superego.

5. Anxiety in small doses (i.e., signal anxiety) is a danger signal that triggers defensive measures designed to avoid awareness and/or behavior geared toward gratification of unconscious wishes in order to avoid an anticipated full-blown traumatic experience of anxiety which would totally overwhelm the ego and flood the organism with an unmanageable amount of excitation.

6. A complete explanation of psychological phenomena should include multiple points of view, or what has been called metapsychology (Rapaport & Gill, 1959): genetic (i.e., developmental), adaptive, dynamic, topographical, economic, and structural. These terms refer, respectively, to the psychosexual stages of development (genetic); the coping devices and defensive measures by which the ego mediates between the motivational drive pressures, external reality, and superego prohibitions (adaptive); the nature of the conflicts involved (dynamic); the relation of mental contents to consciousness (topographical); the energic and quantitative aspects of the dynamic interplay of forces in the mind (economic; now the most discredited aspect of the metapsychology); and the organization of the tripartite psychic apparatus (id, ego, and superego; structural). It should be noted that id, ego, and superego are hypothetical constructs by which the observer organizes the aspects of behavior that are likely to conflict with one another; they are not concrete entities doing battle with one another, even though in the analytic literature it often sounds as if they are.

7. The principle of multiple determination (sometimes misleadingly called overdetermination) refers to the facts of divergent and convergent causality; that is, the same motive can give rise to myriad behaviors and a given behavior is a function of multiple motives (Waelder, 1960).

8. Finally, Freud's notion of a "complementary series" makes room for the joint contribution and interaction of genetic/constitutional and environmental factors as determinants of behavior.

Psychoanalytic ego psychology, aspects of which were clearly implied by Freud, was further developed by Anna Freud (1937), Hartmann, Kris, and Loewenstein (1946), and others. As seen by these theorists, ego capacities (e.g., cognition, delay of gratification, reality testing, and judgment) have an innate, autonomous basis independent of instinctual drives. In Hartmann's (1939) terms, there are "ego apparatuses" that have "primary autonomy" (i.e., originate and evolve independently of the drives) and there are ego functions that achieve "secondary autonomy" (i.e., are implicated at some point in conflict but later function as "conflict-free spheres of the ego"). This theoretical thrust was an attempt to flesh out the ego's role in adaptation and to balance Freud's strong emphasis on the primacy and dominance of the instinctual drives with a recognition that there are behaviors, interests, and motives that are not always or simply indirect expressions or sublimations of sexual or aggressive wishes.

Mahler's (1968) studies of separation–individuation and Jacobson's work on the self (1964) have contributed significantly to our understanding of the development of the self, a topic not directly dealt with in early psychoanalytic writings. In more recent years, issues of self-esteem and disturbances in the sense of self have been a prominent focus of psychoanalytic theorizing, particularly in borderline and narcissistic conditions (Kernberg, 1975, 1980; Kohut, 1971, 1977, 1984). These theoretical developments owe much to Freud's (1914) papers *On Narcissism* and *Mourning and Melancholia* which contain numerous implications for our conceptions of psychosis, character development, identification and loss, and object relations.

PSYCHOLOGICAL HEALTH AND PATHOLOGY

Behavior is dysfunctional or pathological to the extent that the compromise formations among the constituents of the personality are "maladaptive." That is, they create more pain than pleasure, bring the person into significant interpersonal conflict, create undue anxiety and/or guilt and depressive affects, lead to significant inhibitions in personal functioning, and thereby impair the person's capacity to love and/or work. In this view, there is no sharp demarcation between "normal" and "abnormal" functioning.

Stated in the psychoanalytic language of ego psychology, one may ask: How well does the individual adapt to the "average expectable environment"? How adaptive versus maladaptive or pathological are the person's compromise formations? *Pathological compromise formations* refer to outcomes of psychic conflict in which the ego is ineffective in arriving at a solution to the problem of dealing with drive pressures, opposing superego demands, and the requirements of external reality. The appearance of symptoms or the development of ego inhibitions are indications of ineffective coping with inner conflict. For example, the onset of agoraphobia (fear of open spaces) can represent the person's failed defense against the anxiety attached to desires to separate and function in a more autonomous manner, desires that may be experienced as arousing separation anxiety as well as reflecting wishes to rid oneself of the maternal object and thereby induce feelings of guilt. The onset of hysterical blindness in a mother who harbors hostile wishes toward her son, who then has a bad accident because his mother was not watching him, would be understood, in part, as a self-punishment for her hostile wishes. In another example, impotence in a male in relation to certain women but not others may be due to the fact that the women with whom the impotence occurs are unconsciously regarded as incestuous objects, and the impotence is an inhibition of unacceptable and anxiety-ridden Oedipal wishes.

The psychoanalytic formula for the formation of symptoms is that there is a wish that is too strong and/or defenses that are too weak to contain it in a sufficiently disguised form. The outbreak of psychological symptoms is an expression of the "return of the repressed." In this drive–defense model, symptoms appear as a second line of defense to help ward off the awareness and/or expression of wishes (drive derivatives) that are deemed too threatening and/or unacceptable. Symptoms vary with respect to the extent to which they show evidence of the underlying wish *and its attempted gratification* or show more clearly the defensive side of the conflict.

The maintenance of symptoms is due to the *primary* and *secondary* gain they provide. The primary gain is the relative freedom from anxiety and other dysphoric affects (Brenner, 1982) that is achieved while partially satisfying a wish in a compromise form. Secondary gain refers to the fringe benefits of a symptom (e.g., "justifiable" escape from normal responsibilities and feeling that one's dependency needs are more legitimate).

The drive–defense model also is used as part of the explanation for the development of personality or character styles. For example, a pattern of noncommitment in relationships may protect the person against the feared consequences of intimacy in instances in which intimacy might give rise to claustrophobic anxiety, which in turn signifies a sense of danger about what may be seen as an "Oedipal triumph." This term refers to any wish, attitude, or action that signifies (usually on an unconscious, symbolic level), the son's desire to win the competition with his father for his mother's love. Such desires typically are conflicted, due in part to fear of the father's retribution. The daughter experiences a similar conflict vis-à-vis her mother. To avoid this anxiety, the person chooses to enter rela-

tionships that are at some level "known" to preclude the possibility of a serious commitment. When this pattern is repeated, the person may have the conscious experience of feeling frustrated and puzzled at the failure of any of his or her relationships to last, without being aware of the underlying dynamic conflict.

With respect to "choice" of symptoms, Freud, early on, held the simplistic belief that the nature of infantile sexual experience determined the types of symptoms that would appear later. He thought, for example, that a passive sexual experience led to hysterical symptoms, whereas an active sexual experience led to obsessional symptoms. With the abandonment of the *seduction theory* (i.e., the idea that hysterical symptoms would not occur unless the patient had experienced a sexual seduction as a child), Freud came a long way in recognizing that there was no simple correspondence between a particular external event and the type of symptom that might ensue. The question of the "choice" of symptom became as complex as the determinants of personality development and the individual's psychic reality.

It is worth noting that although Freud has been criticized for giving up the seduction theory, Freud clearly never gave up his belief that sexual and other environmental trauma took place. However, and this was decisive for the evolution of psychoanalytic thinking, what was significant for psychological development was what the individual did with what happened to him or her. That is, not everyone reacts to the same external trauma in the same way and individual differences in the way people do react affect and are affected by the conflicts and means of coping and defending they bring to the situation.

It should be apparent thus far that psychoanalytic theory does not make a sharp distinction between symptom neuroses and character neuroses, nor does it posit a sharp dividing line between what is regarded as "normal" versus "pathological." With respect to the distinction between symptoms and character traits, it is true that the former refer to discrete circumscribed impairments in functioning that the patient usually, but by no means always, experiences as ego alien. However, more subtle, behavioral patterns that are not classified as symptoms may and often do cause distress and can be experienced as ego alien. For example, the person who "engineers" one rejection after another in work and/or in love would be seen as having a character style with significant masochistic components. Such a person unconsciously seeks suffering, which is associated with pleasure, even while consciously claiming to want to change. Such a behavior pattern can be ego alien. Thus, the usual formulation that symptoms are always ego alien and that maladaptive character traits are always ego syntonic is too simple.

Since these formulations and the early contributions by Abraham (1927, 1973), Reich (1933), and others, there has been an increasing interest in studying character and character pathology. This interest is due to the apparently growing number of patients who present with character disorders, particularly narcissistic and borderline personalities, rather than symptom neuroses, and to the idea that dealing with symptoms in treatment is less effective if one fails to address the personality in which they are embedded.

By personality or character we mean the unique psychological organization (of traits, conflicts, defensive and coping strategies, attitudes, values, cognitive style, etc.) that characterizes the individual's stable, enduring modes of adaptation across a wide range of conditions encountered in the individual's "average expectable environment" (Hartmann, 1939). The multiple determinants of character include biological, psychological, and sociocultural factors. The complex interactions of these factors are best described in Erikson's (1950) *Childhood and Society*.

Two major psychological paths to character formation are one's identifications with significant others and one's style of coping with and defending against inner conflict. Maladaptive patterns of dealing with conflict tend to become rigidified and repeated in vicious cycles, as will be seen in the case presented later. By definition, personality structure changes at a slow rate. This is one reason why meaningful personality change through psychotherapy generally takes a long time.

THE PROCESS OF CLINICAL ASSESSMENT

The unit of study is the individual or, more specifically, his or her inner world. Although the clinician will want to know a great deal about the individual's actual functioning in different social contexts (family, friends, work groups, etc.), the main relevance of this information is its value in understanding the intrapsychic world of the individual.

The primary means of conducting the assessment of the individual's psychopathology is through the clinical interview. The interview serves simultaneously to assess the prospective patient's suitability and motivation for treatment. In earlier years, if the first few interviews did not reveal any gross contraindications to the start of treatment, clinicians began with a *trial analysis* in order to have an extended period in which to assess suitability for analytic treatment. In recent years, this decision is generally made after two or three consultations.

Referrals for psychological testing are relatively rare, both at the stage of the initial assessment as well as later on. Testing is more likely to be recommended when there is little treatment progress or marked unclarity regarding diagnosis (e.g., if organicity or a learning disability is suspected).

In the course of the clinical interview, the therapist attempts to form an initial picture of the patient's current and past level of functioning, including the nature, onset, duration, intensity, and fluctuation of symptoms. The therapist also begins to get a sense of the patient's character style, his or her principal defenses, and the core, unconscious conflicts presumed to underlie manifest aspects of behavior. The clinician will also want to develop some hypotheses concerning the psychodynamic significance of the current stresses faced by the prospective patient, the manner and effectiveness with which they are handled, and the patient's decision to seek treatment at this time. Part of this broad assessment of the patient's psychopathology and personality functioning includes an appraisal of the person's ego interests, areas of and capacity for pleasure and achievement, and quality of interpersonal relations.

The clinician also attempts to appraise the prospective patient's suitability for psychoanalysis or psychoanalytic psychotherapy. Among the main qualities evaluated are the person's motivation for change, ego resources, including capacity to regress in the service of the ego, and degree of psychological-mindedness. The latter refers to the patient's capacity for self-reflective awareness, for an introspective tuning in on one's inner experiences, fantasies, and dreams. Because analysis requires that the patient oscillate between verbalizing his or her subjective experience and, in collaboration with the analyst, reflecting on the multiple meanings of those experiences, an inability or disinclination to view experience and behavior in psychological terms does not bode well for this form of treatment.

Because an implicit and explicit condition for meaningful introspection, and a value undergirding the therapeutic situation, is self-examination, the capacity to tolerate frustration and not act impulsively is considered a prognostically favorable sign. As indicated earlier, there is a vital collaborative aspect to the analytic work. Therefore, the patient's history of sustained, satisfying interpersonal relationships and reasonably intact reality testing are relevant predictors of the collaborative quality of the prospective therapeutic relationship. This kind of assessment, typically conducted in the course of

several initial interviews, enables the analyst to make a judgment regarding the patient's "analyzability" and is one element in the decision to recommend psychoanalysis versus psychoanalytic psychotherapy.

In addition to the kinds of assessments mentioned, the analyst should also conduct a self-assessment to try to get a sense of whether there are particular personality conflicts, personal biases (e.g., with respect to value systems), or other factors that might preclude the possibility of maintaining the objectivity and attitudes necessary to be helpful to the patient. If there are such potential problems, referral to another clinician is indicated.

Finally, the therapist will need to assess the patient's reality situation to determine whether matters of money, time, and/or immediate crises in the patient's life would interfere significantly with the possibility of a sustained, unhurried exploration of his or her core conflicts. In the event that such factors are present to a strong degree, an alternative approach is recommended (e.g., a delay in the beginning of treatment, crisis intervention, and/or a more supportive, less challenging therapy).

There is no universally accepted, formal psychoanalytic system for diagnosing different varieties of dysfunction (Messer & Wolitzky, 1997). Originally, Freud focused primarily on three symptom pictures: hysterical, obsessional, and phobic. Other psychiatric syndromes soon received attention (e.g., depression, paranoid conditions, bipolar disorder, schizophrenia, and perversions). In recent years, narcissistic and borderline conditions have been the focus of intense interest, as such patients are increasingly common in psychoanalytic practice.

Psychoanalysts have contributed to and generally follow the diagnostic system of the fourth edition of the *Diagnostic and Statistical Manual of Mental Disorders* (DSM-IV; American Psychiatric Association, 1994) even though its successive versions have become increasingly atheoretical and less sympathetic to a psychoanalytic viewpoint. However, many analysts do not place much value on an initial, formal diagnosis beyond the gross classification of the patient as psychotic, borderline, or neurotic. Many, if not most, patients seen in private analytic practices rarely meet all the DSM-IV criteria for a given diagnostic category but frequently approximate, especially as the treatment unfolds, the criteria for several diagnostic categories. That is, rarely do we see pure types and, in any case, the focus is more on the underlying dynamics than on the changing symptom picture. Furthermore, a purely descriptive classification that does not attempt to address etiological and dynamic factors is of limited interest or clinical utility to psychoanalytic clinicians. In general, many analysts have little regard for the DSM classification scheme and view the high rates of comorbidity on Axis I and Axis II as an artifact of the diagnostic system.

There have been several psychoanalytically based attempts to form diagnostic assessments of dysfunction based on dynamic and structural features of personality functioning, particularly when the diagnostic formulation has implications for specific modifications and variations in psychoanalytic approaches to treatment. Here I briefly summarize two examples of a psychoanalytic approach to nosology and the treatment implications that derive from them.

Kernberg (1975), one of the most widely and frequently cited authors in the psychoanalytic world, has concentrated on borderline personality organization and has made notable contributions to the diagnosis of different levels of psychic structure and pathology. His aim has been to understand these conditions from an integrated theoretical perspective that combines British object relations theories, ego psychology, and the work of Mahler (1968) and Jacobson (1964) who were interested in the developmental course of self–object differentiation.

One of the main features of Kernberg's (1975) system is his differentiation of three levels of pathological functioning with re-

spect to four different psychological domains: superego development, object relations, instinctual strivings, and defensive ego operations. With this diagnostic scheme Kernberg distinguishes three levels of psychopathology: neurotic, borderline, and psychotic. Patients designated as psychotic have confused self/object boundaries, that is, they find it hard to keep separate in their mind their mental representations of self and of others. This deficit in differentiation makes adequate reality testing difficult. In borderline personality functioning, self/object differentiation is maintained but the patient cannot integrate mental representations of self and other as both "good" and "bad." This lack of integration is referred to as "primitive splitting." One manifestation of splitting is the tendency to alternate from overidealizing to devaluing the other, which makes the person prone to having unstable interpersonal relationships. Within the category of borderline functioning Kernberg distinguishes "higher," "intermediate," and "lower" levels of functioning. One reason for the development of borderline personality organization, according to Kernberg, is an excess of aggression (due to a combination of a weak ego, strong, innate aggression, and significant external trauma). Borderline patients manifest poor impulse control, poor tolerance of anxiety, and chaotic object relations. So-called structural clinical interviewing involves deliberate trial interpretations of defensive maneuvers that can elicit responses that will enable the clinician to diagnose borderline personalities.

In contrast to those diagnosed as psychotic or borderline, neurotic patients have well differentiated self–other boundaries. They also can better tolerate ambivalence so that they have more integrated "good–bad" mental representations of self and other.

Kernberg's attempt at a precise diagnostic scheme is linked to specific recommendations of how different patients should be treated and what modifications of psychoanalysis should and need not be made in the treatment of borderline conditions. Some therapists suggest mostly supportive therapy with borderline patients. Kernberg, however, believes that the central focus should be on the interpreation of defensive operations that serve to maintain primitive splitting and dissociated ego states (Kernberg, Selzer, Koenigsberg, Carr, & Applebaum, 1989).

Gedo and Goldberg (1973), looking at the entire range of psychopathology, developed a hierarchical organization of therapeutic approaches geared to pathologies at different developmental levels. For example, patients vulnerable to overstimulation require "pacification" (medication, protective environments, etc.), patients susceptible to psychotic states require "unification" (e.g., availability of the therapist as a reliable object), and narcissistic personality disorders need "optimal disillusionment" (titrated confrontation with reality). Interpretation aimed at the resolution of intrapsychic conflict is considered appropriate only for neurotic disorders.

THE PRACTICE OF THERAPY

Basic Structure of Therapy

In what follows, I confine myself to an account of the practice of psychoanalytic treatment as it is usually thought of in relation to neurotic and some high-functioning borderline patients. I do not discuss the modifications that are made with seriously borderline and narcissistic patients, as described by Kernberg (1975) and others (e.g., Bach, 1985).

Before discussing the basic structure of therapy, we have to address the distinction between psychoanalysis and psychoanalytically oriented psychotherapy. There are those who would make a sharp, qualitative distinction between these two forms of treatment and those who prefer to blur the boundaries. In controversies about what should properly be called "psychoanalysis," it has been easiest to fall back on external criteria. The implication is that whenever it

is applicable, psychoanalysis is the treatment of choice. It is regarded as a deeper, more thorough approach to the patient's problems. Other forms of treatment (e.g., supportive psychotherapy) mix the "pure gold of psychoanalysis" with the "copper of suggestion" (Freud, 1919, p. 168). Thus, the common clinical maxim that has guided psychoanalytically oriented clinicians is to be as supportive as necessary and as exploratory as possible, that is to minimize suggestion, advice, and reassurance and to focus on interpretations leading to insight.

Relying on external criteria, psychoanalysis is defined in large part by the frequency of sessions and the use of the couch. Sessions typically are held three or four times per week, for 45 or 50 minutes, over a period of many years. Psychoanalytic psychotherapy usually takes place at a frequency of once or twice a week in the face-to-face position and can last as long as psychoanalysis or may be as short as 12 sessions (e.g., Crits-Christoph & Barber, 1991; Malan, 1976; Messer & Warren, 1995).

A more meaningful distinction between psychoanalysis and psychoanalytic psychotherapy (also called "expressive" or "exploratory" psychotherapy), as well as between these forms of treatment compared with others (e.g., "supportive" psychotherapy), would focus on intrinsic rather than extrinsic features (Gill, 1984). In this regard, the nature of the therapist's focus in psychoanalysis is on the interpretation of transference and resistance (to be described later). Such a focus is considered to be the most emotionally meaningful and therefore most effective way of helping patients become aware of how and why they are reenacting conflicts from the past in the present, particularly in relation to the therapist. Although such explorations go on in psychoanalytic psychotherapy, they are not as prolonged or detailed, nor do they focus as systematically on the past and on the transference.

The range of psychoanalytically informed treatment can be ordered on a continuum from psychoanalysis proper at one end to psychoanalytic psychotherapy (or expressive therapy) in the center to supportive psychotherapy at the other end. These modalities are best regarded as overlapping and distinguishable from one another to the extent that they focus on the interpretation of transference resistances and the less they rely on suggestion and on healing through the direct benefits of the therapeutic relationship per se. The powerful and innovative feature of psychoanalysis proper is the attempt, paradoxical in nature, to use the therapist's authority to free the patient from excessive reliance on suggestion and authority. This is less the case in expressive therapy and even less in supportive treatment, where the therapist capitalizes on his or her authority and uses direct suggestions more freely.

It should be clear that none of the three, overlapping modalities arranged on the continuum outlined previously are pure types; rather, it is matter of emphasis. There are both deliberately supportive and inherently supportive elements in classical psychoanalysis, and interpretations, though not central, are found not only in psychoanalysis and psychoanalytic psychotherapy but in supportive treatments. It also is the case that a treatment that begins with an intent to use one modality will, given certain clinical indications, shift, as least temporarily, to another modality.

In what follows, I focus primarily on psychoanalysis with the understanding that most of what is said is more or less applicable to psychoanalytic psychotherapy.

The Conduct of the Sessions

After the initial consultation sessions and the structuring of the therapy (frequency of sessions, fee, etc), the sessions are deliberately unstructured. If it is not already understood, the analyst asks the patient to free associate, that is, to say whatever comes to mind. Thus, the patient determines the content of the session. The more freely the patient talks, the more he or she is able and willing to suspend the normal inhibitions and editing processes that are part and parcel of our usual dialogues with others, the more introspective and self-disclosing the person will be, and the easier it will be for previously repressed or suppressed feelings and thoughts to come to the surface for analytic scrutiny. This is also the rationale for the use of the couch.

The goal of encouraging the patient to free associate is a mediating or process goal. It allows both patient and analyst to observe when and how the patient engages in defensive maneuvers in the face of actual or anticipated anxiety or other dysphoric affect. In this manner, the patient will get an increasingly clear sense of how his or her mind works and how these workings are shaped by unconscious factors.

Rarely is a time limit imposed on the therapy. The main exception is brief, psychoanalytically oriented treatments in which the patient is explicitly informed that the treatment will last only for a limited number of sessions (see Messer & Warren, 1995, for such approaches).

In individual treatment, significant others in the patient's life typically are not seen by the patient's therapist. Sometimes combined formats are used. For example, a patient in individual treatment may also be seen as part of a couple, family, or group therapy. In these circumstances, it generally is not considered proper practice for the patient's individual therapist to treat the patient in one of the other modalities as well. To do so would interfere with the optimal development and resolution of the transference.

Goal Setting

Stated in general terms, the ultimate goal of treatment is to increase the patient's adaptive functioning by ameliorating the disabling symptoms and crippling inhibitions that have plagued the patient. As the patient gradually reduces the neurotic vicious cycles that characterized his or her prior adaptive efforts, he or she will experience this change as involving an expanded sense of personal agency and freedom. Usually, this goal is assumed to be so basic and obvious as not to require explicit verbalization.

Although this is the patient's presumed goal, it is one that can contradict the patient's often unconscious need to suffer. It is not surprising to a psychoanalytic clinician to observe that after a period of improvement in treatment the patient may deteriorate. Freud called this the "negative therapeutic reaction" and regarded it as a serious obstacle to some treatments.

In the final paragraph of *Studies on Hysteria,* Freud, in response to a patient's query, stated, "No doubt fate would find it easier than I do to relieve you of your illness. But you will be able to convince yourself that much will be gained if we succeed in transforming your hysterical misery into common unhappiness" (Breuer & Freud, 1895, p. 305). At first he thought that this transformation was achieved by "making the unconscious conscious." His later epigrammatic statement of the goal of psychoanalysis, consistent with the replacement of the topographic theory (conscious, preconscious, unconscious) by the structural theory (id, ego, superego), was "where id was, there shall ego be" (Freud, 1933, p. 80). In other words, awareness was still considered a necessary but now a no longer sufficient condition for change. The patient must also be able to accept and to *integrate* previously disavowed, split-off aspects of his or her personality. This is another way of talking about the resolution of conflict. The removal of symptoms is not a direct goal but is expected to occur as a by-product of more adaptive conflict resolution.

At the same time, it should be clear that the resolution of conflict is far from an all-or-none, once-and-for-all matter. In this sense, analysts do not expect to effect a complete and permanent "cure." This point is depicted humorously in a cartoon in which the first picture, titled "Before Therapy," shows a man riding a motorcycle with a monkey on his back; the second picture is captioned "After Therapy" and shows the man riding his motorcycle and the monkey seated in the sidecar. If we can help the patient get the monkey off his back, he will feel considerably less burdened.

Support for this point of view is found in a series of studies by Luborsky and his colleagues (e.g., Luborsky & Crits-Christoph, 1990). They have examined treatment protocols to identify core conflictual relationship themes (CCRTs) based on an assessment of relationship episodes described by the patient. A CCRT consists of a wish expressed by the patient, the response by the person to whom the wish is directed, and the patient's reaction to the response of the other. Patients typically show a few key CCRTs that remain fairly stable over the course of treatment in the sense that the same themes continue to be expressed. What changes is that the patient handles his or her issues in a more adaptive manner and with less subjective distress.

Process Aspects of Treatment

The main strategy in the conduct of psychoanalytic treatment is the analysis of the resistances and transference reactions that emerge from the patient's "free associations." For the most part, readers will have to wait until the "Case Illustration" section for concrete examples of the application of strategies and techniques of treatment.

We can frame our discussion here by citing Gill's (1954) often quoted definition: "Psychoanalysis is that technique which, employed by a neutral analyst, results in the development of a regressive transference neurosis and the ultimate resolution of this neurosis by techniques of interpretation alone" (p. 775). I defer a discussion of neutrality until the next main section of the chapter and focus on the two other key elements of the definition: regressive transference neurosis and interpretation. Gill (1979), 25 years later, claimed that the one defining characteristic of psychoanalysis proper should be the interpretation of transference.

Transference

Freud first mentioned transference in *Studies in Hysteria* (Breuer & Freud, 1895), calling it a "false connection" because the reaction could not be adequately accounted for by the present situation. He saw transference as both a powerful obstacle to and an essential factor in the treatment. Transference can bring to light the patient's hidden and forgotten erotic impulses. At the same time, patients resist awareness of these impulses, particularly when they are directed to the person of the therapist. Freud always emphasized the importance of emotional reliving of the childhood experiences with the analyst so that repressions could be lifted.

As a useful, working definition of transference, one can cite Greenson (1967). Transference is the "experience of feelings, drives, attitudes, fantasies, and defenses toward a person in the present which do not befit that person but are a repetition of reactions originating in regard to significant persons of early childhood, unconsciously displaced onto figures in the present" (p. 155). In describing transference as a "new edition of an old object relationship," Freud (1912, p. 116) was aware that the repetition need not be literal.

Transference reactions to emotionally significant persons in the present are fairly ubiquitous and are not restricted to experiences in analysis. In fact, in everyday life they often are a source of considerable difficulty in interpersonal relationships. What is distinctive about psychoanalytic treatment is that they are *analyzed*.

Freud originally classified transference reactions into three kinds: the positive (erotic) transference, the negative (hostile), and the unobjectionable (i.e., aim inhibited or nonerotic), positive transference necessary for cooperating and collaborating in the analytic work (an attitude that, as we shall see later, is the basis for the therapeutic (Zetzel, 1956) or working alliance (Greenson, 1965). The other characteristics of transference reactions, which essentially follow from Greenson's definition, are that they show evidence of inappropriateness, tenacity, and capriciousness. In this sense, whatever germs of veridicality they may contain, transference reactions are considered inaccurate, distorted attributions about the emotional experience, behavior, intentions, and other aspects of the analyst's behavior. However, as noted earlier, Gill (1994) feels that it is important to realize that so-called transference reactions are not created out of "whole cloth" but are triggered by real qualities of the analyst.

The intense concentration of the patient's core conflicts on the person of the analyst in the form of feelings, fantasies, and marked preoccupation in an increasingly regressive manner has been termed the "transference neurosis," although there is controversy about how frequently a full-blown transference neurosis occurs, as opposed to "transference reactions," and how necessary it is for a good therapeutic outcome.

The term "*regressive* transference neurosis" refers to the enhanced activation of childhood conflicts and attitudes in relation to the analyst. It should be noted that the patient's readiness for the emergence of a regressive transference neurosis (Macalpine, 1950) *also* is facilitated by certain features of the analytic situation (e.g., the relative anonymity of the analyst, the withholding of deliberate transference gratifications, the invitation to free associate, and the supine position of the patient).

In the traditional Freudian account, the analysis of the transference neurosis reveals the *infantile neurosis* (the central conflicts of childhood, whether or not they were clinically manifest at that time). However, Cooper (1987) believes that "the concept of the transference neurosis has lost its specificity and efforts to clarify it no longer expand our vision. The concept should be abandoned" (p. 587). Although most analysts appear reluctant to discard the concept, it is increasingly recognized that (1) not all patients regularly develop a clearly identifiable transference neurosis, and (2) effective analytic work occurs in the absence of a fully formed transference neurosis.

It is sufficient for our present purposes to think in terms of a continuum of intensity of transference reactions. The greater the degree to which the patient's current and infantile conflicts center on the person of the analyst and, correspondingly, the more intense and pervasive the preoccupation with the analyst, the more closely does the patient's state approximate what has been called transference neurosis. As a practical matter, our clinical approach is essentially the same whether we call the patient's reactions a "transference *neurosis*" or refer to them as "significant transference *reactions*." Issues of terminology are not as significant as stressing the affectively charged, vivid reliving of past relationships in the patient's current experience with the therapist that makes eventual awareness of these experiences emotionally meaningful and convincing and gives transference interpretations a particularly mutative impact.

In concluding this section, it should be noted that the therapeutic relationship involves more than bringing the past into the present. It is simultaneously a new experience as well as a reenactment of earlier experiences. The "modernist" view of transference (Cooper, 1987) stresses the aspect of new experience; the "historical" view emphasizes the aspect of reliving the past. In the historical view, the experiencing of the "here-and-now" transference is important not only in its own right but as a path toward the revival and recovery of childhood memories and the interpretive reconstruction of the past. In the modernist view, successfully analyzing the "here-and-now" transference is sufficient. Keep in mind that these are matters of emphasis, not either–or distinctions.

Resistance

As the patient attempts to free associate, there will inevitably be indications of *resistance* both to the awareness of warded-off mental contents and to the behavioral and attitudinal changes that might be attempted based on the awareness of previously repressed fantasies and conflicts. Resistance, following Gill (1982), can be defined as defense expressed in the transference, though Freud (1900) defined it more broadly as "anything that interferes with the analysis."

Because the patient fears the anxiety and/or depressive affect (e.g., humiliation, shame, and guilt) that is anticipated as an accompaniment to the awareness of certain wishes and fantasies, the natural tendency is to defend against and to avoid becoming aware of those mental contents. At the same time, the analytic situation has been deliberately designed to maximize the possibility of such awareness.

Resistance can and does take many forms, both blatant (e.g., a deliberate refusal to say what is on one's mind) and subtle (e.g., filling every silence quickly out of fear that the analyst would be critical of "resistance"). I chose this last example to make two points: (1) The patient's resistance will usually be connected to the analyst, and it is these transference resistances that are the major focus of analytic attention, and (2) patients (and, unfortunately also many therapists) think of resistance as something bad, as something to be overcome. This pejorative connotation doubtless derives from the early days of psychoanalysis in which Freud used hypnosis, pressure techniques, and the insistence on complete candor ("You *must* pledge to tell me *everything* that comes to mind") in the initial formulation of the "fundamental rule." However, as Freud (1912) also said, "The resistance accompanies the treatment step by step. Every single association, every act of the person under treatment must reckon with the resistance and represents a compromise between the forces that are striving towards recovery and the opposing ones" (p. 103).

Thus, resistance naturally and inevitably includes "opposition to free association, to the procedures of analysis, to recall, to insight, and to change" (Eagle & Wolitzky, 1992, p. 124). In this sense, to refer to resistance is to say little more than people defend themselves against anxiety and other dysphoric affects in an analytic situation that fosters free association and the uncovering of repressed conflicts. The underlying sources of the clinical manifestations of resistance, according to Freud (1937), include the constitutional strength of the instinctual drives, rigid defenses, and powerful, repetitive attempts to seek particular, familiar forms of drive gratification.

Finally, it should be noted that the affirmative, as well as the obstructive, aspects of resistance need to be recognized. For instance, resistance can be used in the service of forestalling a feared regression, asserting one's autonomy, or protecting the therapist from one's destructive impulses.

In sum, a major focus of psychoanalysis is the interpretation of transference and resistance, our next topic.

Interpretation

Turning now to interpretation, we may say that interpretation (particularly though not exclusively of the transference) leading to insight has long been regarded as *the* major curative factor in psychoanalytic treatment. In recent years, however, many analysts have given considerable weight to the curative properties of the noninterpretive elements in the therapeutic relationship (e.g., therapist empathy and implicit support), particularly with more disturbed patients.

Interpretation, broadly conceived, refers both to meanings attributed to discrete aspects of the patient's behavior and experience and to constructions that attempt to offer a more comprehensive account of portions of the patient's history.

Schematically stated, the optimal interpretation, though not necessarily presented comprehensively at one time, would take the form of "what you are doing (feeling, thinking, fantasizing, etc.) with me now is what you also are doing with your current significant other (spouse, child, boss, etc.), and what you did with your father (and/or mother) for such and such reasons and motives and with such and such consequences." In the convergence of the past and the present (both in the treatment relationship as well as in other current relationships), the recognition of repetitive, pervasive, and entrenched patterns of relating and of personal functioning can have maximum emotional and cognitive impact.

Although interpretation of transference resistances is "the single most important instrument of psychoanalytic technique" (Greenson, 1967, p. 97), other interventions are necessary prerequisites to interpretation. For example, confrontation and clarification are preparatory to interpretation. *Confrontation* points to the fact of resistance (e.g., "I notice that when you are reminded of your mother, you quickly change the subject"). *Clarification* refers to exploration of why the patient is resisting (e.g., "Talking about your mother that way seems to have made you uncomfortable"). This line of inquiry blends into interpretations of the unconscious fantasies and motives for the resistance (e.g., "You think that wishing to be alone with your mother was wrong and that I will chastise you for feeling that way"). A detailed exposition of these techniques can be found in Greenson (1967).

It should be noted that when Gill (1954) speaks of "interpretation *alone*" (italics added), in his definition cited earlier, he means that although many other interventions occur in psychoanalysis, in addition to confrontation and clarification, the reliance on interpretation leading to insight is presumed to be the key element. The power of the transference is used to resolve the transference through interpretation rather than through suggestion (i.e., the direct manipulation of the transference; for example, praising the patient or telling the patient how to act). At the same time, it is recognized that the effect of interpretations is to some extent carried by the positive transference (*both the aim-inhibited erotic transference and the unobjectionable positive transference*). According to Freud (1940), the positive transference "becomes the *true motive force* of the patient's collaboration . . . he leaves off his symptoms and seems apparently to have recovered merely for the sake of the analyst" (p. 175; italics added).

Thus, the overarching therapeutic strategy is to foster and flexibly maintain the conditions necessary for interpreting the transference. It is believed that a good working alliance (defined later) and an "optimal" degree of transference gratification/frustration will facilitate the desired oscillation between the patient's self-observation and expression of feeling and the analysis of defense and transference. However, there will be occasions, particularly with the so-called nonclassical analytic patient, when one will knowingly and advisedly employ nonanalytic interventions, including advice, active support, suggestions, and so on.

In more recent years, the emphasis is not on interpreting the transference directly but on interpreting defenses against the awareness of the transference. So-called defense analysis focuses on the anxieties and fears that the patient is trying to ward off. Most analysts today agree that defense analysis should start at the "surface" and proceed gradually to "deeper" levels, like peeling the layers of an onion. Some analysts (e.g., Gray, 1994) believe that when the analyst helps the patient become a better observer of his or her own defensive behavior, the patient often will be able to access previously warded-off mental content without much interpretive help from the analyst. Some theorists (e.g., Weiss & Sampson, 1986) stress that feeling safe as a result of the analyst passing tests posed by the patient also will enable the patient to access his or her own previously repressed wishes and fantasies, at times with little or no interpretation from the analyst.

Despite the increased flexibility of analytic technique and the open acknowledgment of the inevitably interactive nature of the analytic relationship (Oremland, 1991), traditional analysts cannot seem to shake the image of being aloof, authoritarian, and technique driven. For example, in the first edition of this book, Greenberg and Cheselka (1995, p. 70) claimed that "There are two different approaches that determine how decisions about technique are made, the technique-driven approach (exemplified by classical psychoanalysis, in which 'correct' technique is clearly specified) and the interaction-driven approach (exemplified by relational psychoanalysis)." These authors further claim that classical psychoanalysts are interested in content while relational analysts are interested in process (i.e., "events that occur in the relationships that are being talked about . . ."). As is the case with many other caricatures of classical psychoanalysis, this depiction has only a germ of truth, namely, the Freudian analyst's expectation that as the analytic material unfolds sexual and aggressive wishes will likely figure prominently in the patient's core conflicts. However, it is bad practice, not dictated by theory, when an analyst of any theoretical persuasion imposes his or her pet theory on the clinical data.

It should be clear that everything that transpires between the patient and therapist, including interpretations, constitutes an interaction. Thus, as Oremland (1991) reminds us, the distinction is really between interactions that emphasize interpretations and interactions that do not. Thus, interpretations are particular kinds of interactions. Therefore, to say that an interpretation is a relational event, as several object relations clinicians have stressed lately, is not a statement that any contemporary Freudian would question.

In fact, from a psychoanalytic perspective, Freudian or otherwise, a vital focus of interpretive work is the patient's experience of an interpretation. The analyst is as interested in this aspect of the process as in the content of the interpretation. For example, does the patient experience an interpretation as an instance of feeling empathically understood (and how does he or she feel if it is not such an instance)? Is the fact and/or the content of an interpretation experienced as a humiliation, a gift, a sexual penetration, or all of the above? Freudian analysts appreciate the recursive nature of the transference (i.e., that often the patient and the analyst are enacting the very theme they are talking about).

By maintaining such a focus on the patient's reaction to the fact as well as to the content of the analyst's interpretation, the analyst reduces the possibility of unanalyzed interactions. Let me illustrate this point with an example, taken from Basescu (1990), that seems to be an instance of an unanalyzed interaction: "One woman said, 'I had a bad weekend. Other people are stable. I'm so up and down. I hide my rockiness.' I said, 'Don't we all.' She: 'You too?' I: 'Does that surprise you?' She: 'Well, I guess not. You're human too.' I understood that to mean she also felt human, at least for the moment" (p. 54).

Wachtel (1993) cites this example approvingly as "a forthright approach to conveying a version of Sullivan's 'we are all much more simply human than otherwise.'" He regards this kind of interchange as "one of the many small increments in reappropriated humanity that in their sum constitute a successful therapy" (p. 217).

The traditional Freudian, as well as many analysts of other persuasions, would view Basescu's remark as a noninterpretive, supportive effort to soothe the patient's self-denigration instead of exploring the meanings of the patient's statement. What does it mean to her that she feels unstable and has a need to hide it? Does she find it shameful? If so, why and in what contexts? Is she envi-

ous of others, including the therapist? Why does she idealize the therapist and what implications does this have for her interpersonal relationships? Is she complaining that the therapist has not yet helped her reach a more stable existence? These are a few of the possible lines of exploration that the analytic therapist would want to pursue in an effort to facilitate an understanding of the motives, origins, and functions of her self-denigration. Unless the patient is in a dire situation, to reassure her by his self-disclosure, to directly dissuade the patient of her self-denigrating attitude and of her idealization of the therapist, is to run the serious risk of not getting to an awareness and an understanding of the patient's underlying conflicts.

A few final comments are in order before we leave the topic of interpretation. The shifting cultural attitude away from a positivistic, objective, knowable reality toward a more relativistic, pluralistic, constructivist stance has had a significant impact on psychoanalysis, particularly with regard to its views of interpretation. This change has been referred to as the "hermeneutic turn" in psychoanalysis. From this perspective, interpretations are regarded much more as constructions than as discoveries of an underlying psychic reality. Parallel to this view is an altered conception of transference–countertransference in which two subjectivities are in constant interaction, in which the transference is decisively shaped by the analyst's countertransference and thus not to be viewed simply as a distortion. Lines of interpretation are considered to be as much the analyst's preferred story lines and narratives as they are veridical readings of the patient's psychic reality (Schafer, 1992). In part, this view is an antidote to an analytic stance in which the analyst thinks that he or she possesses something akin to interpretive infallibility, a countertransference danger that can plague any analyst regardless of theoretical persuasion (Eagle, Wolitzky, & Wakefield, 2001).

Process of Therapy

As noted previously, my focus is on the psychoanalytic treatment of the average expectable neurotic patient. Before proceeding, however, it is important to note that in these days of biologically oriented psychiatry, many therapists have come to believe that there is no inherent contradiction between psychoanalysis and psychopharmacological treatment. Therefore, where there are fairly clear indications of a biological predisposition to aspects of the patient's emotional disturbance or even if the patient's suffering is entirely psychologically based, medication that will take the edge off dysfunctional anxiety and depression actually often facilitates the treatment. Of course, the psychological meanings of taking medication, including the question of whether it is prescribed by the patient's therapist or a psychopharmcologist, will have to be carefully explored, particularly in its transference implications.

According to Freud, psychoanalysis can be likened to chess; the opening moves and the end game are fairly standard, but the long middle phase is not predictable and is open to many variations. In psychoanalytic treatment, clinicians distinguish between an opening phase, the extended, middle phase of "working through," and the termination phase.

Working Alliance

The primary emphasis in the opening phase of treatment is on the establishment of rapport and a good working relationship, the importance of which was recognized early on in Freud's notion of the "unobjectionable positive transference." Subsequently, this aspect of the therapeutic relationship has been called the "working alliance" (Greenson, 1965), the "therapeutic alliance" (Zetzel, 1956), and the "helping alliance" (Luborsky, 1984). Although there are differences in these similar-sounding concepts,

for present purposes I will regard them as equivalent and restrict myself to Greenson's conception.

According to Greenson (1967), the working alliance is the "relatively non-neurotic, rational relationship between patient and analyst which makes it possible for the patient to work purposefully in the analytic situation" (p. 45). The patient achieves this attitude when feeling safe and accepted in the analytic situation and through an identification with, or at least an adoption of, the clinician's analytic stance. This collaborative spirit of inquiry and understanding is part of the alliance between the analyst's analytic attitude and the patient's reasonable, self-observing ego. It is not a once-and-for-all achievement but one that is readily disrupted by the patient's transference reactions as well as the therapist's countertransference reactions.

Analytic interventions, as well as silence, can be experienced as narcissistic injuries caused by the patient's sense of the analyst's failure of empathy. Ruptures in the alliance are not only inevitable but are seen as important and necessary spurs to the therapeutic process because, when recognized, they create the opportunity for repair and the reestablishment of the alliance. From this perspective, the treatment can be thought of as a series of ruptures and repairs that ultimately strengthen the therapeutic bond. Thus, although the ruptures might arouse negative feelings and shake the patient's trust in the analyst, the repairs can restore and solidify it. The patient learns that a relationship can survive some pain and misunderstanding when the analyst is a fair and decent person.

An unwitting transference–countertransference enactment in which the patient and therapist engage in a neurotically based interaction can create a disruption in the alliance. The rupture can take the form of subtle avoidance and withdrawal or be overtly confrontational (e.g., questioning the analyst's competence). In recent years, we have seen an extensive theoretical and research literature on the alliance. The interested reader should consult Luborsky (1984) and Safran and Muran (2000).

Some authors (e.g., Brenner, 1979) have cautioned that an emphasis on promoting and maintaining the alliance runs the risk of providing the patient with unanalyzed transference gratification and is thus counterproductive. However, virtually all analysts would agree that the patient's capacity to listen to, reflect on, and make effective use of transference interpretations requires the presence of a good working relationship. In empirical studies of psychoanalytic psychotherapy, Luborsky and Crits-Christoph (1990) have found that the strength of the helping alliance, measured early in treatment, is a significant predictor of treatment outcome.

How does one foster the treatment alliance? The primary answer is that one listens empathically and nonjudgmentally; is alert to detecting and managing countertransference reactions; explains, to the extent necessary, the rationale for the rules and the framework of the treatment (e.g., why one does not routinely answer questions); and offers interpretations with proper timing, tact, and dosage. By the latter, we mean that we develop a sense of the patient's optimal level of anxiety and his or her vulnerabilities to narcissistic injury (blows to self-esteem). We function in a way that is aimed at not traumatically exceeding these levels. These considerations come under the heading of, for want of a better term, "clinically informed common sense," "clinical wisdom," or "tact" and take precedence over technical rules and precepts for the handling of the opening phase of treatment (or any phase for that matter). Thus, the usual precepts of analyzing defenses before impulses, beginning with the surface, allowing the patient to determine the subject of the session, and so on, are all liable to be suspended if clinical judgment so dictates.

From the aforementioned perspective, the most common and serious technical errors a therapist can make are really not technical per se but are countertransferential attitudes and interventions that reflect rigid, arbitrary, unempathic responsiveness to the patient and that thereby fail to respect the patient's individuality, integrity, and autonomy. Any specific, discrete technical error (e.g., intervening too rapidly and fostering premature closure instead of giving the patient the opportunity to express his or her feelings and thoughts more fully) is considered relatively minor when compared to the danger of retraumatization that can occur if the therapist acts in the manner previously described. Thus, common technical errors such as failing to leave the initiative with the patient; frequent interruptions and questions (especially those that call for a simple "yes" or "no" rather than encouraging exploration); offering farfetched, intellectualized or jargon-filled interpretations; an excess of therapeutic zeal; attitudes of omniscience and grandiosity; dogmatism; the need to be seen as clever; engaging in power struggles with the patient; failure to begin or end the session on time; and being punitive or overly apologetic all derive their potentially adverse effects from the extent to which they express undetected and therefore unmanaged countertransference.

Some analysts recommend explicit techniques for fostering the alliance. For example, the use of the word "we" (if not overdone) can promote a sense of collaboration and bonding. Thus, instead of saying "What did you mean by that?" the analyst could say "Let's try to understand what that meant." This kind of statement encourages an identification with the analytic attitude of reflecting on the meaning of one's experience and behavior. Sterba (1934) offered the distinction between the "experiencing ego" and the "observing ego." In an effective working alliance, the patient oscillates between reporting his experience through free associations and periodically stepping back to observe and reflect on these experiences. This "split in the ego" is essential to the work of self-discovery.

Working Through

In the extended, middle phase of treatment, the focus is on the analysis of transference and resistance with the aim of having the patient "work through" their long-standing conflicts. *Working through* refers to "the repetitive, progressive and elaborate explorations of the resistances which prevent insight from leading to change" (Greenson, 1967, p. 42).

In the early days of psychoanalysis, Freud reported some dramatic "cures" in which hysterical symptoms disappeared, at least temporarily, following the recall of the traumatic memories of the experiences that first gave rise to the symptoms. Patients, even fairly sophisticated ones, often have the fantasy that a single, blinding insight will free them to take the path previously not taken because it was unseen or too frightful to pursue. In fact, as patients become aware of their core conflicts they appreciate that they have been repeatedly reenacting many variations of the same theme in ways that they regard as vital, even though such actions also cause them pain and suffering. Becoming aware of one's patterns of maladaptive living in the context of the transference, recalling their similarity to childhood reactions and modes of relating to significant others, and realizing the unconscious fantasies on which they are based usually is a slow, painstaking, "two steps forward–one step back" process.

Resistance to change often can be slow to dissolve. Maintaining the status quo commonly is seen as the safest course. Fear and guilt concerning the consequences of change (e.g., feelings that one does not deserve to be happy, feeling that changing means that one is abandoning or being disloyal to a parent, and the reluctance to relinquish long cherished fantasies and beliefs) continue to be analyzed in their various, often subtle forms so that the secondary as well as the primary gain of the symptoms or neurotic patterns may be lessened.

Thus, the repeated exploration and elaboration of the patient's key, unconscious conflicts and the defenses against them as they become expressed in the context of the therapeutic relationship and in other aspects of the patient's life are the core of the analytic process. Specifically, the analytic process can be viewed as consisting of numerous sequences of (1) the patient's resistance to awareness and to change, (2) the analyst's interpretation of the resistance, and (3) the patient's responses to the interpretation (Weinshel, 1984).

Termination

Relatively little has been written regarding termination compared with the literature on other aspects of treatment. It is generally agreed that termination should not be forced (as in setting a specific time limit), unilateral, premature, or overdue. It has been claimed that a poorly planned and handled termination phase can practically destroy an otherwise good analysis.

As the work proceeds, therapist and patient periodically implicitly and explicitly assess the degree of progress made toward achieving the therapeutic goals. Ideally, the idea of termination emerges naturally in the minds of both participants as they recognize that the therapeutic goals (both those articulated at the start and ones that developed later on) have been essentially met and that the treatment, therefore, has reached the point of diminishing returns. Unfortunate but realistic reasons for termination include the judgment that little or no progress has been made over a significant period of time.

In any case, actual termination is ideally planned to commence at some specified time after a mutual decision has been made. The rationale for a planned termination phase rather than an abrupt ending includes the idea that separation from the analyst is a significant psychological event that will evoke feelings, fantasies, and conflicts that resonate with earlier separations from or losses of significant others. It is not unusual that once a target date for termination is set, feelings along these lines emerge, feelings that previously had been latent or not dealt with before termination became a reality. Even when the patient initiates the idea of termination, it is not unusual for the analyst's agreement to terminate to be experienced as a rejection and abandonment. In addition, the temporary recrudescence of symptoms in the termination phase is not uncommon, often as an expression of separation fears ("See, I'm not ready to stop treatment").

In summary, the optimal criteria for termination, following Ticho (1972), are the reduction of the transference, the achievement of the main treatment goals, an acceptance (or at least tolerance) of the futility of perfectionistic strivings and childhood fantasies, an increased capacity for love and work (Freud's succinct statement of the goals of analysis), a reduction in the intensity and poignancy of core conflicts, the attainment of more stable and less maladaptive coping patterns, a reduction in symptoms, and the development of a self-analytic capacity. This latter quality is considered an important, new ego function, built on the patient's psychological-mindedness and on his or her identification with and internalization of the analyst's analytic attitude. It should help the person during the posttermination consolidation of the analytic work and subsequently as well. Patient and analyst part on the understanding that the door is open for a return for more analytic work at some time in the future. The analyst goes on analyzing into the last session. Self-understanding is never complete or final. Treatment does not resolve conflict completely, nor is it expected to immunize the patient completely from future psychological difficulties.

THE THERAPEUTIC RELATIONSHIP AND THE STANCE OF THE THERAPIST

The analyst's stance is best described as one in which the primary aim is to maintain an analytic attitude (Schafer, 1983). A major component of the analytic attitude is the analyst's genuine interest in helping the patient, expressed, in part, through the creation of a safe, caring, nonjudgmental therapeutic atmosphere.

Analytic Neutrality

Analytic neutrality is considered an essential feature of the proper analytic attitude. Neutrality is here understood *not* in the sense of indifference but in the sense of *not* taking sides in the patient's conflicts. In other words, the analyst attempts to be objective in the context of offering an empathic understanding of the patient. This stance has also been called a benevolent neutrality or a technical neutrality. As stated by Anna Freud (1954), the analyst adopts a position equidistant between the id, ego, and superego.

In addition, the analyst respects the uniqueness and individuality of the patient and does not attempt to remake the patient to fit any particular image or set of values. The analyst does not exploit the patient to meet his or her own needs. The analyst does not try to rescue the patient, to play guru, to become engaged in power struggles with the patient, to seek the patient's adulation, or to feel critical or impatient toward the patient. The analyst appreciates that patients both seek and are frightened by the prospect of change and that ambivalence is a ubiquitous feature of human experience.

This description may begin to sound like an impossible ideal. It should be kept in mind that it is an ideal to be aspired to with the recognition that one can only approximate it and should not be unduly self-critical when the approximation is inevitably less than one would wish.

The concept of neutrality is closely linked to the idea that the analyst should function like a surgeon, a mirror, or a blank screen, metaphors used by Freud to depict the proper analytic stance as one of optimal abstinence and relative anonymity. These metaphors, which often have been misconstrued and caricatured by critics of psychoanalysis, do *not* mean that the analyst functions with an attitude of a cold, detached, silent observer. Although some analysts undoubtedly have adopted an unnecessarily aloof stance, it is not a stance in the spirit of what Freud meant or did. A neutral stance simply means that the primary, deliberate attitude of the analyst is to analyze and that the analysis is best facilitated by certain conditions. Foremost among these conditions are a genuinely nonjudgmental attitude on the part of the therapist and a situation in which the patient's transference reactions can emerge in a relatively uncontaminated manner. The analytic restraint that the analyst imposes on him- or herself is intended to facilitate the clearer expression of the patient's transference.

Because therapy entails the interaction of two personalities there cannot be a truly "uncontaminated" transference. At the same time, the analyst's technical neutrality and relative anonymity will bring the patient's neurotic contributions into bolder relief. The analyst, of course, gives cues, witting and unwitting, about his or her personality and values from the location and furnishing of the office, the manner of dress, and so forth. However, there is still a large realm of nondisclosure that allows many degrees of freedom for the patient to "construct" the analyst. The patient's appreciation of his or her own needs and motives for making particular attributions or selective readings of the analyst will be more emotionally convincing to the extent to which it is not based on obvious reality cues.

Critics of Freudian analysis not infrequently misconstrue the position described earlier as indicating that Freudian analysts think that they should or somehow can take a position as observers of a process and yet remain outside the interaction. This is obviously impossible and it would be undesirable even if it were somehow possible. What is possible is for the analyst to *subordinate* his or her personality in the service of the analytic work by staying, relatively speaking, in the background in the sense of a certain restraint of one's narcissistic needs or a muted emotional responsiveness of the kind not necessary in an ordinary social relationship. Nonetheless, the patient and the analyst mutually influence one another. The particular transference–countertransference configurations that emerge are unique to each analytic relationship. At the same time, both parties bring to the analytic situation a preexisting set of unconscious conflicts and fantasies, aspects of which are likely to be activated in any, or most, analytic dyads.

Another aspect of the notion of neutrality is the idea of *abstinence,* which means not yielding to the patient's wishes for transference gratification. The rationale for this principle is that providing direct transference gratification (e.g., praise or affection) would at best create a temporary satisfaction but risk reducing the patient's motivation for treatment and make the analysis of the transference and the resistances all the more difficult. The analyst thus imposes a relative deprivation of gratification on both participants in the process. This is not to say that there are no gratifying aspects to the patient's experience of the analytic process. On the contrary there are several silent factors inherent in the situation that can be powerful sources of satisfaction and security. Foremost among these elements is the sense of steady support that comes from the sustained, genuine interest of a benign listener over a long course of regular and frequent contacts. This sense of support has been referred to as a "holding environment" (Winnicott, 1965). This term is a metaphor that derived from Winnicott's (1965) view that the analytic setting bears a similarity to features of the mother–child interaction in which the child is not only literally held as a means of soothing but is cared for and loved more generally and comes to rely on the provision of this protection.

What enables the analyst to provide a good holding environment, an environment that includes a shifting but optimal degree of abstinence with respect to the patient's transference wishes? To answer this question, we have to discuss the concepts of empathy and countertransference.

Empathy

Based on the amalgam of past clinical experience, knowledge of human development, general models of human behavior, and particular psychoanalytic theories, the analyst will listen with "evenly hovering attention" (i.e., not with a preset bias) and will later organize the material in particular ways to develop a working mental model of the patient. This crucial listening process is guided by the analyst's empathy. By empathy we mean that the analyst forms a partial, transient identification with the patient in which he or she attempts to apprehend in a cognitive–affective manner what it is like for the patient to experience his or her world in a particular manner. The analyst tries to become immersed in the patient's subjective experience by imagining, both cognitively and affectively, what the patient's experiential world is like. The analyst oscillates between relating to patients in this way and stepping back as an observer and reflecting on why patients seem to be experiencing their inner world in a particular manner (Schafer, 1959). These reflections serve as the basis for the private clinical inferences made by the analyst which then lead to the actual interpretations made to the patient. Offered with proper timing, tact, and dosage, interpretations attempt to convey empathic understanding and expla-

nation of patients' difficulties (Eagle & Wolitzky, 1997).

Countertransference

Countertransference can be thought of as empathy gone awry. That is, to the extent that the analyst's feelings or actions toward, and understanding of, the patient are influenced by the analyst's unconscious, unresolved conflicts and needs, the analyst is being biased and thereby not functioning in the best interests of the patient.

At first, countertransference was thought of as the direct counterpart to the patient's transference (i.e., as the analyst's transference to the patient's transference, or to the patient more generally). By this definition, countertransference was regarded as an undesirable, potentially serious obstacle to effective treatment. Freud (1910) held that the therapist's countertransference limited the degree to which the patient could progress in treatment. Some authors (e.g., Langs, 1982) go so far as to assert that *all* treatment failures are due to unrecognized and/or unmanaged countertransference reactions.

In more recent years, influenced in large part by work with more disturbed patients, the concept of countertransference has been broadened to include all the analyst's emotional reactions to the patient, not just his or her transference reactions to the patient's transference. This definition has been called "totalistic," in contrast to the earlier "classical" definition (Schlesinger & Wolitzky, 2002). The therapist's emotional reactions, whether based primarily on his or her own conflicts or due mainly to the fact that the patient's behavior would likely evoke the same reaction in virtually all analysts, came to be regarded both as inevitable and as potentially quite useful. They are useful in pointing to feelings that the patient might be "pulling for" from the therapist and therefore can serve as one important guide to the interpretations offered by the therapist. One needs to be careful, however,

and not assume automatically that just because one is feeling a certain way, the patient was trying to evoke that particular reaction. To make such an automatic
assumption (as one unfortunately encounters in some recent psychoanalytic literature) is to ignore the possibility that one's
conflict-based countertransference is responsible for what one thinks the patient is
trying to make one feel.

As noted previously, countertransference–transference enactments are inevitable
even though the analyst has been analyzed.
What is considered crucial is to be able to
recognize such enactments before they become too intense, disruptive, or traumatic
for the patient and to step back, reflect on,
and use one's understanding of them in the
service of interpretation.

Some countertransference reactions are
blatant, but most are subtle and therefore
potentially more insidious. Some are readily
recognized by the analyst; others are
brought to the analyst's attention by the patient. Here is an example from Greenson
(1967) of a subtle kind of countertransference reaction brought to the analyst's
awareness by the patient.

A patient of Greenson, whose symptoms
of depression and stomach ulcers intensified
during an unproductive period in his analysis, also showed changes in his attitude and
behavior toward Greenson. He became
sullen and stubborn in place of his previous
joking and teasing. As Greenson (1967) describes it:

> One day he told me he had dreamed of a
> jackass and then lapsed into a sullen silence.
> After a period of silence on my part, I asked
> him what was going on. He answered with a
> sigh that he had been thinking maybe the two
> of us were jackasses. After a pause he added, "I
> won't budge and you won't either. You won't
> change and I won't change [silence]. I tried to
> change but it made me sick." I was puzzled, I
> had no idea what he was referring to. I then
> asked him how he had *tried* to change. The
> patient answered that he had tried to change
> his political beliefs in accordance with mine.

> He had been a lifelong Republican (which I
> had known), and he had tried, in recent
> months, to adopt a more liberal point of view,
> because he knew I was so inclined. I asked
> him how he knew that I was a liberal and
> anti-Republican. He told me that whenever
> he said anything favorable about a Republi-
> can politician, I always asked for associations.
> On the other hand, whenever he said any-
> thing hostile about a Republican, I remained
> silent, as though in agreement. Whenever he
> had a kind word for Roosevelt, I said noth-
> ing. Whenever he attacked Roosevelt, I
> would ask who did Roosevelt remind him of,
> as though I was out to prove that hating
> Roosevelt was infantile.

> I was taken aback because I had been com-
> pletely unaware of this pattern. Yet, the mo-
> ment the patient pointed it out, I had to agree
> that I had done precisely that, albeit unknow-
> ingly. We then went to work on why he felt
> the need to try to swallow my political views.
> (pp. 272–273)

The prescription for dealing with countertransference reactions is self-analysis, informed by the analyst's own prior training
analysis and clinical supervision, and, if necessary, supplemented by consultations with
colleagues and/or by the resumption of
treatment. In the previous example, Greenson presumably reflected on why he responded to the patient as he did, wondered
whether his response was unique to this patient, whether there were other subtle ways
in which he was critical of the patient, and
so on.

The presumption is that undetected (and
therefore unmanaged) countertransference
reactions always have a detrimental impact
on the treatment. The literature is replete
with clinical vignettes demonstrating that a
bogged-down analysis resumed its forward
thrust following the analyst's awareness of a
countertransference trend and the new interpretation to which it led. Although these
accounts generally are persuasive, it is not
clear how much undetected countertransference the average patient could, in fact,
tolerate and still have a reasonably successful
analysis.

It is also not clear to what extent and under what circumstances the analyst should disclose to the patient the fact of his or her countertransference and the presumed basis for it. Some analysts regard it as essential for the egalitarian spirit of the analytic process and for affirming the patient's sense of reality, whereas others feel that it unnecessarily burdens the patient and should be employed quite sparingly.

Virtually all therapists do agree that the analytic ideal would require that self-analysis be a constant, silent, background accompaniment to the conduct of each analytic session. The process would be heightened at moments when the analyst recognizes a change in the baseline of his or her typical attitudes and reactions to the patient (e.g., a shift in mood or a train of personal associations). Such attention to one's own experience can provide vital data concerning lines of exploration and interpretation that may previously have been avoided.

CURATIVE FACTORS OR MECHANISMS OF CHANGE

Since the inception of psychoanalysis, there has been continual discussion and debate concerning its curative ingredients. By now, it is clear that there is no single factor that can be said to be the major element in therapeutic change for all patients.

Although there are few formal statements of the necessary and sufficient conditions for therapeutic change, there is a general consensus that the conditions conducive to positive outcomes include the following: (1) a person who (a) is suffering emotionally, (b) is motivated to change, (c) shows some degree of psychological-mindedness, (d) has sufficient ego strength, and (e) has a decent enough history of gratifying interpersonal relationships to form and maintain a reasonable working alliance in the face of the inevitable frustrations involved in the treatment; and (2) a therapist who (a) can provide a safe arena and be an effective catalyst

for the patient's self-exploration, (b) can facilitate and maintain the working alliance in the face of its inevitable ruptures, (c) is relatively free of unmanaged countertransference reactions, and (d) provides accurate, empathically based interpretations of transference and extratransference behaviors with the timing, tact, and dosage necessary to facilitate insight into the unconscious conflicts that influence the patient's symptoms and maladaptive patterns of behavior.

These conditions are expected to promote increased self-understanding, self-acceptance, and some inner reorganization of the personality (i.e., so-called structural, as opposed to merely behavioral, change). The patient is freed from excessive reliance on maladaptive defenses, becomes less anxious and guilt ridden, and is more effective in work, in love, and in play.

Broadly speaking, the curative factors created by the foregoing conditions have been divided into two main categories—insight and the relationship. This is a potentially misleading distinction because insight based on interpretation can only take place in the context of a relationship. Thus, an interpretation leading to an emotionally meaningful insight can be, and often is, simultaneously experienced as a profound feeling of being understood (perhaps the strongest expression of a solid holding environment). Nonetheless, the distinction between insight and relationship factors is retained in order to assign relative influence to the element of enhanced self-understanding versus the therapeutic benefits of the relationship per se. Among the benefits of the latter one can include the support inherent in the therapeutic relationship, the experience of a new, benign object relationship with a significant person (i.e., one who does not recreate the traumatic experiences that the patient suffered in relation to the parents), and identification with the analyst and the analytic attitude, including a softening of superego self-punitiveness and feeling understood and supported, even by interpretations that arouse some degree of anxiety.

Among most traditional analysts, these relationship elements are regarded as necessary, but secondary, background factors which give interpretations their mutative power. In some contemporary views, particularly some versions of object relations theory and Kohut's self psychology, the relationship is regarded as directly therapeutic in its own right, and at times the primary curative factor. Kohut (1984), for example, argues that the main impact of interpretations is that they strengthen the empathic bond between patient and therapist.

Some writers have suggested that a comprehensive theory of curative factors would have to consider that the relative therapeutic efficacy of insight and relationship factors might depend on the type of patient being treated and the stage of treatment. The generalization has been offered that, relatively speaking, patients whose early history was marked by serious disturbances in the mother–child relationship would benefit more, relatively speaking, from the healing aspects of the relationship, whereas patients who struggle primarily with Oedipal problems would find insight a more potent factor.

All analysts believe that insight is most effective when it is emotionally meaningful and includes both current and past experiences. Thus, as noted earlier, an insight in which the patient sees how he or she is repeating in the here-and-now transference to the analyst an experience that occurs with contemporary significant others and that took place with one or another or both parents is more convincing, in part, because of the convergence of these three domains. Such insights both presuppose a degree of change and point the way to further changes. The patient, for example, can recognize the tendency to invite, rebuff, or undermine him- or herself in certain ways. Although this awareness does not automatically result in behavioral change, it can set the stage for it.

There are many examples in the literature of the relative emphasis on the pa-

tient–therapist relationship and on insight. A good contemporary example of an emphasis on the healing power of the relationship is seen in the writings of the Boston Process Group (e.g., Lyons-Ruth, 1998). Basing themselves on studies of early infant–mother interaction and processes of attunement to each other's subjective states, these authors look for analogous processes in the psychoanalytic situation. One of their key concepts is "implicit relational knowing" (Lyons-Ruth, 1998) that derives from shared "moments of meeting." These "moments" of attunement constitute new ways of being together. An example might be the patient's realization that the analyst is genuinely interested in listening to and responding to what the patient is saying and by this interest the analyst is expressing the attitude that the patient is a person of worth. This experience contrasts with the patient's internalized way of relating to those perceived to be in authority. For instance, a patient recalls that the clear rule, particularly at the family dinner table, was that his parents expected silence from the children during dinner unless specifically asked to speak. As an adult in treatment, this patient can have the experience of the analyst as a new object and engage in new, experiential learning. That is, he can realize that it is permissible, even desirable, to speak freely to an interested listener. This experience does not preclude interpretation (e.g., "I have the feeling that you fell silent just now because you were not sure that I was really interested in what you were starting to say and that this feeling reminds you of how it felt at the family dinner table when you felt you were getting the message that you should be seen but not heard."). The implicit message in this interpretation is that the analyst is in fact interested in what the patient has to say. Whether such messages generally are better conveyed implicitly and/or noninterpretively is an interesting empirical question.

A major example of the emphasis on insight is seen, for example, in the work of

Gray (1994), who advocates "close process monitoring." In this approach, the analyst is particularly alert to moments in the session when the patient's associations and behavior suggest that anxiety signals have become active and defenses have been instigated to ward it off. The patient is encouraged to become an observer of this process and (implicitly) to refrain from it in order to uncover the warded-off, anxiety-laden mental contents. Insight into unconscious conflicts is still the goal, but the analyst is less active in interpreting these conflicts than analysts were in the past.

Those, like Gray, who see themselves as facilitators of the patient's self-analysis find it important to minimize the role of suggestion in the treatment. Freud was troubled by the specter of suggestion for at least two reasons. First, despite rare disclaimers, Freud needed to use the data from the consulting room for the evidential basis for his theories. To the extent that the patient accepted Freud's interpretations out of transferentially based compliance, the results could not be taken as validation of theoretical claims. Second, Freud's concern about mixing the "pure gold" of psychoanalysis with the "copper of suggestion" was based on wanting to liberate the patient, as much as possible, from reliance on authority (both parental and analytic). The concept of technical neutrality was formulated with this aim in mind. The uniqueness of psychoanalysis proper was the ideal that the lifting of repression and the integration of previously disavowed wishes would be liberating by virtue of the truths it revealed and not due to the subtle, hidden, hypnotic-like, suggestive influence of the positive transference to the analyst as a parental authority. Keeping this suggestive influence to an irreducible minimum is an attempt to approximate as much as one can the "pure gold" of psychoanalysis, in contrast to what Freud called the "copper of suggestion." Freud (1905) claimed that there was "the greatest possible antithesis between suggestive and analytic technique" (p. 260). The clear, but untested, implication of Gray's approach is that is leads to superior long-term outcomes, at least for those for whom it is deemed suitable.

TREATMENT APPLICABILITY AND ETHICAL CONSIDERATIONS

Psychoanalysis originated as a novel treatment for adults with neurotic afflictions, although even in the early days the patients seen by Freud and his colleagues often were more seriously disturbed.

Individuals seeking psychoanalysis or psychoanalytic psychotherapy usually do so at a time of anticipated or actual loss, typically the loss of an important personal relationship. Other common reasons for entering treatment at a particular point include the outbreak of symptoms (e.g., panic attacks), diminution of self-esteem, and the unavailability of usual social or emotional supports at times of life transition (e.g., graduating from college, being fired from a job, or the birth of a child). The latter normal life changes often create significant stress which, when superimposed on chronic, unresolved conflicts, can give rise to disabling symptoms. In other words, patients typically seek treatment in a state of disequilibrium.

Social Class

Psychotherapy in general, and psychoanalysis in particular, has long been criticized as limited to a small segment of the population. The so-called YAVIS syndrome refers to the typical psychotherapy patient as Young, Affluent, Verbal, Intelligent, and Socially Mobile. Psychoanalytic patients have been depicted as those who are wealthy and without significant personal problems (i.e., "the worried well"; Doidge, 1999; Kaley, Eagle, & Wolitzky, 1999). According to this view, psychoanalysis is a personal journey of self-exploration for the narcissistically self-indulgent rather than an experience of encounter with painful truths about oneself by individuals who are troubled and dysfunctional in their relationships and in their work. While attempts were made early on to apply psychoanalytic understanding to work with underprivileged and disadvantaged populations (e.g., Aichorn, 1935), it is by and large true that unmodified, intensive psychoanalytic treatment in this country is an expensive proposition, particularly in these days of managed care.

However, it is not the case that those in psychoanalysis are merely the "worried well." For example, Doidge (1999) found that in a study of Canadian patients, 82% had tried less intensive forms of therapy before they entered psychoanalysis. The characteristics of this sample included the following: almost 25% had been sexually and/or physically abused and a similar percentage had suffered traumatic separation in childhood. With respect to formal DSM diagnoses on Axis I, 11.9% showed substance abuse or dependence, 64.8% had a mood disorder, 48.9% had an anxiety disorder, 23.3% had a somatoform disorder, and 43.4% had a sexual dysfunction disorder. Many patients had more than one disorder. Slightly over 70% of the patients studied were diagnosed as having one or another Axis II personality disorder. The findings from this Canadian study are consistent with those in other studies (Doidge, 1999).

Types of Patients and Patient Pathology

Patient Populations

Freud never intended that psychoanalysis have a broad range of application and realized that it would require significant modification to be employed more widely. Over the years, psychoanalytically oriented approaches have been developed for the treatment of children, adolescents, couples, groups, and families. A separate chapter would be required to begin to do justice to the range and complexity of the factors involved in these treatment applications.

Range of Pathology

It should be pointed out that in the past, psychoanalytic treatment, in one variation or another, was tried with schizophrenic patients. Federn (1952), Searles (1965), Fromm-Reichmann (1950), Sechehaye (1951), and Rosenfeld (1965) were among the more prominent clinicians and theorists who pioneered this most taxing approach. In more recent years, however, the practice of dynamic psychotherapy, and particularly psychoanalytic therapy, with schizophrenics seems to have diminished substantially in favor of drug therapy and other forms of intervention (e.g., supportive therapy, social skills training, behavior therapy, family therapy, and community treatment programs). However, there still are a few residential treatment centers in which psychoanalytic therapy is practiced with seriously disturbed patients, some of whom are schizophrenic but most of whom are severe borderline personalities. Blatt and Ford (1999) reported substantial therapeutic gains with long-term, intensive, psychoanalytically oriented treatment with seriously disturbed, treatment-resistant inpatients. The psychoanalytic treatment of severe borderline and narcissistic conditions is more frequently carried out on an outpatient basis (Kernberg et al., 1989).

Cultural Factors

Psychoanalytic psychotherapy has certain inherent features and values that sets boundaries on its range of application. It assumes that the prospective patient (1) is curious and interested in the nature of his or her inner life; (2) is capable, or potentially capable, of psychologically minded introspection; (3) sees one's self as the main source of suffering, despite environmental obstacles and difficulties; (4) is motivated to change; (5) has a decent enough history of past relationships that would allow for trust in the therapist; (6) can tolerate the delay and frustration involved in a slow, introspective process in which direction, suggestion, advice, and structure are deliberately kept to a minimum; and (7) has adequate reality testing. These are some of the main indications for treatment. Cultural factors can influence the degree to which patients show these qualities.

In addition to assessing the foregoing characteristics, one also needs to consider variations in cultural values and practices. For example, although psychoanalytic therapy is used with groups, it is used mainly as an individual therapy focused primarily on individual pathology. Collectivist cultures do not value this approach and might find group, family, or community approaches more compatible (Markus & Kitayama, 1998). Second, psychoanalytic treatment encourages the free expression of emotions so that cultures that value restraint of emotion would find this central feature incompatible. Third, people from some cultures are less inclined to take the initiative and expect the therapist to be more active and to provide more structure than is typical in psychoanalytic treatment. Fourth, sociocultural differences between patient and therapist also need to be considered.

In summary, I believe it is fair to say that the bulk of psychoanalytic psychotherapy, and virtually all of psychoanalysis proper, is applied to upper-middle-class individuals in major urban centers who do not rely primarily on third-party payments and can afford private fees, even if it means having two or three sessions per week instead of the four or five that were more common in the past. At the same time, psychoanalytic approaches have informed many other treatment approaches.

Ethical Considerations

Although practitioners have a natural inclination to recommend to patients the kind of treatment they have been trained to con-duct, ethical considerations require caution. For example, standard psychoanalysis is not the treatment of choice for patients whose reality situation is so dire and overwhelming as to preclude prolonged, leisurely introspection, nor should it be recommended to someone whose sole aim is to overcome a specific habit (e.g., smoking). In general, the ethical issues relevant to psychoanalysis are those germane to psychotherapy in general (e.g., not exploiting the patient's emotional vulnerability).

Matching Patients with Therapeutic Modalities and with Therapists

With respect to the question of matching patient and treatment, there is general agreement that neurotic patients are suitable for either psychoanalysis or psychoanalytic psychotherapy and that borderline patients are best suited for psychoanalytic (or expressive) psychotherapy. In addition, there has been increasing attention to the issue of patient–therapist match, with respect to personality, cognitive style, gender, and ethnicity.

RESEARCH SUPPORT

For most of its history psychoanalysis has based its theories almost exclusively on the case study method. Few analysts were trained in research methodology. Conducting an analysis was seen as simultaneously doing research. Conceptions of therapeutic action were based on accumulated "clinical wisdom"—an amalgam of the received wisdom of their supervisors and teachers, theory, and common sense. In recent years, analysts have begun to supplement clinical insights and claims with more systematic, empirical inquiries focused on the process and outcome of treatment, spurred partly by increasing demands for accountability.

The several available meta-analytic studies of psychotherapy outcome (in which the results of many studies are combined statistically) did not include studies of long-term psychoanalytic treatment. Furthermore, they used outcome criteria (e.g., symptom reduction) that do not reflect the kinds of personality changes aimed for in psychoanalytic treatment.

The few outcome studies of long-term psychoanalytic treatment reviewed by Bachrach, Galatzer-Levy, Skolnikoff, and Waldron (1991) have a number of methodological weaknesses; most notably, none of them employed a control group. Yet, what kind of control group could feasibly and ethically be employed in a study of long-term treatment? An untreated group, a wait-list control, or an attention-placebo control obviously are inappropriate.

The most ambitious long-term treatment and follow-up study ever undertaken, is the Menninger Foundation Psychotherapy Research Project (PRP), initiated more than three decades ago. Five books and more than 60 articles have been based on this project, including follow-up studies and a detailed write-up of each of the cases (Wallerstein, 1986).

In the PRP study, 42 patients were seen in either psychoanalysis (22) or psychotherapy (20). Overall, the outcome for the two groups was similar; about 60% of patients showed at least moderate improvement. Most of the patients in psychoanalysis required modifications in the treatment and all the treatments contained more supportive elements than originally intended. In fact, half of the 42 patients showed positive therapeutic changes without evidence of having obtained insight into their core conflicts. By the criteria of durability and effective coping in the face of conflict and stress, the supportive elements were no less significant than insight in generating structural change. Wallerstein (1986) concludes that there has been "a tendency to overestimate the necessity of the expressive-analytic treatment mode, and of its central operation via conflict resolution based on interpretation, insight, and working through, to achieve therapeutically desired change" (p. 723).

It is hard to draw definitive conclusions from this one study, even though these patients were followed carefully for many years after treatment. Many of these patients had failed in prior treatments and about one-third of those who received psychoanalysis had to be hospitalized at some point during their treatment. (Bachrach, Galatzer-Levy, Skolnikoff, & Waltzer, 1991). This suggests that psychoanalysis probably was not the treatment of choice in the first place. The challenging question of importance of interpretation and insight relative to other presumed therapeutic ingredients (e.g., provision of a safe, supportive atmosphere) remains to be answered and is likely to vary from patient to patient.

Based on a detailed review of the PRP and the only three other large-scale studies (the Columbia Psychoanalytic Center Research Project, the Boston Psychoanalytic Institute Prediction Study, and the New York Psychoanalytic Institute Studies), Bachrach and colleagues (1991) concluded that "the majority of patients selected as *suitable* for analysis derive substantial therapeutic benefit: improvement rates are typically in the 60–90% range, and effect sizes, when they have been calculated, are significant" (p. 904). The main predictor of outcome was initial ego strength. Appropriate comparison groups are needed to evaluate these findings.

Since the first edition of this book there has been an impressive proliferation of empirical research on the process and outcome of psychoanalytic treatment. The best single source of information concerning this research is the recently published *Open Door Review of Outcome Studies in Psychoanalysis* (Fonagy, 2002). This compendium of treatment research contains a review of some 80 different studies being conducted all over the world, as far away as New South Wales. Given the dearth of psychoanalytic treatment research in the 20th century and the historical resistance to research among most analysts, we are witnessing a remarkable shift, even if one wants to argue that it is happening because analysts can no longer avoid the pressures of accountability in the era of managed care, rival psychotherapies, and psychopharmacological interventions. At this stage, most of the studies are naturalistic, without control groups, randomized assignment of patients (although this requirement is debatable) and other desiderata of an ideal research design. However, some of the studies do include the important feature of evaluation at various time points, including long-term follow-up.

It obviously is impossible to summarize here the 80 or so studies in the *Open Door Review* or the few dozen that have preceded it. But just to give a flavor of the work being done I refer to the studies by Sandell and colleagues (2000). Among the findings of this series of studies are that (1) the outcomes for psychoanalysis were superior to those for analytically oriented psychotherapy; (2) classical analysts achieved better results with psychoanalysis than with psychotherapy; (3) psychoanalytic psychotherapy and psychoanalysis, compared with various kinds of short-term treatments and a no-treatment control group, showed greater symptom reduction and social adjustment at 1- and 2-year follow-up; (4) over seven time periods of evaluation, the benefits of treatment, compared to a waiting-list control, increased over the period from prior to treatment to long-term follow-up, from roughly 30% to 55% for a psychotherapy group (with effect sizes ranging from 0.4 to 0.6) and from 10% to 75% for the psychoanalysis group (with effect sizes ranging from 0.4 to 1.5, a very large effect size); and (5) better results were achieved by more experienced psychoanalysts, especially females, and with greater session frequency during treatment Unfortunately, the outcome measures in these studies (e.g., the Symptom Checklist-90, which focuses on symptoms) are not those that index the kinds of personality change described by the theory. For a promising beginning to specify and operationalize, on an experience-near level, what is meant by "structural change," see the work by Wallerstein (1991).

In any event, these data provide some encouragement for the claims made by analysts on the basis of their clinical experience. Together with other studies summarized in the *Open Door Review* (Fonagy, 2002), it is reasonable to offer the overall statement that the majority of these studies report positive results for psychoanalysis and psychoanalytic psychotherapy. For the most part, the studies not only aim at assessing outcome but also attempt to look at the process of change in the hope of specifying the mechanisms of change. Within the next 10 years we ought to have much more solid evidence concerning the degree and nature of therapeutic change based on psychoanalytic treatment. To what extent we finally have empirical confirmation of accumulated clinical wisdom and to what extent we have new insights leading to revisions of theories of therapeutic action remain to be seen. It is also unclear to what extent findings from research on psychoanalytic process and outcome support one school of thought over another and to what extent the research findings affect the actual practice of psychoanalysts.

CASE ILLUSTRATION

At the request of the editors, I have not selected a case that proved to be an outstanding success. On a scale including "deterioration," "no change," "minimal improvement," "mild improvement," "moderate improvement," and "marked improvement," I chose a case that showed a moderate degree of improvement. Obviously, I can only present a highly condensed account of some aspects of the case.

Mr. T started treatment at the age of 27. He had been referred to the university counseling service because he was on the verge of being dropped from the university for an increasingly long string of incompletes that began in his freshman year (age 18) and snowballed such that he was adding new incompletes at a faster rate than he was undoing the backlog of those he had already accumulated. In every realm of his life he showed extreme procrastination and lateness.

The patient grew up in a midwestern, upper-middle-class Jewish family. He was favored over his brother, 2 years his senior. His father, a person of seemingly indefatigable energy, was a successful attorney who also was actively involved in the life of his community. The boy was awed and envious when witnessing the respect and esteem accorded his father. His admiration of and identification with his father was one important basis for (1) his feeling that he wanted to be similarly recognized as well as his serious doubts that he ever would be held in such high regard, and (2) his belief that to devote his energies exclusively to only *one* major goal or project was to forgo the possibility of successfully competing with his father.

His parents, particularly his mother, led him to believe that he had the ability, the potential, and the *obligation* to achieve greatness as an adult; all that was required was the proper motivation. These messages became internalized and contributed to his sense of having a special destiny that he ought to fulfill. Together with the model of his father described previously, this sense of a duty to perform, combined with his perfectionistic strivings, motivated him to overextend himself and contributed to his procrastination. He never completed any project until faced with a truly unavoidable deadline. Not surprisingly, Mr. T felt himself to be the passive victim of an unremitting barrage of environmental impingements and hassles (e.g., bills and taxes that he was expected to pay on a timely basis) and interpersonal expectations, which he experienced as onerous obligations (e.g., being on time for therapy sessions and dates).

He experienced his mother as an extremely demanding, controlling, manipulative, opinionated, intolerant, and unempathic person who derived sadistic pleasure from taking advantage of her power over him. For example, she often would be the last mother to arrive to pick him up after school.

Given the entrenched nature of Mr. T's behavioral problems and his characterological difficulties, I recommended, after three or four initial interviews, that we embark on psychoanalysis at a frequency of four sessions per week. I reviewed with him the material of the initial interviews and summarized the main presenting issues to be dealt with: his severe procrastination and his problems with time; his feelings of anxiety, depression, and low self-esteem; his turbulent, sticky relationship with his mother; and his difficulties with women, his problems in concentration, his need to take on more than he could handle, and the problems generated by this tendency.

We then turned to the contractual aspects of our working relationship; we agreed on a fee and arranged a schedule. I informed him about my usual vacation times and told him about my fee policy regarding missed sessions: I would charge him for missed sessions but would try to arrange make-up sessions when I could. I then offered a brief description of how I thought we could best work together. Because he had no prior experience in treatment, save for the three sessions in the college counseling service (and a few sessions when he was an unhappy high school student), I invited him to feel free to say what comes to mind without editing or withholding any thoughts or feelings that he might regard as tangential or irrelevant. I added that my role would be to facilitate his self-exploration by making comments and observations from time to time.

The treatment involved an elaboration of the themes and conflicts outlined previously. In the interest of brevity, I restrict my account almost exclusively to his problems with time and with concentration. Fairly quickly, these issues began to be expressed in his relationship with me. For instance, the patient had a great deal of difficulty getting to the sessions on time. Not infrequently, he would arrive *exactly* at the midpoint of the session, seemingly without conscious intent to do so. On a couple of occasions he arrived with 2 or 3 minutes left, explaining that the idea of missing the session altogether was more troubling than the frustration of traveling 40 minutes each way for 2 or 3 minutes of his session with me. Once on the couch, he showed little awareness that the end of the session was approaching, continuing to talk in a way that made my stopping the session feel to both of us like an intrusive interruption rather than a somewhat natural ending.

Time was a bitter enemy in *every* aspect of his life. He would resist doing things until he inevitably was coerced into action, even though he consciously hated being coerced. In addition to his precarious academic standing based on his long list of incompletes, his telephone and electrical service were regularly threatened with termination for delinquent payment of bills; he was never on time to a date, a dance, a concert, or other activities.

Transitions from one activity to another were extremely difficult for him. He recalled that as a child, he had a strong resistance to going to sleep, exceeded by his even more powerful resistance to getting up on time to go to school. For Mr. T, simply to be awake and conscious was to automatically feel a profound sense of the impingement of reality and an aversive sense of burden and responsibility in relation to all his unfinished daily tasks, to say nothing of the grand accomplishments that were on his future agenda. So profound were his yearnings to be free of these pressures that to stand up straight and carry himself erect, as opposed to being in a slouched or supine position, often felt extremely effortful and was experienced as a hardship to be endured and resented.

The patient experienced the passage of time during which he managed to avoid chores, school assignments, or other obligations as but a temporary reprieve from feeling coerced. He realized that his ability to resist the passage of time was an expression of his need for freedom. Because his procrastinating stance was an invitation to others to pressure him, it was hard to relax. His sense of his mother constantly nagging him was never far from his awareness.

Material relevant to the patient's problems with time emerged over many months and became one main focus of the analysis. These problems were intimately intertwined with his problems in concentration. I draw on this material from several points in the treatment to create a composite vignette in order to illustrate some of the technical precepts that guided my overall approach to this patient and to demonstrate the actual interventions derived from these precepts.

By my listening, by my periodic, general requests for elaboration of his associations (e.g., "What comes to mind?"), by occasional, specific, but open-ended questions designed to elicit further associations, I attempted to understand and to interpret the meanings of his behavior and experiences in relation to time and to the matter of concentration as expressions of unconscious, core conflicts, particularly as they were expressed in the transference.

Some months into the analysis I pointed out to the patient that he had been late a lot, something that, of course, he knew. He replied that it was difficult for him to get anywhere on time, that I should, therefore, not take it personally, and that he did not keep track of time enough to focus on when he would have to leave to show up on time. The tone of his remarks suggested to me that he took my observation as a criticism. Rather than respond directly to the content of what he said, I focused on the affect-laden manner of his reply. The technical precept guiding this choice was the idea of emphasizing the implicit, affective aspects of the "here-and-now" transference.

From the perspective of technique, my reference to his lateness is what Greenson (1967) would call a *confrontation*. It conveys the message: "Both the fact of your repeated lateness and your affective-cognitive response to my calling attention to it are matters of psychological import that we might profitably examine together."

By inquiring whether he might have experienced my observation as a criticism I was engaging in the technical intervention that Greenson calls *clarification*. As indicated earlier, confrontation and clarification are preparatory to *interpretation,* which searches for the *meanings* of behavior and experience. My confrontation and clarification already hint at the possibility of a transferential response while trying to maintain a positive working alliance by implicitly suggesting that we look at our interchange. As the therapist, I also need to be aware of why and how I am choosing to intervene at the time I do: What attitudes, affects, and conflicts might have been activated in me, including the questions of how I feel about his lateness (e.g., Am I irritated and sounding critical in the content, tone, syntax, or other aspects of my remarks?). In short, I need to monitor, manage, and get interpretive clues from my own countertransference reactions.

Not surprisingly, the patient replied that he did feel somewhat chastised by my comment and that it reminded him of a similar reaction to the female therapist he saw initially and who referred him to me. His thoughts next turned to his mother and her almost invariable lateness in picking him up from elementary school in the afternoon. He felt angered at what he felt was the power differential and double standard in their relationship; she constantly chided him for being late in getting ready for school, yet she apparently had no compunction about keeping him waiting in all sorts of situations (e.g., she would drag him to stores and would take her time shopping while he waited impatiently and with much frustration). After listening to him elaborate these memories and feelings, I interpreted one meaning of his lateness with me to be a desire to keep me waiting as his mother had kept him waiting, to right the humiliating, infuriating wrong that he felt she had imposed upon him. This desire for revenge was expressed in this manner both with me and with others. I later rephrased and amplified my interpretation by stating that he wished to reverse roles with me by having me suffer helplessly as he had and that he found this desire to be legitimate in some sense. But, I added, it also was something he felt was wrong, just as his mother regarded his attempts to defy her as evidence of his badness and lack of respect for her. I wondered whether he heard his mother's critical voice in my observation of his lateness and whether his feeling criticized by me was something he seemed to feel was in some sense justified and in some sense unfair. In making this kind of interpretation I was communicating the view that while he bitterly resented his mother's accusations and criticisms, he also felt that they had a certain degree of merit and that this contributed to his feeling that he was being a "bad boy."

Variations and elaborations of this line of *interpretation* were offered repeatedly in contexts in which issues of control, autonomy, and a sense of obligation were prominent in the patient's associations and in a host of childhood memories and in his current behavior. For instance, he would graciously accept a dinner invitation, but as the hour of his expected arrival approached, he increasingly felt the invitation to be a burden. What began as a freely chosen, pleasant anticipation became transformed into an onerous obligation. He felt similarly about our sessions.

As indicated earlier, the patient's problems with time were closely linked to his difficulties in concentration. For example, it was evident that Mr. T had a great deal of difficulty listening to my comments and interpretations. Not infrequently, he would remark, "Could you say that again? I completely lost track of what you said." Rather than simply repeat what I had said, I asked what came to mind about his not retaining it in the first place. He replied, "As you know, I've always had trouble paying attention to what I'm doing. I can't concentrate and often don't realize that I'm not concentrating until some time later. If I'm reading an assigned chapter in a textbook I find that after a few pages I turn to some unassigned portion of the text and I start to read without any problem in concentration or in remembering what I read. Of course [said with a knowing chuckle], if the unassigned portion became the assignment I would wander to some other part and forget what I had read. I engage in my shutdown procedure without realizing it at the time." I then said, "It seems that you often experience what I say in here as carrying the demand that you pay attention and do your 'homework' here immediately." The patient, struggling to retain my comment, replied that he did feel that it was coercive to pay attention to what I had to say. In this context, as earlier in relation to the issue of time and being kept waiting by his mother, he again recalled ignoring his mother's entreaties to do his homework and struggles with his mother around toilet training and cleanliness training in general. The patient spontaneously acknowledged that there was something gratifying in defying what he felt was required or expected. For example, he again recalled times at which his mother thought that he was in his room studying and he was playing instead, feeling good (but also guilty) that he was getting away with something.

We were able to see that not hearing what I said was not some meaningless, momentary memory lapse but a significant here-and-now transference marker of his conflict between obedience and defiance. When I spoke, his mind "wandered to the unassigned portion" and he engaged in his "shutdown procedure" with me. His emotional insights into the nature, origins, and pervasiveness of this conflict were facilitated by so-called genetic transference interpretations linking his resistance to aspects of the analytic process to his struggles with his mother.

It should be emphasized that what I am describing here is a *tiny* fragment of a long, often arduous process. It is not that the pa-

tient and analyst suddenly arrive at one all-encompassing, blinding insight in which everything heretofore cloudy and obscure gels such that long-standing conflicts suddenly become fully and forever resolved. This image, still a common fantasy, is a holdover from the rapid, usually short-lived, dramatic "cures" in the early days of psychoanalysis in which the retrieval of an unconscious, traumatic memory appeared to play an immediate, decisive role. In fact, the process is one in which insights are gained, lost, and regained. There are strong resistances against translating insight into action. This is why analysts talk about the importance of "working through." At times, working through is written about as though it were a special process or phase within the analysis. It is more accurate to say that working through *is* the analysis, as analyses usually are characterized by variations on a few central themes.

In summary, the diagnostic picture that emerged over the course of treatment was that Mr. T had an obsessive–compulsive character structure, with narcissistic, depressive, and passive–aggressive features. Dynamically, his core conflicts centered on (1) his passive wishes in relation to his mother and his guilt over such wishes, as well as his autonomous strivings to free himself from enmeshment with his mother; (2) his rage at, and desire to defy, parental authority and his feeling that he should obediently yield to it in order to be a good boy; and (3) his Oedipal rivalry with his father, contributing to his grandiose wishes to be mother's favorite through some great achievement, along with his indentification with and love for his father and his desire not to hurt him. Although these conflicts interacted with one another in synergistic ways, it was the second conflict listed that was the most significant one and the one that contributed most to his impaired functioning. That is why I focused on this aspect of his personality in this brief presentation. It should be noted, however, that the three conflicts listed previously, originating, respectively, from the oral, anal, and phallic stages of psycho-sexual development, interact; that is, the same behavior can simultaneously express aspects of each conflict and the conflicts themselves are related to one another.

I shall illustrate briefly. One particularly prominent manifestation of Mr. T's obsessive–compulsive style was his severe preoccupation with the idea of lost or missed opportunities, particularly with respect to his search for the perfectly gratifying female. He would always arrive at a dance late and then be unable to let go of the idea that the girl of his dreams had been there and left.

In general, whatever he had or was experiencing at a given moment was, by definition, at least mildly disappointing; perfection was an elusive, future possibility for which he had to keep his options open. When he opened a gift-wrapped package he was invariably disappointed because, however nice the gift was, it immediately stirred his fantasy of the perhaps truly special contents of the other package that was still gift-wrapped.

This material was elaborated in further sessions and eventually led to interpretations to the effect that he was seeking a blissful merger with a perfect, omnipotent woman who would immediately recognize and happily satisfy all his needs, without his having to verbalize them; that he had a marked sensitivity to feeling controlled and trapped by a powerful woman; and that he constantly yearned for an elusive, special, but unattainable woman. Thus, conflicts at the oral, anal, and phallic/Oedipal levels, respectively, were expressed in the foregoing clinical material as well as in his difficulties in making commitments to a woman and to his career.

The reenactment, eventual understanding, and working through of these conflicts in a context of empathy and support contributed to a much greater sense of personal agency and to increased self-esteem based on a diminution of the superego pressures that he fulfill his alleged potential for greatness. Eventually, his battles with time diminished. He made considerable progress in coming to terms with his rage against his mother and his fear and guilt about relinquishing her as a manipulative, persecutory object. There was a reduction in his anger and in the self-directed aggression he practiced on himself in atonement for his guilt over his defiant rage and "misbehavior." He also came to uncouple the idea of his success with the notion of his father's demise. In these ways he freed himself to take more genuine control over his own life.

The treatment lasted for 8 years. The patient finished college, obtained an advanced degree, and, after several turbulent relationships with women modeled on the conflicts in his relationship with his mother, became engaged to a woman who was refreshingly different from his mother. However, relative to others he had a lower threshold for feeling coerced by others and still showed a tendency to procrastinate.

What one hopes to achieve in psycho-analysis is nicely captured in McDougall's (1985) quasi-poetic chararacterization of the ideal psychoanalytic outcome:

> Psychoanalysis is a theater on whose stage all our psychic repertory may be played. In these scenarios the features of the internal characters undergo many changes, the dialogues are rewritten and the roles recast. The work of elaboration leads analysands to the discovery of their internal reality and their inner truth, once all the different parts of themselves and all the people who have played important roles in their lives have had a chance to speak their lines. Accounts are settled with the loved-hated figures of the past; the analysands now possess them in all their aspects, good and bad, instead of being possessed by them, and now are ready to take stock of all they have received from those who brought them up and of what they have done with this inheritance. Whatever their conclusions may be, they recognize their place in this inner universe and claim that which is their own. (p. 284)

CURRENT AND FUTURE TRENDS

Pulver (1995) has divided the evolution of theoretical and technical approaches to psychoanalytic treatment into three main historical eras: the Early Period, which emphasized the uncovering of so-called id material; the Classical Period, which began in 1923 with the publication of *The Ego and the Id,* which focused on the analysis of ego defenses and was dominant until the late 1950s, and the Contemporary Period, which made more room for a consideration of pre-Oedipal deficits and pathology and emphasized the interactive nature and healing power of the analytic relationship,

Analysts in the Classical Period were said to view the analyst as an observer who was an objective, impartial interpreter and arbiter of the patient's distortions of reality, as though the analyst could somehow take a position outside the interaction. In the current climate, the patient and analyst are seen as interactive participants in a relationship in which each party influences the subjective experiences of the other. The analyst has a less privileged position as the arbiter of "truth" and the conveyor of insight, although, in my view, sensible Freudian analysts of earlier eras operated in this fashion. Freud's use of the metaphors of the "surgeon" and the "mirror" or "blank screen" were misleadingly taken to justify an attitude of aloofness, austerity, and reserve that is not necessary to implement what Freud really had in mind, namely, to create an unstructured situation that facilitated and highlighted the unfolding of the patient's dynamics.

Other characteristics of the Contemporary Period, particularly among Freudian analysts, include (1) the continued emphasis on unconscious, conflicted motives and fantasies; (2) a focus on generating insights primarily through interpreatation of the transference, especially the "here-and-now" transference (Gill, 1982, 1994) in a manner that recognizes the analyst's contribution to the way the transference evolves and is experienced by the patient; (3) understanding the patient's pathology in terms of the dynamic equilibrium between conflicted sexual and aggressive wishes and conflicts; (4) an increased blurring of the distinction between psychoanalysis proper and psychoanalytic psychotherapy and between "transference neurosis" and "transference reactions"; (5) being more attuned to the subjective, interactive nature of the therapeutic relationship, including the importance of patient–therapist match and the inevitable transference-countertransference enactments; (6) looking more closely at the countertransference reactions as a basis for information about the patient and a greater tendency toward intentional, judicious disclosure of countertransference reactions; (7) greater recognition that the presumed curative elements do not operate in the same manner for all patients or even for the same patient at different stages of treatment; and (8) dispensing with Freud's metapsychological concepts, particularly the untenable notion of psychic energy.

Within this Freudian common ground, Freudian analysts differ among themselves in the extent to which they (1) emphasize the here-and-now transference, relative to historical and extratransference interpretations; (2) focus on close analysis of the patient's defenses (what one might term the "ego-psychological" Freudians [e.g., Gray, 1994]); (3) incorporate concepts and therapeutic approaches from self psychology and object relations theories (referred to by Ellman, 1998, as the "self and object Freudians"); (4) deliberately foster and safeguard the therapeutic alliance; (5) in a related vein, make room in their conception of therapeutic action, for the importance of the analyst as a "new," as well as an "old," object; (6) relax the rule of abstinence in balancing the ratio of spontaneity and restraint, particularly with more disturbed patients; and (7) focus not only on the patient's defenses but also on their underlying unconscious fantasies and conflicts (what

Ellman, 1998, refers to as the "structural Freudians," e.g., Brenner, 1982).

Despite these changing conceptions, the Freudian approach to treatment has been criticized on a number of grounds, including its alleged limitations when applied to seriously disturbed narcissistic and borderline patients (Druck, 1989). It also has been claimed that the theory of technique that derives from the Freudian view is limited, even with neurotic patients. Underlying many criticisms of traditional theory is the view that Freudian theory and the tripartite, structural theory of mind (id, ego, superego) fails to account adequately for the richness and variety of human motivation and experience (Sandler, 1988). Furthermore, the emphasis on sexual and aggressive drives, on tension reduction, and on the depiction of human beings as more apt to seek a regressive path rather than a more progressive alternative reflect a generally pessimistic view of the human condition. It assumes, for example, that patients prefer the stagnating safety of familiar patterns of behavior and that they will be more inclined to seek from the analyst the satisfaction of dependent and sexual wishes than the more independent direction of insight, risk taking, and potential satisfaction with suitable objects in the real world. Adherents of object relational theories and of self psychology regard the focus on the vicissitudes of sexual and aggressive conflicts as failing to capture patients' concerns with issues of selfhood and of interpersonal relationships. There are rebuttals to these points, but there is insufficient space to present them here. In any event, a major challenge for Freudians, as well as for all psychoanalysts, is the integration of the essential insights that each approach has to offer into an internally consistent, comprehensive theory of personality and of therapy.

A related challenge for the future is for analysts to engage in further process and outcome studies to see if the innovations in theory and practice over the last 40 years constitute true progress or merely reflect shifts in fashion dictated by charismatic clinicians and changes in the *Zeitgeist*. In waiting for more evidence of the relative effectiveness of different analytic approaches, one sees indications of more modest claims and aims with respect to analytic goals and outcomes and a greater respect for alternative analytic approaches. We no longer speak of cures but of therapeutic changes. Conflicts are not forever eliminated but become more manageable, transferences are not fully resolved, we analyze resistances rather than overcome them, we do not doggedly pursue buried, childhood memories, dreams are no longer considered *the* royal road to the unconscious, and we no longer talk of a singular, "correct" technique.

SUGGESTIONS FOR FURTHER READING

Storr, A. (1979). *The art of psychotherapy*. New York: Methuen.—A clear introduction to the basic principles, concepts, and techniques of psychoanalytic psychotherapy.

Wallerstein, R. S. (1986). *Forty-two lives in treatment: A study of psychoanalysis and psychotherapy*. New York: Guilford Press.—An exhaustive account of the theory, research, and treatment of patients in the Menninger Foundation Psychotherapy Research Project. Reading the 42 cases will give the reader an excellent sense of the nature of psychoanalytically oriented treatment.

Wolitzky, D. L., & Eagle, M. (1997). Psychoanalytic theories of psychotherapy. In P. L. Wachtel & S. B. Messer (Eds.), *Theories of psychotherapy: Origins and evolution* (pp. 39–96). Washington, DC: American Psychological Association.—A comparative account of the theory and technical aspects of the main psychoanalytic approaches to treatment.

REFERENCES

Abraham, K. (1927). *Selected papers on psychoanalysis*. London: Hogarth Press.

Abraham, K. (1973). *Selected papers on psychoanalysis*. London: Hogarth Press.

Aichhorn, A. (1935). *Wayward youth*. New York: Viking Press.

American Psychiatric Association. (1994). *Diagnostic and statistical manual of mental disorders* (4th ed.). Washington, DC: Author.

Bach, S. (1985). *Narcissistic states and the therapeutic process*. New York: Jason Aronson.

Bachrach, H., Galatzer-Levy, R., Skolnikoff, A., & Waldron, S. (1991). On the efficacy of psychoanalysis. *Journal of the American Psychoanalytic Association, 39*, 871–916.

Basescu, S. (1990). Show and tell: Reflection on the analyst's self-disclosure. In G. Stricker & M. Fisher (Eds.), *Self-disclosure in the therapeutic relationship* (pp. 47–59). New York: Plenum Press.

Bernheim, H. (1886). *De la suggestion et de ses applications à la thérapeutique* (2nd ed., 1887). Paris.

Blatt, S. J., & Ford, R. Q. (1999). The effectiveness of long-term, intensive inpatient treatment of seriously disturbed, treatment-resistant young adults. In H. Kaley, M. N. Eagle, & D. L. Wolitzky (Eds.), *Psychoanalytic therapy as health care* (pp. 221–238). Hillsdale, NJ: Analytic Press.

Brenner, C. (1979). Working alliance, therapeutic alliance and transference. *Journal of the American Psychoanalytic Association, 27*(Suppl.), 137–157.

Brenner, C. (1982). *The mind in conflict*. New York: International Universities Press.

Breuer, J., & Freud, S. (1895). Studies on hysteria. *Standard Edition, 2*, 1–305. London: Hogarth Press, 1955.

Charcot, J. M. (1882). Physiologie pathologique: Sur les divers états nerveux determines par l'hypnotization chez les hystériques. [Pathological physiology: On the different nervous states hypnotically induced in hysterics]. *CR Academy of Science Paris, 94*, 403–405.

Cooper, A. M. (1987). Changes in psychoanalytic ideas: Transference interpretation. *Journal of the American Psychoanalytic Association, 35*, 77–98.

Crits-Christoph, P., & Barber, S. P. (1991). *Handbook of short-term dynamic psychotherapy*. New York: Basic Books.

Derogatis, L. R. (1994). *SCL-90: Administration, scoring, and procedures manual*. Minneapolis, MN: National Computer Systems.

Doidge, N. (1999). Who is in psychoanalysis now? Empirical data and reflections on some common misperceptions. In, H. Kaley, M. N. Eagle, & D. L. Wolitzky (Eds.), *Psychoanalytic therapy as health care* (pp. 177–198). Hillsdale, NJ: The Analytic Press.

Druck, A. (1989). *Four therapeutic approaches to the borderline patient: Principles and techniques of the basic dynamic stances*. Northvale, NJ: Jason Aronson.

Eagle, M. (1987). Theoretical and clinical shifts in psychoanalysis. *American Journal of Orthopsychiatry, 57*(2), 175–184.

Eagle, M., & Wolitzky, D. (1992). Psychoanalytic theories of psychotherapy. In D. K. Freedheim (Ed.), *History of psychotherapy: A century of change* (pp. 109–158). Washington, DC: American Psychological Association.

Eagle, M., & Wolitzky, D. L. (1997). Empathy: A psychoanalytic perspective. In A. C. Bohart & L. S. Greenberg (Eds.), *Empathy reconsidered* (pp. 217–244). Washington, DC: American Psychological Association.

Eagle, M., Wolitzky, D. L., & Wakefield, J. (2001). The analyst's knowledge and authority: A critique of the "new view" in psychoanalysis. *Journal of the American Psychological Association, 64*(2), 457–490.

Ellman, S. (1998). The unique contribution of the contemporary Freudian position. In C. S. Ellman, S. Grand, M. Silvan, & S. J. Ellman (Eds.), *The modern Freudians* (pp. 237–268). Northvale, NJ: Jason Aronson.

Erikson, E. H. (1950). *Childhood and society* (rev. ed.). New York: Norton, 1963.

Fairbairn, W. R. D. (1941). A revised psychopathology of the psychosis and psychoneurosis. *International Journal of Psychoanalysis, 22*, 250–279.

Federn, P. (1952). *Ego psychology and the psychoses*. New York: Basic Books.

Fonagy, P. (2002). An open door review of outcome studies in psychoanalysis [Online]. Available: *www. ipa. org. uk/research/complete. htm*

Freud, A. (1937). *The ego and the mechanisms of defence*. New York: International Universities Press.

Freud, A. (1954). Problems of technique in adult analysis. *Bulletin of the Philadelphia Association for Psychoanalysis, 4*, 44–69.

Freud, S. (1900). The interpretation of dreams. *Standard Edition, 4*, 1–338; *5*, 339–627. London: Hogarth Press, 1953.

Freud, S. (1901). The psychopathology of everyday life. *Standard Edition, 6,* 1–310. London: Hogarth Press, 1960.

Freud, S. (1905). On psychotherapy. *Standard Edition, 7,* 255–268. London: Hogarth Press, 1953.

Freud, S. (1910). The future prospects of psychoanalytic therapy. *Standard Edition, 11,* 139–151. London: Hogarth Press, 1957.

Freud, S. (1911). Formulations on the two principles of mental functioning. *Standard Edition, 12,* 218–226. London: Hogarth Press, 1958.

Freud, S. (1912). The dynamics of transference. *Standard Edition, 12,* 97–108. London: Hogarth Press, 1953.

Freud S. (1914). On narcissism: An introduction. *Standard Edition, 14,* 73–102. London: Hogarth Press, 1957.

Freud S. (1919). Lines of advance in psychoanalytic therapy. *Standard Edition, 17,* 135–144. London: Hogarth Press, 1955.

Freud, S. (1923). The ego and the id. *Standard Edition, 18,* 12–66. London: Hogarth Press, 1961.

Freud S. (1926). Inhibitions, symptoms and anxiety. *Standard Edition, 20,* 77–174. London: Hogarth Press, 1959.

Freud S. (1933). The dissection of the psychical personality. *Standard Edition, 17,* 57–81. London: Hogarth Press, 1964.

Freud S. (1937). Analysis terminable and interminable. *Standard Edition, 23,* 216–253. London: Hogarth Press, 1964.

Freud S. (1940). An outline of psycho-analysis. *Standard Edition, 23,* 144–207. London: Hogarth Press, 1964.

Fromm-Reichmann, F. (1950). *Principles of intensive psychotherapy.* Chicago: University of Chicago Press.

Gedo, J., & Goldberg, A. (1973). *Models of the mind: A psychoanalytic theory.* Chicago: University of Chicago Press.

Gill, M. M. (1954). Psychoanalysis and exploratory psychotherapy. *Journal of the American Psychoanalytic Association, 2,* 771–797.

Gill, M. M. (1979). The analysis of transference. *Journal of the American Psychoanalytic Association, 27,* 263–288.

Gill, M. M. (1982). *Analysis of transference.* New York: International Universities Press.

Gill, M. M. (1984). Psychoanalysis and psychotherapy: A revision. *International Journal of Psycho-Analysis, 11,* 161–179.

Gill, M. M. (1994). *Psychoanalysis in transition: A personal view.* Hillsdale, NJ: Analytic Press.

Gray, P. (1994). *The ego and the analysis of defense.* Northvale, NJ: Jason Aronson.

Greenberg, J., & Cheselka, O. (1995). Relational approaches to psychoanalytic psychotherapy. In A. S. Gurman & S. B. Messer (Eds.), *Essential psychotherapies* (pp. 55–84). New York: Guilford Press.

Greenson, R. R. (1965). The working alliance and the transference neurosis. *Psychoanalytic Quarterly, 34,* 155–181.

Greenson, R. R. (1967). *The technique and practice of psychoanalysis* (Vol. 1). New York: International Universities Press.

Hartmann, H. (1939). *Ego psychology and the problem of adaptation.* New York: International Universities Press.

Hartmann, H., Kris, E., & Loewenstein, R. M. (1946). Comments on the formation of psychic structure. In *Papers on psychoanalytic psychology (Psychological Issues, 4,* Monograph No. 14, pp. 27–55). New York: International Universities Press.

Holt, R. R. (1989). *Freud reappraised: A fresh look at psychoanalytic theory.* New York: Guilford Press.

Jacobson, E. (1964). *The self and the object world.* New York: International Universities Press.

Janet, P. (1907). *The major symptoms of hysteria.* New York: Macmillan.

Kaley, H., Eagle, M. N., & Wolitzky, D. L. (Eds.). (1999). *Psychoanalytic therapy as health care.* Hillsdale, NJ: Analytic Press.

Kernberg, O. (1975). *Borderline conditions and pathological narcissism.* Northvale, NJ: Jason Aronson.

Kernberg, O. F. (1980). *Internal world and external reality.* New York: Jason Aronson.

Kernberg, O. F., Selzer, M. A., Koenigsberg, H. W., Carr, A. C., & Appelbaum, A. H. (1989). *Psychodynamic psychotherapy of borderline patients.* New York: Basic Books.

Kohut, H. (1971). *The analysis of the self.* New York: International Universities Press.

Kohut, H. (1977). *The restoration of the self.* New York: International Universities Press.

Kohut, H. (1979). The two analyses of Mr. Z. *International Journal of Psycho-Analysis, 60,* 3–27.

Kohut, H. (1984). *How does analysis cure?* Chicago: University of Chicago Press.

Langs, R. J. (1982). Countertransference and the process of cure. In S. Slipp (Ed.), *Curative factors in dynamic psychotherapy* (pp. 127–152). New York: McGraw-Hill.

Luborsky, L. (1984). *Principles of psychoanalytic psychotherapy: A manual for supportive–expressive (SE) treatment.* New York: Basic Books

Luborsky, L., & Crits-Christoph, P. (1990). *Understanding transference: The CCRT method.* New York: Basic Books.

Lyons-Ruth, K. (1998). Implicit relational knowing: its role in development and psychoanalytic treatment. *Infant Mental Health, 19*, 3, 282–289.

Macalpine, I. (1950). The development of the transference. *Psychoanalytic Quarterly, 19*, 501–539.

Mahler, M. (1968). *On human symbiosis and the vicissitudes of individuation: Vol. I. Infantile psychosis.* New York: International Universities Press.

Malan, D. (1976). *The frontier of brief psychotherapy.* New York: Plenum Press.

Markus, H. R., & Kitayama, S. (1998). The cultural psychology of personality. *Journal of Cross-Cultural Psychology, 29*, 63–87.

McDougall, J. (1985). *Theaters of the mind.* New York: Basic Books.

Messer, S. B., & Warren, C. S. (1995). *Models of brief psychodynamic therapy: A comparative approach.* New York: Guilford Press.

Messer, S. B., & Wolitzky, D. L. (1997). The traditional psychoanalytic approach to case formulation. In T. D. Eells (Ed.), *Handbook of psychotherapy case formulation* (pp. 26–51). New York: Guilford Press.

Mitchell, S. (1988). *Relational concepts in psychoanalysis.* Cambridge, MA: Harvard University Press.

Oremland, J. (1991). *Interpretation and interaction.* Hillsdale, NJ: Analytic Press.

Pine, F. (1990). *Drive, ego, object, and self.* New York: Basic Books.

Pulver, S. (1995). The technique of psychoanalysis proper. In B. E. Moore & B. D. Fine (Eds.), *Psychoanalysis: The major concepts* (pp. 5–25). New Haven, CT: Yale University Press.

Rapaport, D., & Gill, M. M. (1959). The points of view and assumptions of meta-psychol-ogy. *International Journal of Psycho-Analysis, 40*, 153–162.

Reich, W. (1933). *Character analysis: Principles and techniques for psychanalysis in practice and training* (3rd ed.). New York: Orgone Institute Press.

Rosenfeld, H. A. (1965). *Psychotic states.* London: Hogarth Press.

Safran, J. D., & Muran, J. C. (2000). *Negotiating the therapeutic alliance: A relational treatment guide.* New York: Guilford Press.

Sandell, R., Blomberg, J., Lazar, A., Carlsswon, J., Broberg, J., & Schubert, J. (2000). Varieties of long-term outcome among patients in psychoanalysis and long-term psychotherapy: A review of findings in the Stockholm Outcome of Psychoanalysis and Psychotherapy Project (STOPP). *International Journal of Psychoanalysis, 81*(5), 921–942.

Sandler, J. (1988). Psychoanalytic technique and "Analysis terminable and interminable." *International Journal of Psycho-Analysis, 69*, 335–345.

Schafer, R. (1959). Generative empathy in the treatment situation. *Psychoanalytic Quarterly, 28*, 342–373.

Schafer, R. (1983). *The analytic attitude.* New York: Basic Books.

Schafer, R. (1992). *Retelling a life.* New York: Basic Books.

Schlesinger, G., & Wolitzky, D. L. (2002). The effects of a self-analytic exercise on clinical judgment. *Psychoanalytic Psychology, 19*(4), 651–685.

Searles, H. (1965). *Collected papers on schizophrenia and related subjects.* London: Hogarth Press.

Sechehaye, M. A. (1951). *Symbolic realization.* New York: International Universities Press.

Sterba, R. (1934). The fate of the ego in analytic therapy. *International Journal of Psychoanalysis, 15*, 117–126.

Sullivan, H. S. (1953). *The interpersonal theory of psychiatry.* New York: Norton.

Ticho, E. (1972). Termination of psychoanalysis: Treatment goals and life goals. *Psychoanalytic Quarterly, 41*, 315–333.

Wachtel, P. L. (1993). *Therapeutic communication: Principles and effective practice.* New York: Guilford Press.

Waelder, R. (1960). *Basic theory of psychoanalysis.* New York: International Universities Press.

Wallerstein, R. S. (1986). *Forty-two lives in treat-

ment: A study of psychoanalysis and psychotherapy. New York: Guilford Press.

Wallerstein, R. S. (1990). Psychoanalysis: The common ground. *International Journal of Psycho-Analysis, 71,* 3–20.

Wallerstein, R. S. (1991). Assessment of structural change in psychoanalytic therapy and research. In T. Shapiro (Ed.), *The concept of structure in psychoanalysis* (pp. 241–261). Madison, CT: International Universities Press.

Weinshel, E. M. (1984). Some observations on the psychoanalytic process. *Psychoanalytic Quarterly, 53,* 63–92.

Weiss, J., & Sampson, H. (1986). *The psychoanalytic process: theory, clinical observation, and empirical research.* New York: Guilford Press.

Winnicott, D. W. (1965). *The maturational processes and the facilitating environment.* London: Hogarth Press and Institute of Psycho-Analysis.

Zetzel, E. R. (1956). Current concepts of transference. *International Journal of Psycho-Analysis, 37,* 369–378.

3

Relational Approaches to Psychoanalytic Psychotherapy

REBECCA C. CURTIS
IRWIN HIRSCH

HISTORICAL BACKGROUND

Relational approaches to psychoanalytic psychotherapy represent a paradigm shift consistent with developments in science and the humanities in the 20th century. One of the benefits of this approach is that it allows a rapprochement with current mainstream cognitive and social psychology. It is difficult to describe relational approaches in a unitary way. What is inherent in the concept is the view that each individual asked to describe it will present a subjective view that differs somewhat from the next "expert's" view.

Freud had developed the psychoanalytic method in a culture that increasingly looked to science as a source of orientation in a world in which technology and industrialization had led to major changes in people's lifestyles. The science of the 19th century was that of objective observation. The observer of mental processes in psychoanalysis was to be this sort of neutral, impartial scientist at work, like an archeologist looking for deeper and deeper layers of unconscious facts in the patient's mind. Essentialism and positivism are other terms that characterize the natural science model that reflected much of psychoanalytic thinking for at least the first half of the 20th century.

Images of the world were jolted in the 1920s and 1930s by Einstein's relativity theory, quantum physics, and Heisenberg's uncertainty principle. Quantum physics emphasized interconnections and mutual interactions and Heisenberg demonstrated that phenomena were always affected by being measured. The ideal of the totally objective observer in the hard sciences was demonstrated to be impossible. If the observer were also a participant in the world of particle physics, then the analyst was certainly a participant in interactions with a patient, and the influence of the analyst would have to be taken into account in that situation as well. Nonetheless, this ethos did not filter down to psychoanalysis until the late 1940s, heralded then by Harry Stack Sullivan's model of the therapist as both an observer and an unwitting participant in the dyad.

The ideas of the individual as embedded in relationships and the therapist as a participant observer were taken up in the United States by Sullivan (1953) in his development of what was first called "interpersonal psychiatry." Unlike many psychoanalysts who worked with rather well-functioning patients, Sullivan developed many of his ideas from working with male schizophrenics. Sullivan joined forces with several prominent psychoanalysts who were also interested in social and cultural influences on personality development—Karen Horney, Erich Fromm, Frieda Fromm-Reichmann, and Clara Thompson—eventually forming with the three latter therapists what became know as the Interpersonal School of Psychoanalysis. Clara Thompson (as well as Melanie Klein) had been analyzed by Freud's colleague Sandor Ferenczi. Ferenczi was known as an analyst's analyst and was sent difficult patients other analysts could not help. Whereas Freud was considered the "father" of psychoanalysis, Ferenczi was considered the "mother." He was known for his focus on early developmental and often pre-Oedipal, nonverbal interactions between mother and child, prioritizing such engagement over Freud's emphasis on the unfolding of phase-specific innate drive states as the building blocks of human personality. Ferenczi also experimented with various new techniques, including conceptualizing the psychoanalytic relationship as mutually constructed. Ferenczi and Sullivan both had considerable influence on the development of relational psychoanalysis, the former more indirectly, through his impact on analysands such as Clara Thompson, Melanie Klein, and Michael Balint (cf. Aron & Harris, 1993). Thompson became a consolidating figure within the Interpersonal School, while Klein and Balint were key to the development of different aspects of object relations theory. Although there are important differences among these traditions, all basically share the view that relationships with caretakers are the most central features in any

effort to understand development of personality. With respect to the therapeutic relationship, all three traditions highlight various ways, beyond objective observation, that therapists both unwittingly and purposefully interact with their patients (Hirsch, 1987). Perhaps partly because some of these analysts were working with patients more disturbed than their classical counterparts, these analysts deviated early on from the standard Freudian technique of the time.

Around the same time as Sullivan was developing his interpersonal psychiatry in the United States, W. R. D. Fairbairn (1952) in Great Britain was arguing that people were primarily motivated to seek other people. This position, too, was in contrast to the classical Freudian belief that people were motivated primarily by sexual and aggressive drives and derivatives of these drive states. He developed, simultaneously with, but independent of, Klein and Balint, an "object relations theory of psychoanalysis," drawing from the philosophical tradition of "subjects" (people) and the "objects" they observed. For Fairbairn, the term "objects" referred to the internalization of experiences with other people—what cognitive psychologists might call internalized "representations" of others.

In 1983 Merton Gill published a paper arguing for a "person" point of view in contrast to Freud's energy discharge model of the mind. He proposed the term "person" because "interpersonal" carried too heavily the weight of Sullivanian thinking, and "object relations" failed to distinguish between the work of Klein where an instinct-oriented model was still present to a degree, and the work of Balint and Fairbairn, where the relations with early caretakers were dominant. In 1983, Greenberg and Mitchell also published a volume titled *Object Relations in Psychoanalysis,* followed by Eagle's (1984) *Recent Advances in Psychoanalysis.* Greenberg and Mitchell (1983) argued that a paradigm shift had taken place in psychoanalysis such that relations with others "constitute the fundamental building blocks of mental life" (p. 3) in contrast to Freud's emphasis on the unfolding of bio-logically based, prewired psychosexual stages of development. All the approaches Greenberg and Mitchell included under the "relational" umbrella have in common the focus on relationships, external and inter-nalized, as the primary way of understand-ing human development and personality organization. Although the clearest expres-sion of this paradigm initially came in the work of Harry Stack Sullivan and W. R. D. Fairbairn, other key psychoanalytic theo-rists, such as D. W. Winnicott, Margaret Mahler, Edith Jacobsen, and Hans Loewald, are viewed as moving psychoanalysis toward this emphasis, some without breaking com-pletely with their Freudian framework. Edgar Levenson (1972), a major contributor to the interpersonal tradition, had already described paradigm shifts from Freud's work-machine model, to the information/communication model, and from this to the organismic model found in biology where every element has connections with many other elements, so that influence can flow in several directions. Levenson emphasized the interpersonal entanglements into which the analyst could be drawn by the patient. Far from the objective scientist or the "blank screen" of the Freudian analyst, the therapist in the interpersonal/relational ap-proach was a subjectivity all of its own in-teracting with the other subjectivity—the patient. Participant observation is not a *pre-scription* of how therapists should relate—it is a *description* of what is inevitable in any two-person interaction. When in the pres-ence of another, one cannot *not* participate, as quiet and subtle as such engagement might be (Greenberg, 1991). In all relational perspectives, the presence of the other is in-escapable in both human development and in the therapeutic relationship. The second "person" cannot be removed from any as-pect of interaction.

More recently, from the 1980s to the pre-sent, the relational approach has been repre-sented in the works of such contemporary writers as Neil Altman, Lewis Aron, Beatric Beebe, Jessica Benjamin, Philip Bromberg, Jody Davies, Muriel Dimen, Mary Gail Frawley, Emmanuel Ghent, Jay Greenberg, Adrienne Harris, Irwin Hirsch, Irwin Hoff-man, Donnel Stern, and Robert Stolorow, among others (cf. Mitchell & Aron, 1999; Skolnick & Warshaw, 1992). This body of writing builds on the contributions of earli-er innovators from the Interpersonal tradi-tion (e.g., Erich Fromm, Harold Searles, and Benjamin Wolstein), the varieties of object relation theorists (e.g., Heinrich Racker, Wilfred Bion, and D. W. Winnicott), and the development of self psychology originally spearheaded by Heinz Kohut and his col-leagues in Chicago.

Greenberg and Mitchell suggested that the interpersonal approach of Sullivan and his colleagues (Horney, Fromm, Fromm-Reichman, and Thompson) lacked a well-developed theory of intrapsychic processes, whereas the varieties of object relations ap-proaches (Winnicott, Fairbairn, and Klein) lacked sufficient focus on modes of describ-ing actual interpersonal relations. These ap-proaches complement each other, with the interpersonal tradition originally focused more on external relations (and realities) and the object relations tradition focused more on internalized relationships. By this time in history, however, both traditions address and have integrated the fundamental notion that unconscious processes or internalized worlds consist largely of internalized relational con-figurations (Mitchell, 1988, 1993).

In the United States, Heinz Kohut (1971, 1977, 1984) also developed many ideas that were in considerable harmony with Fer-enczi's original view of the analyst as an em-pathic observer, and with theories of devel-opment that have much in common with object relations theorists such as Balint and Winnicott. Robert Stolorow and others (At-wood & Stolorow, 1984; Orange, Atwood, & Stolorow, 1997; Stolorow & Atwood, 1992) have tried to extend Kohut's self psychology and integrate it into the intersubjective ethos long held by Interpersonal psychoanalysts

and their contemporary relational counterparts (Benjamin, 1998).

In 1991 a new journal, *Psychoanalytic Dialogues: A Journal of Relational Perspectives* was
begun and became a forum for comparing
and contrasting the numerous traditions
that lie within the large relational umbrella:
interpersonal, varieties of object relational
(Fairbairn, Winnicott, and Klein), self psychological, intersubjective, and postmodern
feminist thinking. The relational approach
continues to inspire excitement, with an International Association for Relational Psychoanalysis and Psychotherapy, founded by
Stephen Mitchell, holding its first meeting
in 2002, with Lewis Aron serving as its first
president.

Relational approaches have been influenced by other intellectual trends in the
20th century, particularly postmodernism
and constructivism (see Neimeyer &
Bridges, Chapter 8, this volume). Postmodern thinking is characterized by a loosening
of hierarchies and categories in the pursuit
of knowledge, with an emphasis on subjective perception (in contrast with the ability
to discern absolute truth), and considering
cultural contexts as opposed to searching
for essential qualities. Constructivism emphasizes the aspects of reality that are created by our perceptions. A view that social reality is largely constructed stands in priority
to a view that reality is discovered by one
party about a second party which is then
viewed as an absolute truth. Relativism (the
idea that criteria of judgment are relative)
and perspectivism (the idea that reality is
known only in terms of the perspectives of
it seen at a particular moment) dominate
relational thinking, including both therapists' interactions with, and their efforts to
understand the psyches of, their patients.

THE CONCEPT OF
PERSONALITY

Because relational approaches draw from
some disparate theoretical frameworks,
there is not a unified concept of personality.
Generally, it is thought that individuals develop relatively stable patterns of being in
the world. Their ways of being are intimately connected to the internalization of
identifications with significant caretakers,
much of which lies outside the boundary of
consciousness. Many relational therapists
believe that people tend to construct unconsciously their contemporary world to
conform to the familiarity of past experience. In other words, people are inclined to
repeat their key early experiences; the current relational world tends to become an
updated version of earlier life.

The particular approach of Sullivan centered around the *self-system* (whereas other
theorists might discuss concepts such as
psychic structure or "character"). For Sullivan (1953), personality is the entire functioning of a person. The *self* refers to the organization of experience within the
personality and is largely a composite of internalized experiences with others. Anxiety-free experiences as an infant with the
caretaker, usually the mother, lead to the
experience of the *good me,* whereas anxiety-
filled experiences lead to the *bad me.* Some
experiences, however, are so traumatic that
they cannot be integrated at all. These experiences Sullivan refers to as the "not me."
They are experiences felt as dread or as horror, such as in a nightmare. Concerns with
the lack of integration of positive and negative experiences in persons suffering from
disorders of the self are a central theme in
many relational writings.

Although Winnicott had differentiated a
true self from a *false self,* most relational analysts view the self as socially constructed.
People are seen as having different
thoughts, feelings, and ways of acting in the
presence of different people and when
alone in different contexts. All these multiple self-states are viewed as real, including
one or more that may be oriented toward
pleasing others instead of being considered
"false" (Bromberg, 1998; Davies, 1998;
Mitchell, 1993). The person is never con-

ceived of as an isolated being in relational thought: "There is no such thing as a baby," Winnicott (1964) had stated, "only a nursing couple" (p. 88). A person is not a closed system. Winnicott was trying to convey the idea that there were properties of a dyad that transcend the attributes of each individual person. Similarly, relational analysts refer to their approach as a *two-person psychology* because these properties of the relationship between two people must always be taken into account in efforts to understand the individual. Thomas Ogden (1994), a contemporary Kleinian analyst, for example, has referred to the space between the analyst and the patient as the "analytic third," in other words, the reflective space of psychoanalysis being another presence in the room. Other relational analysts such as Altman (1995) have suggested that the culture is always a third party present in the relationship between two people.

Sullivan's theory of personality was influenced by developments in the cognitive science of his time. His model of the self is one not dominated by the repression of unacceptable impulses. Instead, he posits a lack of connection, or dissociation of experiences, that would be so conflictual as to be overwhelming if held in consciousness simultaneously. Such awareness may be disorganizing because it is incongruous with the current and stable organization of experience. Experiences that are out of awareness or unconscious are critically important to relational psychoanalysts, as they are to psychoanalysts of all traditions. Atwood and Stolorow (1984) described three realms of unconscious processes. The first is the *prereflective unconscious.* These experiences are not a by-product of defensive activity. They are simply the organizing principles that unconsciously shape a person's experiences. In this sense, prereflective unconscious processes are similar in some ways to what cognitive psychologists refer to as procedural memory. The *dynamic unconscious* "consists in that set of configurations that consciousness is not permitted to assume, because of

their association with emotional conflict and subjective danger" (Atwood & Stolorow, 1984, p. 35). *Unvalidated unconscious* experiences are those experiences that never evoked the required validating responsiveness from others. These experiences were simply never able to become articulated. When failure to evoke validating attunement from caretakers occurs, people may be prone to become disorganized or to develop psychosomatic symptoms. Such experiences are quite similar to what Donnel Stern (1983, 1997) has called "unformulated experience," and what cognitive psychologists have described as *implicit* perceptual and memory processes. Stolorow and Atwood have explained these three realms of unconscious processes by the use of an analogy to a building. Consciousness corresponds to the part of the building above ground. The dynamic unconscious corresponds to the basement, the prereflective unconscious to the architect's blueprint, and the unvalidated unconscious to the unused bricks and other such materials.

For Sullivan, the self-system developed out of a sense of anxiety. Anxiety may lead to selective inattention regarding experiences that are inconsistent with a person's dominant views or ways of being. To the extent the person is anxious, the person's flexibility in attending to incongruous information and responding becomes more rigidified. For Fairbairn as well, the representations of the self developed out of anxiety.

A dissociative view of the mind also prevails in relational thinking (cf. Bromberg, 1998; Curtis, 1996a; Davies & Frawley, 1993). Fairbairn (1929/1994), in his only recently published medical thesis, had argued that repression was a specific type of dissociation. Dissociated states may manifest themselves by physical symptoms, such as tics or somatic symptoms. Trauma may lead to a dissociation of experiences, such that a person may seem numb or intellectualized when discussing a traumatic event all the while experiencing signs at other times that something is amiss. People do not feel con-

flicted about dissociated experiences because they are not aware of them simultaneously with other states. Experiences that are
"repressed" or pushed out of awareness, on
the other hand, were experienced as conflict at the moment of repression. Internal
conflict, nonetheless, is an ever-present aspect of the human condition. The wish to
risk knowing oneself and to change as a
person is in ubiquitous conflict with the
wish to remain ignorant of one's self and
maintain a stable equilibrium.

In place of Freud's sexual and aggressive
motivations as the central force that moves
people, Sullivan conceptualized the need to
satisfy tendencies toward security, tenderness
(intimacy), and lust. When these needs cannot be met, they can undergo what he called
a "malevolent transformation," leading to aggression and perhaps cruelty. Overall, in relational theories, aggression is not seen as instinctual. It is viewed as learned, stemming
from either frustration or identification with
a familiar aggressor. To the extent that the
parent is empathic and is able to try to take
the baby's perspective or to reflect on the
baby's functioning (cf. Beebe & Lachman,
2002: Fonagy, 2001; Stern, 1985), the child is
likely to feel soothed when anxious and to
be more likely eventually to satisfy its desires.
Infant researchers, such as Beebe, have observed that caretakers, who can match the
rhythm of their infants in a sort of dance-like
interaction are able to help the baby regulate
his or her emotions.

Sexuality, though instinctually based, is
viewed as an important medium in which
relational struggles are played out. The form
of one's sexuality is developed through relational interaction. Sexuality provides the
imaginative elaboration of bodily functions.
It is a "powerful medium in which emotional connection and intimacy is sought,
established, lost, and regained" (Mitchell,
1988, p. 107).

Relational analysts have been among the
strongest critics of Freudian theories regarding the development of sexuality since
Freud expressed them. Karen Horney
(1926) and Clara Thompson (1942) both
criticized his notions of female sexuality, arguing that penis envy was related to the
cultural advantages given to men. Castration anxiety in the literal sense has been
seen as more related to the real, threatening
statements given to boys in Freud's turn-of-
the-century European culture than as a universal phenomenon per se. However, "castration" fears in the sense of feelings of
threat and/or helplessness, are seen as something universal. Robert Stoller (1985) argued that castration anxiety was "existence
anxiety" (p. 20n) and that men "do not fear
loss of genitals per se (castration anxiety) as
much as they fear to lose their masculinity
and—still more fundamental—their sense
of maleness" (p. 35). "Masochistic" tendencies in women have been viewed as a consequence of a lack of recognition of a girl's
subjectivity by the father, not as a consequence of an adjustment to a sense of having been "castrated" (Benjamin, 1988).

Relational analysts think that the development of heterosexuality needs as much
explanation as the development of homosexuality or bisexuality—there are no universal causalities for either. In addition, homosexuality and bisexuality are viewed as
normal variants, not as pathological. This is
also true for much of other sexual behavior,
which had historically been referred to as
"perversions" (Dimen, 2001; Dimen &
Goldner, 2002; Drescher, 1998).

Aggression comes from being aggressed
upon and from frustration, not from an inborn drive that must be discharged. People
have the impulse to hurt when they are
harmed, but if empathy is learned through
the experience with a loving caretaker, the
impulse to hurt another can be contained.
Although all people have aggressive feelings, when loving feelings outweigh aggressive ones, relationships are easier to maintain. The desire to hurt others by people
who have been neglected or harmed is not
to be underestimated (Harris, 1998).

Relational theory has sometimes been criticized for reducing human motivation to a single drive—that for relationships. Yet Greenberg (1991), for example, has posited two broad categories of basic needs—one for security or safety; the other for effectance. This thinking is built on the work of Erich Fromm (1964) who described a universal human conflict between enmeshment in what is safe and familiar, and the wish to expand oneself—to separate from what is known and familiar. Both Fromm's and Greenberg's thinking is important to many relational therapists and reflects a dimension of experience that transcends simply relationship seeking.

A theory of five motivational systems in the work of Joseph Lichtenberg, Frank Lachmann, and James Fosshage (1992) has been incorporated into much of relational thinking. These five systems are the need for (1) regulation of physiological requirements, (2) attachment and affiliation, (3) exploration and assertion, (4) responding aversively through withdrawal and antagonism, and (5) sensual enjoyment and sexual excitement. Relational analysts are more likely to think about desires than drives (Benjamin, 1988, 1995). Desire is "experienced always in the context of relatedness" (Mitchell, 1988, p. 3).

Personality formation begins in the early stages of infancy, or even in the uterus. Relational analysts have embraced the recent work of attachment researchers (Mitchell, 2000), following in the tradition begun by the psychoanalyst John Bowlby (1969). It is thought that infants develop expectations that others will be available to them emotionally to the extent the early caretaker is. Infants and their caretakers communicate nonverbally by "eye contact, proxemics, conversational rhythms, games and signaling" (Beebe, Jaffe, & Lachmann, 1992, p. 66). The infant develops expectancies of characteristic interaction sequences that become generalized in the first year of life at the time the ability to abstract information develops.

Daniel Stern (1985) referred to the infant's capacity to internalize interactions and to generalize them, similar to what Bowlby had called *internalized working models*. The unconscious organizing structures early in life are believed to play a major role in the way other people are integrated into one's life. The open communication patterns of securely attached children and their parents provide a greater ability to flexibly revise working models of self and others than are more closed patterns of communication.

These internalized interactional patterns provide a model of development that is largely drawn from infant research, and it is quite different from much of Freudian developmental theory. Still, it is acknowledged that there are often self-critical and self-punitive tendencies among children reared by benign parents (Sandler & Sandler, 1987). Aggressive fantasies on the part of the child may produce guilt when parents are benign. Some relational analysts have been drawn to Kleinian theories of development, theories that place a central emphasis on innate aggression and its projection. Mitchell (1988) and others have noted that Klein's theories were not taken from the observations of normal infants and children but from interactions of older and more disturbed children.

Although Oedipal dynamics, a central theme in the Freudian tradition, are examined and may well be a significant source of conflict, problems in living arise for a larger variety of reasons. For example, personality continues to develop during the elementary school years when the formation of a close friendship may mitigate or modify earlier troubled engagements with caretakers. Like Freudian theory, relational theory assumes that conflicts within the personality are inevitable. Symptoms are not only rooted in conflicts between wishes and fears or between people and society but, as well, between conflictual relational configurations that have been internalized from a life history of self–other interactions.

PSYCHOLOGICAL HEALTH AND PATHOLOGY

Sullivan preferred the term "problems in living" over other nomenclatures for psychiatric disorders. Fromm criticized the conformist personality he saw in American culture and was scathing in his attack on the "marketing personality." Joyce McDougall (1978, p. 156) coined the term "normopath" and Christopher Bollas (1987, p. 137) referred to the "normatic personality," both terms referring to people who conform to the values of a society to the extent that their individual vitality is stifled. Thus, the problems in living for relational psychoanalysts do not correspond neatly with the *Diagnostic and Statistical Manual of Mental Disorders* of the American Psychiatric Association. Nonetheless, relational analysts do make assessments regarding the level of functioning, and may even prescribe medication or refer patients for medication evaluations if they believe that psychotherapy alone is insufficient to help a particular patient. They are, however, quite critical of the "disease" model inherited from medicine. They do not expect to uncover a pathogen—a single repressed wish, for example. Instead, they view personality patterns as having been largely learned in social situations, and as having been reasonable, adaptive ways of coping in those situations (e.g., attachment styles learned largely in infancy and childhood). (Obviously, the temperaments with which infants are born also play a role.) If troubled ways of being are learned, new ways of relating also can be learned. There exists an inherent optimism in a way of thinking that emphasizes personality as a function of experiential learning, not as biologically driven.

Relational analysts make note of patients' strengths and help patients become more aware of their strengths and how to appreciate them. At the same time, relational analysts are looking at the gaps in patients' resources and helping them become aware of these deficits. A patient with an obsessive style who avoids feelings and provides endless details might be asked, for example, "What are you feeling?" or "Can you tell me what is the most important thing that happened?" Problems in relating to others are obviously often a core focus, for much of what can be called psychopathology is expressed in the broad arenas of love and work.

Flexible ways of relating are signs of health, whereas rigid ways of being are signs of inhibition and anxiety. Symptoms are always viewed as communications (Phillips, 1988). They do not simply reflect illness or pathology. According to Adam Phillips, the healthy child has a "flexible repertoire of symptoms" (p. 50).

A number of relational analysts have made important contributions to the understanding of severe disturbances. In particular, Sullivan, Freida Fromm-Reichmann, and Harold Searles worked successfully with schizophrenics before the advances of psychotropic medications. One of Fromm-Reichmann's patients, Hannah Greenberg (1964), documented her treatment in a popular novel and film, *I Never Promised You a Rose Garden*. For Sullivan, the self in the schizophrenic has lost control of awareness and has lost the sense of a consensually validated self. For Searles (1979), treating schizophrenic patients simply as unformed or egoless people is profoundly condescending. Sullivan, Fromm-Reichmann, and Searles all subscribed to an ethos characterized by Sullivan's attitude that we are all more simply human than otherwise. They argue that although schizophrenics are more difficult to work with, they are not essentially different from others.

Classical psychoanalysis emphasized the meanings patients made of their internal and prerelational experiences and focused on patients' fantasies based on such experiences. The relational tradition has paid more attention to what has actually happened and fantasy based on that experience. Whereas Freud once theorized that many of the stories he heard of incest and the sexual abuse of women, for example, were wishes and fantasies, the interpersonalists and relational analysts believed the stories could be based on something that really occurred. Traumas, especially those stemming from betrayal by parents, relatives, and other people in positions of authority, affect feelings and expectations in current situations in ways that fantasies not founded on experiences do not. Relational analysts, more so than their Freudian colleagues, are mindful of the impact of what actually happens, that is, the social and cultural contributions to problems in living.

Health does not simply represent having better feelings about one self (self-esteem) and others. By allowing more experiences into awareness a person may also notice more threatening experiences when they exist. Health means a greater tolerance for such anxiety-provoking experiences, in addition to tolerance for desired, exciting experiences. Psychic health, as much as anything, refers to the ability to assimilate new experience, to transcend the identifications and the constraints of the past.

THE PROCESS OF CLINICAL ASSESSMENT

Relational therapists make informal assessments of patients in all interactions, even as they are gathering a history of the patient. Assessments are made at both the interpersonal and intrapsychic levels, consistent with the origins of the approach. Of particular note are the interactional styles of the patient, styles of coping and defense, the range of emotions, cognitive abilities, feelings about one self and others, and conflicts and inhibitions that may block the patient from achieving his or her goals. Self-experiences in the presence of different people are of interest, so that both the therapist and patient can get a sense of different internalized relational configurations and the behaviors that ensue. Diagnostic categories are known to the therapist, but categories eliminate the

unique qualities of the individual that are of interest to the relational therapist. Such categories are used to the extent that they are required for records and are useful in summarizing characteristics of the patient but are generally viewed as too restrictive and stereotyping, especially in regard to personality disorders (Westen, 2002).

Assessments are made at the individual, dyadic, and systemic levels. Although the individual is the primary focus of attention, the therapist is monitoring continually what is transpiring in the therapeutic dyad and is cognizant of the cultural context as well. If the therapist thinks that couple or family therapy would be of benefit, such treatment (usually with a different therapist) is recommended.

Circumstances surrounding the problems the patient presents are elicited. The events and feelings preceding a problem, the overall context in which it occurs, and any secondary gains the problem may provide are given serious consideration. A detailed inquiry is made into any problems, such as substance abuse, that will require specialized treatment. In the case of potential danger to self and others, inquiry into matters related to the likelihood of such events is conducted and a judgment is made. Relational therapists working in hospital or clinic settings will use any formal assessments usually conducted in that setting. Therapists in private practice refer patients for psychological, neuropsychological, or medical assessments when appropriate.

THE PRACTICE OF THERAPY

In the practice of psychotherapy, relational analysts draw from the rich literature of case studies and theory in psychoanalysis, although their practice may differ somewhat from that of their classical forebears. The relational emphasis is distinct from that of some other contemporary approaches, particularly from psychotherapies focused largely on symptom reduction. For relationalists, the unique experiences and meanings of people's existence are of special interest. This contrasts with an interest in the *general* characteristics of all patients with a particular psychiatric diagnosis, and with the application of a standard technique that is relevant to everyone. As Benjamin Wolstein (cited in Hirsch, 2000) has said, "Every therapist is unique, every patient is unique, every dyad is unique" (p. 225). Indeed, most relational therapies prefer the term "approach," to the more technical word "technique."

Basic Structure of Therapy

Relational therapists usually prefer to meet with patients more than one time each week, although this often may not be possible. Rarely would a relational therapist set a time limit unless the therapist is working from one of the models of brief therapy consistent with this approach (see Hoyt, Chapter 10, this volume). Most relational therapists would hope for frequent sessions with the therapist in order for the interpersonal interactions (transference) that the patient finds problematic with others to emerge with the therapist. These problematic interactions may take some time to occur, or a meaningful level of intimacy to develop. Although the treatment is most likely to be individual, family or group therapy may be used in conjunction with individual treatment. Despite sessions generally being unstructured, the relational therapist becomes more active if life-threatening or treatment-threatening issues occur.

Goal Setting

Traditionally, the goal of psychoanalytic treatment has been to increase awareness and through this process to effect a broadening of the organization of experience so that a person is more flexible and less rigid. Enrichment of experience takes priority over symptom reduction, and optimal functioning in the arenas of love, work, and play

is of interest to relational therapists, as it is to all psychoanalytic therapists. In many ways, the precise goals of the therapy are not known in advance, because the hope is that the patient will feel opened up to new experiences and, in this process, formulate new goals. Ultimately, however, the patient sets the goals, and the patient is certainly free to choose less ambitious aims than what most analytic therapists prefer. In this sense, the patient and therapist begin a journey, but the destination is not determined.

If the therapist has reservations about a goal the patient expresses, the therapist has an obligation to express a dissenting opinion or to attempt to arrive at a mutually compatible goal. The relationally oriented therapist has a responsibility to explain in the first meeting or first set of meetings something about the way he or she works if the patient comes from a background that is likely devoid of such knowledge. For example, if the patient comes to the therapist saying that he would like to work more hours each week and is already working an 80-hour week, the therapist might question this goal and suggest an alternative, such as exploring what makes working so many hours so important.

Despite the ambitious aims of most analytic therapies, patients often want help first and foremost with symptom reduction. Increased awareness of when the symptom occurs, what covaries with it, and what other problems the symptom might reduce or disguise likely will help with symptom reduction. Addressing life-threatening and treatment-threatening behaviors will take priority over other goals. Certain other behavioral problems may also take priority, such as a substance abuse problem that will neutralize any benefit psychoanalytic therapy may offer. Relational analysts vary in the extent to which they would refer a patient for behavioral and other auxiliary treatments or integrate such treatments into their own approach.

Although relational therapists must be respectful of the patient's goal of reducing symptoms, they are usually thinking of the symptoms in the broader characterlogical and cultural context. Not only are the therapists noticing what symptoms are present; but they are also cognizant of what is missing. They are thinking of what the symptoms may communicate, how they have been adaptive, what they may symbolize, and with what they may coincide. A man who presents with a problem of premature ejaculation may have impulse-control problems in other areas; a man who has retarded ejaculation may procrastinate elsewhere. The partner may be anxious and/or undermining of the patient's confidence. The man may prefer not to be involved with this partner or may prefer a partner of another sex. To the extent that therapists conceive of the presenting problem as embedded in a larger picture, they will listen to the patient's communications with an open mind or inquire in a more structured manner to have a more nuanced picture of the whole person.

In helping the patient achieve whatever goals he or she has articulated, the therapist also has ideas about how best to achieve these goals. This reflects the two-person situation described previously. As already noted, the therapist will likely have in mind the traditional psychoanalytic goal of helping the patient work, love, and play more freely. Sullivan (1953) stated that treatment is aimed at "increasing a patient's skill in living" (p. 175). Relational analysts will have in mind a variety of desired outcomes such as the tolerance of uncertainty and emotions, arousing of curiosity, becoming more aware of one's impact upon others, increasing the capacity for self-reflection, mourning of losses and lost possibilities, separation from embeddedness in the past, and finding richer meaning in life. "Self-actualization," a term developed by humanist psychologists, is one way to characterize the broadest aim of most psychoanalytic psychotherapists.

In many cases, the patient will prioritize the treatment goals. The therapist, however, may think it likely that the patient's goals

are linked with other goals that the patient has not considered important. For example, a woman who wishes to stop her bingeing and purging may insist that she does not wish to have closer personal relationships. The therapist may be wondering, however, how the patient can stop turning to food for comfort without an alternative and might suggest that the food is her most comfortable "relationship." The relational therapist is likely thinking about the overall possible adaptive purposes a symptom may be serving, and that an attempt to remove the symptom without the patient developing an alternative way of fulfilling a longing or desire may not be effective. In this way the relational therapist is not simply trying to remove the symptom without understanding its meaning.

Process Aspects of Treatment

Some relational therapists object to the use of the word "technique" because it connotes the idea that the therapist always knows exactly what he or she is doing, as one might in a procedure closer to natural science. Relational therapists do not work in the same way—the unique personality of each therapist plays a significant role in how one relates to patients (cf. Hoffman, 1998). Though decidedly there is no standard relational technique, relational therapists do have some characteristic ways of working. Free association, interpretation, inquiry, empathy, observation, and the analysis of defense and transference are some of the major types of interventions used by relational therapists—actually by all analytic psychotherapists.

As noted, different relational approaches and different therapists emphasize differing ways of being with patients. Therapists likely will be more active with more disturbed patients. Traditionally, psychoanalysts have tried to facilitate a patient coming up with his or her own solutions to problems through increased awareness and less rigid and defensive ways of being. But psychotherapy is inherently interactional. Psychoanalysts have attempted to avoid "transference cures," or having the patient simply adopt the therapist's ways of being or belief system out of a liking, identification with, and/or respect for the therapist. Traditionally, techniques such as reassurance and particularly suggestion were to be avoided largely because of the danger of influencing patients to conform to the values of the therapist. Because relational analysts recognize the interactive nature of the therapeutic relationship, however, they recognize that some of these processes may inevitably seep into the interaction to some extent. Indeed, questions may contain an element of suggestion. For example, the question "How is it that you didn't pay your taxes?" suggests that it might have been a good idea to pay taxes. Reassurance is often given nonverbally, by "uh-huh," and by further commentary on a topic that may be of interest to the therapist. Because autonomy and self-actualization of patients is an ideal, therapists must always be vigilant about their inevitable subtle influence on their patients. Ideally, all influence is addressed in the dyad, in order that the patient's conformity and idealization of the therapist is not mistaken for true change. Among the more dangerous aspects of therapy is the possibility that patients change in accordance with therapists' desires alone. This is known as *transference cure* or *false self* accommodation.

History Taking and Inquiry

Some relational analysts begin therapy by gathering a thorough developmental history. This history includes the background of the parents and grandparents, such as their place of birth, ethnicity, race, and religion. Also noted are the way the parents met, birth order of siblings, childbirth, preschool years, and relationships through childhood and adolescence. Sullivan suggested that therapists conduct a "detailed inquiry" into all the areas of the patient's life, though this need not be in the beginning of treatment, and

may, indeed be quite gradual. Other relational therapists inquire in less detail, perhaps speaking very little with patients. These therapists may prefer entering a state akin to that of reverie at times, attempting to sense what the patient is experiencing without impinging. For most it is important to strike a balance between therapeutic reserve and impassioned interest. Curiosity is a vital characteristic, but excessive questioning may take up too much room in the therapeutic dyad. The relational therapist may ask questions, often to look not only at what the patient says but also at what the patient omits. The therapist's inferences about what may be taking place are also posed as questions. The therapist will ask, "Could it be that . . .?" or say, "I wonder if. . . .

Silence and Free Association

Most relational therapists are concerned with giving the patient space so that the patient's own experience and ways of interacting can emerge. This is accomplished largely through the process of patients' free association, unless the lack of structure leads to a detrimental degree of anxiety. The relational therapist may remain relatively silent in order to encourage the patient to speak. One of the strengths of a psychoanalytic approach is that the patient's unique and idiosyncratic way of perceiving the world is encouraged by a therapeutic attitude that emphasizes reserve. The therapist's attitude of remaining in the background allows the patient to emerge into the foreground

Sullivan cautioned therapists that too much anxiety would impede treatment. The therapist should not interfere too much with the patient's "security operations," lest the patient become more rigid or paralyzed by overwhelming anxiety. For this reason, an atmosphere of safety and predictability is created, with a clear frame of treatment in terms of the starting and ending times of sessions, and, if possible, a regular meeting time each week. The therapist is often thinking of creating an environment in which the patient can feel "held" or "contained," to use Winnicott's terms. In this tradition, the therapist attempts to be neither neglectful nor impinging. Sullivan had suggested, similar to findings by learning theorists, that a moderate level of anxiety or arousal is also desired in the therapy situation, with too little arousal not leading to much new learning and too much arousal leading to performance of the already dominant response, in this case, the previously learned maladaptive response.

In this relatively nonstructured situation, the patient's own unique experiences are most likely to come into relief. The therapist will note the sequence of topics discussed, attempting to help the patient provide concrete, vivid examples if the patient tends toward generalities and abstractions. The therapist will also note when the patient has difficulty continuing. Paying close attention to process in this way keeps both parties seeing how defenses may emerge and, as well, patterns of interaction.

Relational analysts acknowledge that they are often providing a "corrective emotional experience," a term first used by Alexander and French (1946). Many types of experiences can lead to change, and elements of the relationship may be curative in and of themselves (Thompson, 1950). Those who speak of the relationship as mutative usually refer to a sequence of unwittingly living through old and "bad" experience with the patient, examining this experience, and evolving something new. At best, this new experience may become internalized by the patient. Fromm-Reichmann (1959) has been clear, however, that childhood deprivations cannot be remedied in treatment simply by giving the adult what the child lacked. Mitchell (1988) also cautioned against what he called the "developmental tilt" in psychoanalysis—the idea that simply providing an experience with a good type of parental figure that the patient did not have as a child will repair the early deficiencies. Unfortunately, meaningful change is not that easy. Epstein (1977) has suggested

that therapists often wish to be the good parent that the patient did not have, but it is in unwittingly being the "bad parent" that the patient is most helped. Salubrious new experience can only develop in a context in which old experience is first repeated, perhaps mourned, and let go of.

Analysis of Defense and Resistance

For relational therapists, resistance to change, and therefore to the therapeutic process, is universal. Every patient who comes to treatment wishes both to change and to remain embedded in his or her old world. Remaining stationary requires limiting awareness of dissociated internal experience. Anxiety is likely whenever what was dissociated in the first place is reactivated in the therapeutic process. The therapist's task is to help the patient feel safe enough to experience these dissociated aspects of self in a way that begins their integration into self-experience. The extent to which relational therapists point out how the patient is avoiding experience varies, yet Curtis, Knaan-Kostman, and Field (cited in Curtis & Qaiser, in press). found that when interpersonal analysts rated which of 68 analyst behaviors they had found most helpful in their own analysis, the item "helped me experience feelings I was avoiding" was rated the most helpful. Some therapists, in acknowledgement of the patient's sense of vulnerability, simply wait for the defenses to wither away.

Fosshage (1997) has differentiated "empathic-centered" and "other-centered" listening. Therapists vacillate between these two perspectives at times—either reflecting empathic immersion in the patients' point of view (e.g., Kohut) or taking the position of the other (being the observer of the patient; e.g., Wolstein). By empathizing with patients' experiences and reflecting them, however, the therapist actually may be joining the patient's defenses or resistance, a technique originally suggested by Spotnitz (1985) with disturbed patients. For example, the therapist, in the empathic-centered mode might reflect the patient's experience with parents and say, "They were very cruel."

Another form of resistance is "resistance to the awareness of transference" (Gill, 1982). Some patients resist the idea that patterns are occurring with the therapist that have occurred with other people outside the treatment. For therapists hoping to use the important leverage of the here-and-now situation in the session, this form of resistance will necessitate the therapist's persistently pointing out interactional phenomena until patients are able to see how a pattern is occurring in the relationship with the therapist.

Analysis of Transference

The aim of transference analysis is an illumination of the patient's subjective reality. Although the patient is bringing into the relationship with the therapist expectations from previous relationships, it is not assumed that the patient is totally distorting reality and/or that the therapist knows the objective "truth" about reality (Hoffman, 1983). The analyst is not believed to be a "blank screen" onto which the patient simply projects his or her own view of reality, but instead, another subjectivity, albeit a reserved one. The patient's experiences are explored in terms of their plausible meaning, not simply as distortions. Given the relative ambiguity of the therapist's reserved stance, there are many possible ways any given patient may experience the therapist's participation. There are also many different feelings patients may have toward their therapist. Having one set of feelings or interpretation of the therapists' attitude in preference to another always reflects meaningful data about what patients bring from their past to present.

As patterns of interaction and selective attention emerge that have worked to reduce anxiety for the patient in the past, the patient not only may see the therapist in ways that

he or she has seen an important person in the past but also may elicit responses from the therapist that have been elicited from others. In this way, patients' transferences often become actualized, reflected in the core relational notion that people tend to construct their contemporary world to conform to the past. It is crucial from the relational perspective that the therapist not simply interpret these responses as the patient's projections but accept responsibility for what indeed may be a *mutual* enactment in the transference–countertransference matrix. For example, in the interpersonal tradition when the therapist is accused of being cold and uncaring, the therapist needs to inquire with true curiosity how he might be cold. Lichtenberg, Lachmann, and Fosshage (1996) recently referred to this process as "wearing the attribute," implying that it is plausible that the therapist may indeed be acting icily, thereby repeating jointly with the patient interactions from the latter's past. As treatment progresses the patient may become attuned not only to aspects of the therapist that reflect old relational processes but to interactions that reflect something new (Levenson, 1983). Greenberg (1986) makes this point succinctly: "If the analyst cannot be experienced as a new object, analysis never gets under way; if he cannot be experienced as an old one, it never ends" (p. 98).

Mutual Enactment

Perhaps the most radical, albeit logical, extension of the relational view of the therapist as a subjective participant in the therapeutic process is the concept of mutual enactment (see Hirsch, 1996). Prior to the introduction of the therapeutic model of participant observation, a split existed between the subjectively participating patient and the presumably objectively observing therapist. The therapist's role was conceived of as analogous to that of a scientist, capable of viewing the mind of the patient with objective clarity. In this one-person psychology model, the patients were viewed as effectively enacting his or her internalized past (transference) in the context of a therapeutic relationship where therapists were uninfluenced by either their emotion or personal history. The term "enactment" referred only to transference—the subjective patient living out core internal conflicts in the presence of an objective therapist. The therapist's task was to see veridically and to understand the patient's past through the lens of here-and-now experience. The power of the therapeutic process lay in the patient's emotional engagement with the therapist, and in that context, transferring to the therapist affects and perceptions that lingered from past history. Essential to this earlier one-person model was the therapist's ability to control countertransferential feelings in order that the patient's experience be similar to that of a "pure culture" in a biology laboratory, free of influence from the other person in the dyad. Although this still may be viewed as a worthy therapeutic aim were it truly possible, many contemporary analytic therapists no longer believe that therapists are able to neutralize their subjectivity. In other words, therapists also unconsciously enact their subjectivity in the context of an intersubjective relationship, and countertransferential enactments are inevitable, much as are transferential enactments.

The concept of participant observation, based largely on Heisenberg's uncertainty principle, liberated many therapists from the unrealistic expectancy of achieving a most literal therapeutic neutrality and objectivity (cf. Mitchell, 1997), free from countertransferential enmeshment. From this newer relational point of view, analytic therapists should attempt to be both neutral and objective, and to refrain from purposefully influencing patients, while simultaneously recognizing that enactment of one's subjectivity is inevitable. Much of therapist's engagement is not purposeful; unwitting participation, for better or for worse, is inevitable. This is not considered a premeditated technique; it is a natural occurrence in any two-person interaction (Ghent, 1992).

Countertransference, subjectivity, unwitting participation, and enactment all can refer to more or less the same phenomenon—unconsciously based interaction that is unintended yet unavoidable. One can find examples of this in any segment of clinical interaction. As originally documented by Racker (1968), therapists are always feeling one thing or another at any given moment of engagement with patients, and such feelings cannot fail to have an impact on patients. Once viewed as feelings that patients are unlikely to notice, therapist countertransference, for better or for worse, is now considered to be expressed in the form of subtle nonverbal, tonal, and attitudinal actions that inevitably affect patients. These countertransferential feelings may be consciously experienced affects or may lie outside the therapist's awareness. In either case they inevitably register consciously or unconsciously with patients (Hoffman, 1983). A therapist may be bored or disinterested in a patient, excited and deeply involved, furious and enraged, profoundly empathic and tender, sexually aroused, and so on. All such feelings are translated into subtle expressions that either consciously or unconsciously affect patients. Therapists' feelings are influenced by patient's interactions and affective states, and likewise, patients are reciprocally influenced (i.e., influence is mutual, ongoing, and unavoidable). Most relational therapists agree that close attention must be paid to how patients are affected by their therapists, and that patients always should be encouraged to express their sentiments about such engagement.

The concept of mutual enactment follows logically from this intersubjective way of thinking about analytic therapeutic process. One can no longer look at transference enactment outside the context of the transference–countertransference matrix. One of the ways that therapists express the unconscious aspects of their countertransference is in the context of what some have referred to as actualization of patients' transferences. This is not as complicated as it may sound initially. For example, I (IH) found myself often bored and disinterested with a withdrawn and reserved man. He entered therapy to address his chronic underachievement in work and failure to develop enduring love relations. His life history was highlighted by increasing disinterest on the part of his parents as each of three younger sisters was born. His father in particular was inattentive, and, when he was involved, tended to be impatient and critical. This extremely intelligent man developed a pattern of emotional withdrawal in order to hibernate from disappointing interactions, and severe underachievement both to elicit attention and to pay back, passive–aggressively, his highly educated parents for their insensitivities toward him. My patient brought these relational patterns into his current world and, of course, into the transference–countertransference matrix. He withdrew from me and sabotaged our efforts, and I unwittingly responded by reciprocal withdrawal and my own anger-based disinterest. In some fundamental ways my patient's life history was relived in therapy—relived not only through transference enactment but through an unconscious mutual enactment with his therapist. At some point, ideally either patient or therapist becomes aware of such unwitting mutual interactions and addresses them in the verbal realm of the therapy.

This rather simple and everyday example captures the essential aspects of what many relational therapists believe is an ongoing part of every therapeutic relationship. What is talked about in the therapy actually begins to be relived between the two participants, and there is always a significant element of unconscious process on both sides. Actualization of transference refers to patients living out their core internalized experience in a context in which the therapist, always unwittingly, lives out the reciprocal role of the significant others in the patient's life history. In other words, I became the critical and disinterested parents

for him, expressing unwittingly a facsimile of his key life experience with significant others. It should be no surprise that my patient developed relationships in his current life outside therapy that resembled both his life history and his relationship with me. This is, of course, why he so egregiously sabotaged in his own work and induced both his supervisors and his lovers to become angry and impatient and, ultimately, to withdraw and fire him or leave him. The aim of therapy is to view this interaction *in vivo*, discuss it, and by so doing arrive at a new configuration. If all works well in therapy, this new and explored interaction becomes part of the patient's internal experience, altering both his expectancies about life with others and the way he constructs his life.

Essential to this view of therapy is a developmental theory emphasizing that experience, internalized through core developmental interaction with significant others, becomes part of what is expected from life with others and essentially how life with others also tends to be constructed. The template laid down by repeated self–other experience is what is best known, familiar, and comfortable, even if highly unsatisfying. The most natural way to proceed in life is to unconsciously repeat past experience, and to shape contemporary life to conform to the past. Psychopathology, therefore, can be defined not only as a function of troubled early experience but as a carrying forward of that experience into present living. People choose, albeit unconsciously, to construct contemporary life in close facsimile to the past. This is fine when one's developmental years were rich and loving, but not so fine when they were characterized by the kind of rejection experienced by my patient.

Every patient who enters psychotherapy is expressing a wish to change, although there exists a part of the patient that wishes to repeat the past (i.e., stay loyal to the patient's internalized family). This universal conflict between adhesion to the comforts of what is most known and separation and individuation from internal objects is core to what is played out in the therapeutic interaction. It is inevitable, as with my patient, that old and "bad" internalized experience is mutually enacted between therapist and patient. Looking at therapy through this lens, it is impossible for therapists to be only a "good" object. Therapists get drawn into reliving old and "bad" interactions (i.e., mutual enactments), and this seemingly unfortunate occurrence may be turned into therapeutic gold when it is recognized and examined. If therapists fail to see these enactments, or fail to encourage patients to express their feelings about the therapists' participation, enactments may congeal into destructive therapeutic impasses. When enactments become visible to both therapy participants, this experience becomes the richest source of discussion and, according to the relational model, the most likely route to therapeutic change. As Levenson (1983) has said, therapists must become part of the problem before they can help patients separate from their internalized pasts.

Interpretation

Although a relational therapist may suggest a possible meaning to feelings, thoughts, or events, such a communication is viewed only as a hypothesis, rather than a truth about the patient's mental life. Interpretations may be provided in order to deconstruct or reframe the patient's usual understanding. They are provided in a collaborative manner to help patients make more sense of their lives and to expand consciousness. Interpretations explain current life by examining historical antecedents. They reflect the fundamental psychoanalytic value that self-awareness is preferable to mystification. To understand the way one is helps a person feel that he or she is not controlled by external forces but by conflicts that currently lie within the psyche.

Analysis of Dreams

Dreams hold significance for relational analysts, just as they do for other psychoanalysts from Freud forward. The interpersonalist Fromm (1951) had traced the importance of dreams through history and described the lack of value given to them in Western industrialized cultures. Recently, Lawrence (1998) has revived Fromm's tradition of discussing dreams in groups in a process he calls "social dreaming". Freud, of course, believed dreams to be the "royal road to the unconscious." Relational analysts are especially curious about the connection of the dream to the patient's life. The dream is viewed as an urgent message to oneself to examine something that might lead to trouble if unexamined. In the context of analytic psychotherapy, there are often transferential implications to the dream. The dream might reveal feelings that have arisen in the therapeutic interaction but have yet to be addressed. Other relational analysts will investigate the different experiences of the self represented in the dream using the Gestalt technique of asking the patient to "become" each object and person in the dream. Some recent relational writers have criticized this approach from within for the relative neglect of the significance of dream analysis (Blechner, 2001; Lippmann, 2000). They recommend placing dreams back into the heart of psychoanalysis.

Encouraging Experiences in the Moment

Relational therapists might ask patients to imagine being in a situation in the moment in order to help them experience a situation fully. Comments such as "Imagine being there right now" are used. Such interventions are especially likely when the patient is describing an event but having difficulty recalling parts of it, or when the patient is avoiding the affect associated with the event. Similarly, relational therapists may emphasize experiences going on in the moment with the therapist, as described elsewhere in this chapter. Lichtenberg, Lachmann, and Fosshage (2002) have referred to such moments as "now moments."

Technique with Children and Families

Approaches to these modalities are beyond the scope of this chapter. For a more thorough exploration of relational child psychotherapy, see Altman, Briggs, Frankel, Gensler, and Pantone (2002). For further discussion of family therapy from this perspective, see Gartner (1995), Gerson (1996), and Wachtel (1994).

Technical Errors

All choices in therapy have advantages and disadvantages. Because relational approaches can vary so much from one tradition to another, within each tradition, and from one practitioner to another, it is often difficult to get agreement on what is and is not a technical error. The term "error" suggests that there are right and wrong ways of conducting therapy. This relational flexibility is, on the one hand, quite liberating for therapists, yet there is always the risk that such an attitude can be exploited by an "anything goes" approach. When most everything is viewed as contextual, one can justify most anything. Nonetheless, psychoanalytic therapists of most persuasions agree about basic boundary issues such as a set amount of time for each session, stability of fee among patients, no social contact outside therapy hours, and avoidance of advice giving or imposition of values. Though there may be exceptions when even these basic boundary issues are breached, they stand as "rules of thumb" for analytic therapists of all stripes.

Aside from issues related to basic boundaries, some common possibilities for error are as follows: imposition of a preferred theory on the patient's verbalizations, thereby failing to understand the unique individuality of each patient; a rush to interpretation before the patient has the chance to fully

express him- or herself; failure to inquire about patient statements; withholding observations that may be illuminating; imposing so many observations that the patient becomes the secondary party in the interaction; assuming or insisting that a particular interaction is transferential, despite the patient's insistence that it is not; and failing to address transferential material when it may be vividly present in the interaction.

Another common error is the provision of an intellectual explanation or understanding without an experience-near or emotional insight. Some have called this the easiest activity for a therapist to perform, as it comes closest to the brand of academic learning with which so many professionals are at home. In most instances, such activity avoids the necessary emotional encounter required for meaningful change to occur. Still another "error" can be frequently pointing out problematic behaviors or defenses to the extent that the patient feels unduly criticized. It is important for all therapists to acknowledge how particular interactional patterns that have developed were adaptive—the only ones possible in a past situation—or how they were indeed rewarded in previous situations.

By becoming highly active, a relational therapist may foreclose the space and ambiguity for the patient's idiosyncratic perceptions and experiences to emerge, including transferential ones. By the therapist's being too inactive, the patient may remain repetitive or "stuck" longer than if the therapist had intervened. It is difficult to determine in advance which approach will benefit the patient more, and there is no uniform prescription for how to relate to all patients.

Wachtel (1993) has described a number of "errors" in the therapist's wording of communications and ways for therapists to express themselves in a more helpful fashion. It is less blaming, for example, to point how a defense was useful in the past than to say simply that a patient is being defensive in a particular way. Wachtel (1997) has also described some ways to avoid what he considers "errors" from a relational perspective by using techniques from nonpsychoanalytic approaches, as have Frank (1993, 1999) and Curtis (1996b).

Termination

Termination will depend on achieving the patient's goals, although the particular style of termination will be reflective of and coordinate with the interaction up to that point. Therapeutic goals often change; at times the goals initially set will be achieved, but new goals will emerge. Although a particular patient may still have goals to pursue for which a therapist might be helpful, the patient and therapist at some point may realize that the patient is able to pursue for which goals largely on his or her own. In regard to psychoanalysis, Witenberg (1976) stated, "Analysis never terminates. It is visits-to-the-analyst that terminate" (p. 336). One goal of any analytic therapy is to help the patient become his or her own therapist. Certainly the therapist could provide an opinion about the advisability of termination, but ultimately the decision rests with the patient.

Termination brings up feelings of attachment, separation, and loss. Sometimes symptoms will reappear when a termination date is set. Because intense feelings may arise, a termination date is set well in advance. Some relational therapists taper off sessions, in order for patients to see how they manage on their own. Others may schedule an appointment a month or so after the second-to-last meeting. Therapists will help patients focus upon what they have done themselves in order to bring about change. Some relational therapists may engage in additional activities at termination. The patient's previous stressors and dominant and new ways of responding may be reviewed (Curtis, 2002). Some therapists will inquire as to what was helpful and hurtful in the treatment. As expressed throughout this text, there is no standard relational procedure for termination, and much depends on the idiosyncrasies of each unique dyad.

THE THERAPEUTIC RELATIONSHIP AND THE STANCE OF THE THERAPIST

An intense therapeutic relationship is considered essential to change. Otherwise, the therapist would not be able to help a patient face fears and wishes that had been too frightening to face during a whole lifetime. By trial and error, the relational therapist must find a balance between the safety of the old and the danger of the new. An alliance is created between the patient and therapist through the rapport, empathy, support, reflection, and the patient's sense of being known. A good example of a supportive comment would be that of Fromm-Reichmann (1959) when working with a disturbed woman. The patient, apparently envious of Fromm-Reichmann, saw the label inside Fromm-Reichmann's coat from the Best Department Store in Washington, DC. Seeing the label, the patient commented, "Best, best, best—you have the best of everything." Fromm-Reichmann supportively answered, "I hope you'll be shopping again soon at Garfinkel's" (referring to an even fancier store in Washington) (p. 181).

Different relational approaches have different basic stances; most conceive of the relationship as mutual but asymmetrical (Aron, 1996). Mutuality does not imply equality. The relationship is considered mutual because there is inevitably mutual influence, recognition, and empathy. The relationship remains asymmetrical, however, because the therapist does not purposefully disclose personal information anywhere near to the extent that the patient does. If the therapist were to take on a role similar to that of the patient, the relationship would blur into one similar to a friendship.

Countertransference

Though the concept of mutual enactment represents the most radical view of how countertransference works in relational psychoanalytic therapy, the key concept of countertransference is inherent in all relational perspectives. As noted, the interpersonal wing of relational thinking, starting with Sullivan's (1953) conception of participant observation, has always placed countertransference at the heart of analytic therapy. If therapists' unwitting or inadvertent participation is inevitable, it becomes incumbent upon all therapists to become as aware as possible of all feelings related to their patients. Feelings that remain out of awareness are more likely to intrude into the therapeutic relationship in ways that might be harmful. As much as interpersonal/relational therapists believe that all of the therapist's affects intrude into the therapeutic space and can potentially lead to useful mutual enactments, there is value, too, in using one's countertransference in a conscious way.

Conscious countertransferential feelings are often a therapist's strongest source of data in efforts to understand patients (Wolstein, 1975). As subjective as such data are, a therapist is in a prime position to speculate about the way patients are with others, by experiencing the feeling of otherness in the context of the therapeutic dyad. To give an example, one lonely man entered therapy with the complaint that women seemed unresponsive to him. It quickly became apparent to me (IH) that everything about this man's demeanor smacked of coldness, aloofness, and self-absorption. Although of the same gender as he, I assumed that the women he pursued found him as offputting as I did. Using my own feelings of boredom, disinterest, and reciprocal withdrawal, I pointed out to him how I perceived him, suggesting prospective girlfriends might be feeling something similar. Had I not been aware of my feelings and their import, I might have acted out my countertransferential disinterest and essentially abandoned my patient emotionally. Countertransferential awareness provided the dual reward of controlling the possibility of my abandoning my patient and making him aware of the way he relates to others. Some relational therapists are more cautious about sharing their countertransferential observations than are others, believing that such input might be experienced as too imposing. Those relational therapists are more likely to use countertransferential data only as a source of valuable information about the patient, and as a way to exert some control over countertransferential acting out. Evenly hovering attention to both oneself and to the patient (and to the interaction) has become a prima facie value for most relational therapists.

The type of countertransference just discussed, "concurrent countertransference" (Racker, 1968), has been central to those relational therapists identified with the interpersonal tradition. Those more influenced by Melanie Klein (1957/1975), alternately referred to as "Kleinians" or Kleinian object relationists, emphasize the type of countertransference that Racker called "concordant." That is, countertransferential affects, also termed "projective identifications" (Bion, 1967), are experienced by the therapist as feelings projected into him or her by the patient, because they are too frightening for the patient to tolerate. This is less magical a process than it sounds at first reading, and it is indeed, a part of everyday interactional experience. Everyone has become anxious when in contact with another who is highly anxious, or angry with someone who is quietly seething. Patients do not, of course, literally put their feelings inside their therapists but unconsciously communicate difficult affects to therapists with the consequence that the latter can understand these feelings firsthand, and constrain patients' anxiety about living with frightening affects. This unconscious communication is picked up by the therapist, who unconsciously identifies with the patient's feeling, now being held inside the safety of the mind of the therapist. Once the therapist becomes aware of the projectively identified feeling, he or she can both reduce the patient's anxiety by experiencing the feeling with less anxiety and can better know the patient firsthand by experiencing the same feeling.

Here is an illustration of this process. For a number of years, I (IH) worked with a highly articulate and intelligent college professor who spent a portion of his session time berating me for my inadequacies in helping him and attempting to humiliate me for the many weaknesses he perceived me to have. His presenting complaint was an inability to feel happy, regardless of his achievements and his sexual conquests. My patient's way of relating to me closely resembled the way his father had interacted with him. Throughout his childhood he was the butt of his father's sadistic teasing and put-downs, regardless of how hard he tried to make his father proud of him. This relentless persecution was unceasing, lasting until the day his father died. I feared that my patient would remain this way with me until one of us died. My patient could not be happy because he internalized his father's sadistic and competitive assaults, and no one could tolerate a close relationship with him because he identified with his hateful father. My primary feeling state when with this man resembled the way he felt with his father. My patient showed me firsthand what it was like to be him, and to live with his hidden sense of abject humiliation. This gave me a clear sense of what it was like inside my patient's skin beneath his most defensive attacking ways. I was then able to convey to him what I imagined he felt and what it was like to live with his father. My ability to conceptualize this feeling enabled me both to refrain somewhat from retaliation and to withstand his assaults. As one might imagine, this interactional pattern did not cease with a single interpretation, although it helped give both of us a framework to make more sense of my patient's life, and it aided me not to drown in my patient's attempted humiliations.

Countertransference tends to be less central in the tradition that represents the Winnicottian (Winnicott, 1971) stream under the relational umbrella (interpersonal and Kleinian object relations theory are the first two streams discussed), because the basic therapeutic model is conceived of as a mother–child dyad, or a "holding environment." With regard to countertransferential feelings, therapists are normally advised to serve as "containers" for their patient's difficult affects, "holding" them until the patient might prove ready to expose his or her feelings. The notion of therapist as container is similar to that described by Kleinians (the origins of these two traditions are similar), although the therapist in the Winnicottian tradition is far more likely to contain patients' feelings than is the Kleinian. Patients tend to be viewed more from their regressive child self-states, and the therapeutic atmosphere is maternal and protective. Countertransferential feelings, both concurrent and concordant, are less likely to be translated into verbal observations or questions than with interpersonal or Kleinian relational therapists. Patients are generally viewed as requiring an unchallenging and maternal environment, with the therapist allowing the patient's internal state to emerge in this safe environment. Therapists are encouraged to be aware of their own feeling states but to subsume these affects into efforts toward a holding environment.

The newer tradition of self psychology (Kohut, 1984) bears great similarity to the Winnicottian object relationists in its basic view of the patient–therapist interaction. From this perspective, the primary therapeutic intention is toward empathic immersion in the patient's experiences. The role of the therapist is to channel his or her own self-experience into the greater good of optimally attuning to the patient. Otherness, or the concurrent countertransference of the interpersonal tradition, is eschewed as too therapist-centered—an abandonment of efforts at immersion in the patient's experiential world. Like its Winnicottian counterpart, Kohut's self psychology conceptualizes patients as suffering from early deficiency and analytic psychotherapy as an opportunity to regrow the patient. Empathy is the food that patients lacked, and when provided with enough consistency by the attuned therapist, empathic attunement will allow the patient to come closer to his or her potential. Self psychologists are well aware that perfect empathic attunement is impossible and lapses in attunement are both inevitable and potentially beneficial. Similar to the holding environment, patients are expected to be hurt and/or angry when the therapist fails. These breaches on the therapist's part are never premeditated. When accepted by the therapist as inevitable and natural, countertransferential misattunement can be helpful to the patient's growth via recognition that life is disappointing as well as gratifying, under the best of conditions.

As we have seen, the therapeutic use of countertransference differs from one relational tradition to the other. Nonetheless, every relational perspective holds that therapists are always "countertransfering," and that affective neutrality is impossible. Given this assumption, awareness of countertransference is always preferable to absence of awareness, even when such feelings are not revealed by the analyst directly. For those who more actively share their countertransference feelings with patients, the therapist's awareness of both concurrent and concordant versions represents an ideal.

Self-Disclosure

Whereas classical psychoanalysis is known for the lack of deliberate self-disclosure on the part of the analyst, relational analysts may disclose their feelings in the moment with a patient, or provide other information, usually only after asking the patient the reasons for the question. Tauber and Green (1959) made the controversial suggestion that an analyst might decide to tell a patient a dream the analyst had about the patient. For example, one morning before a patient came in, the therapist (RC) woke up dreaming that the patient brought a bag of golf clubs to the session. The therapist did not mention the dream to the patient in that session but continued to think about it. Not getting anywhere that seemed to make any sense in that session, the therapist decided to mention it to the patient at the following session. The patient responded immediately, "I think of golf as what people do when they have nothing else to do. I've been taking it easy in here, lately. That is what your dream is about."

Recently, Davies (1994) and Ehrenberg (1992) have addressed the potential value of judicious affective countertransference disclosures. Davies (2002) gave the following example of such disclosure. A patient had been pushing to schedule a session earlier during the coming week. Davies was getting annoyed. The patient stated, "You're cold and unfeeling and ungiving. You've never been there for me, not ever. I mean, sometimes you pretend, but it's just skin-deep. Down deep inside you, where I can see, it's justice. The least you could do is admit it." Davies responded, "Sometimes we hate each other, I think. Not always. Not even usually. But sometimes we can get to this place together. I guess we're gonna have to see where we can get from here. Neither of us likes it much. It just is." Whereas in the classical Freudian approach self-disclosure was taboo, among relational therapists it exists as one option. Some therapists self-disclose fairly liberally, while others rarely if ever do so. Disclosure is not a part of any standard relational approach, but judicious disclosure is among the interactional options.

CURATIVE FACTORS OR MECHANISMS OF CHANGE

New experiences and the development of new meanings of experiences are the major factors leading to change according to the relational approach. Although new experiences include an increase in awareness of previously unconscious data, they often also include a new relational configuration with the therapist as well. Some relational theorists think that the relationship may be curative in and of itself. To examine here-and-now interactions, certainly a fair degree of warmth and empathy is called for on the part of the therapist. The therapist must not, however, act in a way that is so kind and gratifying that it will deprive the patient of the freedom to feel anger that will likely arise in the context of a more ambiguous and reserved therapeutic situation. For most analytic therapists, analysis of transference–countertransference matrices is viewed as a major way of conveying to patients a sense of being understood. The extent of the analysis of the relationship with the therapist (the transference–countertransference matrix) is a major variable distinguishing psychoanalytic treatments from other treatments.

Gill (1982, 1983) criticized his contemporaries for spending too much time on the past, when the real leverage in psychoanalysis, he believed, came from discussions of the relationship between the two therapy coparticipants. Since that time, there has been an increasing focus on the analysis of transference, with most relational analysts noting that the analyst has transferences as well and, therefore, can never be simply an objective observer of the patients' transferences. Because the notion of an objective knowledge of the "truth" by an impartial observer largely has been abandoned, analysis of the contributions of both parties to mutual patient–therapist enactments has become an integral part of the change process.

Early in the history of the interpersonal–relational tradition, many interpersonalists emphasized extratransferential analysis over analysis of the transference. Sullivan had noted that it was too anxiety provoking, especially for disturbed patients, to discuss the relationship in the "here and now." Therefore, therapists could help patients deal with experiences in other relationships in their lives and by so doing, at least in some cases, the patient and therapist might communicate implicitly about their own

relationship. In contrast, Searles (1965, 1979) worked with schizophrenic patients in a way that brought explanation of the transference–countertransference matrix into the very center of the work. He is among a group of analysts that helped shift the focus from extratransferential relationships to the here and now of the therapeutic interaction. That said, relational therapists can be quite different from one another and may have different emphases in their work. For instance, strengthening the "healthier components" of a patient's personality is considered a major curative factor. For some, engaging in this manner may enable the patient "to better cope with his deficiencies and defects" (Szalita, 1964, p. 176).

Certainly, analytic therapists have always relied on insight to bring about change. Insight may be about the relationship with the therapist, about matters outside the relationship, and especially about the impact of life history on current functioning. Such insights at best are not simply cognitive realizations—they are profoundly emotional, especially when focused on the here-and-now relationship between the two therapeutic participants. Some relational therapists consider insight alone to belong to the classical Freudian model. In the relational paradigm, change results not from excessive focus on insight into "the truth" but from the expansion of awareness of a wider set of interactional patterns and experiences visible within the transference–countertransference matrix. The patient has new experiences of self and others as hidden or disavowed aspects are noticed and reclaimed. Incorporation of these experiences into the person's self-representation is also considered an expansion of awareness. Increased tolerance of uncertainty and anxiety allows conflictual ways of being to be held in awareness simultaneously. Living with paradox may be seen as one sign of "health." New self-organizing processes and meanings emerge from previously unformulated experiences.

Mourning lost possibilities is considered to be another curative factor by relational psychotherapists. Many patients must grieve the loss of good relationships with parents or aspects of family relationships on which they missed out. Patients may also have missed opportunities that must be mourned, or they may benefit from coming to grips with the reality that all choices foreclose other possibilities. When impossible goals are fully mourned, more energy is available for the possible ones.

Expansion of awareness, openness to new experiences, new meanings of experiences, and new self-organization occur in a situation of safety. Some analysts have called such a state "regression." The word "regression" is misleading, however, in that a person does not "regress" to an earlier level of functioning but instead feels a sense of safety with the therapist such that the patient feels held or contained, or as if there is a "primary substance' to "carry the patient" that cannot be destroyed (Balint, 1968, p. 167). In this relaxed state, all may be experienced—rational and irrational. One's worst fears are experienced in a state of relative safety. In this relaxed state, the patient's internal representations and internalized patterns may become more flexible. In this state patients feel truly recognized by another person who is not imposing his or her own needs; they have a better opportunity to give up old repetitive patterns and begin anew. The limitations of the therapist are recognized. Unfulfilled desires are tolerated. Those that never will be satisfied are mourned. The anxiety regarding the uncertainty of whether desires will be fulfilled is also tolerated. For some relational analysts, this experience is akin to that of love—not of romantic or brotherly love, but more that of the Greek *agape,* which refers to the idea of a god's love for his or her children. Reports by relational analysts of what was most helpful in their own treatments revealed that it was the therapist helping them to become aware of experiences they were avoiding and to experience irrational thoughts and feelings (cf. Curtis & Qaiser, in press).

TREATMENT APPLICABILITY AND ETHICAL CONSIDERATIONS

Relational psychoanalytic therapy is applicable to a wide variety of patients, including very disturbed patients. As with any verbal therapeutic endeavor, it is most likely to be effective with patients who are self-reflective, verbal, and willing to examine their own contributions to their problems in living. Psychoanalytic therapists, however, adjust their interventions with patients who are not ideal candidates for analytic therapy and engage in a form of treatment that may lead up to psychoanalysis. This is one advantage of an approach to therapy that builds on the individual's uniqueness and eschews a standardized technique. For example, with patients who externalize their problems or who are narcissistic, the therapist may need to emphasize reflective and empathic modes of intervention. With children or patients who are less verbal, modifications in the technique are required (e.g., the therapist might decide to talk more with a seriously disturbed patient who is mute). For patients who may come from a cultural background in which it is inconceivable that a professional will not provide professional direction or advice, the therapist may want to meet the patient's wishes to some extent and attempt to examine the consequences of these interventions later. Wachtel, (1997), Frank (1991, 1993, 1998), and Curtis (1996b) have described using adjunctive therapies in relational treatments. Relational therapists have described adjustments in this approach in working with inner city (Altman, 1995, 2000; Wachtel, 1999), bilingual (Perez Foster, 1996), and deaf patients (Kolod, 1994).

If a patient comes for treatment exclusively for a specific behavioral problem such as substance abuse, a phobia, sexual misconduct, or smoking, the patient might be referred for a behavioral treatment specifically dealing with this problem (see Anthony & Roemer, Chapter 6, this volume). A therapist might decline to treat a child alone, however, if the child would benefit more were the whole family in treatment. Psychoanalytic approaches are useful for anyone who has the inclination or the patience for self-examination—individuals who seek to live more fulfilling lives or to become more enriched in their work, relationships, and avocations.

Relational therapists must be clear with patients seeking symptom reduction about the manner in which they work and the length of time the treatment may take. Problems ensue if the therapist overvalues fantasy and fails to inquire or be sufficiently concerned about external realities (e.g., losing a job or physical health). Relational therapists face similar ethical considerations as do other types of therapists, namely, the lack of knowledge of techniques from other theoretical orientations that may be more effective for particular problems or the overuse of an approach they prefer even when they know that other approaches have been shown to be more effective. There is a body of research that suggests that symptoms dominated by substance abuse may be best alleviated through treatments established by groups such as Alcoholics Anonymous or by a period of residential treatment and that phobias caused by traumatic experiences are best treated with behavioral therapies. Even Freud (1918/1953) recommended behavioral exposure for phobias. In additional areas of dysfunction where many research findings have suggested that a biological component plays a large role, (e.g., bipolar disorder, schizophrenia, and Crohn's disease), many believe that medications must be employed in addition to "talk therapy." Some relational therapists, indeed, are disinclined to employ psychoanalytic therapy in the foregoing sorts of situations where research literature points to other approaches that

have been effective. On the other hand, many other relational therapists would argue that the research literature has not shown the relational approach to be less valuable than other therapies—the research to compare them is yet to be done. Relational therapists view all symptoms in the whole context of personality. As extremely difficult as the work might be with schizophrenics or alcoholics, for example, some relational therapists undertake it without adjunctive treatments if they have the time and the patience.

RESEARCH SUPPORT

Although there is considerable support for the effectiveness of psychoanalytic treatments (Wolitzky, Chapter 2, this volume), these tend not to include relational psychoanalytic psychotherapy. Due to the lack of funding for studies of psychoanalytic psychotherapy in the United States, such research support will come increasingly from Europe where governments reimburse patients for psychoanalytic treatment and fund research for studying its effects. Recently, in Sweden, Sandell and colleagues (2000) followed more than 400 patients in analytically based psychotherapy over 3 years. Some of the analysts in this study likely held an object relations orientation. This study showed progressive improvement in measures of symptoms and morale the longer the patients were in treatment. It is interesting to note that the use of a classical analytic stance (i.e., the nongratifying style Freud advocated) was found to be counterproductive.

In the United States, most of the research on psychoanalytic therapies has been conducted on brief treatment (Messer, 2001). Messer and Warren (1995) have categorized a number of such short-term therapies as relational approaches. Interpretation of the patient's core conflictual relationship theme (CCRT) in Luborsky's supportive–expressive therapy has been found to be related to better outcomes (Crits-Christoph, Cooper, & Luborsky, 1988), including improvement in symptoms (Barber, Crits-Christoph, & Luborsky, 1996). Although this research was not designed from within the "relational" approach to psychoanalysis, the outcome data support it. Safran and Muran (2000) report preliminary evidence that brief relational therapy is more effective than cognitive-behavioral and ego-psychological (supportive) treatment for patients with whom therapists find it difficult to establish a therapeutic alliance.

Patients with mixtures of anxiety, depression, low self-esteem, and interpersonal problems have shown significant improvement in brief psychodynamic or cognitive-behavioral treatments of 20 sessions (Piper, Joyce, McCallum, & Azim, 1998). Other studies have found similar results for therapies of 8 and 16 sessions with depressed patients, with more sessions resulting in greater improvement for severely depressed patients (see Messer, 2001). Interpersonal therapy of 15-week duration was found to be more effective for patients with obsessive personality styles, whereas cognitive therapy was more effective for patients with avoidant patterns (Barber & Muenz, 1996). Depressed patients in two forms of brief psychodynamic therapies showed improvement over a wait-list control group (Winston et al., 1994). It should be noted that the applicability of the results of these brief therapies for long-term relational therapy is unknown.

There is considerable support for relational models of the mind, personality, and change. Relational theory, to some extent, has developed as a consequence of this knowledge. In recent years, cognitive psychologists have published many studies supporting the idea of implicit, or what they call "nonconscious," factors in attention and memory (Westen, 1998). Whereas there is support for psychoanalytic ideas about defensive attention and memory, knowledge about the Freudian idea of *repression* per se is inconclusive (Holmes, 1990). There is,

however, much more support for the concept of dissociation (Kihlstrom, Barnhardt, & Tataryn, 1992), a broader idea of disconnections explained earlier in this chapter. Relational ideas about the mental representations of self, other, and relationships are similar to those found in a large body of research by social and cognitive psychologists (Westen, 1998).

There is also research evidence for the existence of transferential processes (Andersen & Cole, 1990; Fried, Crits-Christoph, & Luborsky, 1992; Glassman & Andersen, 1999). Although the evidence regarding the effectiveness of transference interpretations is mixed, positive therapy outcome has been found to be related to accurate transference interpretations in low dosages for high-functioning patients (Messer, 2001; Ogrodnicuk & Piper, 1999). Progress in therapy was also found to be related to therapist adherence to a psychodynamic focus formulated in object relations terms (Messer, Tishby, & Spillman, 1992).

Attachment research has been influential in relational theories of development (Mitchell, 2000). The study of attachment processes within the psychoanalytic tradition began with the work of John Bowlby (1969, 1988). Bowlby was excluded, along with Sullivan and Fairbairn, from what was then mainstream psychoanalysis. Bowlby (1969) challenged Freud's view that hunger led infants to seek out their caretakers, describing instead an autonomous instinctual attachment system relatively independent of the drives related to hunger, sex, and aggression. For Bowlby, the need for attachment was primary, whereas for Freud it was secondary.

Attachment patterns have been studied by Ainsworth (Ainsworth, Blehar, Waters, & Wall, 1978) in infants, by Main (2001), and by a plethora of other researchers using a variety of measures of adult attachment styles (e.g., Bartholomew & Horowitz, 1991; Hazan & Shaver, 1987). Various patterns of insecure attachments styles have been linked with many forms of psychopathology (cf. Livesley, Schroeder, & Jackson, 1990; Parkes, Stevenson-Hine, & Marris, 1991). Both attachment style (Fonagy, 2001; Levy, 2002) and representations of self and other (Blatt, Stayner, Auerbach, & Behrends, 1996) have been found to change during psychotherapy, which is consistent with the relational psychoanalytic approach.

CASE ILLUSTRATION

Scott, age 26 when he started treatment, presented a symptomatic history of poorly controlled anger, initially in the form of adolescent brawling and more currently expressed in extreme impatience, intolerance, arrogance, and provocative argumentativeness. His physically violent bullying behavior culminated in his suspension from high school for part of his senior year, despite being near the top of his class in grade-point average. Although he gained admission to an Ivy League college, his suspension cost him acceptance to his most coveted school. After he finished college, where he excelled in varsity wrestling and largely reformed his physically bullying ways, Scott accepted training positions at one, then a second, top-tier investment banking firm. In both instances his technical performance was exemplary, yet he was fired for his surly and belligerent manner. He began therapy depressed about his unemployed status, wishing to prevent further self-destructive aggression.

Scott is extremely ambitious, placing far greater import on his career than on his love life. He acknowledged that his short temper had interfered with romantic involvements with women, and that he had not yet had a long-term love relationship. This did not particularly disturb him, as he had a network of male buddies with whom he drank, gambled, and competed in sports, and he rarely felt lonely. His relations with his parents were fractious. They were quite involved with one another, although this was punctuated by frequent and ugly verbal

brawls and periods of estrangement. It was his mother who urged him to consider psychotherapy. Parenthetically, she had a long and highly satisfactory experience in her own analytic psychotherapy, at a point in life when she struggled in her marriage, and as a mother to her only child. Scott was a most reluctant patient, having little predisposition toward cessation of destructive action and for self-reflection. Despite his high intelligence, he lived in a universe of action and reaction. Thinking about things that were highly personal was viewed as inefficient at best, or as soft and effeminate at worst.

Scott, an only child, is Central American by birth, abandoned in the street by his mother and adopted from an orphanage at about 1 year of age by upper-class Caucasian parents in California. He is short, squat, and brown-skinned with distinct Native Indian features. He was raised with privilege in an affluent suburb by parents whom he describes as basically devoted and loving. He notes that his father, a successful businessman, is a highly competitive person, loses his temper readily, argues frequently and holds fierce grudges. His mother, who is a housewife, is described as more even tempered, although is not readily bullied by her husband or son. She has had a rich social life that was focused around country club activity and philanthropic causes. Scott described her as beautiful and vain, placing strong emphasis on physical appearance. Both parents noticed early their adopted son's high intelligence and expected from the beginning that he would be a high achiever.

Scott, on the surface, at least, identified with the noblesse oblige outlook of his family's white Anglo-Saxon Protestant cultural background. He showed virtually no interest in his own personal or cultural heritage and had never traveled to Central America or researched his biological beginnings. He was rarely conscious of his racial characteristics except when rebuffed by the tall, light-skinned, blond women he uniformly desired. Parenthetically, Scott's mother is fair in complexion and taller by 3 inches than he. Scott's early dreams in therapy were replete with imagery suggesting both a strong sense of difference and an inclination toward hypervigilance based on danger. In his first dream after entering therapy he spoke of being in a room where it was his task to kill scorpions that were continuously emerging from cracks in the walls of his costly Manhattan apartment. Despite his lack of overt curiosity about his origins, the tenor of his dreams suggested that in his unconscious life, he lived between his two worlds.

My earliest contacts with Scott left me feeling shut out, intimidated, and angered. It took many telephone messages to finally speak and make an initial appointment with him. When we did meet I found Scott cold, terse, with clipped speech, and impatient with my initial questioning. He was business-like, neither reflective nor curious, and rarely elaborated on answers to my queries. He did not expand on his reported dreams or initiate dialogue. It looked as if he could not wait to leave the session and appeared bored and restless. After asking him what it was like to be with me and getting a noncommittal answer, I observed that it seemed to me that he was generally angered and/or bored by my presence—barely tolerant of my existence. He replied that he was neither, but that this experience was simply uncomfortable and unfamiliar. When I pressed, referring to the evidence for my statement (e.g., his terseness, restlessness, disengagement, and annoyed and bored facial expressions), he became angry, declaring that he had already answered what I had asked and why was I trying to provoke him. I backed off, realizing only much later that this reflected the first of my many unwittingly enacted, countertransference withdrawals from him.

My informal assessment of Scott after 1–2 months of twice-weekly analytic psychotherapy was of a young man who dealt with his anxieties and vulnerabilities largely through denial and aggressive activity. I assumed that Scott's pervasive anger and competitiveness reflected a partial identification with his father, feelings of being physically unappealing to his mother, and an unconscious effort to avoid emotional recognition of feelings associated with his having been abandoned, orphaned, and adopted. His profound lack of reflectiveness, despite his education and cultured background, underscored the degree to which self-examination was threatening. Scott felt a sense of well-being to the extent that he engaged successfully in the male world of sports and academic or business competition. Literally or figuratively beating another man helped him avoid recognition of his internal sense of profound tenuousness and fragility, the legacy of early rejection followed by the vulnerability of adoption. Those whom Scott was able to defeat carried for him the weakness within himself that he feared facing. He tried hard not to recognize that he looked different from his peers, for this too was a reminder of both the impoverishment and abandonment that characterized his early life. He felt that he was his parents' biological child, denying the almost inevitable adoptee's anxieties of once again being unloved or discarded.

Scott's lifelong efforts to leap aggressively over his vulnerabilities helped him to achieve considerably and to feel a sense of external, if not internal, strength. On the other hand, Scott appeared throughout his life to engage in self-destructive actions and, by so doing, repeat his core experience of being abandoned. This occurred most dramatically in his being kicked out of high school and in his recent firings, and on a more everyday level through initiating parental rejection via argument and initiating sexual abandonments through the choice of girls and women who would be unlikely to find him appealing. The absence of a viable career at the time of the initial consultation represented a great threat to him. Minus external success and avenues for competitive achievement, Scott was having difficulty avoiding the affective experience of depression, fear of aloneness, and abject weakness and helplessness. It would take having to face such a danger to catapult this highly defended man into a probing analytic therapy.

It should be noted that I felt that there was no utility in arriving at a formal diagnosis, nor do I at this point almost 20 years later, in writing about this patient. From a relational perspective, a description of the patient's internal and external life including core conflicts mitigates the necessity for a formal diagnosis. Although I use the traditional designation, "patient," I do not consider psychological problems to reflect illness. I view psychotherapy patients, as well as psychotherapists, and those people who never even consider entering psychotherapy, as functioning on a continuum between optimal and minimal. Symptoms are problematic, but they are also adaptive and usually reflect a compromise to forestall facing something more threatening. Symptoms, like anxiety in general, are a signal to people that they are not living to their fullest in the broad domains of love and work. If one is sufficiently troubled by this (or if someone in the person's interpersonal environment becomes alarmed), analytic psychotherapy affords the opportunity to attempt to live one's life closer to one's potential. When a psychotherapy patient begins such a journey, the therapist's description of the total person, including conflicts and adaptations to them, is a richer alternative to an illness and diagnostic model. In psychology, problems in living are never adequately captured by a diagnostic designation as in illness or medicine.

Regarding Scott, I originally formulated that his unconsciously motivated, intermittent failures led him to a point where he ran the risk of being overwhelmed by vulnerabilities for which he chronically tried to overcompensate. The absence of romantic love in his life was more salient to him when he lost his work—the arena of life

that helped him maintain his psychological equilibrium. With both deficient love and work relationships, Scott was beginning to feel depressed and anxious that the world he built, which was based on denial and acting out, would come falling down on him. His key internal conflict revolved around, on the one hand, attachment to an internalized past highlighted by abandonment and impoverished experience and fear of being orphaned by his adoptive parents, and, on the other, the wish to embrace securely his new world of opportunity. Scott's inability to address his extraordinary vulnerability, terror, and absence of caretaking guaranteed that he would unconsciously repeat or live out these themes in his contemporary life. He would be unlikely to embrace many of the opportunities afforded to him without recognizing that internal forces were pulling him toward repeating his most basic and primitive relational attachments. His extreme anger and aggressivity both protected him from experiencing weakness and vulnerability and guaranteed that the abandonments of the past would be repeated. Scott unconsciously controlled his abandonments by bringing them on himself. Because his aggression and hardheartedness served this dual purpose, I believed initially that emotional connection with Scott would be difficult.

Although Scott was indeed quite emotionally distant, speaking with my recalcitrant patient about his life in a way that was new to him nonetheless appeared to translate into some quick, palpable results. I was very pleased that after only 2 months of therapy Scott found a good new job and seemed to be controlling his anger and brusqueness with colleagues. However, it was not long after this development that his sense of urgency about therapy diminished, and he began to become more overtly bored and disinterested in our venture. The time in our sessions moved slowly, and there was abundant silence. I felt generally inhibited, although too tense about Scott's angry and critical eye to be bored. After a couple of months more of this trying work, Scott failed to show up for a session without calling. I was convinced (and somewhat relieved) that he had quit. When he arrived for his next session he said that he had had an emergency business meeting. When I asked why he had not called, he stated that he knew he was going to see me again in 2 days anyhow. The next time he canceled he called in advance and asked for an alternate time. I returned his message asking him to confirm the time I offered and his 1-plus day-late return message was barely understandable: "Hi, that's okay." He did not leave his name on the message or engage in any other social amenity. When I questioned him about taking so long to call back and then not leaving his name on my answering machine, he was dismissive and said that I was wasting his time with such small and petty interests. He was most likely simply busy at work, he said.

At about this time Scott began to yawn increasingly during sessions and these yawns were becoming noisier and his hands were failing to cover his mouth. My own feelings ranged from a sense of invisibility, to identifying with the high school kids this thick-necked wrestler had beaten up, to the angry and retaliatory feeling that I was with someone who was uncivilized, and whom I would like to have disappear from my life. I asked him if he were aware of his increasingly loud and uncovered yawns, and he responded that he must be suffering the effects of long work hours and early morning sessions. At this juncture I told Scott, probably with an edge to my voice, that his manner on the telephone, the yawning, and his general absence of social decorum was striking, and that given his social background this had psychic significance. I added that I thought he was trying to get me to boot him out of treatment. To my surprise at the time, these observations were not met with a totally slammed door. I became freer in pointing out both subtle and gross interactional nuances, especially his interactions with me that tested my toler-

ance and provoked my wish to abandon him. Though Scott was still combative, this series of interactions proved to be a turning point in our 5-year psychotherapy.

Any psychotherapy that goes too smoothly is suspect. Everyone's core internalized conflicts and experience are deeply embedded, and the process of change involves many repetitions of such experience before there is a gradual evolution to greater flexibility in living. Therefore, even though Scott became more receptive to my observations, and more willing to reflect on himself, he still remained an angry and guarded young man for much of the duration of our work. His conflicts around attachment to his core identity as an abandoned child in an impoverished and violent society, and his fear of fully recognizing these vulnerabilities and terrors, continued to have an impact on his life even as we addressed these issues, both inside and outside the transference–countertransference matrix. Within our relationship, there were as many moments of self-protective anger, boredom, emotional withdrawal, coldness, and acting-out behaviors (e.g., missing sessions and not returning phone calls), as there were moments of receptivity to my questions, observations, and interpretations. More commonly than otherwise, I felt abandoned or battered by my patient.

This feeling could be viewed as a projective identification, or "concordant countertransference," as described earlier. These phenomena refer to the adaptive tendency, in a relationship of intimacy or intensity, to identify with the internal processes of the patient. In analytic therapy it becomes a way of using the therapist's experience to better know the patient. Scott gave me difficult feelings to contain within myself, and I experienced firsthand some semblance of what it was like to live with battering and constant fear of abandonment.

For much of our work together I never knew whether Scott would show up for any given session or quit treatment. He often canceled sessions, sometimes without calling before or afterward, and frequently threatened to quit. I sometimes imagined that he had been in an accident and was injured or dead. I was normally off balance with him. He was frequently scathingly critical, dismissive, and icy cold. I began to speculate with him that perhaps he was physically beaten as a baby, prior to his adoption. Over time this hypothesis became plausible, although he did not recover specific memories.

We spoke of his father's intense temper, piecing together his fear that such rage provoked fears that he had not before articulated, both of being abandoned and of being physically injured. He began, tentatively, to address his feeling that his mother found him physically unattractive. In addition to identifying with Scott's deepest fears and humiliations, I often felt the other side of the equation—the wish that he would go away or, at times, even die. He provoked enormous rage in me, and I continually struggled not to withdraw emotionally not to ask him to leave treatment during periods when he missed sessions or otherwise withdrew and/or demeaned me. This is "concurrent transference," and it refers to the therapist's feeling toward the patient some facsimile of what significant others feel when with the patient. Addressing his evocation of such feelings, we gradually arrived at Scott's becoming aware of his own stimulus value (i.e., what it is like to engage with him). It helped Scott see, for example, how he both intimidated and enraged his parents and provoked his bosses to fire him. Indeed, Scott did drop out of therapy for brief periods over the 5 years, and such interludes dovetailed with his feeling vulnerable to and sensing my wishes to abandon him.

This sequence tended to run as follows: Scott appears involved with me and working productively, I feel a reciprocal warmth and affection, Scott misses sessions and/or becomes verbally sadistic with me, I interpret this sequence of vulnerability and attack to him, but it has no visible impact on

his attitude (or he just becomes angrier and colder), I feel initially impotent, and then a quiet but nonverbally detectable wish for him to go away, Scott angrily walks out of a session saying he'll never return, or just fails to show up for a number of sessions and does not return my calls. Sequences such as this occurred six or seven times over our 5 years together, though less frequently in our final year. I credit Scott's feeling reasonably understood by me, and my relative resilience in the face of his assaults, for his returning to see me after each time he quit. Nonetheless, the durability of our therapy was touch-and-go for the better part of it.

Scott's life outside sessions, unsurprisingly, paralleled our relationship. He continued to clash periodically with, and to behave arrogantly and nastily to, colleagues and bosses alike, resulting in his eventually losing the job he found shortly after he started therapy. Indeed, he was fired from still another good job before he settled in and endured with his current one. In parallel, Scott's relationship with his parents remained volatile until near the end of psychotherapy. At one point his rage was so intense that his parents did not speak with him for 4 months. This breach and others tended to coincide with Scott's being frightened by his growing awareness of feelings of dependence and weakness, and his rageful and highly provocative response to such affects. Scott's love life remained barren until near the end of therapy, when he began to date a young woman who appeared to be a good match for him. Prior to this, Scott would inevitably engage with women in one of two ways: He would pursue tall, blond, slender women who showed absolutely no interest in him, or he would begin to date a woman who seemed to like him and would soon turn on her in a nasty and abusive manner.

Scott and I agreed to terminate therapy at a time that his relational patterns had improved. Both of us agreed that he was getting along better with others. I thought this reflected a change in his internal relational configurations and at least a partial resolution of internal conflict. If his changes were judged to be only behavioral or external, there would be little optimism that there was potential for these changes to endure meaningfully. Near termination, Scott seemed more inclined toward self-reflection and less inclined toward action. He was able to be more open, vulnerable with and generous toward me, his parents, a girlfriend, and his coworkers. His rage and protective, yet self-destructive, provocations subsided considerably. This does not mean that my patient became "a sweetheart"; he remained at termination a moody young man and often a difficult person for others to be with. He could still be cold, emotionally withdrawn, nasty, sarcastic, arrogant, and difficult to embrace. As might be expected, some of Scott's most abrasive ways returned and were manifest in the transference, as we began to discuss termination. Fortunately, we were able to say good-bye on a note of relatively mutual warmth and affection. Scott is not a new person. He is someone who has faced some of his dreaded vulnerabilities and is open to a wider range of affective experiences with others, and within himself. I will not be surprised if he returns to therapy at a point at which he experiences internal conflict in relation to some new level of personal intimacy or personal enrichment.

As might be clear by now, I view the mutative action of psychoanalytic therapy to lie in the exploration of the mutually developed interaction between patient and therapist. The power of my work with Scott lay in my focus on elucidating the nature of the ongoing shifts in our relationship and how this paralleled both key historical and contemporary relational configurations. Emotional insight, or expanded awareness, a key ingredient in any psychoanalytic therapy, emerges often from examining the therapeutic relationship, and working backward to understanding life history. Insight, at its best, helps people see how early identifications and internalized objects, and the internal conflicts in relation to them, unconsciously guide

contemporary life. Over the course of therapy with Scott, he became far more curious about his history and more willing to face painful and heretofore unconscious experience. He traveled, with a close male friend, to his country and city of origin, although to my knowledge he has not yet tried to find his biological parents. He became able to articulate that his father's rages scared him as a child and provoked fears of once again being placed for adoption.

Scott spoke of a vague sense that his mother seemed affectionately inhibited with him—that she did not seem to appreciate his male body as did the moms of some of the kids with whom he grew up. He was able to discuss feeling pained by this, though as a child he did everything possible to prevent his becoming aware of such affects. More and more he recognized how defensive his anger was, and how it often served both to compensate for weakness and vulnerability and to provoke the very abandonment he feared would occur. He was able to tell me that he now sometimes allowed himself to own his origin as a Central American peasant, and to speculate that some of his physically violent behavior reflected his then unarticulated connection with how he imagined his biological parents to be. Scott's evolution as a person, though still far from optimal, reflects the value of an analytic psychotherapy that emphasizes the examination of the here-and-now interaction between patient and therapist as central to the development of self-reflection and to new internalized experience.

CURRENT AND FUTURE TRENDS

Although relational analysts are especially interested in transference–countertransference configurations and enactments "in the moment," the pendulum often swings in an opposite direction after a trend is pursued in depth for a long period. The patient–therapist relationship is of great interest to therapists from many orientations, partly in reaction to the movement toward empirically supported treatments that have emphasized techniques at the expense of the relationship (e.g., Messer & Wampold, 2002). If, as we predict, research continues to accumulate showing the importance of the relationship to all forms of treatment, relationally oriented therapists will also likely look more closely at the specifics particular to psychoanalytic treatments that are important to the change process.

The current trend in relational psychoanalysis has been toward a hermeneutic perspective—that is, away from a natural science way of viewing intrapsychic and interpersonal phenomena. This is in harmony with postmodern sentiments that emphasize subjectivity and intersubjectivity in contrast to positivism, essentialism (i.e., a philosophical approach emphasizing essence, often the biological, over existence, or the psychological) and the quest for objective truth (e.g., Neimeyer & Bridges, Chapter 8, this volume). To appeal to the general public and to insurance companies that support psychotherapy, however, psychoanalytic therapies will need to demonstrate their effectiveness. It should be noted, however, that theories emphasizing the irreducible subjectivity of mutual interaction do not readily lend themselves to traditional scientific research. The unfortunate isolation of psychoanalysis from psychology is a major obstacle to the further development of this approach and much effort and creative thinking will be required to bridge this gap and to design studies that can address relational approaches.

Although in earlier eras the emphasis on sexuality may have distinguished psychoanalytic treatments from other forms of therapy, as the acceptance of diversity in sexual longings and behaviors has become more widespread in Western culture, this focus has become less distinctive. Instead, the emphasis on aggressive feelings in psychoanalytic treatment continues to distinguish it from other treatments. Such feelings, especially desires to hurt others, are still socially unacceptable and the source of conflict for many people. Relational therapies, drawing on the work of Winnicott, have emphasized the need for the patient to be able to express destructive urges and to experience the therapist surviving the expression of such affects.

Within the relational approach to psychotherapy, the experiences of people with gay, lesbian, and bisexual orientations, not previously viewed in psychoanalytic literature as healthy sexual choices, are being integrated into the understanding of "normal" development and of therapeutic practice. Such a trend is part of the overall direction to eschew the pathologizing of difference and to accommodate more diverse backgrounds than those that were originally part of the Victorian culture from which psychoanalysis was derived.

Relational psychoanalysis will likely continue to reflect major trends in the sciences, humanities, and the culture at large. It is not possible to predict the extent to which psychoanalytic thinking will become more integrated into and influence the thinking of psychologists, nonanalytic psychotherapists, and the culture in general. The focus of Western culture on efficiency, productivity and their measurement is somewhat antithetical to the contemplative, reflective nature of psychoanalytic approaches, and their valuing of the subtle examination of relationships and of inner life. Yet to the extent that human fulfillment remains important, patients will likely turn to such approaches in their attempts to enjoy more fully their love relationships, work, and play.

SUGGESTIONS FOR FURTHER READING

Books

Benjamin, J. (1988). *Bonds of love: Psychoanalysis, feminism, and the problem of domination.* New York: Pantheon.—Describes how women become masochistic from being treated as objects rather than subjects of desire. It demonstrates a feminist perspective derived from Hegelian philosophy.

Lionells, M., Fiscalini, J., Mann, C. H., & Stern, D. B. (1995). *Handbook of interpersonal psychoanalysis.* Hillsdale, NJ: Analytic Press.—Includes a complete review of all aspects of interpersonal psychoanalysis—basic psychological processes, development, psychopathology, therapy process, and technique.

Mitchell, S. A., & Aron, L. (Eds). (1999). *Relational psychoanalysis: The emergence of a tradition.* Hillsdale, NJ: Analytic Press.—Includes seminal articles regarding relational psychoanalysis.

Research

Safran, J. D., & Muran, J. C. (2000). *Negotiating the therapeutic alliance: A relational treatment guide.* New York: Guilford Press.—Provides an overview of research on the therapeutic alliance and offers a model of brief relational psychotherapy.

Westen, D. (1991). Social cognition and object relations. *Psychological Bulletin, 109,* 429–455. —Review of research supporting the relational conceptualization of representations of self, others, and social causality.

Readings with Case Studies

Blechner, M. J. (1992). Working in the countertransference. *Psychoanalytic Dialogues, 2,* 161–180.—A case example followed by commentaries.

Davies, J. M., & Frawley, M. G. (1993). *Treating adult survivors of childhood sexual abuse.* New York: Basic Books.—Many case examples and profiles of various types of patients who have been sexually abused, including patterns of transference–countertransference configurations that emerge over time.

REFERENCES

Ainsworth, M. D. S., Blehar, M., Waters, E., & Wall, S. (1978). *Patterns of attachment.* Hillsdale, NJ: Analytic Press.

Alexander, F., & French, T. M. (1946). *Psychoanalytic therapy.* New York: Ronald Press.

Altman, N. (1995). *The analyst in the inner city: Race, class, and culture through a psychoanalytic lens.* Hillsdale, NJ: Analytic Press.

Altman, N. (2000). Black and white thinking: A psychoanalyst reconsiders race. *Psychoanalytic Dialogues, 10,* 589–606.

Altman, N., Briggs, R., Frankel, J., Gensler, D., & Pantone, P. (2002). *Relational child psychotherapy.* New York: Other Press.

Andersen, S., & Cole, S. W. (1990). "Do I know you?" The role of significant others in social perception. *Journal of Personality and Social Psychology, 59,* 384–399.

Aron, L. (1996). *A meeting of minds: Mutuality in psychoanalysis.* Hillsdale, NJ: Analytic Press.

Aron, L, & Harris, A. (Eds.). (1993). *The legacy of Sandor Ferenczi.* Hillsdale, NJ: Analytic Press.

Atwood, B., & Stolorow, R. (1984). *Structures of subjectivity.* Hillsdale, NJ: Analytic Press.

Balint, M. (1968). *The basic fault.* London: Tavistock.

Barber, J. P., & Muenz, L. R. (1996). The role of avoidance and obsessiveness in matching patients to cognitive and interpersonal psychotherapy: Empirical findings from the Treatment for Depression Collaborative Research Program. *Journal of Consulting and Clinical Psychology, 64,* 951–958.

Barber, J. P., Crits-Christoph, P., & Luborsky, L. (1996). Effects of therapist adherence and competence on patient outcomes in brief dynamic therapy. *Journal of Consulting and Clinical Psychology, 64,* 619–622.

Bartholomew, K., & Horowitz, L. M. (1991). Attachment styles among young adults: A test of the four-category model. *Journal of Personality and Social Psychology, 61,* 226–244.

Beebe, B., Jaffe, J., & Lachmann, F. M. (1992). A dyadic systems veiw of communication. In N. Skolnick & S. Warshaw (Eds.), *Relational approaches to psychoanalysis* (pp. 61–82). Hillsdale, NJ: Analytic Press.

Beebe, B., & Lachmann, F. M. (2002). *Infant research and adult treatment: Co-constructing interactions.* New York: Other Press.

Benjamin, J. (1988). *Bonds of love: Psychoanalysis, feminism and the problem of domination.* New York: Pantheon.

Benjamin, J. (1995). *Like subjects, love objects.* New Haven, CT: Yale University Press.

Benjamin, J. (1998). *The shadow of the other: Intersubjectivity and gender in psychoanalysis.* Florence, KY: Taylor & Francis/Routledge.

Bion, W. R. (1967). Notes on memory and desire. *Psychoanalytic Forum, 2,* 271–280.

Blatt, S. J., Stayner, D. A., Auerbach, J. S., & Behrends, R. S. (1996). Change in objects and self-representations in long-term, intensive, impatient treatment of seriously disturbed adolescents and young adults. *Psychiatry: Interpersonal and Biological Processes, 59,* 82–107.

Blechner, M. J. (2001). *The dream frontier.* Hillsdale, NJ: Analytic Press.

Bollas, C. (1987). *The shadow of the object: Psychoanalysis of the unthought known.* New York: Columbia University Press.

Bowlby, J. (1969). *Attachment and loss (Vol. 1).* New York: Basic Books.

Bowlby, J. (1988). *A secure base.* New York: Basic Books.

Bromberg, P. (1983). The mirror and the mask: On narcissism and psychoanalytic growth. *Contemporary Psychoanalysis, 19,* 359–387.

Bromberg, P. (1998). *Standing in the spaces.* Hillsdale, NJ: Analytic Press.

Crits-Christoph, P., Cooper, A., & Luborsky, L. (1988). The acccuracy of therapists' interpretations and the outcome of dynamic psychotherapy. *Journal of Consulting and Clinical Psychology, 56,* 490–495.

Curtis, R. (1996a). The "death" of Freud and the rebirth of free psychoanalytic inquiry. *Psychoanalytic Dialogues, 6,* 563–589.

Curtis, R. (1996b). A new world symphony: Ferenczi and the integration of nonpsychoanalytic techniques into psychoanalytic practice. In P. L. Rudnytsky, A. Bokay, & P. Giampieri-Deutsch (Eds.), *Ferenczi's turn in psychoanalysis.* New York: New York University Press.

Curtis, R. (2002). Termination from a psychoanalytic perspective. *Journal of Psychotherapy Integration. 12,* 350–357.

Curtis, R., & Qaiser, M. (in press). The training analysis: Historical perspectives and empirical research. In J. Geller, J. Norcross, & D. Orlinsky (Eds.), *The therapy of therapists: Patient and therapist perspectives.* New York: Oxford University Press.

Davies, J. M. (1994). Love in the afternoon: A relational reconsideration of desire and dread in the countertransference. *Psychoanalytic Dialogues, 2,* 153–170.

Davies, J. M. (1998). Multiple perspectives on multiplicity. *Psychoanalytic Dialogues, 8,* 195–206.

Davies, J. M. (2002, January). *Whose bad objects are these, anyway? Repetition and our elusive love affair with evil.* Paper presented at the International Conference on Relational Psychoanalysis and Psychotherapy, New York.

Davies, J. M., & Frawley, M. G. (1993). *Treating adult survivors of childhood sexual abuse.* New York: Basic Books.

Dimen, M. (2001). Perversion is us? Eight notes. *Psychoanalytic Dialogues, 11,* 825–860.

Dimen, M., & Goldner, V. (2002). *Gender in psychoanalytic space: Between clinic and culture.* New York: Other Press.

Dimen, M., & Harris, A. (2001). *Storms in her head: Freud and the construction of hysteria.* New York: Other Press.

Drescher, J. (1998). *Psychoanalytic therapy and the gay man.* Hillsdale, NJ: Analytic Press.

Eagle, M. (1984). *Recent developments in psychoanalysis.* New York: McGraw-Hill.

Ehrenberg, D. (1992). *The intimate edge.* New York: Norton.

Epstein, L. (1977). The therapeutic function of hate in the countertransference. *Contemporary Psychoanalysis, 13,* 442–460.

Fairbairn, W. R. D. (1952). *Psychoanalytic studies of the personality.* London: Routledge.

Fairbairn, W. R. D. (1994). Dissociation and repression. In E. F. Birtles & D. E. Scharff (Eds.), *From instinct to self: Selected papers of W. R. D. Fairbairn* (pp. 13–79). Hillsdale, NJ: Jason Aronson (Original work published 1929)

Fonagy, P. (2001). *Attachment theory and psychoanalysis.* New York: Other Press.

Fosshage, J. (1997). Countertransference as the analyst's experience of the analysand: Influence of listening perspectives. *Psychoanalytic Psychology, 12,* 375–391.

Frank, K. A. (1991). Action techniques in psychoanalysis. *Contemporary Psychoanalysis, 26,* 732–756.

Frank, K. A. (1993). Action, insight and working through: Outline of an integrative approach. *Psychoanalytic Dialogues, 3,* 535–578.

Frank, K. A. (1999). *Psychoanalytic participation: Action, interaction, and integration.* Hillsdale, NJ: Analytic Press.

Freud, S. (1918). Lines of advance in psychoanalytic theory. *Standard Edition, 17,* 159–168. London: Hogarth Press, 1953.

Fried, D., Crits-Christoph, P., & Luborsky, L. (1992). The first empirical demonstration of transference in psychotherapy. *Journal of Nervous and Mental Diseases, 180,* 326–331.

Fromm, E. (1951). *The forgotten language.* New York: Rinehart.

Fromm, E. (1964). *The heart of man.* New York: Halpern Row.

Fromm-Reichmann, F. (1959). Some aspects of psychoanalytic psychotherapy with schizophrenics. In D. M. Bullard (Ed.), *Psychoanalysis and psychotherapy: Selected papers of Frieda Fromm-Reichmann* (pp. 176–193). Chicago: University of Chicago Press. (Original work published 1952)

Gartner, R. (1995). The relationship between interpersonal psychoanalysis and family therapy. In M. Lionells, J. Fiscalini, C. H. Mann, & D. B. Stern (Eds.), *Handbook of interpersonal psychoanalysis* (pp. 793–822). Hillsdale, NJ: Analytic Press.

Gerson, M.-J. (1996). *The embedded self: A psychoanalytic guide to family therapy.* Hillsdale, NJ: Analytic Press.

Ghent, E. (1992). Paradox and process. *Psychoanalytic Dialogues, 2,* 135–159.

Gill, M. M. (1982). *Analysis of transference* (Vol. I). New York: International Universities Press.

Gill, M. M. (1983). The point of view of psychoanalysis: Energy discharge or person? *Psychoanalysis and Contemporary Thought, 6,* 523–552.

Glassman, N. S., & Andersen, S. M. (1999). Activating transference without consciousness: Using significant-other representations to go beyond what is subliminally given. *Journal of Personality and Social Psychology, 77,* 1146–1162.

Greenberg, H. (1964). *I never promised you a rose garden.* New York: Henry Holt.

Greenberg, J. R. (1986). Theoretical models and the analyst's neutrality. *Contemporary Psychoanalysis, 22,* 87–106.

Greenberg, J. (1991). *Oedipus and beyond: A clinical theory.* Cambridge, MA: Harvard University Press.

Greenberg, J., & Mitchell, S. A. (1983). *Object relations in psychoanalytic theory.* Cambridge, MA: Harvard University Press.

Harris, A. (1998). Aggression: Pleasures and dangers. *Psychoanalytic Inquiry, 18,* 31–44.

Hazan, C., & Shaver, P. (1987). Romantic love conceptualized as an attachment process. *Journal of Personality and Social Psychology, 52,* 511–524

Hirsch, I. (1987). Varying modes of analytic participation. *Journal of the American Academy of Psychoanalysis, 15,* 205–222.

Hirsch, I. (1996). Observing-participation, mutual enactment, and new clinical models. *Contemporary Psychoanalysis, 32,* 359–383.

Hirsch, I. (2000). Interview with Benjamin Wolstein. *Contemporary Psychoanalysis, 36,* 187–232.

Hoffman, I. Z. (1983). The patient as interpreter of the analyst's experience. *Contemporary Psychoanalysis, 19,* 389–422.

Hoffman, I. Z. (1998). *Ritual and spontaneity in psychoanalysis.* Hillsdale, NJ: Analytic Press.

Holmes, D. S. (1990). The evidence for repression: An examination of sixty years of research. In J. L. Singer (Ed.), *Repression and dissociation* (pp. 85–102). Chicago: University of Chicago Press.

Horney, K. (1926). The flight from womanhood: The masculinity complex in women as viewed by men and by women. *International Journal of Psychoanalysis, 12,* 360–374.

Kihlstrom, J. F., Barnhardt, T. M., & Tataryn, D. J. (1992). The psychological unconscious: Found, lost, and regained. *American Psychologist, 47,* 788–791.

Klein, M. (1975). *Envy and gratitude.* New York: Delacorte Press. (Original work published 1957)

Kohut, H. (1971). *The analysis of the self: A systematic approach to the treatment of narcissistic personality disorders.* Madison, CT: International Universities Press.

Kohut, H. (1977). *The restoration of the self.* Madison, CT: International Universities Press.

Kohut, H. (1984). *How does analysis cure?* Chicago: University of Chicago Press.

Kolod, S. (1994). Lack of a common language: Deaf adolescents and hearing parents. *Contemporary Psychoanalysis, 30,* 634–650.

Lawrence, W. G. (Ed.). (1998). *Social dreaming @ work.* London: Karnac Press.

Levenson, E. A. (1972). *The fallacy of understanding.* New York: Basic Books.

Levenson, E. A. (1983). *The ambiguity of change.* New York: Basic Books.

Levy, K. (2002, April). *Changes in attachment organization during the long-term treatment of pa-*

tients with borderline personality disorder. Paper presented at the annual meeting of the Society for the Exploration of Psychotherapy Integration, San Francisco.

Lichtenberg, J. D., Lachmann, F., & Fosshage, J. (1992). *Self and motivational systems: Toward a theory of psychoanalytic technique.* Hillsdale, NJ: Analytic Press.

Lichtenberg, J., D., Lachmann, F., & Fosshage, J. (1996). *The clinical exchange: Techniques derived from self psychology and motivational systems.* Hillsdale, NJ: Analytic Press.

Lichtenberg, J. D., Lachmann, F., & Fosshage, J. (2002). *The spirit of inquiry: Communication in psychoanalysis.* Hillsdale, NJ: Analytic Press.

Lippman, P. (2000). *Nocturnes: On listening to dreams.* Hillsdale, NJ: Analytic Press.

Livesley, W. J., Schroeder, M. L., & Jackson, D. N. (1990). Dependent personality disorder and attachment problems. *Journal of Personality Disorders, 4,* 131–140.

Main, M. (2001). Categories of infant, child adult attachment: Attention stress. *Journal of the American Psychoanalytic Association, 48,* 1055–1096.

McDougall, J. (1978). *Plea for a measure of abnormality.* New York: International Universities Press.

Messer, S. B. (2001). What makes brief psychodynamic therapy time efficient? *Clinical Psychology: Science and Practice, 8,* 5–22.

Messer, S. B., Tishby, O., & Spillman, A. (1992). Taking context seriously in psychotherapy research: Relating therapist interventions to patient progress in brief psychodynamic therapy. *Journal of Consulting and Clinical Psychology, 60,* 678–688.

Messer, S. B., & Warren, C. S. (1995). *Models of brief psychotherapy.* New York: Guilford Press.

Messer, S. B., & Wampold, B. E. (2002). Let's face facts: Common factors are more potent than specific therapy ingredients. *Clinical Psychology, 9,* 21–25.

Mitchell, S. A. (1988). *Relational concepts in psychoanalysis.* Cambridge, MA: Harvard University Press.

Mitchell, S. A. (1993). *Hope and dread in psychoanalysis.* New York: Basic Books.

Mitchell, S. A. (1997). *Influence and autonomy in psychoanalysis.* Hillsdale, NJ: Analytic Press.

Mitchell, S. A. (2000). *Relationality: From attach-ment to intersubjectivity.* Hillsdale, NJ: Analytic Press.

Mitchell, S. A., & Aron, L. (Eds.). (1999). *Relational psychoanalysis: The emergence of a tradition.* Hillsdale, NJ: Analytic Press.

Ogden, T. (1994). *Subjects of analysis.* Northvale, NJ: Aronson.

Ogrodniczuk, J. S., & Piper, W. E. (1999). Use of transference interpretations in dynamically oriented individual psychotherapy for patients with personality disorders. *Journal of Personality Disorders, 13,* 297–311.

Orange, D. M., Atwood, G. E., & Stolorow, R. D. (1997). *Working intersubjectively: Contextualism in psychoanalytic practice.* Hillsdale, NJ: Analytic Press.

Parkes, C. M., Stevenson-Hinde, J., & Marris, P. (Eds.). (1991). *Attachment across the life cycle.* London: Routledge.

Perez Foster, R. (1996). The biligual self: Duet in two voices. *Psychoanalytic Dialogues, 1,* 99–122.

Phillips, A. (1988). *Winnicott.* Cambridge, MA: Harvard University Press.

Piper, W. E., Joyce, A. S., McCallum, M., & Azim, H. F. A. (1998). Interpretive and supportive forms of psychotherapy and patient personality variables. *Journal of Consulting and Clinical Psychology, 66,* 558–567.

Racker, H. (1968). *Transference and countertransference.* New York: International Universities Press.

Safran, J., & Muran, J. C. (2000). *Negotiating the therapeutic alliance: A relational treatment guide.* New York: Guilford Press.

Sandell, R., Blomberg, J, Lazar, A., Carlsson, J., Bromberg, J., & Schubert, J. (2000). Varieties of long-term outcome among patients in psychoanalysis and long-term psychotherapy. *International Journal of Psychoanalysis, 81,* 921–942.

Sandler, J., & Sandler, A. M. (1987). The past unconscious, the present unconscious, and the vicissitudes of guilt. *Interntational Journal of Psychoanalysis, 68,* 331–342.

Searles, H. (1965). *Collected papers on schizophrenia and related subjects.* New York: International Universities Press.

Searles, H. (1979). *Countertransference and related issues.* New York: New York Press.

Skolnick, N. J., & Warshaw, S. C. (1992). *Relational concepts in psychoanalysis.* Hillsdale, NJ: Analytic Press.

Spotnitz, H. (1985). *Modern psychoanalysis of the schizophrenic patient: Theory of the technique.* New York: Human Sciences Press.

Stern, D. (1985). *The interpersonal world of the infant.* New York: Basic Books.

Stern, D. B. (1983). Unformulated experience. *Contemporary Psychoanalysis, 19,* 71–99.

Stern, D. B. (1997). *Unformulated experience: From dissociation to imagination in psychology.* Hillsdale, NJ: Analytic Press.

Stoller, R. (1985). *Observing the erotic imagination.* New Haven, CT: Yale University Press.

Stolorow, R., & Atwood, G. (1992). *Contexts of being.* Hillsdale, NJ: Analytic Press.

Sullivan, H. S. (1953). *The interpersonal theory of psychiatry.* New York: Norton.

Szalita, A. (1964). Discussion of Sheiner. *American Journal of Psychoanalysis, 24,* 174–178.

Tauber, E. S., & Green, M. (1959). *Prelogical experience.* New York: Basic Books.

Thompson, C. (1942). Cultural pressures in the psychology of women. *Psychiatry, 5,* 331–339.

Thompson, C. (1950). *Psychoanalysis.* New York: Grove Press.

Wachtel, E. F. (1994). *Treating troubled children and their families.* New York: Guilford.

Wachtel, P. L. (1997). *Psychoanalysis, behavior therapy, and the relational world.* Washington, DC: American Psychological Association.

Wachtel, P. L. (1999). *Race in the mind of America.* London: Routledge.

Westen, D. (1998). The scientific legacy of Sigmund Freud: Toward a psychodynamically informed psychological science. *Psychological Bulletin, 124,* 333–371.

Westen, D. (2002, April). *The nature and origins of character.* Paper presented at the annual meeting of the Psychoanalytic Division of the American Psychological Association, New York.

Winnicott, D. W. (1964). *The child, the family, and the outside world.* Reading, MA: Addison-Wesley.

Winnicott, D. W. (1971). *Playing and reality.* Middlesex, UK: Penguin.

Winston, A., Laikin, M., Pollack, J., Samstag, L. W., McCullough, L., & Muran, J. C. (1994). Short-term psychotherapy of personality disorders. *American Journal of Psychiatry, 151,* 190–194.

Witenberg, E. (1976). Termination is no end. *Contemporary Psychoanalysis, 12,* 335–338.

Wolstein, B. (1975). Countertransference: The analyst's shared experience and inquiry with his patients. *Journal of the American Academy of Psychoanalysis, 3,* 77–89.

4

Person-Centered Psychotherapy and Related Experiential Approaches

ARTHUR C. BOHART

The focus of this chapter is person-centered psychotherapy and experiential psychotherapies related to it. These experiential psychotherapies are focusing-oriented psychotherapy (Gendlin, 1996), process–experiential psychotherapy (Greenberg, Rice, & Elliott, 1993), and Gestalt psychotherapy (Yontef, 1995). Focusing-oriented psychotherapy and process–experiential psychotherapy have roots in person-centered theory and practice. Gestalt psychotherapy (Yontef, 1995) does not. I consider Gestalt psychotherapy briefly in this chapter because its philosophy is similar to person-centered theory, and Gestalt ideas and procedures play an important role in process–experiential psychotherapy. Person-centered and experiential therapies are members of a larger family of "humanistic" psychotherapies, which also includes existential therapy (Schneider, Chapter 5, this volume).

"Person-centered therapy" refers to a theoretical view of the nature of human beings and their interactions originally developed by Carl Rogers in the 1940s and 1950s (Brodley, 1988), and to a philosophy

of how to relate to human beings in growth-producing ways, both inside and outside psychotherapy. Rogers first developed his ideas in the form *of client-centered therapy* and later changed the name to "person-centered" when he expanded the practice of his ideas to other realms of human interaction, such as education and international conflict resolution. I first describe the general person-centered perspective on human beings, psychopathology, and therapeutic change. I then describe the specific therapeutic practices of person-centered, focusing-oriented, process–experiential therapy, and Gestalt therapy.

HISTORICAL BACKGROUND

Several influences led Carl Rogers to begin to develop the person-centered view of humans and therapy. As a youth, Rogers spent much of his time on a farm where he was particularly interested in the processes of facilitating growth, and where he studied scientific experimentation with respect to agriculture. Growth facilitation and a hypothesis–testing, experimental attitude toward both life and theoretical constructs are basic characteristics of Rogers's views.

Later, when Rogers was already working as a child guidance counselor, he was exposed to the ideas of Otto Rank. Rankian ideas that influenced Rogers included an emphasis on creativity and potential, the aim of therapy as acceptance of the self as unique and self-reliant, the belief that the client must be the central figure in the therapeutic process and that the client is his or her own therapist, and an emphasis on present experience in therapy (Raskin & Rogers, 1989).

Another influence was the *Zeitgest* of the 1930s (Barrett-Lennard, 1998), the "Roosevelt years." Some of the features of these times that Barrett-Lennard speculates influenced Rogers include a focus on empowering people, on learning through trial and error, and on openness to new thought and solutions. Roosevelt also emphasized participation in appraisal and decision making by those affected. He encouraged and accepted divergent thinking and pressed for the integration of opposites. His supervision style was a supportive one in which he tried to release the creativity of his subordinates. Roosevelt held an optimistic view of human nature in that people were to be treated as basically trustworthy and reasonable, even if their behavior was not always rational.

However, for Rogers, the most formative influences came from his experience with clients:

> I had been working with a highly intelligent mother whose boy was something of a hellion. The problem was clearly her early rejection of the boy, but over many interviews I could not help her to this insight. . . . Finally I gave up. I told her that it seemed we had both tried, but we had failed, and that we might as well give up our contacts. She agreed . . . and she walked to the door of the office. Then she turned and asked, "Do you ever take adults for counseling here?" When I

replied in the affirmative, she said, "Well then, I would like some help." She came to the chair she had left, and began to pour out her despair about her marriage, her troubled relationship with her husband, her sense of failure and confusion. . . . Real therapy began then, and ultimately it was very successful. This incident was one of a number which helped me to experience the fact . . . that it is the *client* who knows what hurts, what directions to go in, what problems are crucial. (Rogers, 1961a, pp. 11–12)

Rogers formulated an early version of person-centered therapy, "nondirective therapy," in the 1940s. This stage was characterized by a fundamental emphasis on the therapist's nondirectiveness: The goal was to create a permissive, noninterventive atmosphere. The major therapeutic "interventions" were acceptance and clarification. In the 1950s, empathic understanding of the client increasingly came to be emphasized. In the 1960s the emphasis shifted to the congruence or genuineness of the therapist.

Rogers's interests later expanded beyond the field of psychotherapy. He began to work increasingly in group settings to facilitate growth in nonpatient populations and, in his last years, focused his energy on using the group format to foster world peace. He studied the potential of bringing together warring political factions to promote open, constructive dialogue. Groups were run, for instance, with blacks and whites from South Africa and with Protestants and Catholics from Northern Ireland. The person-centered perspective was also extended to education (Rogers, 1983) and medicine (cf. Levant & Shlien, 1984; Lietaer, Rombauts, & Van Balen, 1990).

There have been many other innovations and derivations that have flowed from the person-centered philosophy, including communication skills training (Goodman, 1984). Programs for training parents, leaders, and teachers and for enhancing relationships have been devised (Gordon, 1984; Guerney, 1984).

One of the most important innovations was Gendlin's (1970) concept of experiencing, which led to the development of focusing-oriented psychotherapy (Gendlin, 1996). Another important innovation was the attempt to translate person-centered ideas into the language of cognitive science (Wexler & Rice, 1974), a precursor of process–experiential psychotherapy (Greenberg et al., 1993).

Types of Clients with Whom the Approach Was Originally Developed

Person-centered therapy was developed from work with a wide range of clients in a number of different settings. Carl Rogers's first clinical work was at a psychoanalytically oriented child guidance clinic in Rochester, New York, where he began to develop his approach with underprivileged children and their families. Later, at the University of Chicago Counseling Center, he and his colleagues saw clients from both the community and the college campus. Person-centered therapists worked with problems of all types, including depression, anxiety, personality disorders, and psychosis. During the late 1950s a major research project with schizophrenics resulted in additions to both theory and practice.

Research Tradition

Carl Rogers has been called the "father of psychotherapy research" and was the first to record psychotherapy interviews for research study. During the 1940s and 1950s, Rogers and his graduate students carried out a series of studies on psychotherapy research, and many studies have been conducted since then. This tradition continues with several of the most important current psychotherapy researchers affiliated with the person-centered tradition, such as Leslie Greenberg, Robert Elliott, Laura Rice, William Stiles, David Rennie, and Eugene Gendlin.

THE CONCEPT OF PERSONALITY

Personality as Process

Is personality fixed, like the structure of a building or a sculpture, or is it constantly changing, more like the improvisations of a melody as played by a jazz musician? Person-centered theory holds that personality is relatively fluid and evolving, rather than like a fixed inner structure that "holds us up" much as the structure of a building bolsters it. People are "structures-in-process." Person-centered theory does not deny that structures, such as traits, may exist. Nor does it deny that there is continuity in personality over time. Of greater importance is that personality structures are continually *evolving*, even while they may stay the same in some respects (Bohart, 2001). People change all the time, most of the time making small, subtle adjustments, sometimes major ones. As an analogy, consider the coastlines of the continents from the viewpoint of a space satellite. They look the same as they did 20 years ago. Yet from a closer perspective they are continually changing. Similarly, personality structures may stay "the same" over time, although a closer look reveals that their manifestations have shifted (Cantor, 1990; Caspi, Elder, & Herbener, 1990). Caspi and colleagues (1990), for instance, found that men who were dependent in childhood still showed signs of it as adults but in different forms (e.g., being interpersonally nurturant themselves or stable marital partners). Dependency had evolved into more mature ways of relying on and maintaining supportive relationships. The theoretical ideas of Carl Rogers and Sigmund Freud are also examples of structure-in-process: Their perspectives continually evolved and grew, although neither fundamentally ever shifted his perspective.

This emphasis on personality as process is compatible with a view of personality traits as action strategies rather than as fixed characteristics (Cantor, 1990). It is also compatible with Gestalt psychotherapy. The following description of the person-centered view of personality, therefore, focuses on aspects of the person as a living process: moment-by-moment living, learning, growth, creativity, future orientation, interaction, the self-in-context, agency, the multiplicity of personal reality, communication, self–self relationships, experiencing and feeling, and the self-as-process.

Moment-by-Moment Living

It is commonly held that our personality traits, core schemata, and the like determine how we will act in a given situation. The "reappearance hypothesis," as Anderson (1974) has referred to it, holds that "the individual learns and stores percepts, images, memories, and acts, which then are simply reactivated upon need or demand as exact replicas or duplicates of those earlier events" (p. 30).

By contrast, person–centered theory emphasizes the moment-by-moment nature of personal functioning. General frames, personality traits, or rules that people use to help. themselves cope in a given situation are never specific enough to concretely determine what the individual actually does. Behavior in any given situation is a creative application of the general structure to the specific circumstances in that particular situation, always resulting in something slightly new and different than before.

Neisser (1967), a cognitive scientist, has noted concerning the reappearance hypothesis that "this assumption is so ingrained in our thinking that we rarely notice how poorly it fits experience. If reappearance were really the governing principle of mental life, repetition of earlier acts or thoughts should be the natural thing, and variation the exception. In fact, the opposite is true" (p. 282). Similarly, Epstein (1991), a radical behaviorist, has noted, "The behavior of organisms has many firsts, so many, in fact, that it's not clear that there are any seconds. We continually do new

things, some profound, some trivial . . . when you look closely enough, behavior that appears to have been repeated proves to be novel in some fashion. . . . You never brush your teeth exactly the same way twice" (p. 362),

As an example of this principle, I believe that one of my personality traits is a capacity for empathy, and one of my values is being empathic. Yet, as I interact with my clients I am continually challenged to find new situation-sensitive ways to be empathic that differ from how I tried to be with prior clients or even with the same clients at an earlier point in therapy. And I do not always succeed, and have to try again. My personality traits, general beliefs about empathy, and prior experience act only as rough guides to influence the continually improvisatory nature of the decisions I make with each new and different person.

Gestalt psychotherapy also emphasizes the importance of living life moment by moment. For Gestalt therapists, individuals are able to most effectively make decisions when they are fully in touch with all relevant information in a given moment. This includes having no blocks to awareness of the situation itself, nor blocks to inner awareness. For both person-centered theory and Gestalt theory, moment-by-moment living, also sometimes called living-in-the-here-and-now, or being "present-centered," does not mean "eat, drink and be merry for tomorrow you shall die," or any such endorsement of an impulsive hedonistic approach to life. Rather, it means that even in making effective and responsible long-range choices for both self and society, I do it best if I am open to all the information available in the moment and realize that I can only do now what I can do now.

Learning Potential

To function fully, people have to learn continually on a moment-by-moment basis. They incorporate feedback to make adjustments as they interact with persons or tasks.

For instance, therapists must continue to learn from one moment to the next as they try out approaches with clients. Therefore, people function most fully when they are operating intelligently, and person-centered therapy has been found to work by strengthening clients' ability to think clearly and intelligently (Van Balen, 1990; Zimring, 1990). Learning operates to constantly flesh out generalized beliefs, concepts, schemata, constructs, and operating traits. This will lead over time either to gradual evolution of these broader, longer-term frameworks or, on occasion, to major, significant shifts. From a Gestalt perspective, enhancing a person's capacity for awareness and for contact with both self and situation facilitates the person's capacity to make intelligent choices and to learn.

Growth Potential

Carl Rogers originally discussed an *actualizing tendency* in living things and later expanded this idea by suggesting that it was merely an individual form of a broader formative tendency found in the universe at large. This formative tendency is for things (such as crystals, as well as living creatures) to move toward greater order, complexity, and interrelatedness. This process includes the subprocesses of differentiation and integration.

On the level of the individual person, the actualizing tendency is the inherent tendency of individuals to develop by forming more differentiated and integrated personal life structures. This does not necessarily mean that people are basically "good." Shlien and Levant (1984) note that "we are basically both good and bad. . . . What is fundamentally assumed is the *potential to change*" (p. 3).

I think of the actualizing tendency as the person's inherent *self-righting* tendency (Masten, Best, & Garmazy, 1990). Based on their research on children who grow up and survive in adverse circumstances, these authors suggest that "studies of psychosocial resilience support the view that human psychological development is highly buffered and self-righting" (p. 438). Recently, following Carl Rogers, a colleague and myself have argued that it is people's capacities for self-righting that are the primary force in psychotherapy (Bohart & Tallman, 1999).

Emphasis on Creativity

To be fully functioning, individuals will be creative in everyday life because each situation is a little different from the past and presents the challenge to creatively incorporate old learning into what is different and new about this particular situation. In the course of any given day, people are continually exploring and discovering new ways of being and behaving, even though many of these new ways represent relatively minor creative adjustments.

Future Orientation

An organism that is continually exploring and learning will be oriented toward the future and toward its open possibilities. Humans are forward looking in that their behavior is guided by what they imagine will be there in the next moment more so than by what is there in this moment. Even being effectively present in the here and now is, like a surfer riding a wave, based on having a sense of what may be immediately coming next. The basketball player Larry Bird once noted that he was always playing "one step ahead" of what was actually happening.

It is our anticipation of where we want to go, how likely we think it is that we can get there, our estimation of our talents and skills for getting there, and what we believe the obstacles will be that determine our behavior. Shlien (1988) has argued that "the future is more important than the past in determining present behavior." The past influences us because we use it to make predictions about the future, not because it gets "wired" into us and then mechanistically drives behavior.

Interaction

Humans are inherently interactional. Human beings are not little self-encapsulated "shells" or monads, moving around like automobiles on a freeway. Persons are always "persons-in-contexts," and their behavior arises both from their personalities and from their relationships in their "ecological niches." It is meaningless to talk about individuals as if they were completely free of contexts. A person's ecological niche includes the family and other interpersonal situations as well as the broader network of neighborhoods, social support networks, and cultural variables and values. Also included are occupational and economic circumstances, religious and political affiliations, and so on. There is a continual dynamic interplay between self and situation. We "configure ourselves," so to speak, partially in response to what is important and present in each moment. Thus, some "sides" of ourselves come out in some situations, and other sides in other situations. This is a "field" view of human behavior and is compatible with a systems perspective (see Kaslow & Gurman, Chapter 11, this volume). Gestalt therapy is also a field view.

Selves-in-Context, Autonomy, and Individualism

For Carl Rogers, becoming autonomous was a major goal of human development, as it has been for most theories of personality developed in the West. Rogers thought that the fully functioning person had an internal locus of control and operated on the basis of personally chosen values rather than by rigidly conforming to the dictates of society.

However, the emphasis on a separate, bounded, autonomous self that "self-actualizes" could be seen as a reflection of largely Western, white male values. Some person-centered theorists have recently criticized the emphasis on individualism and autonomy in Rogers's work as well as

in Western thought in general (Holdstock, 1990; O'Hara, 1992). They note that these values are highly specific to Western culture and are even more specifically masculine in nature. They have noted that in other cultures the boundary of the self does not stop at the skin of the person but is extended to the family or the group. Fluid boundaries are emphasized over the firm self-boundaries emphasized in Western psychology. The determinants of behavior are seen as located in a field of forces, which includes the self, in contrast to Western psychology in which causes are located inside the individual.

What O'Hara (1992) argues for is the view of a self-in-context, which stresses the interconnected, interdependent nature of humans. Barrett-Lennard (1993) has noted that "individual selves are only one of the forms human life takes; other forms include relationships, families and living communities" (p. 1). O'Hara and Wood (1983) note that in some of the large group experiments conducted by person-centered theorists in recent years, "the individual achieves an integration with all of his or her own inner world. Individuals achieve integration with other group members and with the collective mind [as well]. . . . The individuals do not lose their identity to the group, they integrate the I with the 'We'" (p. 109).

Agency

I believe that the operative ingredient in Rogers's emphasis on *autonomy* is a sense of *agency:* A sense that one can confront challenge. A sense of ableness or effectance may be more important than a sense of self-sufficiency. Because challenge is an inherent part of doing most things worthwhile in life (careers, relationships, childrearing), having a sense of ableness that one can confront and cope with challenges is fundamental to effective functioning (Dweck & Leggett, 1988). An orientation toward confronting challenges leads to a focus on the process of doing more so than on the outcome and means that failure is viewed as information to learn from rather than as information about one's inadequacies.

Multiple Personal Realities

The recognition that different cultures have different concepts of the self is part of a larger recognition that personal and social realities are fundamentally multiple. Individuals and cultures find many different viable but workable ways of constructing personal realities. Individuals, based on their cultural background, gender, and history, live in different "perceptual universes" (O'Hara, 1992). Therefore, therapists must respect the growth potential available within each person's personal perceptual universe rather than try to impose an objectively "correct" way of being on them. This belief makes person-centered theory particularly compatible with the increasing importance of respecting cultural diversity. From a person-centered point of view, what is most fundamental is to respect the personal realities of clients and work from within their framework. Person-centered theory, therefore, would be philosophically compatible with the work of a therapist who might use folk healing methodologies compatible with a client's cultural or religious beliefs (Comas-Díaz, 1992).

Communication

Person-centered therapists assume that there is some "sense" in each individual's perceptual universe. Therefore, facilitating communication among different people's perceptual universes, such as those between therapist and client, is more important than judging who has the correct view. Open sharing of feelings and perspectives in a mutually respecting and accepting atmosphere will facilitate movement toward congruence among the parties involved and mobilize the "wisdom of the group or dyad." This is an important process for cou-

ples, families, and the workplace and between ethnic groups and among nations.

Congruent Self–Self Relationships

An open *internal* process of communication in which all aspects of the self are respected and listened to is equally important. Open, "friendly" listening to all aspects of thoughts, feelings, and experiences (including any internalized "voices" from parents and society) allows one's "internal community within" to move toward creative synthesis. All internal voices may have something to contribute.

Congruence is precisely this inner openness (Lietaer, 1991). Congruence does not always mean inner harmony. An inner sense of harmony comes and goes. However, if one is being congruent—open and receptive to all inner voices—the creative synthesizing process of the individual can move forward. The Gestalt words for the same process are *contact* and *awareness*—the person is in contact with and aware of their inner experience.

Experiencing, Feelings, and Emotions

Person-centered therapists value both intellectual, rational thinking and feelings and experience as important sources of information about how to deal with the world creatively.

Experiencing is a different, more fundamental way of knowing self and world than is rational, conceptual thinking. Experiencing is also different from emotion (Bohart, 1993). Experiencing is the immediate, nonverbal sensing of patterns and relationships in the world, between self and world, and within the self. It includes what is often called "intuitive knowing." However, there is nothing mysterious about it. We can sense or perceive relationships that we cannot easily describe in words. People can, for instance, sense or "feel" when a human face is drawn out of proportion long before they can cognitively and intellectually identify what is wrong with it (Lewicki, 1986).

The meanings that are acquired through direct experiencing are much more powerful than meanings acquired through conceptual thought. The *experience* of feeling loved in a relationship is a complex, whole-bodied sense of interaction that has much more to it than any intellectual or conceptual description can convey. Infants can tell from their interactions with their mothers whether the latter are empathically attuned to them. This does not mean they have a "concept" of empathic attunement. Rather, they sense immediately an attuned pattern of interaction between themselves and the mother (Stern, 1985). Gendlin (1970) believes experiencing can be more complex than conscious verbal–conceptual thought and is the source of creativity. We can sense more complex patterns experientially than we can put into words. Einstein, for instance, had a nonverbal sense of relativity theory before he had spelled it out in concepts. Internally we have a "felt sense" of how our lives are going and how each specific situation is presenting itself to us. It is at the level of felt sense that therapeutic change must take place, according to Gendlin. Therapy must lead to a directly felt shift in how we relate to the world, rather than merely to intellectual change.

Feelings

Person-centered therapists have been well-known for advocating "getting in touch with" and "trusting" feelings. Feelings, from a person-centered view, are more than emotions. Although we can feel anger and sadness, we also feel or sense complex meaning patterns. To be aware of feelings, therefore, is to be aware of both emotions and of sensed patterns of relationships between self and world at a given moment. We can "feel that something is wrong in our relationship" and "feel that our life is out of balance." To "trust one's feelings" means to listen to them as a source of information. It does not mean to do what they say.

A client came to me after seeing another therapist. Her problem was that she was *feeling* that her husband did not love her. Yet intellectually, when she thought about it, she could identify no logical reason for that feeling. Her husband claimed he loved her, and the other therapist had concluded that she was misperceiving the situation based on childhood problems with her father. A month or two after she had started to see me her husband suddenly announced that he was leaving her. He admitted that he had been having an affair for months and was in love with someone else. Clearly my client's feeling had been based on the apprehension of a set of subtle changes in her husband's manner of relating, which were so subtle that her intellectual, rational side could not identify them. If she had been able to trust her feelings, she would have explored her experience more carefully and might have been able to identify the subtle cues involved.

Feelings are not always correct, however, and sometimes we are misled because something "feels right" when it is not. It could have been that my client's feelings about her husband were wrong. If, in that case, she had been able to trust her feelings, she would have been able to continuously check them against her ongoing experience with her husband and would have discovered they were wrong. The legacy from her childhood was not so much that she projected lack of love onto her husband but that she had learned to distrust her feelings.

Person-centered theorists believe that fully functioning people use *all* their faculties. They use both their ability to think rationally and problem-solve and their ability to experientially sense what is personally meaningful to the self. Either source of information can be mistaken: Full functioning takes both into account.

Emotions

As I have pointed out, for a person-centered therapist, "getting in touch with feeling" does not necessarily mean getting in touch with emotion. Furthermore, neither person-centered theory nor Gestalt theory is accurately described as a "cathartic" theory. Catharsis is the idea that emotions are like fluids. They build up inside and must be expressed and discharged for the sake of mental health. The idea of catharsis—that sheer venting of emotions is helpful—is not compatible with research findings (Elliott, Greenberg, & Lietaer, in press). In both person-centered theory and Gestalt theory, accessing emotion is important because emotion is an important part of the body's self-regulatory capacities (Greenberg et al., 1993). Expression of emotion in psychotherapy may be useful, but it is useful because of its informational value more so than because of its cathartic value. Process–experiential psychotherapy particularly has emphasized the self-regulatory functions of emotion (Greenberg et al., 1993).

The Self as Process

For person-centered theory, the self is not an internal thing or agent but the experience of oneself as a whole person in any given moment. At the same time, we form concepts of ourselves to help us organize our knowledge about reality, just as we form concepts of other things. The self-concept is a knowledge structure we use as a "map" to help us navigate reality (Shlien, 1970). It is multidimensional, but there are two aspects of prime importance: the "real self-concept" and the "ideal self-concept." The real self-concept is our image of who we think we actually are, and the ideal self-concept is our image of who we would like to be or think we should be. When they are fully functioning, people hold both aspects of the self-concept tentatively, in the sense that maps may need to be revised to deal with change. It is not healthy to have too firm a self-concept, as selves are growing and changing, and one must be able to modify one's self-concept to incorporate

new experience just as one must revise other concepts to fit with experience.

Theory of Development

Although Rogers offered some views on psychological development, person-centered theory has not emphasized it. However, person-centered theory implies a view of development. First, the infant at birth is an active, curious, exploratory organism, interested in learning about the world and intrinsically interested in developing its own capacities. The child will listen to and learn from all its experiences: parents, peers, relatives, teachers, neighbors, cultural stories, and so on. It will be particularly interested in learning that results from its own efforts and exploratory activity.

As a growing organism, the child will not be "finished" within the first few years of life. Whereas in psychoanalytic theory early experience is "foundational," seen as the primary shaping influence on all later constructions of personal reality, person–centered theory assumes that people continually develop. As they do so, they incorporate what was learned earlier into broader and more inclusive frameworks for understanding themselves and their world. This view is more compatible with Piaget's theory than with Freud's. In Piaget's view, development is an expanding process in which later stages involve a transcending and reorganizing of what has come before. Earlier ideas and experience are retained but are incorporated in newer, more sophisticated constructions of reality in such a way that the form in which they were originally learned is altered. Freudian models view development as being like a pyramid, with early learnings forming a broad base for what comes later. Person-centered theory sees development more like a series of Chinese boxes. Early childhood is like the smallest box, which gets incorporated into the next largest box, and so on. Each new developmental experience forms a broader and more coherent framework for personal integration than the previous one.

Furthermore, humans are more oriented toward exploring and confronting challenge than they are toward avoiding pain and frustration. Psychodynamic theorists assume that humans have a "ubiquitous tendency to avoid pain" (Strupp & Binder, 1984, p. 32) and that children commonly avoid, deny, and repress painful experiences or emotions. In contrast, I am constantly amazed by my clients' courage and persistence in confronting pain and challenge and their attempts to master them. Children also repeatedly face up to painful events and frustrating experiences in attempts at mastery. Humans only avoid pain and frustration when they feel incompetent to deal with them (Bandura, 1986), as might occur with overwhelming experiences such as early childhood abuse.

When One Is Functioning Fully

Rogers and his colleagues developed a Process Scale to measure change in therapy from "dysfunctional" to more "fully functional" ways of being. Rogers describes the scale thus: "it commences at one end with a rigid, static, undifferentiated, unfeeling, impersonal type of psychologic functioning. It evolves through various stages to, at the other end, a level of functioning marked by changingness, fluidity, richly differentiated reactions, by immediate experiencing of personal feelings, which are felt as deeply owned and accepted" (Rogers, 1961b, p. 33). When people are functioning fully they are therefore fluid and flexible: holding constructs tentatively, testing them against experience, open to and accepting of feelings, listening to and learning from feedback, dialoguing with themselves and their surroundings, and experiencing themselves as able to direct their own lives.

Fully functioning simply means that, at a given moment, a person is operating as an evolving process. This does not mean the person is fulfilled, content, or even happy (Rogers, 1961a). Nor is there such a thing as a "fully functioning *person*" who is always

operating optimally. Even when functioning fully, people may periodically feel blocked, incompetent, inadequate, or frustrated. However, being in process they struggle with problems, try to learn, and continue onward.

PSYCHOLOGICAL HEALTH AND PATHOLOGY

From a person-centered perspective, abnormal behavior is likely to arise if a person is unable to operate in an ongoing, evolving way. Psychological problems are neither faulty beliefs or perceptions nor inadequate or inappropriate behavior per se. As humans confront challenges in life they will periodically misperceive, operate on mistaken beliefs, and behave inadequately. Dysfunctionality occurs if we *fail to learn* from feedback and therefore remain stuck in our misperceptions or inadequate behavior. Dysfunctionality is really a failure to learn and change. There are three interrelated explanations in the person-centered literature for how this occurs: incongruence, failure to be in process, and difficulties in information processing.

Incongruence

The most pervasive view of dysfunctionality in the person-centered literature is that abnormal behavior arises from a disparity between aspects of the self-concept and experience. For example, Janet was a premed student I knew in college. Her self-image was that she would be a doctor. Yet she was experiencing classes in biology and chemistry as alien and unfulfilling, and this disparity troubled her.

However, it is not disparity per se that creates dysfunctionality but how the person responds to and tries to resolve the disparity. All people experience such disparities periodically. If constructs are held tentatively, one will be able to work toward integrating disparate aspects of the self, and it is from such integration that creativity arises. However, if any aspects of the self-concept are held rigidly, integration and synthesis will be blocked.

People learn to hold parts of their self-concept rigidly when parents, teachers, or culture impose *conditions of worth* on them. That is, they are made to feel that they are worthwhile only when they conform to others' standards and values. This leads to the adoption of rigid "shoulds" about how they are supposed to be. When incongruence between rigid shoulds and experience occurs, people are unable to challenge their shoulds and so may respond by trying to ignore their experience or by misinterpreting it. Being unable to listen to their own experience, they disempower themselves. They then must rely exclusively on the rigid shoulds to guide their choices. And when that does not resolve anxiety and incongruence they feel helplessness and may become depressed. Janet had been "programmed" for years by herself, her parents, and her teachers to become a doctor. To follow this program she had to ignore any inconsistent feelings, which is what she did with her feelings toward her chemistry and biology classes. This appeared to affect her personality as well: I experienced her as a distant and guarded person. One day, however, she came to class and was different: open, warm, and friendly. She told me she had made a major personal decision and had changed her major to art. She disclosed that she had finally begun to listen to her experience and had realized that she really did not want to be a doctor. Trusting that part of her experience allowed her to "open up" in other ways.

Janet's problem was that she was holding her belief that she was to be a doctor rigidly. When she was able to hold it tentatively and evaluate it against her experience, she chose to change her major. However, she could have gone in the opposite direction: choosing to become a doctor even though she did not like chemistry and biology. What was important was that she be open to question and challenge her constructs.

Incongruence can come in many shapes and forms. Some people have generalized negative self-concepts and judge themselves harshly in all areas. This may lead to serious problems, such as antisocial behavior or personality disorders. Others may feel incongruent only in specific areas—for instance, being unable to accept an emotion such as anger.

Failure to Be in Process

This view can be thought of as an extension of the idea of incongruence. As Rogers's thought evolved, he focused more and more on the idea that dysfunctionality related to the degree to which a person was not functioning as a person in process. A person at the low end of the Process Scale, for instance, is described as functioning in a "rigid, static, undifferentiated, unfeeling" way (Rogers, 1961b, p. 33).

Gendlin (1969) also held that psychopathology resulted from a failure to be in process. Individuals who are experiencing psychological problems are not "focusing." That is, they are not attending inwardly to the flow of their experience in a manner that promotes creatively working on their problems. Instead of engaging in internal empathic listening, they harshly criticize their own feelings and reactions by lecturing themselves, analyzing themselves, or trying to "self-engineer" (Gendlin, 1970). In extreme cases, such as with schizophrenia (Gendlin, 1967), individuals may come to feel that their own inner life is so chaotic and "sick" that they turn away from it altogther, assuming that there is nothing there to be trusted.

Information-Processing Views on Dysfunction

In 1974, Wexler and Rice published a seminal volume presenting several information-processing perspectives on person-centered therapy. The ideas of Rogers and Gendlin were recast in the language of cognitive psychology. Individuals are held to develop schemata for organizing information about the world. Full functioning consists of continual assimilation of information into these schemata, creating more differentiated and integrated knowledge structures. Psychopathology results from rigid, undifferentiated systems of schemata that fail to integrate new information. An important process in the creation of more differentiated and integrated knowledge structures is that of *attention*. Failure to productively attend to new information results in the rigid persistence of old knowledge structures (Anderson, 1974).

Greenberg and colleagues (1993) have developed an integrative cognitive theory of personal functioning based in person-centered theory. For them a person's experience in a given moment is a product of a complex integration of cognitive schemata, motivation, and action tendencies. These are synthesized and result in both a holistic sense of the person in a given situation and specific emotional reactions, which organize the person for action. Psychological problems occur either because individuals fail to attend to and symbolize their own internal reactions or because their reactions come out of rigid "emotion schemes" (*not* "schemata").

These authors particularly emphasize the importance of emotional reactions in human functioning. Emotions reflect action tendencies, which inform people as to how they are experiencing a given moment. Therefore, the failure to be aware of or to access emotional information interferes particularly with adaptive capabilities. This failure may lead to a persistence in dysfunctional reactions and an inability to flexibly choose new behaviors to meet the demands of a situation.

Interactive View of Psychopathology

Psychological problems are not viewed as entities *within* the person but are considered to exist in interaction with life situations and are transactions with the world. Problems develop when people encounter situations that challenge their abilities to respond in flexible, integrative, problem-solving ways. Some people have been less prepared by life than others to effectively process and learn in situations that pose a challenge. However, any of us is capable of becoming temporarily dysfunctional if we encounter a challenge that overwhelms our resources to cope. Extreme stress due to economic circumstances or illness may disrupt our ability to openly relate to and integrate problematic experience. Being part of a group that is operating dysfunctionally, such as a family or a committee at work, might also disrupt that ability.

Gestalt View of Dysfunction

The Gestalt therapy view of psychopathology is similar to the person-centered view. People develop dysfunctional behavior when they are not aware of themselves as beings-in-process and when they are blocked from creatively and intelligently learning and coping with situations. Gestalt emphasizes the concepts of contact and awareness: people behave dysfunctionally when they are not in full contact with themselves and their environments, and when they are not aware. Contact and awareness allow people to operate as learning, growing processes.

THE PROCESS OF CLINICAL ASSESSMENT

Person-centered and experiential therapists generally do not find traditional diagnosis or assessment procedures useful. Such procedures encourage an "outside" perspective on the client, as if the client is being put under a microscope and dissected. This is antithetical to the person-centered empathic stance in which the therapist tries to feel him- or herself into the client's unique experience. Categorizing people tends to bias the therapist toward treating the individual as a member of a *class* rather than as a unique being. As a person-centered thera-pist I am interested in understanding and relating to Jack or Carolyn, not Jack-the-borderline or Carolyn-the-narcissist. How-ever, because the mental health field uses diagnostic labels, person-centered therapists will sometimes employ them for commu-nication purposes (as I have done in this chapter).

Process–experiential therapists (Green-berg et al., 1993) do make "process diag-noses" in therapy. A process diagnosis is an assessment by the therapist of the presence of some dysfunctional emotional scheme that the client needs to change, and of the client's readiness to work on it, at a given moment in therapy. It is important to note that the therapist does not focus on the con-tent of this emotional scheme (e.g., anger toward one's father) but merely on evidence that the client is experiencing some block in the process of resolving a personal prob-lem. Process–experiential therapists look for "markers," which are specific verbal, behav-ioral, or emotional signs that a client is struggling with a particular kind of emo-tional-processing problem. For instance, a marker for a "problematic reaction point" is that clients are describing an incident in which they found themselves reacting to some situation or person in a way that puz-zles them. This puzzlement may consist of feeling that their reactions to the situation or person were unreasonable, dysfunctional, exaggerated, or unexpected. A process diag-nosis of a specific kind of marker will sug-gest to the therapist what kind of procedure could be best used at that moment to foster and deepen the client's exploration. Process diagnoses are attempts to formalize or sys-tematize, based on research, the intuitions of therapists that at a given moment in therapy a particular type of response is called for.

THE PRACTICE OF THERAPY

Person-centered therapy in its traditional or "pure" form is highly nondirective. The therapist's goal is primarily to be a compan-ion on the client's journey of self-discovery. By being a certain kind of companion, namely, a warm, empathic, and genuine one, the therapist provides an atmosphere in which the client's own thrust toward growth can operate.

However, in the 1960s a trend developed among some person-centered therapists to treat person-centered therapy more as a philosophy of therapy than as a specific way of doing it. It was argued that if therapists were warm, empathic, and genuine and re-spected the client's own growth process, they could be more active and even use techniques from other therapies (Holdstock & Rogers, 1983). For many, person–cen-tered therapy became a philosophy in the context of which therapists could practice in eclectic ways. As a result, some modern person-centered therapists have incorporat-ed behavioral, hypnotic, Gestalt, and con-frontational techniques into their practice. Natalie Rogers (Toms, 1988) includes art and dance in her "person-centered expres-sive therapy." Similarly, Gendlin's focusing-oriented therapy and Greenberg et al.'s process–experiential therapy hold that the therapist can systematically try to facilitate exploratory processes that help clients grow. Other, more traditional person-centered therapists (Brodley, 1993) disagree with this development. They believe that to use any technique systematically is to violate the basic "nondirective attitude" of following the client and letting the client find his or her own pathway to growth.

Philosophy of Therapy

Person-centered and experiential therapies are based on the belief that it is the clients who "heal" themselves and who create their own self-growth (Bohart & Tallman, 1999). Growth and healing happen from within the person, though external processes can facilitate or retard that growth. As analogies to the person-centered view, plants and children both grow themselves, though farmers and parents can foster or retard that growth.

Person-centered and experiential therapies are relatively unique in how much they emphasize the self-righting, self-healing tendencies of the person. Although there are other approaches that agree that humans have positive potential within, they believe people may not use this potential unless guided to do so by the therapist. This may be because clients are presumably so motivated by their desires to avoid pain and to gain security that they avoid dealing with issues that will unlock that potential. Or, it is because they are trapped in faulty thinking from which they must be freed by the therapist. The therapist becomes the "expert guide" on what issues the client needs to face in order to grow.

In contrast, the job of the person-centered therapist is to provide optimal conditions under which the intrinsic self-organizing and self-transcending capabilities of the person can operate. Under supportive conditions, the client's thrust toward growth will override any tendencies toward avoidance of pain. People are adept at facing up to and bearing a great deal of pain while continuing to function, as long as they feel they have a chance of productively mastering painful circumstances. They will only avoid pain and seek security at the expense of growth if they feel helpless (Dweck & Leggett, 1988) or low in self-efficacy (Bandura, 1986) to deal with the pain.

Consider the example of my daughter when she first learned to swim. Initially, she was frightened and went slowly, first paddling around with a life vest on for several months. I did not try to cajole or pressure her to "face her fears" and to go farther, as some parents might have done. One day she spontaneously decided to take off the life vest and to try swimming on her own. I trusted her process, and she was motivated eventually to face her fears in order to move forward, but in her own time.

Therapists do not have to make clients face up to even extremely repressed, painful experiences such as those of early childhood abuse. If conditions are provided under which clients can begin to begin to develop a sense of self-efficacy in their own capacity for self-righting and growth, they will come to want to face up to such experiences when necessary for their continued development. At that point such experiences will begin to emerge slowly as a part of the process of self-healing.

Person-centered therapists take clients where they are when they come into therapy. If the client's problem is that he or she is chronically feeling tense, the person-centered therapist will work with what the client focuses on and will not assess whether there are "deeper issues" to confront. This is due to person-centered therapists' belief that clients' development of their capacities for self-direction and self-regulation are the most important aspect of therapy and that clients will move deeper on their own when necessary. Gestalt therapists, however, are more likely to confront clients if they appear to be stuck.

Basic Structure of Person-Centered and Experiential Therapies

Person-centered and experiential therapists are flexible in how the therapy interaction is structured. Although they most typically meet with the client for a 1-hour session on a once-a-week basis, person-centered therapists modify this format if needed to conform to the needs of working with a particular client. A client might be seen either more or less than once a week, sessions might last either longer or shorter than 1 hour, and meetings might or might not be held in the therapist's office. Gendlin (1967) talks about taking hospitalized patients for a walk down to the hospital cafeteria as therapy. I worked with a young hospitalized "paranoid" client by meeting with him on the hospital lawn.

Although at least several sessions will typically be needed, person-centered and experiential therapists believe that occasionally, important change can occur in a single session. There is no meaningful "average length" that can be prescribed for person-centered therapy. I have seen clients for 1 session and for well over 100 sessions.

Person-centered and experiential therapists might use any or all of individual, couple, family, or group therapy formats. The choice would be jointly decided by the therapist and all participants.

Goal Setting

Person-centered and experiential therapists believe that it is the client who knows what hurts and what needs to be changed (though this knowing is often of a felt, intuitive nature). Therefore, these therapists do not set goals for what changes clients need to undergo in order to improve (e.g., "become more assertive," "stop thinking irrationally," or "get out of your dysfunctional relationship"). Rather, the goal is to provide the conditions under which the client's own intrinsic tendencies to confront problematic experiences, explore them, extract new and important meanings, and creatively reorganize ongoing experience in more productive ways can operate.

Why can't the therapist simply tell the client "the answer"? I argued earlier that people live in different perceptual universes of which therapists can know only little bits. In a famous film of Carl Rogers working with Gloria (Shostrom, 1965), Gloria's problem was that she had lied to her daughter about the fact that she was having sexual relationships although she was not married. She wanted Rogers to tell her whether or not to tell her daughter the truth. Rogers refused to do so and helped Gloria arrive at her own answer. In watching the film, some of my students have expressed frustration: Why can't Rogers just tell her to be honest?[1]

One reason is that only Gloria knows the true subtleties and complexities of her life and of her relationship with her daughter. Only Gloria knows the intricate "web" of

relationships that constitutes her "ecological niche." What might seem wise from an outside perspective might not be wise from an inside one. Therefore, only Gloria will know how, ultimately, to reorganize and synthesize all the factors in her perceptual universe to provide a solution that is "ecologically wise" within that universe. By "ecologically wise" I mean a solution that best takes into account this complex web of relationships. If Rogers were to give generalized advice ("Yes. It's better to be honest."), it might work. However, it also is possible that if Gloria simply followed this advice without working out its "ecological wisdom" within her universe, it might backfire.

Although all person-centered and experiential therapists agree on not setting goals for *what* the client needs to change, they differ on whether to have goals regarding *how* to best help the client find his or her own answers. Traditional person-centered therapists set no goals for their clients or for the therapy process at all. Although traditional person-centered therapists believe that therapy leads to outcomes such as people being more open to experience, more fluid, and more differentiated, they believe that these changes will best occur if they do not try to make them happen but rather focus on how they can best be present with their clients. That is, traditional person-centered therapists' goals are ones they set for *themselves:* to be empathic, accepting, respectful, and congruent. The therapist, in some sense, works on *him- or herself* in therapy rather than on the client. If the therapist feels that he or she is not understanding the client, the therapist struggles to do so. If the therapist feels incongruent, he or she struggles to be more so.

Focusing-oriented and process–experiential therapists do not adopt this nondirective attitude as thoroughly as do person-centered therapists. They believe that the therapist can have "process" goals; that is, they hold that helping facilitate certain kinds of processes of exploration with clients can more efficiently help clients find their own answers. I describe this process in more detail when I discuss these two therapies later.

Techniques and Strategies

Person-Centered Therapy

For person-centered therapy, the establishment of a facilitative therapeutic relationship is itself the therapeutic technique and strategy. The process of "being with" the client in the sense of accepting the client as he or she is, entering imaginatively into the client's world of perception and feelings, and being authentic is sufficient for the facilitation of a process of change.

What the therapist primarily does is express his or her struggles to understand the client's experience. This will often come out in the form of "reflection." Reflection is a way of responding in which the therapist tries to express his or her attempt at understanding what the client is experiencing and trying to say. Therapists can reflect feelings, meanings, experiences, emotions, or any combination thereof. They often go beyond what the client has explicitly *said* to try to grasp what the client is also experiencing but has been left unsaid. However, the therapist tries to grasp only what is within the client's current range of awareness of experiencing. The therapist does not try to grasp possible unconscious aspects of the client's experience. This is the main theoretical difference between a reflection and a psychodynamic interpretation. Following is an example of a reflection compared to an interpretation:

Client: "I'm feeling so lost in my career. Every time I seem to be getting close to doing something really creative, which would lead to a promotion, I somehow manage to screw it up. I never feel like I am really using my potential. There is a block there."

Reflection: "It's really *frustrating* to screw up and kill your chances; and it feels like it's

something in *you* that's making that happen again and again,"

A psychodynamic interpretation: "It sounds like every time you get close to success you unconsciously sabotage yourself. Perhaps success means something to you that is troubling or uncomfortable, and you are not aware of what that is."

Notice that this interpretation might in fact be true but is an attempt to bring to the client's attention something that is not currently in the client's awareness. This is the key difference between reflections and interpretations.

For person-centered therapists it is important to react in a therapeutically spontaneous manner to whatever is happening in the moment between themselves and the client. Although reflection has been the traditional form for expressing empathy, spontaneous expressions of empathy may take many other forms (Bozarth, 1997) such as the self-disclosure of the therapist's own experience in "resonance" to client experience. At a given moment, the sense of sharing between therapist and client might also lead the therapist to spontaneously suggest a technique. Person-centered therapists are not banned from suggesting techniques. It is *how* they suggest techniques that is important. A technique would only be suggested when to do so is to further the process of being together with the client in a real, empathic relationship (Bohart & Rosenbaum, 1995). It is not an attempt to "do anything" to the client or "make anything happen." The client is always free to reject the technique. However, techniques are used relatively infrequently by person-centered therapists.

Focusing-Oriented Psychotherapy

Gendlin's (1996) focusing-oriented psychotherapy is based on the idea that change arises from tuning into and working with a "bodily felt sense." Research has shown that clients grow when they are actively referring inwardly to their experience and feelings and articulating that experience in words (Hendricks, 2002). They are less likely to grow if they talk about their problems in distanced intellectual ways or focus externally on the situations in their lives. Based on this premise, focusing-oriented psychotherapists try to facilitate this experiencing process in psychotherapy in three basic ways. First, they use a variant of empathic responding—"experiential" responding (Gendlin, 1968). Experiential responses specifically focus on the felt aspects of the client's present experience and often rely on metaphors. An experiential response to our aforementioned client might be, "It sounds like you're feeling really up against it, like up against a big wall, which you're trying to push aside and you don't know how to."

A second technique used by experiential therapists is the sharing of their own immediate experience in the therapy relationship with their clients (Gendlin, 1967). The therapist focuses on his or her own immediate experience in the situation and tries to explicate it in words. This helps clarify the nature of what is going on between therapist and client and provides a model for clients of how to relate inwardly to their own experience. For instance, the therapist might say to a silent, sad client who has just suffered a loss, "Part of me wants to reach out and contact you, and talk to you about the loss, and part of me feels like I just want to sit in silence with you and keep you company in your pain. I'm not sure what you want but I want you to know that I'm here if you want to talk, and I'm here even if I just stay silent with you for a while."

The third technique is "focusing" (Gendlin, 1996). Clients are asked to focus inwardly and to "clear a space" by imagining that they have set all their problems aside for the moment. Then they take one problem and try to focus on how all the problem feels inside. Although people can think about only parts of a problem at any given moment, they can feel all those parts together. They then wait and listen to see whether some words or concepts come from the feeling. This process often leads to a "felt shift" in which the sense of the problem reorganizes so that the person can get a better "handle" on what the crux of it is.

Any concept or technique from other therapies might be used by a focusing-oriented therapist if it helped facilitate contacting, exploring, and articulating inner experiencing. Experiential therapists have used Gestalt role playing, body techniques, cognitive techniques, and relaxation. They can talk about psychoanalytic ideas if these concepts help clients directly refer to their immediate felt experience. Thus, Gendlin's theory of experiencing has provided a theoretical rational for eclectic therapeutic practice (Gendlin, 1996).

Gestalt Psychotherapy

Gestalt therapy developed independently of person-centered therapy and is not a direct "relative" of it. However, I briefly review it because process–experiential psychotherapy is an integration of person-centered and Gestalt therapy.

Philosophically, Gestalt therapy shares much in common with person-centered theory (C. Rogers, personal communication, April 1971). However, at the level of practice it is considerably different. Gestalt psychotherapy was co-developed by Fritz Perls, Laura Perls, and Paul Goodman, although Fritz Perls, because of his charismatic persona, has popularly gotten most of the credit for being its "founder," or "finder," as he often referred to it.

Gestalt therapy emphasizes awareness and contact. A person who is in full contact with his or her environment and his or her self on an ongoing basis is able to make effective choices. If there is awareness and contact the organism has the capacity to organize and reorganize itself spontaneously for effective functioning. Gestalt therapy is a field theory. It holds that the organism is a system and exists in a systemic relationship with its environment. The person *is* an interaction: There is a fluidity between self and world, so that the person is in continuous dialogue or contact with his or her world. Therefore he or she has the capability to organize and reorganize him- or herself so that the "self" is appropriately functional at given moments.

As with person–centered therapy, Gestalt emphasizes growth. It does not focus on specific symptom removal. The process of Gestalt therapy is based on developing the client's capacities for maintaining ongoing direct contact and awareness. This leads to the individual's being able to make effective choices and to be "response-able" (responsible). The Gestalt therapist facilitates this by providing an empathic, responsive, and responsible here-and-now relationship, and through suggesting various experiments designed to help clients explore their capacities for contact and awareness.

Gestalt is famous for some of the "techniques" that Gestalt therapists often use. However, for the Gestalt therapist these are not really "techniques." There is no "script" or schema for using a given technique. Nor is any specific outcome expected. Rather, they are experiments in awareness. What is chosen is what emerges as relevant based on the ongoing therapy interaction. Gestalt therapists do not make plans in advance for sessions. They are "disciplined improvisors" and may use techniques from any approach if they are used as exploratory experiments.

Among the many experiments Gestalt therapists have devised, the most well-known are those that involve "chair work." Following from the goal of helping clients learn how to stay in contact, Gestalt therapists believe that sometimes "just talking" about a problem can allow the person to stay *out* of contact. To bring them into contact with the immediacy of experience, they will have clients enact role-plays. For instance, with the "empty chair," the client may be talking about a problem with "the other person." The Gestalt therapist will have the client imagine that the person is sitting in an empty chair across from him or her and then speak directly to that person, thus bringing the client into fuller contact with the immediacy of experiencing that other person. Then the client is asked to switch chairs and role-play the other person's side, and to continue switching chairs to continue the dialogue.

That this can create immediacy of experiencing was brought home forcefully to me when I was a graduate student. One client was a man who had a psychotic mother. At one point he expressed some anger toward his mother. He described an incident in which he had seen her try to choke his brother when he was a little child. He described the incident in an emotional, but relatively controlled fashion. I asked him to role-play a dialogue with her. As he expressed his anger and hurt directly toward his mother in the role-play he broke into deep sobs. He was confronting it in a much more emotionally immediate way than he had ever done before. This led him to realize how deeply hurt, angry, and frightened he had been by his mother's behavior. It also helped him realize how he blocked himself from fully experiencing closeness.

With Gestalt therapy in mind, let us turn to process–experiential therapy.

Process–Experiential Psychotherapy

Process–experiential psychotherapy (Greenberg et al., 1993) has been developed by Leslie Greenberg and his colleagues. It is an integrative psychotherapy based in a person-centered view of the nature of the human being that also draw on ideas from both cognitive theory and Gestalt psychotherapy. It is a member of a larger class of integrative emotion-focused psychotherapies (L. Greenberg, personal communication, March 18, 2002), which also includes another therapy developed by Greenberg and his colleagues, specifically "emotion-focused therapy" (Greenberg & Johnson, 1988). I focus on process–experiential psychotherapy here.

Carrying forward work by Wexler, Rice, and others (cf. Wexler & Rice, 1974), process–experiential therapists (Greenberg et al., 1993) view clients' problems as a result of the failure to productively explore certain classes of cognitive–affective information. The goal of the process–experiential therapist is to facilitate different types of cognitive–affective operations in the client at different times to best enhance deeper exploration. The job of the therapist is (1) to select the intervention that will best facilitate work on a given emotional task at a given moment, and (2) to systematically guide the client through the operations involved in the chosen intervention. Different client behaviors serve as therapeutic markers to guide the therapist in choosing which intervention to use.

Greenberg and colleagues (1993) identify five basic therapeutic markers. I briefly describe three herein. The first is a "problematic reaction point." A problematic reaction point refers to the client's having behaved in some way that strikes the client as exaggerated, inappropriate, or unexpected. For instance, the client may have said something in anger about which he or she feels ashamed. The therapist uses "evocative unfolding" and guides the client to explore both "edges" of the problematic experience: the situation in which the problematic reaction occurred and the person's inner experience at the time. Evocative unfolding consists of empathic responses designed to be highly vivid and emotionally evocative (e.g., "That superioristic smirk on his face really made you boil"). This process leads clients to discover how they were construing the situation and how that led to their reaction. Typically, clients feel better when they realize that their behavior, no matter how dysfunctional, had some "sense" behind it, and this discovery allows for the possibility of new options to develop. Often clients also spontaneously recognize how this way of construing a situation has played a role in other problematic situations in their lives.

The second client marker is that of an experienced "split": The client is in conflict about something. Usually there is a "should" side saying "do this," and a "want" side saying "I don't want to." With this marker, the Gestalt two-chair exercise (Yontef, 1995) is used. The client role-plays both sides, speaking from the "should" side and then switching chairs to speak from the "want" side. The client goes back and forth until some integration is reached. This integration occurs because both sides begin to see some "sense" in the other side. Changes in the "should" side particularly facilitate integration because the should side moves from talking in "shouldistic" language to expressing hopes and fears. Instead of "You should study harder," it says, "I'm worried that if you don't study harder you won't achieve your goals."

A third marker occurs when the client has "unfinished business" with another person. For this problem another version of the Gestalt two-chair exercise is used. Clients role-play dialogues between themselves and the other person, taking both roles. This role-play allows the client to arrive at a personal resolution with the emotional problems created by the relationship with the other person. For instance, a sexually abused daughter role-plays a dialogue between herself and her father. In her chair she expresses her rage, guilt, and sadness over what her father has done to her. She may play her father as someone whom she can ultimately come to forgive, or she may play him as an "unrepentant bastard." In either case she becomes able to let go of her guilt and of the past and reclaim a sense of her own worth and potency.

Process of Therapy

For each of the previously described therapies, the therapeutic process is one of staying closely with the moment-to-moment "flow" of what is happening in the session. Therapists focus on what clients bring up to talk about and do not try to guide the conversation toward topics the therapist thinks are important. For instance, Gloria shifted topics several times over the course of her half-hour session with Carl Rogers. He stayed with her shifts, and it is clear that there was a kind of intuitive wisdom to these shifts as they led Gloria to deepen her exploration.

What is talked about is not nearly as important as the moment-by-moment process: Are clients relating to themselves in a productive, self-evolutionary way no matter what is being talked about? The process of therapy will have, therefore, its own intrinsically structured flow, and clients will often recycle topics several times before they are resolved.

From person-centered and experiential perspectives, "resistance" is not a useful concept. What other therapists call resistance may be defined as occurring when the *therapist* thinks the client should be talking about something, feeling something, or doing something other than what the *client* is doing. When clients are "resisting" they are trying to follow what they feel will best help them maintain or grow at that time. As with anything else the client is doing, person-centered and experiential therapists will "respect the resistance" and try to empathize with "where the client is coming from" at that moment. If an experiential therapist were to use a technique at that point it would be used in an experimental way to see if it helped the client move forward. It would not be used to "break through" the resistance. This is the best way to facilitate the process of moving forward. Clients will grow out of resistance if the therapist remains in empathic and genuine contact but may get stuck in resistance if therapists (or anyone else) relate to them in a "superior" manner—correcting them or imparting "truth" to them.

Because person-centered and experiential therapists invest so much trust in clients' ability to direct their process of growth, termination of therapy is rarely a problem. In my experience, clients are motivated to move away from being dependent on the therapist and to "try their wings" when they are ready. They do not need to be "fully healed" with all problems resolved (who is?) in order to try to live on their own. Problems are a part of life and clients sometimes leave because they now feel they can manage the problems on their own. Sometimes clients ease themselves into termination by deciding to come every other week instead of every week for a time, before they decide to stop altogether. In other instances, clients just decide they are ready to stop.

When a client decides to stop therapy, the therapist and client talk over the decision. If the therapist has reservations about the client's terminating, he or she may express them, especially if the client asks for the therapist's opinion. But contrary to the "expert therapist" model, in which clients are sometimes told that they are avoiding or resisting because they want to stop therapy, a person-centered therapist would confine him- or herself to a *personal* self-disclosure (e.g., "I worry that we didn't quite work through that issue, and I wonder if it might bother you again, but you know I'm here if you ever do feel a need for further work").

Virtually all the errors a person-centered therapist or an experiential therapist could commit would come out of failing to be warm, empathic, and genuine; imposing an agenda upon the client; or failing to be in touch with the unfolding moment-by-moment process. Even Carl Rogers was capable of committing an error. Raskin (1991) has pointed out that, early in the interview with Gloria, the value Rogers placed on people trusting their own organismic wisdom interfered with his ability to empathically hear all of Gloria's concern about being honest with her daughter, although he did become more empathic later on. Zimring (1991) has pointed out that so-called transferential reactions in which the client begins to focus on the therapist rather than on his or her own experience occur when the therapist is not being sufficiently empathic.

THE THERAPEUTIC RELATIONSHIP AND THE STANCE OF THE THERAPIST

The therapeutic relationship is the single most important factor in both person-centered and experiential approaches. According to Carl Rogers (1957), the three primary conditions of a good therapeutic relationship are unconditional positive regard or warmth, empathy, and genuineness or congruence. Rogers postulated that these basic relationship conditions were "necessary and sufficient" for therapeutic growth to occur, although Bozarth (1993) has recently suggested that these conditions are sufficient but not absolutely necessary because the self-actualizing tendency may sometimes facilitate growth even without a therapeutic relationship.

The implications of Rogers's (1957) statement were (and are) radical: It is the relationship which is the "healing" element in therapy. Techniques, theoretical points of view, and even professional training have nothing to do with making therapy work. Strupp and Hadley (1979), for instance, found that untrained college professors chosen for their sensitivity were, on the average, as therapeutic as professional therapists.

Warmth or unconditional positive regard has also been called "acceptance," "respect," "liking," "prizing," or even "nonpossessive love." The quality is a basic attitude of liking, respecting, or prizing directed at the client as a whole person. It rests on a distinction between the client as a person and the client's behavior. Just as good parents continue to like and prize their children even while disliking specific behaviors (e.g., writing on the walls with crayons), the person-centered therapist continues to prize the client as a person even when the client's behavior is dysfunctional. Unconditional regard does not mean the person-centered therapist conveys support or approval for dysfunctional behavior.

Holding an attitude of unconditional positive regard toward others precludes nei-ther feeling angry at them nor setting limits. Good parents set limits while prizing and respecting their children. Good relationships in which both partners generally like and prize one another include times when either or both of the participants become angry with one another. Good therapy relationships as well may include moments in which the therapist must set limits (e.g., if the client is tearing up the therapist's office), or in which the therapist may experience anger or dislike toward some of the client's behavior. I will discuss how this is handled when I discuss genuineness and congruence.

Feeling liked and prized as people, clients begin to feel safe to explore their experience and to take a more objective look at their behavior. Clients are able to distinguish between their intrinsic worth as persons and the dysfunctionality of current ways of experiencing and behaving. Bozarth (1997) has held that unconditional positive regard is the core healing element in therapy.

Empathy is the ability to intuit oneself inside the client's perceptual universe, to come as close as one can to seeing and feeling as the client sees and feels. From an "outside" perspective, client behavior often seems irrational, self-destructive, manipulative, narcissistic, rigid, infantile, or egocentric. However, from an "inside" perspective behaviors that seemed dysfunctional and irrational from the outside usually make "sense" in terms of how the client is experiencing the world. This does not mitigate the behavior's dysfunctionality. Rather, it suggests that from within the client's skin, there is a "positive thrust" underlying it (Gendlin, 1967).

A client of mine was arrested for exposing himself to his 13-year-old stepdaughter. As I struggled to understand him from inside his perceptual universe it became clear that he felt totally helpless and impotent in his dealings with this girl whom he experienced as ignoring him and consistently treating him with disrespect. Exposing himself was an extreme (albeit dysfunctional) reaction to one particularly hurtful show of disrespect on her part, and a way of his expressing his helplessness, anger, and rage. I later describe what happened in this case.

There are a number of different positive therapeutic effects of empathy. First, the experience of being known seems to be intrinsically therapeutic. When I feel fully known by someone, it is as if I feel I come into focus. I feel better able to sort things out and to make choices for myself. Second, finding that there is some sense in my experience, even when I have acted dysfunctionally, makes me feel generally less crazy or dysfunctional. I begin to have some confidence in my own inner experience. Increased confidence allows me to look at things more carefully and to confront painful experience.

Third, therapist empathy provides a model for a "friendly" way for clients to listen to their own experience. This friendly listening lets clients accept and hear meanings that they were previously afraid of because they seemed "unfriendly" to the self, thus allowing them to begin to find more productive and less dysfunctional ways of dealing with those feelings and meanings. As my client began to listen to his own experience in a friendly manner, he began to realize there was some "sense" in his impulsive act of exposing himself to his stepdaughter. He decided that what he wanted to do was to develop more proactive and less hurtful ways of asserting himself and expressing his anger, which is what we worked on.

Genuineness or congruence refers to the degree to which a therapist is "being him- or herself" in therapy. Being oneself does not mean that one acts out one's feelings or says whatever is on one's mind. Genuineness and congruence are matters of *inner* connection (Lietaer, 1991). They have to do with the degree to which therapists are in touch with the flow of their inner experience, and the extent to which their outward behavior reflects some truly felt aspect of their inner experience. For instance, as I listen to my client describe his exposing himself to his stepdaughter, I may experience both empathy for him and dislike of what he did. At one moment in therapy it may feel more congruent to express my empathy; at another moment to let my client know I disliked his action. Being genuine does not mean that I "dump" what is on my mind at any given moment into the therapy session.

Lietaer (1991) has distinguished between congruence and *transparency*. Congruence is attending inwardly to one's experience and working to sort out its meanings. Transparency is the open self-disclosing of what is within the therapist. Person-centered therapists value self-disclosure in therapy. However, self-disclosure should be "sensitively relevant" to what will promote the therapeutic process. Rogers has argued that therapists should only self-disclose their reactions when (1) they are persistent, and (2) they are getting in the way of the therapeutic relationship itself.

Gendlin (1967) has noted that therapists must self-disclose in more effective and productive ways than does the person in the street. The way people in the street are "honest" is often to label, criticize, and judge (e.g., "You're boring"). If I have a reaction to my client (such as anger) which I wish to share, I first must work with it myself before I self-disclose. I tune inwardly and try to sort out the degree to which my reaction is "mine" from the degree to which it belongs in the relationship. If I conclude that it belongs in the relationship, I will share it. However, I then share it as my reaction, not as the "truth."

Genuineness as a Basis for Therapeutic Eclecticism

From the 1960s on, many person-centered therapists increasingly emphasized genuineness as the most important of the therapeutic conditions, although only in the context of warmth, empathy, and a belief in the client's intrinsic self-directive capacities. For many, the emphasis on genuineness provided a basis for eclectic therapeutic practice. First, it encouraged therapists to find their own styles for expressing empathy instead of expressing it primarily in the form of reflection. Responding empathically in the moment might sometimes mean backing off and allowing the client some distance, being silent, asking a question, sharing a thought or feeling, or even suggesting a technique. Genuinely expressed empathy became a matter of tuning in and timing rather than a specific kind of response.

One of my clients, for instance, did not experience reflections as empathic, and I soon gave up sharing my understanding with him in that way. He felt more comfortable with my expressing my own reactions to what he said, and he experienced me as "really understanding him" when I responded in that manner. With other clients my empathy has sometimes come out in a light, humorous way of interacting.

Second, the emphasis on genuineness provided a philosophical basis for therapists to disclose their views, share their opinions, and suggest techniques. If I as a therapist have an opinion or a thought or know of a technique and I deliberately withhold it in order to "play my role as a nondirective therapist," then I am not being genuine. The issue is not whether a technique is suggested but how. Is it suggested as the expert trying to fix the client or as one human sharing his or her own experience with another human? In the latter, the implicit message is: This is something from my experience that you may find useful; however, it is up to you to evaluate its usefulness and to use it if you wish. With this modification, many person-centered therapists have incorporated hypnosis, dream-work, Gestalt techniques, and behavioral techniques. One can even confront.

How can one confront while still being person-centered? After all, confrontation often entails the provision by a therapist of an alternative perspective to the client. Some

therapists hold that confrontation is particularly important with clients who are "in denial." However, this sets the therapist up as the expert on the client's experience. Although person-centered therapists might also "confront," they do so from a completely different philosophical base. When I provide an alternative perspective on the client to the client my goal is to share my perspective, not to "impart truth." Clients may accept what I say, reject what I say, or alter what I way. All three have happened productively. In addition, I do not provide such perspectives until the relationship has progressed to the point where the client knows that he or she has the right to disagree with me.

In sum, the shift toward genuineness allowed many person-centered therapists to practice in a more flexible, eclectic way that suited their individual personalities. It also allowed greater flexibility in "tailoring" the relationship to suit different clients. However, as was true in the advent of focusing-oriented and process–experiential therapy, this change has not been welcomed by some person-centered therapists, who believe that clients grow best when they are in the company of someone who empathically follows the client's lead in self-exploration and self-growth.

Transference and Countertransference

Many person-centered therapists such as Shlien (1984) and myself do not find the concepts of transference and countertransference either meaningful or therapeutically helpful. These terms originate m psychoanalytic theory. Transference refers to the tendency of the client to read things into the therapist's behavior based on the client's past experience (primarily with parents). Countertransference refers to the tendency of the therapist to read things into the client's behavior based on the therapist's past experience and unresolved problems.

My view is that these concepts are not helpful because they do not make meaningful distinctions between different kinds of experiences. To understand the present we *always* "transfer" past experience onto it. We are "transferring" right now when we read these words as if they were in "English." Whenever we use past experience to interpret the present there is the possibility of error. For instance, in some other cultures people stand much closer to one another when they talk than they do in our culture. Based on our past experience we might misinterpret someone from such a culture as being intrusive or overly familiar were we to meet them. We might continue to feel uneasy around them, even when we know intellectually that we are just dealing with a cultural difference. We might also make dysfunctional decisions about the person based on our erroneous interpretation.

The key is not whether we use our past experience to understand the present—we always do that. It is whether or not we attend to the *discrepancies* between what is new and different in the present from our past experience and use that to learn and to adjust our perceptions. Clients often appear to persist in their "misreadings" of the therapist, but that is not because they are "transferring." Rather, their ability to openly listen to corrective information, both from others and from their own inner experiencing, has been compromised by a lack of self-trust. As they come to trust themselves and the therapist, and as they learn how to listen to their feelings, they become better and better at correcting misreadings of situations.

Therapists also always "countertransfer" (i.e., they use preconceptions based on their past experience to try to understand their present client). Therapists' preconceptions arise from far more than the therapist's personal problems. They are also based on cultural norms and stereotypes, and on the therapist's professional training. Therapists countertransferentially see clients through the eyes of both psychiatric diagnoses and their pet theories. For a psychodynamic therapist, *seeing* a client's response as trans-

ference may be an example of the therapist's countertransference!

As I have already noted, therapists' personal reactions can be productively used in therapy if they are expressed therapeutically and owned as the therapists' own reaction rather than presented as objective truth about the client. Therapists need to listen to clients to see whether their perceptions and reactions are fitting with the client's experience. In other words, therapists need to notice discrepancies between their perceptions of their clients and their clients' actual reactions, whether these perceptions are based on theory, cultural background, or personal experience.

What is important is that both therapists and clients engage in a process of getting to know what is unique and different about this person and this situation compared to the past. The question is: Is the individual exploring preconceptions in order to modify them over time and truly get to know this person or situation? This process is crucial for effective coping in life. This is the process the therapist must develop for him- or herself and the process that person-centered therapy models for the client through its emphasis on acceptance and open exploration.

The concepts of transference and countertransference grow out of a traditional medical view of psychotherapy in which the personal is kept separate from the professional. However in person-centered theory the personal *is* the professional in an important sense. If I, as the therapist, have a personal reaction to my client, the issue is how can I use that therapeutically, not "can I eliminate it?" If I have a similar unfinished problem that my client has, this will harm my therapeutic relationship only if it blinds me to how my client is uniquely experiencing the problem. On the other hand, I can use my struggle with the problem to help me empathize. There is no need to resolve the problem in order to be therapeutic as long as I continue to check my perceptions and listen. Sometimes it is therapists who have resolved their problems who are *most* likely to impose *their* solutions on the client.

CURATIVE FACTORS OR MECHANISMS OF CHANGE

For person-centered and experiential therapies, therapy is more a process of creation than of repair. Some therapies focus on repairing damage from the past. However, for person-centered and experiential therapy the focus is on forging creative new ways of synthesizing old experience, which carry one forward beyond old ways of being. As part of that process, old traumatic experiences will be related to in new ways, allowing them to be worked through and more productively incorporated into personal functioning. A person who was abused as a child may come to appreciate and value the processes whereby she managed to preserve herself and survive. She may gain from that a sense of strength rather than one of weakness. She may use her experience to develop her own sensitivity and capacity for caring. Working through past trauma is therefore not really repairing damage as much as it is learning how to assimilate and reorganize traumatic experience in order to mobilize potential.

Because the therapy process is creative, therapists will often have no idea of the new solutions that will emerge from the therapy process. Mahoney (1991) and others have talked about Ilya Prigogine's research in chemistry and physics, which has found that systems confronted with disorganization will sometimes spontaneously jump to entirely new, more sophisticated levels of organization. Person-centered and experiential therapists believe this is what often happens in therapy.

The therapist does not therefore have to be the expert who knows the answer. Rather, the therapist must be a "process expert" who can facilitate this creative process. In developmental psychology those who follow the Piagetian approach do not believe that children can be taught to go from one developmental level to another. Yet if children who are at the same developmental level are brought together to discuss a problem, their collaboration often moves both of them to a higher level (Perret-Clermont, Perret, & Bell, 1991). Similarly, person-centered and experiential therapists try to provide a dialogical and exploratory *process* that will result in the emergence of new, creative, and more sophisticated ways of functioning. Two heads are better than one, even if neither "knows" the solution—or even the path—in advance.

The provision by person-centered and experiential therapists of an engaged, experientially supportive, and empathic relationship will provide a "conflict-free zone" that mobilizes the client's "critical intelligence." Clients will begin to become curious about their own experience and perceptions and begin to explore them. This exploratory process will lead to the creative synthesis of incongruencies between different thoughts and perspectives or thoughts and experiences. It will lead to clients learning to incorporate and include all their experience. Clients will feel free to try out new behaviors, and to fail with them, before they refine them so that they become truly effective.

A sense of *efficacy* develops: I can learn and change and move my life forward. One learns that one can struggle with something one is up against and make some productive accommodation with it, no matter how awful the problem. For instance, a client may learn to live productively even if paralyzed. One learns that life is a process of continual confrontation of problems and challenges and of moving onward—the goal of life is not necessarily personal fulfillment or happiness, in contrast to what some other humanistic therapies hold.

Person-centered and experiential therapists do not explicitly teach life skills, as do some behavioral approaches. Nevertheless, the process is one in which such skills as learning to explore and to listen to one's experience, as well as good communication skills, are modeled and experienced. The client learns that there is something valuable and trustworthy in everyone's experience and that it is better to listen to others than it is to impose one's will and values upon them. Dialoguing in an open, cooperative way about mutual problems is the best way to find a solution and mobilizes the "wisdom of the group." Respecting different ways is not only interpersonally important but fosters the creativity that comes from openness to difference.

Focusing-oriented, process–experiential, and Gestalt therapists would all agree with the previous description. In addition, each specifically emphasizes a mechanism of change. Process–experiential therapy stresses a process of accessing emotion which allows for the restructuring of emotion schemes. Focusing-oriented therapy stresses the importance of clients tuning into the bodily felt sense of their problems and turning that felt sense into words. This leads to a creative unfolding process which produces a bodily shift in how the problem is experienced, acompanied by a bodily felt reorganization of the problem in a new, more productive way. Gestalt therapy emphasizes the importance of removing blocks to contact and awareness, which then frees up the person's intrinsic capacities for creative growth.

Insight

The acquiring of insight is not a primary change mechanism in person-centered or experiential therapy, although clients often may attain it. Change often occurs without insight (Meyer, 1981). It is the direct experience of the therapy relationship itself that has the most impact. *What* one learns about oneself is less important than *the changes that come about in how* one relates to oneself, to others, and to problematic experience. These are complex, lived, whole-bodied changes that occur in an experiential man-

ner rather than being guided "from above" by insight.

Because *self*-exploration is the important key, interpretations are generally not used in person-centered therapies. The therapist does not try to bring "news" to the client or to give the client insights.

The Role of the Therapist's Personality

I have previously described how the therapist's ability to be congruent and to be a real person in therapy is crucial to the change process. Good therapists would seek out their own therapy whenever it appeared that their problems or personalities were getting in the way of providing a therapeutic environment for the client.

Factors That Limit the Success of Person-Centered and Experiential Therapies

Practically all the factors that limit the success of person-centered and experiential therapists have to do with whether the client is willing to actively engage in the tasks of therapy. First, although person-centered and experiential therapists have developed ways of working with unmotivated clients (e.g., Gendlin, 1967), effectiveness is limited by low client motivation. Clients who are in therapy against their will, such as those who are court-referred or adolescents brought by their parents, are more difficult to work with. The establishment of a good relationship becomes even more central with such populations.

Second, clients with whom it is difficult to establish a relationship will limit the effectiveness of person-centered and experiential therapy. Some clients labeled with "borderline personality disorder," for instance, are difficult to work with not because their personality structure is primitive but because some have difficulty staying with the frustrations that are a normal part of the working environment of therapy. If a strong therapeutic alliance can be formed, I believe these clients can be worked with effectively.

It has been asserted at times that person-centered therapy in particular is not useful with "nonverbal" clients. However, person-centered therapists have had success with nonverbal schizophrenics (Gendlin, 1967). Prouty (1990) recently developed techniques for working with both severely regressed schizophrenics and persons with mental retardation. Sometimes when people talk about nonverbal clients what they mean are lower-class clients. Aside from the fact that this is a "classist" position and that lower-class people are every bit as verbal as anyone else, Lerner (1972) has found evidence that person-centered therapy can help with lower-class clients as well.

Aspects Shared with Other Approaches

A number of aspects of person-centered and experiential therapies are shared by other approaches. The emphasis on the relationship has been adopted by most therapy approaches. Empathy is now valued by virtually all approaches, although different therapies mean different things by it (Bohart & Greenberg, 1997). The idea of using one's personal reactions in therapy rather than trying to exclude them is now being emphasized in psychoanalytic object relations therapy and in some of the newer behavior therapies (e.g., Kohlenberg & Tsai, 1991). Therapist self-disclosure has become more highly emphasized by many psychodynamic therapists as well. The importance of accessing emotion and experiencing is becoming more and more emphasized in cognitive therapy.

TREATMENT APPLICABILITY AND ETHICAL CONSIDERATIONS

Person-centered and experiential therapies have been used with a wide range of client problems, including alcoholism, schizophrenia, anxiety disorders, and personality disorders. They have also been used with individuals with a mental handicap and the elderly (cf. Lietaer et al., 1990). Process–experiential therapy has been successfully applied to the treatment of depression (Greenberg & Watson, 1998). Focusing-oriented therapy has been used with a variety of problems, including borderline personality disorders and cancer (cf. Greenberg, Elliott, & Lietaer, 1994). A number of person-centered therapists have been developing models for working with families and couples (cf. Levant & Shlien, 1984; Lietaer et al., 1990). Emotionally focused therapy (Johnson & Boisvert, 2002), a variant on process–experiential therapy, is an empirically supported approach for couples. Person-centered therapy was originally developed in a child guidance clinic and person-centered play therapy has been used successfully with children (Bratton & Ray, 2002).

With children, a good relationship in which the child learns that he or she is valuable, understandable, and acceptable through the therapist's empathy, congruence, and acceptance is even more a primary change agent than in adult psychotherapy. The therapy format is one in which the child and the therapist play, and feelings are talked about in that context. Similarly, establishing a good therapeutic bond is the primary treatment goal with adolescents. Many adolescents are in therapy against their will and do not trust adults. Establishing a trustful empathic relationship in which the therapist is willing to be open is already therapeutic, regardless of what issues are talked about. Santen (1990) has also used focusing with traumatized children and adolescents.

The philosophy of person-centered and experiential therapies makes them particularly appropriate for work with women, minorities, people of different cultural backgrounds, or people of alternative sexual orientations. This is because the therapist is not an "expert" who is going to impose the "right way of being" on the client but, rather, is a "fellow explorer" who tries to enter the life world of the client in a curious, interested, accepting, and open way. The therapist tries to work from the frame of reference of what the client thinks is important. Paradoxically, this might lead the therapist to become somewhat more directive with a client who might want directiveness based on his or her cultural background, at least until the client become comfortable taking the "reins" into his or her own hands.

Working with people who come from experiential backgrounds different from the therapist, however, imposes a particular burden on therapists to continually check to make sure their perceptions of their clients' experience are not being colored by their own backgrounds and preconceptions. Despite *philosophically* being compatible with working with people of diverse cultural backgrounds, person-centered and experiential therapists, as all therapists, must be careful that their *implicit* cultural assumptions do not color what they do (Johnson, 2001). O'Hara (1996) has analyzed a film of Carl Rogers working with a woman and has pointed out how Rogers's implicit cultural assumptions, particularly about autonomy, interfere with his hearing her. Johnson (2001) has argued that person-centered, experiential, and other humanistic therapists, because of their philosophical commitment to respect diversity, may paradoxically overlook how their implicit cultural assumptions may shape their beliefs about autonomy, expression of emotion, authenticity, empathy and so on.

None of the person-centered therapies discussed in this chapter would be the treatment of choice for problems where the teaching and learning of specific skills is important, as is the case in sex therapy. I would refer clients if there were specific skills that I do not have that could help them. Certain problems are best treated by behavioral methods, for instance. I would not require a

client to obtain medication, but with certain kinds of problems (such as major affective disorders), I would make the client aware of the availability of medication and tell the client that there is a good possibility that his or her problem would be alleviated by it.

As a person-centered therapist I would neither recommend nor not recommend that potential clients enter therapy. I would talk it over to help the client arrive at his or her own decision.

There are no particular ethical issues unique to the use of person-centered or experiential therapy. However, the egalitarian, democratic stance of the therapist, along with the belief in clients' self-healing potential, can sometimes create a disparity with the perspectives of other professionals. The problem is that person-centered and experiential therapists do not adopt an "expert" stance vis-à-vis the client. Although they may have expertise, they share it with their clients in a collaborative, nonauthoritarian way and do not prescribe treatment for the client. For instance, they would not decide for a client who had been sexually abused as a child that the number-one priority of therapy must be working with the abuse (as many abuse therapists hold). Yet the field of psychotherapy is currently increasingly adopting a "medical" view in which the therapist is the "expert/professional" who decides on the course of treatment. Because a crucial part of person-centered and experiential therapy is to trust the client's judgment, if a client chose not to explore his or her childhood abuse, the therapist would go along with that decision. This might bother therapists who believe it is the expert professional's role to decide what focus is best.

This does not mean a person-centered or experiential therapist would go along with any decision a client made. There are cases when a person-centered or experiential therapist has to choose to impose his or her judgment upon the client, though this is avoided as often as possible. Person-centered and experiential therapists have loyalties to society as well as to their clients and would take action to protect others from a client's choices if necessary. As a member of society I would also make a personal choice to have an acutely suicidal client hospitalized, even against my client's judgment. However, I would take the responsibility for my decision—I did it because I wanted to save the client's life—rather than because I the expert know what is "best for" my client.

Generally there are a number of different indicators that a person-centered or experiential therapist might look for as signs that therapy is being effective. These indicators include greater client access to and acceptance of feelings and experiencing; a greater sense of client self-acceptance and self-trust; signs of the client showing more initiative in making personal choices; signs that the client is beginning to relate more as an equal to the therapist; more client comfort with personal self-disclosure; and signs that the client can better tolerate, face up to, and continue to try to master adversity. Gestalt therapists would particularly look for signs that the client was better able to stay in immediate contact in the therapy hour. Ultimately, because client-centered and experiential therapists place their trust in clients' increasing capacities to know their own experience, the single most important criterion of effectiveness is the client's own judgment that he or she is making progress.

RESEARCH SUPPORT

Research on Therapy Outcome

Elliott (2002) conducted a meta-analysis of research on experiential psychotherapies. Ninety-nine therapy conditions were examined; 53 were of person-centered/nondirective psychotherapy, 24 were of process–experiential psychotherapy and emotionally focused therapy for couples, and 7 were of Gestalt therapy. The remaining 15 were on a variety of other experiential psychotherapies. An overall "effect size" for how much change experiential therapies brought about was calculated. This was 1.06, where a large effect size is considered to be 0.80 or higher. Comparing these therapies to cognitive-behavioral therapy, Elliott concluded that these therapies are equivalent to cognitive-behavioral therapy in effectiveness.

Analyzing these findings by type of psychotherapy, the overall effect size for the effectiveness of person-centered therapy compared to control groups that did not receive psychotherapy was 0.80. For process–experiential psychotherapy it was 0.86, for emotionally focused therapy for couples it was 1.59, and for Gestalt therapy it was 1.05. The conclusion is that there is substantial evidence for the effectiveness of these psychotherapies. There is less evidence on focusing-oriented psychotherapy. However, there is evidence that focusing can be effective for coping with cancer, dealing with weight problems, and working with public speaking anxiety (cf. Greenberg et al., 1994). There have also been studies finding focusing to be effective with prison inmates, the elderly, health-related concerns, and stress management (Hendricks, 2002).

Other evidence (Elliott, 2002; Elliott et al., in press) indicates that person-centered and experiential therapies are effective for problems of depression, anxiety, "mixed neurotic" problems, schizophrenia and personality disorders, health-related problems, problems of minor adjustment, and relationship problems. Bratton and Ray (2002) have concluded that humanistic play therapy, particularly person-centered, for children has empirical support for its effectiveness. In most of these areas the evidence is strong enough to meet criteria for "empirically supported therapy" (Chambless & Hollon, 1998; see below).

Research on Therapy Process

Rogers emphasized two qualities of importance to successful therapy: the active self-healing agency of the client and the therapeutic relationship. Rogers hypothesized that clients have the capacities to heal themselves if they have a warm, empathic, and supportive relationship within which they can engage in the kind of self-exploration/self-examination process which leads to personal evolution. What is the evidence for this proposition?

Bohart and Tallman (1999), Duncan and Miller (2000), and Wampold (2001) all have concluded after reviewing the literature that therapy is primarily a process of mobilizing clients' capacities for change. For instance, client involvement is one of the best predictors of change in therapy. In addition, there is evidence that humans have more capacity for resilience and self-change when confronted with personal problems than once thought (Bohart & Tallman, 1999). Finally, Rennie (2002) has found that clients are highly active and agentic in how they pursue their aims in therapy, picking and choosing what they want to use from therapists' communications, subtly trying to influence the therapist if they feel the therapist is off-track, and so on. In sum, Rogers's faith that clients have considerable capacities for self-healing, and that it is they who make therapy work, has received research support.

Second, research has generally shown that the single most important thing that therapists provide is the therapeutic relationship (Bozarth, Zimring, & Tausch, 2002). In keeping with Rogers's hypothesis, the relationship seems to be a stronger predictor of outcome than the use of therapeutic techniques (Bohart, Elliott, Greenberg, & Watson, 2002). Rogers's (1957) hypothesized that the necessary and sufficient conditions for psychotherapy to work were the therapist's level of warmth, empathy, and genuineness. It has not been shown that these conditions specifically are necessary and sufficient, although there is evidence linking them to psychotherapy outcome. Of the three, the strongest links to outcome are for empathy and acceptance/positive regard. Recently, Bohart and colleagues (2002) performed a meta-analysis of studies relating empathy to therapy outcome. An effect size of 0.32 was found, suggesting a moderate relationship between empathy and outcome.

Farber and Lane (2002) similarly studied all the research on positive regard and concluded that that also bore a positive relationship to therapeutic outcome. For instance, for 16 recent studies, the average effect size of the relationship of positive regard to various positive indices of therapeutic progress was 0.33 (calculated from their published data). This again suggests a moderate relationship. Recently, Miller (2000), after reviewing research on recovery from addictions, has concluded that love may be the best explanation for what causes change. In particular, Miller stresses the acceptant quality of love: the client experiences acceptance "*as he or she really is*" (Miller, 2000, Internet version, p. 6, italics in the original).

The research on congruence/genuineness and self-disclosure is more ambiguous. Klein, Kolden, Michels, and Chisholm-Stockard (2002) have reviewed the research and have found a weaker but still positive relationship between therapist genuineness and therapeutic outcome. They found that of 61 relationships studied, 20 showed a significant relationship and 41 were nonsignificant but not negative. This suggests that genuineness sometimes bears a positive relationship to therapeutic outcome and sometimes does not. The evidence on self-disclosure is similar (see also Hill & Knox, 2002), although recently Barrett and Berman (2001) conducted a study in which they deliberately had therapists self-disclose either a lot or a little. They found that high self-disclosure was related to greater symptom reduction and greater liking by clients for the therapist.

Another hypothesis about therapy process has concerned the role of experiencing and emotion in facilitating change. Gendlin (1996) has emphasized the importance of the client's tuning into his or her own experiencing process, which is supported by evidence. Hendricks (2002) concludes that 50 studies have found that the client's level of "focusing" (the degree to which the client is tuning into his or her experience) is correlated with therapy outcome. With regard to emotion, there is evidence that emotional activation is also important in facilitating change in many therapeutic conditions (Elliott et al., in press).

In conclusion, Rogers's two major hypotheses—concerning the importance of the client's self-healing capacities and the importance of the relationship—have both received research support. Focusing and emotional activation are also important factors in bringing about change.

CASE ILLUSTRATION

Marcie, age 38, came for therapy because of a serious relationship conflict. She had been engaged to marry Sam, but a few weeks before the marriage she had called it off. This had happened because a man with whom she had had a prior relationship, Jack, had reappeared in her life. Marcie was a nurse who had previously been married. This marriage had been brief and stormy and had ended when she was 26. Since then she had been in and out of a series of relationships.

During the initial meeting Marcie related that she loved Sam, but was feeling torn between Sam and Jack. About 2 years previously she had had an intense relationship with Jack. She had been in love, but Jack had eventually broken off the relationship. This had led to depression and a brief hospitalization. She had eventually met Sam through a mutual friend. Sam was a 45-year-old high school teacher, quiet, solid, and stable. He and Marcie liked many of the same things, such as jogging and hiking.

Marcie had not had a lot of stability in her life. Her father had been an explosive

man who had physically abused her and her older brother. Her mother was a traditional housewife who managed the children and tried to keep the family together. After Marcie left home in her early 20s she had met a man at a singles bar who seemed exciting and charismatic. They plunged into a passionate relationship which culminated in marriage 3 months later. The marriage had lasted only 2 years. They started to fight and eventually her husband had left her for another woman.

Marcie blamed herself for the failure of her marriage. She said that she had intimacy problems and problems with commitment. She reported that about 9 months into the marriage she herself had had a brief affair with a coworker. She blamed this affair on her impulsivity. Marcie had broken off the affair shortly after it had started but had felt immensely guilty. She wondered whether her guilt had affected her marriage. Even though she did not think her husband had ever explicitly known about the affair, he had probably sensed something was wrong and this may have led to their fights.

After the failure of her marriage Marcie had had a number of other stormy relationships. She reported that she would get attracted quickly and get involved too soon. She said she had picked a variety of "losers." One man had been older, had never been married, and had lived with his mother. Several men, initially charming, had turned out to be playboys. Another man had wanted her, but he had been overly possessive. Still another man, who she had thought promising, had been getting over a prior relationship. She had not been able to stand the ambiguity of waiting around to find out if he would ever be emotionally available.

Jack was a successful businessman who loved the arts. They attended operas, concerts, and art shows together. Jack's second divorce had happened about 2 years previously. He was loving and kind but reported that he was not interested in getting married again. Marcie found it maddening that they got along so well but that he would not make a commitment. Eventually they had broken up because Jack had found her "too clingy."

Marcie reported a history of moodiness and emotional instability. She was prone to depression and when she got depressed it was hard to get out of it. She had been suicidal in the past, although she was not now. She had been in and out of psychotherapy and had been on various psychotropic medications. One therapist, exasperated with Marcie's unstable relationship behavior and suicidal feelings when she was in her late 20s, had told her that she was a "borderline personality disorder." To her that meant she was a fundamentally flawed person.

The presenting problems as defined by Marcie were as follows: First, she felt deeply confused as to what to do about Jack and Sam. Sam was waiting for her, but she was not sure how long he would wait. Second, Marcie believed that this conflict represented a deeper issue: that she had commitment problems. Third, she wondered if she indeed had a borderline personality disorder. Specifically she worried about her "impulsivity." Next, Marcie was moderately overweight and was hoping that if she could master her impulsivity she could learn to control her eating.

From my person-centered/experiential perspective I did not focus on whether Marcie was a "borderline personality disorder" with intimacy and impulsivity problems. My goal was to listen to and relate to her as a person struggling to make her way through that complicated and difficult thing called "living." I was hoping that by empathically connecting with her she would be able to mobilize her own internal resources for self-change, growth, and coping. I was much more interested in focusing on, appreciating, and understanding her concrete lived experience, including her concrete choices, than I was on abstract diagnostic categories such as "borderline personality disorder." Accordingly, in the first session we started where Marcie wanted to start—her relationship with Jack.

A few weeks before her scheduled marriage to Sam, Jack had reappeared in her life. He had called her and they had met for dinner. He said he wanted to resume their relationship. He did not explicitly offer commitment, but he said he missed Marcie and he was now open to the possibility. Marcie was tempted. Specifically, she felt sexually tempted. Marcie had held off sexually that night, but she was unsure whether she would be able to hold off if she saw Jack again.

Marcie began to explore her relationship with Jack. As she did so, I empathically reflected her experience. Jack had been loving at times, but he was inconsistent. Sometimes he was close; other times he was distant and closed. Marcie had blamed this on herself. She thought she must be doing something that blocked his being able to make more of a commitment to her. She had tried repeatedly to be open, caring, and loving, but Jack had grown more distant and finally had broken off the relationship.

Marcie then said: "I'm tired of being alone, Dr. Bohart. I'd really like to be married. But I want to make the right decision for myself. Sam is very consistent and trustworthy. But I loved Jack so much, and now he says he's ready for a committed relationship. I'm afraid that when I see him again I might go to bed with him and get involved with him again just 'cause it feels so good to get his attention. But I really think I need to meet with him and give myself the chance to find out what I want to do. My head is saying that Sam is better for me. But I feel so drawn to Jack. I don't know what to trust or what to believe." I empathized with the dilemma Marcie was feeling: "It feels so lousy to be alone. You'd really like to have someone to love you. And suddenly here are two possibilities. Sam seems to love you, but here Jack is again. And there's a lot of unfinished business with Jack. You're not sure if he isn't the right one for you." Marcie then went on to speculate: "But maybe this is all just my problem with intimacy. Maybe I'm just afraid of getting involved with Sam so that now, when Jack reappears, I find an excuse to back away from Sam." I empathized with this too: "You really doubt your own motives. You don't know if your interest in Jack is legitimate or if it comes out of intimacy problems." I added on an empathic speculation: "That must feel awful paralyzing." She said, "Yes! That's the trouble—I don't know what is really legitimate about my own feelings."

Later in the session Marcie asked me whether I thought she should break up with Sam and get reinvolved with Jack. I certainly did not know and disclosed my empathic sense of her confusion: "If I were in your shoes I think I'd feel as confused as you. The scary part for me would be the fear I might make make a wrong choice. I sense that may be true for you but I'm not sure. And you don't even know what's drawing you back to him or whether or not it can be trusted."

As I continued to empathically respond, Marcie continued to focus on her ambivalence. She accessed a growing sense of danger about getting reinvolved with Jack. She began to trust a funny feeling that something was "wrong with the picture." Maybe it was the way in which Jack had hesitated when he said that he was now more open to the possibility of a committed relationship? With a more differentiated sense of her own experience, Marcie was able to listen and explore when she met with Jack that night. She discovered that she did indeed have reservations as to how much she could trust him. Further, she was able to identify one of the sources of that distrust as a sense that Jack had possibly come back to her because he was lonely. Another source of the distrust was that Marcie had an increasingly clear sense that the relationship with him had been, and would likely continue to be, imbalanced, with her taking care of him but not with him taking care of her. With these in mind she was able to forego getting sexually reinvolved with Jack, thus giving herself time to figure out what she wanted to do.

As Marcie continued to explore her feelings both in therapy and in two other meetings with Jack, she increasingly came to realize that she could trust herself to reliably explore her own perceptions and come to intelligent, considered judgments. Ultimately she chose not to get reinvolved with Jack. Furthermore, she began to realize that her "impulsivity" was sometimes a lack of self-trust. Because she had felt she could not trust her capacity to explore her perceptions and make reliable judgments, she had tended to "leap" without looking (because she did not trust her capacity to look). Often it was fear and desperation, born out of her lack of trust in her judgmental capacity, that led her to make impulsive choices.

Evocative Unfolding

As she began to trust her capacity for choice, Marcie also began to focus on the self-perception that she had an "evil tendency" inside to sabotage a relationship whenever it began to get too serious. She brought up the example of ruining her first marriage by having an affair. She was self-critical and could not understand why she had done this. For her it was a problematic reaction point. She had always attributed it to her impulsivity. I suggested it might be interesting to go back to the moment she actually chose to commence the affair. I suggested the evocative unfolding technique.

In the evocative unfolding procedure the therapist helps the client to reenter a situation in which a problematic reaction occurred in as much vivid, experiential detail as possible. Then, using highly vivid empathic reflections the therapist helps the client explore his or her reaction. As we worked to get a vivid sense of the circumstances surrounding her decision to begin this first affair, Marcie remembered that she had gone home with a colleague after an office party when her husband was out of town. As she worked toward the fateful moment when she decided to go back to the colleague's apartment, she began to unpack her memory in more detail. Memories flooded back of the feeling of deep connection and intimacy she had experienced talking to the colleague at the party. He had really listened to her. She remembered how her feelings about her marriage had gushed out. She had not realized how lonely and abandoned she had been feeling. She remembered telling him that her husband drank. For the two previous nights he had been completely unavailable: sitting on the couch drinking himself into a stupor. This had been going on for months. This pattern had made her doubt the marriage, but she had pushed these doubts aside, unable to trust her perceptions either that there was something wrong or that it was not her fault. The sense of connection with the colleague felt so good that when he asked her if she wanted to leave the party and get a drink somewhere else she had agreed. They had gone to a bar and one thing had led to another. The affair was brief; her colleague wanted her to leave her husband for him. However, she felt too guilty and she had ended it.

Realizing that there was some sense in her "impulsive" decision to have an affair did not make Marcie approve of her behavior. Rather, it led to a more realistic evaluation of it. She realized that it still was not probably the best way to handle the situation, but she also realized that it made sense given the circumstances. She felt more forgiving toward herself. She also began to evaluate other examples of her "dysfunctional" behavior in relationships and began to discover that, on a finer-grained look, there had been some "wisdom" in those choices as well. She began to shift her self-perception from "There is something horribly wrong with me" to "I am a sensible person, although I don't always make the best choices."

Empty-Chair Technique

In an early session Marcie had mentioned that her father had physically abused her.

Many therapists would have become directive at that point and focused Marcie's attention on the abuse. This is an example of being *content directive*—the therapist decides what content the client will focus on. In contrast, I followed Marcie's process. I believed that as she explored the topics of immediate relevance to her, and as she gained more and more of a sense of self-trust and self-efficacy, she would come to explore the abuse experience if and when it became meaningful for her to do so.

At one point Marcie started talking about her feelings of negative self-worth. She brought up an example of feeling self-critical because she had no children and it was probably too late to do so. She knew that her parents saw her as a failure because of this. Her father particularly had been critical of her for not having been able to get in a stable marriage and have children. I suggested the empty-chair procedure as a possible aid to help her explore and understand her feelings vis a vis her father. She sat facing an empty chair. She was to imagine that her father was in the empty chair. Then I had her switch chairs and begin a dialogue by role-playing her father. As her father she forcefully expressed criticisms: "You really have mismanaged your life. Here you are age 38 and you're not even married yet. Furthermore, you cannot even manage your own emotions. You ended up in the hospital a while ago. You really need to get your act together."

Then Marcie switched chairs. In the other chair she assumed a demeanor that reminded me of a beaten child. She was unable to defend herself. She stopped the exercise and began to spontaneously explore her abuse experiences with her father. He had a volatile temper, and more than once he had hit her—hard. There had been bruises, but in those days teachers did not report suspected child abuse, and Marcie had been too ashamed to say anything to anyone. He was also extremely critical. As Marcie explored this she began to become directly aware of how her attention in that relationship had been so exclusively focused on pleasing her father and avoiding his wrath that she had not had any left over to focus on what *she* wanted or what *she* thought, thereby paralyzing her own ability to think critically. As she focused on her reactions of fear and fright she also began to recognize directly how she had lost a sense of herself in that relationship.

Several sessions later Marcie suggested trying the empty chair again. Over a period of two more sessions, Marcie used this procedure to work out her feelings toward her father. She cycled through several emotions. First, she expressed fear and hurt toward him. Then she accessed anger and was able to say assertively that she would not let his criticisms paralyze her any more. This fit in with her developing sense of herself as being able to trust herself and make her own judgments. As this sense grew stronger Marcie began to access some sadness toward her father. It was almost as if she went through a process of mourning the relationship she wished she had been able to have with her father but never had and never would have. Finally she began to feel some forgiveness toward him and acceptance of who he was.

A Theoretical Note

It would be instructive to contrast a person-centered view of how Marcie's childhood affected her with a psychodynamic view. A psychodynamic view might assume that Marcie's pattern of poor relationships with men was due to her choosing men, albeit unconsciously, in order to re-create the kind of relationship she had with her father. However, from a person-centered perspective Marcie was not trying to re-create her relationship with her father. Rather, her motives were the same motives everyone has in trying to form a relationship: wanting intimacy, sharing, sex, and support.

Yet she had impulsively and prematurely entered dysfunctional relationships, and when she had left them, she criticized herself for intimacy problems, overlooking problems in the relationships themselves. Why? From a person-centered perspective, her childhood experiences with her father had created an extreme form of self-distrust in Marcie. She was afraid of men and unable to trust her feelings and critically evaluate the men with whom she got involved. Having no sense of self-trust, she had leapt into relationships without "looking" carefully. The result was that she had chosen several poor partners, usually basing her decision on some superficial characteristic that seemed initially promising. Even if she had fortuitously made a good choice, her fear and her lack of self-trust made her think all problems were her fault. This fear paralyzed her ability to discuss and solve problems that did come up in the relationship.

As Marcie began to trust her own feelings and judgmental capacity, she became more and more adept at evaluating what was going on in her life in terms of whether or not it was truly meeting her needs. A distinct felt shift had occurred. She now had a direct sense of herself trying to take care of herself in relationship contexts rather than of herself as a negative force ruining her relationships. She began to feel more proactive and more hopeful about making good choices in the future.

Conclusion

I saw Marcie 35 times on a once-a-week basis over a period of about 10 months. In general, how did she do and why did we terminate? Did we stop because she was completely cured, no longer showing any borderline symptoms, as slim as she wanted to be, no longer depressed, relationship problems all solved, and safely ensconced in a new, more rewarding relationship with Sam?

Things did not turn out *this* rosy. Generally, in terms of her presenting problem, Marcie's conflicts over Jack had been resolved. She had increased trust in her capacity to form a good relationship, and she and Sam were working on their relationship. Sam had waited for her, but Sam had been injured by the process, so there was work to do to reestablish trust. Marcie still was bothered by mood instability. She still got easily depressed and had a hard time fighting out of it, although she handled it better now than she had in the past. However, she was better able to avoid making impulsive choices. On the other hand, she still was overweight.

As is typical of my experience with person-centered therapy, termination was not a problem. At first Marcie chose to cut down from once a week to once every 2 weeks. Then she decided to go for a while without coming in. She eventually came in once or twice more. Then, several months later I heard from her by phone that she was doing okay and that she and Sam seemed to be working out their problems. She would come back "if needed." It has now been several years since that telephone call and I have not seen her again.

I do not believe Marcie was "cured" or that she may never again need therapy. I would have liked to work with her longer to consolidate the gains she had made and to explore more thoroughly the impact of her early abuse. I would have preferred to work with her and Sam as a couple (Sam had rejected this idea). However, I trusted Marcie to take care of herself and to return if she felt the need to. I knew she would still be bothered by depression. However, when she left she seemed better able to ride out and transcend these periods rather than to sink into them.

CURRENT AND FUTURE TRENDS

Person-centered and other experiential psychotherapies continue to have wide influence. In a poll conducted by Smith (1982), Carl Rogers was rated the most influential psychotherapist, even over Freud. Although only a small minority of practicing therapists identify themselves as person-centered, experiential, or Gestalt, most therapists cur-

rently consider themselves to be eclectic, and over a third of those combine person-centered and other humanistic–experiential approaches with some other orientation (Norcross & Prochaska, 1988). The influence of the person-centered and other experiential approaches is increasing in Europe, and Bankart, Koshikawa, Nedate, and Haruki (1992) have noted that "among Japanese psychotherapists the work of Carl Rogers is probably more highly regarded than [that of] any other Western theorist . . ." (p. 144). The work of Greenberg and his colleagues (1993) has been one of the major influences in reintroducing psychotherapists to the importance of emotion in therapy. Process–experiential psychotherapy has spawned a vigorous group of young theorists and researchers who are expanding its use into new realms and contributing to our understanding of the process of change in therapy. With the publication of a major book on research on humanistic psychotherapy (Cain & Seeman, 2002) has come a resurgence of interest in person-centered and other experiential approaches.

Another new development is the appearance of two integrative models for therapy practice which are squarely based in assumptions that person-centered and experiential therapists share. These are the "client as active self-healer" approach of Bohart and Tallman (1999) and the "client-directed" approach of Duncan and Miller (2000). Both models build on the idea that clients are active, creative agents in therapy and that therapy must work from within their frames of reference. Techniques and procedures will work only if they jibe with how the client is construing the problem. In addition, Bohart and Tallman emphasize the importance of providing clients with "empathic workspaces," where they feel supported to do their own creative thinking. Duncan and Miller propose a set of criteria for choosing procedures that will be compatible with clients' frames of reference. Miller and Rollnick (2002) have recently integrated person-centered and cognitive-behavioral approaches to create "motivational interviewing," an approach to treating addictions that has received considerable empirical support.

At the same time, person-centered and experiential approaches face threats. These approaches are among a larger group of psychotherapies that are discovery oriented. This group includes psychodynamic, narrative, feminist, and some systemic therapies. The focus of discovery-oriented therapies is on facilitating client exploration and discovery, whether it be of the past, of present experience, of self-in-relationship, or of how one constructs meaning in one's life. Client solutions are *emergents* that arise from this discovery process. As such they are not solutions dictated in advance by therapists. Further, person-centered and experiential psychotherapies believe that by facilitating growth, clients can "grow out of" their psychopathology. Their focus, therefore, is on mobilizing client resources rather than on symptomatology.

Discovery-oriented therapies in general, and person-centered and experiential therapies in particular, find themselves at odds with the dominant model of practice, which is patterned after medicine. In the "medical model" of psychotherapy, the therapist plays a role similar to that of a physician in medicine: someone who is the expert on the client's condition, who diagnoses the client's problem and decides on a treatment plan for the client that will "fix" his or her symptoms. As with medical disorders, it is assumed that different specific "treatments" will be needed to "cure" different "disorders." The problem is that this model dominates the current field of psychotherapy practice, even though research does not support it (Wampold, 2001). Some licensing boards require therapists to diagnose and write "treatment plans" under threat of losing their licenses.

However, person-centered and experiential therapies, as practiced in their pure forms, are not "treatments." The therapy interaction is a dialogical process between two (or more) intelligent beings working together to help one (or more) of those beings resolve problems. Person-centered and experiential therapists view clients as the ultimate experts on what they need to do to change. The idea that the therapist selects the "treatment" for the client's pathology is antithetical to these approaches. Even when an experiential therapist suggests a procedure, such as chair work or focusing, it is not viewed as a "treatment" for patient "conditions" but rather as an experiment or tool that clients can use to enhance their own natural self-healing capacities.

The incompatibility between the dominant medical model and how many person-centered or experiential therapists prefer to practice creates strain. Making matters worse, a task force of the Clinical Psychology Division of the American Psychological Association in 1995 set about defining a narrow set of criteria for evaluating research studies based squarely in the medical model view of psychotherapy. This movement has become the "empirically supported treatments" (EST) movement (Bohart, 2002; Chambless & Hollon, 1998). Only therapies that had been researched in a particular way were to be considered "empirically supported." The criteria included requirements that were incompatible with the "pure" practice of person-centered and many other experiential psychotherapies, such as that they be manualized. Writing a manual for the practice of person-centered therapy is philosophically a contradiction in terms. Yet if the research study did not manualize the therapy it could not be considered empirically supported. It was no surprise that on early lists of EST, nearly 100% were cognitive-behavioral. The potential danger of the EST movement was the loss of legitimization in the current field of practice—this despite the fact that using equally legitimate but broader criteria, all the bona fide major brands of therapy should be considered empirically supported (Wampold, 2001).

The threat to person-centered and experiential therapies has been mitigated by findings from research studies that have used manualized versions of person-centered and other experiential psychotherapies. Elliott and colleagues (in press) conclude that experiential therapies have met the EST criteria for efficacy for many disorders. Nonetheless, many person-centered and experiential therapists continue to believe that the EST movement poses a threat. It potentially constrains the effective practice and development of these therapies in ways that are more intrinsic to their actual natures (Bohart, 2002).

Nonetheless, I believe that the person-centered and experiential approaches to therapy will continue to play an important role in the further development of psychotherapy practice. A new young group of students and practitioners continue to display interest in them, and many clients are drawn to them. They have carved out a meaningful and enduring place alongside other effective approaches such as psychodynamic and cognitive-behavioral therapies.

NOTE

1. Although, interestingly, in the last 2 years some students have begun to say the opposite: that Rogers should tell her *not* to tell her daughter about her sex life because it is a "boundary violation." The interesting point is how much "truth" according to social convention has changed in the last 30 years. From a person-centered point of view, only Gloria will ultimately be able to decide what is the best thing for her particular relationship with her daughter. The goal is to facilitate her in making this decision intelligently. In fact, Gloria did tell her daughter about her sex life and it was a productive experience (John Shlien, personal communication, April 2001).

SUGGESTIONS FOR FURTHER READING

Cain, D. J., & Seeman, J. (Eds.). (2002). *Humanistic psychotherapies: Handbook of research and practice.* Washington, DC: American Psy-

chological Association.—This comprehensive volume summarizes research on each of the approaches covered in this chapter, as well as on humanistic therapy with children, group therapy, relationship variables, the self, and emotion.

Farber, B. A., Brink, D. C., & Raskin, P. M. (Eds.). (1996). *The psychotherapy of Carl Rogers: Cases and commentary.* New York: Guilford Press.—Cases of Carl Rogers with commentaries by eminent psychotherapists from person-centered and other psychotherapeutic traditions.

Gendlin, E. T. (1996). *Focusing-oriented psychotherapy: A manual of the experiential method.* New York: Guilford Press.—This book gives details on practicing focusing-oriented psychotherapy and gives extensive case history material.

Greenberg, L. S., Rice, L. N., & Elliott, R. (1993). *Facilitating emotional change: The moment-by-moment process.* New York: Guilford Press.—This book on process–experiential psychotherapy has detailed case histories at the end.

Lietaer, G., Rombauts, J., & Van Balen, R. (Eds.). (1990). *Client-centered and experiential psychotherapy in the nineties.* Leuven, Belgium: Leuven University Press.—A comprehensive collection of articles on theory, research, and practice of person-centered, process–experiential (before it was named that), and focusing-oriented psychotherapies.

Roberts, A. (Ed.). (2000). *From the radical center: The heart of Gestalt therapy: Selected writings of Erving and Miriam Polster.* Cleveland, OH: Gestalt Institute of Cleveland Press.—A collection of articles by two of the most eminent Gestalt therapists. Includes case material.

REFERENCES

Anderson, W. (1974). Personal growth and client-centered therapy: An information processing view. In D. A. Wexler & L. N. Rice (Eds.), *Innovations in client-centered therapy* (pp. 21–48). New York: Wiley.

Bandura, A. (1986). *Social foundations of thought and action: A social-cognitive analysis.* Englewood Cliffs, NJ: Prentice-Hall.

Bankart, C. P., Koshikawa, F., Nedate, K., & Haruki, Y. (1992). When west meets east: Contributions of eastern traditions to the future of psychotherapy. *Psychotherapy, 29* 141–149.

Barrett, M. S., & Berman, J. S. (2001). Is psychotherapy more effective when therapists disclose information about themselves? *Journal of Consulting and Clinical Psychology, 69,* 597–603.

Barrett-Lennard, G. T. (1993). The phases and focus of empathy. *British Journal of Medical Psychology, 66,* 3–14.

Barrett-Lennard, G. T. (1998). *Carl Rogers' helping system: Journey and substance.* Thousand Oaks, CA: Sage.

Bohart, A. C. (1993). Experiencing: The basis of psychotherapy. *Journal of Psychotherapy Integration, 3,* 51–67.

Bohart, A. C. (2001). A meditation on the nature of self-healing and personality change in psychotherapy based on Gendlin's theory of experiencing. *The Humanistic Psychologist, 29,* 249–279.

Bohart, A. C. (2002). A passionate critique of empirically supported treatments and the provision of an alternative paradigm. In J. C. Watson, R. N. Goldman, & M. Warner (Eds.), *Client-centered and experiential psychotherapy in the twenty-first century: Advances in theory, research and practice* (pp. 258–277). London: PCCS Books.

Bohart, A. C., Elliott, R., Greenberg, L. S., & Watson, J. C. (2002). Empathy. In J. C. Norcross (Ed.), *Psychotherapy relationships that work: Therapist contributions and responsiveness to patients* (pp. 89–108). New York: Oxford University Press.

Bohart, A. C., & Greenberg, L. S. (1997). Empathy and psychotherapy: An introductory overview. In A. C. Bohart & L. S. Greenberg (Eds.), *Empathy reconsidered: New directions in psychotherapy* (pp. 3–32). Washington DC: American Psychological Association.

Bohart, A., & Rosenbaum, R. (1995). The dance of empathy: Empathy, diversity, and technical eclecticism. *The Person-Centered Journal, 2,* 5–29.

Bohart, A., & Tallman, K. (1999). *How clients make therapy work: The process of active self-healing.* Washington, DC: American Psychological Association.

Bozarth, J. D. (1993). Not necessarily necessary but always sufficient. In D. Brazier (Ed.), *Beyond Carl Rogers: Toward a psychotherapy for the 21st century* (pp. 287–310). London: Constable.

Bozarth, J. (1997). Empathy from the framework of client-centered theory and the Rogerian hypothesis. In A. C. Bohart & L. S. Greenberg (Eds.), *Empathy reconsidered: New directions in psychotherapy* (pp. 81–102). Washington, DC: American Psychological Association.

Bozarth, J. D., Zimring, F. M., & Tausch, R. (2002). Client-centered therapy: The evolution of a revolution. In D. J. Cain & J. Seeman (Eds.), *Humanistic psychotherapies: Handbook of research and practice* (pp. 147–188). Washington, DC: American Psychological Association.

Bratton, S. C., & Ray, D. (2002). Humanistic play therapy. In D. J. Cain & J. Seeman (Eds.), *Humanistic psychotherapies: Handbook of research and practice* (pp. 369–402). Washington, DC: American Psychological Association.

Brodley, B. T. (1988). Responses to person-centered versus client-centered? *Renaissance, 5,* 1–2.

Brodley, B. T. (1993). Response to Patterson's "Winds of change for client-centered counseling." *Journal of Humanistic Education and Development, 31,* 139–143.

Cantor, N. (1990). From thought to behavior: "Having" and "doing" in the study of personality and cognition. *American Psychologist, 45,* 735–750,

Caspi, A., Elder, G. H., & Herbener, E. S. (1990). Childhood personality and the prediction of life-course patterns. In L. E. Robins & M. Rutter (Eds.), *Straight and devious pathways from childhood to adulthood* (pp. 13–35). New York: Cambridge University Press.

Chambless, D. L., & Hollon, S. D. (1998). Defining empirically supported therapies. *Journal of Consulting and Clinical Psychology, 66,* 7–18.

Comas-Díaz, L. (1992). The future of psychotherapy with ethnic minorities. *Psychotherapy, 29,* 88–94.

Duncan, B. L., & Miller, S. D. (2000). *The heroic client: Doing client-directed, outcome-informed therapy.* San Francisco: Jossey-Bass.

Dweck, C. S., & Leggett, E. L. (1988). A social-cognitive approach to motivation and personality. *Psychological Review, 95,* 256–273.

Elliott, R. (2002). The effectiveness of humanistic therapies: A meta-analysis. In D. J. Cain & J. Seeman (Eds.), *Humanistic psychotherapies: Handbook of research and practice* (pp. 55–82). Washington, DC: American Psychological Association.

Elliott, R., Greenberg, L. S., & Lietaer, G. (in press). Research on experiential psychotherapies. In M. Lambert, A. Bergin, & S. Garfield (Eds.), *Handbook of psychotherapy and behavior change* (5th ed.). New York: Wiley.

Epstein, R. (1991). Skinner, creativity, and the problem of spontaneous behavior. *Psychological Science, 2,* 362–370.

Farber, B. L., & Lane. J. S. (2002). Positive regard. In J. C. Norcross (Ed.), *Psychotherapy relationships that work: Therapist contributions and responsiveness to patients* (pp. 175–196). New York: Oxford University Press.

Gendlin, E. T. (1967). Therapeutic procedures in dealing with schizophrenics. In C. R. Rogers, E. T. Gendlin, D. J. Kiesler, & C. B. Truax (Eds.), *The therapeutic relationship and its impact* (pp. 369–400). Madison: University of Wisconsin Press.

Gendlin, E. T. (1968). The experiential response. In E. Hammer (Ed.), *Use of interpretation in treatment* (pp. 208–227). New York: Grune & Stratton.

Gendlin, E. T. (1970). A theory of personality change. In J. T. Hart & T. M. Tomlinson (Eds.), *New directions in client-cen-tered therapy* (pp. 129–174). Boston: Houghton Mifflin. [Reprinted from P. Worchel & D. Byrne (Eds.). (1964). *Personality change.* New York: Wiley.]

Gendlin, E. T. (1996). *Focusing-oriented psychotherapy: A manual of the experiential method.* New York: Guilford Press.

Goodman, G. (1984). SASHAtapes: Expanding options for help-intended communication. In D. Larson (Ed.), *Teaching psychological skills: Models for giving psychology away* (pp. 271–286). Monterey, CA: Brooks/Cole.

Gordon, T. (1984). Three decades of democratizing relationships through training. In D. Larson (Ed.), *Teaching psychological skills: Models for giving psychology away* (pp. 151–170). Monterey, CA: Brooks/Cole.

Greenberg, L. S., Elliott, R., & Lietaer, G. (1994). Research on humanistic and experiential psychotherapies. In A. Bergin & S. Garfield (Eds.), *Handbook of psychotherapy and behavior change* (4th ed., pp. 509–542). New York: Wiley.

Greenberg, L. S., & Johnson, S. M. (1988). *Emotionally focused therapy for couples.* New York: Guilford Press.

Greenberg, L. S., Rice, L. N., & Elliott, R. (1993). *Facilitating emotional change: The moment-by-moment process.* New York: Guilford Press.

Greenberg, L. S., & Watson, J. (1998). Experiential therapy of depression: Differential effects of client-centered relationship conditions and process–experiential interventions. *Psychotherapy Research, 8,* 210–224.

Guerney, B. G. (1984). Contributions of client-centered therapy to filial, marital, and family relationship enhancement therapies. In R. F. Levant & J. M. Shlien (Eds.), *Client centered therapy and the person-centered approach: New directions in theory, research, and practice* (pp. 261–277). New York: Praeger.

Hendricks, M. N. (2002). Focusing-oriented/experiential psychotherapy. In D. J. Cain & J. Seeman (Eds.), *Humanistic psychotherapies: Handbook of research and practice* (pp. 221–252). Washington, DC: American Psychological Association.

Hill, C. E., & Knox, S. (2002). Self-disclosure. In J. C. Norcross (Ed.), *Psychotherapy relationships that work: Therapist contributions and responsiveness to patients* (pp. 255–2650). New York: Oxford University Press.

Holdstock, T. L. (1990). Can client-centered therapy transcend its monocultural roots? In G. Lietaer, J. Rombauts, & R. Van Balen (Eds.), *Client-centered and experiential psychotherapy in the nineties* (pp. 109–121). Leuven, Belgium: Leuven University Press.

Holdstock, T. L., & Rogers, C. R. (1983). Person-centered theory. In R. J. Corsini & A. J. Marsella (Eds.), *Personality theories, research, and assessment* (pp. 189–228). Itasca, IL: Peacock.

Johnson, S., & Boisvert, C. (2002). Treating couples and families from the humanistic perspective: More than the symptom, more than solutions. In D. J. Cain & J. Seeman (Eds.), *Humanistic psychotherapies: Handbook of research and practice* (pp. 309–338). Washington, DC: American Psychological Association.

Johnson, Z. (2001). Cultural competency and

humanistic psychology. *The HumanisticPsychologist, 29,* 204–222.

Klein, M. H., Kolden, G. G., Michels, J., & Chisholm-Stockard, S. (2002). Congruence. In J. C. Norcross (Ed.), *Psychotherapy relationships that work: Therapist contributions and responsiveness to patients* (pp. 195–216). New York: Oxford University Press.

Kohlenberg, R. J., & Tsai, M. (1991). *Functional analytical psychotherapy: Creating intense and curative therapeutic relationships.* New York: Plenum Press.

Lerner, B. (1972). *Therapy in the ghetto.* Baltimore: Johns Hopkins University Press.

Levant, R. F., & Shlien, J. M. (Eds.). (1984). *Client-centered therapy and the person- centered approach: New directions in theory, research, and practice.* New York: Praeger.

Lewicki, P. (1986). *Nonconscious social information-processing.* New York: Academic Press.

Lietaer, G. (1991, July). *The authenticity of the therapist: Congruence and transparency.* Paper presented at the 2nd international conference on Client-Centered and Experiential Psychotherapy, Stirling, Scotland.

Lietaer, G., Rombauts, J., & Van Balen, R. (Eds.). (1990). *Client-centered and experiential psychotherapy in the nineties.* Leuven, Belgium: Leuven University Press.

Mahoney, M. (1991). *Human change processes.* New York: Basic Books.

Masten, A. S., Best, K. M., & Garmazy, N. (1990). Resilience and development: Contributions from the study of children who overcome adversity. *Development and Psychopathology, 2,* 425–444.

Meyer, A.-E. (Ed.). (1981). The Hamburg Short Psychotherapy Comparison Experiment. *Psychotherapy and Psycho-somatics, 35,* 81–207.

Miller, W. R. (2000). Rediscovering fire: Small interventions, large effects. *Psychology of Addictive Behaviors, 14,* 6–18 (Internet version, pp. 1–15).

Miller, W. R., & Rollnick, S. (2002). *Motivational interviewing: Preparing people to change* (2nd ed.). New York: Guilford Press.

Neisser, U. (1967). *Cognitive psychology.* New York: Appleton-Century-Crofts.

Norcross, J. C., & Prochaska, J. O. (1988). A study of eclectic (and integrative) views revisited. *Professional Psychology: Research and Practice, 19,* 170–174.

O'Hara, M. M. (1992, April). *Selves-in-context: The challenge for psychotherapy in a postmodern world.* Invited address at the Conference of the Society for the Exploration of Psychotherapy Integration, San Diego, CA.

O'Hara, M. M. (1996). Rogers and Sylvia: A feminist analysis. In B. A. Farber, D. C. Brink, & P. M. Raskin (Eds.), *The psychotherapy of Carl Rogers: Cases and commentary* (pp. 284–300). New York: Guilford Press.

O'Hara, M. M., & Wood, J. K. (1983). Patterns of awareness: Consciousness and the group mind. *The Gestalt Journal, 6,* 103–116.

Perret-Clermont, A.-N., Perret, J.-F., & Bell, N. (1991). The social construction of meaning and cognitive activity in elementary school children. In L. B. Resnick, J. M. Levine, & S. D. Teasley (Eds.), *Perspectives on socially shared cognition* (pp. 41–62). Washington, DC: American Psychological Association.

Prouty, G. F. (1990). Pre-therapy: A theoretical evolution in the person-centered/ experiential psychotherapy of schizophrenia and retardation. In G. Lietaer, J. Rombauts, & R. Van Balen (Eds.), *Client-centered and experiential psychotherapy in the nineties* (pp. 645–658). Leuven, Belgium: Leuven University Press.

Raskin, N. J. (1991, August). *Rogers and Gloria: Listening, respectful, and congruent-Response to Weinrach.* Presentation as part of a symposium on "Carl Rogers and Gloria— Interpreting or listening therapist?" at the annual convention of the American Psychological Association, San Francisco.

Raskin, N. J., & Rogers, C. R. (1989). Person-centered therapy. In R. J. Corsini & D. J. Wedding (Eds.), *Current psychotherapies* (4th ed., pp. 155–194). Itasca, IL: Peacock.

Rennie, D. L. (2002). Experiencing psychotherapy: Grounded theory studies. In D. J. Cain & J. Seeman (Eds.), *Humanistic psychotherapies: Handbook of research and practice* (pp. 117–144). Washington, DC: American Psychological Association.

Rogers, C. R. (1957). The necessary and sufficient conditions of therapeutic personality change. *Journal of Consulting Psychology, 21,* 95–103.

Rogers, C. R. (1961a). *On becoming a person.* Boston: Houghton Mifflin.

Rogers, C. R. (1961b). The process equation of

psychotherapy. *American Journal of Psychotherapy, 15,* 27–45.

Rogers, C. R. (1983). *Freedom to learn for the 80's.* Columbus, OH: Merrill.

Shlien, J. M. (1970). Phenomenology and personality. In J. T. Hart & T. M. Tomlinson (Eds.), *New directions in client-centered therapy* (pp. 95–128). Boston: Houghton Mifflin.

Shlien, J. M. (1984). A countertheory of transference. In R. F. Levant & J. M. Shlien (Eds.), *Client-centered therapy and the person-centered approach: New directions in theory, research, and practice* (pp. 153–181). New York: Praeger.

Shlien, J. M. (1988, September). *The future is more important than the past in determining present behavior.* Paper presented at the 1st international conference on Client-centered and Experiential Psychotherapy, Leuven, Belgium.

Shlien, J. M., & Levant, R. F. (1984). Introduction. In R. F. Levant & J. M. Shlien (Eds.), *Client-centered therapy and the person-centered approach: New directions in theory, research, and practice* (pp. 1–16). New York: Praeger.

Shostrom, E. L. (Producer). (1965). *Three approaches to psychotherapy* [Film]. Orange, CA: Psychological Films.

Smith, D, (1982). Trends in counseling and psychotherapy. *American Psychologist, 37,* 802–809.

Stern, D. N. (1985). *The interpersonal world of the infant: A view from psychoanalysis and developmental psychology.* New York: Basic Books.

Strupp, H. H., & Binder, J. L. (1984). *Psychotherapy in a new key: A guide to time-limited dynamic psychotherapy.* New York: Basic Books.

Strupp, H. H., & Hadley, S. W. (1979). Specific versus nonspecific factors in psychotherapy: A controlled study of outcome. *Archives of General Psychiatry, 36,* 1125–1136.

Toms, M. (1988, January/February). Expressive therapy: Creativity as a path to peace. A conversation with Natalie Rogers. *New Realities,* 13–17.

Van Balen, R. (1990). The therapeutic relationship according to Carl Rogers: Only a climate? A dialogue? Or both? In G. Lietaer, J. Rombauts, & R. Van Balen (Eds.), *Client-centered and experiential psychotherapy in the nineties* (pp. 65–86). Leuven, Belgium: Leuven University Press.

Wampold, B. E. (2001). *The great psychotherapy debate.* Mahwah, NJ: Erlbaum.

Wexler, D. A., & Rice, L. N. (Eds.). (1974). *Innovations in client-centered therapy.* New York: Wiley.

Yontef, G. (1995). Gestalt therapy. In A. Gurman & S. Messer (Eds.), *Essential psychotherapies* (pp. 261–303). New York: Guilford Press.

Zimring, F. (1990). Cognitive processes as a cause of psychotherapeutic change: Self-initiated processes. In G. Lietaer, J. Rombauts, & R. Van Balen (Eds.), *Client-centered and experiential psychotherapy in the nineties* (pp. 361–380). Leuven, Belgium: Leuven University Press.

Zimring, F. (1991, August). *Rogers and Gloria: Genuine and prizing but insufficiently empathic.* Presentation as part of a symposium on "Carl Rogers and Gloria—Interpreting or listening therapist?" at the annual convention of the American Psychological Association, San Francisco.

5

Existential–Humanistic Psychotherapies

Kirk J. Schneider

HISTORICAL BACKGROUND

Existential humanism is rooted in the deepest recesses of recorded time. All who addressed the question "What does it mean to be fully and subjectively alive" have partaken in the existential–humanistic quest. Existentialism derives from the Latin root *ex-sistere,* which literally means to "stand forth" or to "become" (May, 1958, p. 12), whereas humanism originates in the ancient Greek tradition of "knowing thyself" (Grondin, 1995, p. 112). Together, existential humanism embraces the following three values: (1) freedom (e.g., to know oneself), (2) experiential reflection (e.g., to discover what one is becoming), and (3) responsibility (e.g., to act on or respond to what one is becoming).

Although existential humanism has its roots in Socratic, Renaissance, Romantic, and even Asiatic sources (Moss, 1999; Schneider, 1998b; Taylor, 1999), it was not until the mid-19th century that existential philosophy, as such, was formalized. With the advent of Soren Kierkegaard's (1844/1944) *Concept of Dread,* a new era had dawned in which freedom, experiential reflection, and responsibility played an increasingly pivotal philosophical and therapeutic role. In Kierkegaard's thesis, freedom emerges from crisis, and crisis from intellectual, emotional, or physical imprisonment. In Kierkegaard's time, this imprisonment often took the form of acquiescence to the Catholic Church or to objectifying trends in science. In one of the most damning oppositions to social objectification (and doctrinaire living) ever waged, Kierkegaard called for a complete transformation of values. We must move, Kierkegaard exclaimed, from a mechanized or externalized life to one that is centered in the subject, and that struggles for the truth of the subject. It is only through facing and grappling with our selves, Kierkegaard elaborates, that consciousness can expand, deepen, and seek its vibrant potential.

Writing at about the same period, but with an even feistier style, Friedrich Nietzsche (1844–1900) traced the devitalization of conventional culture to the dominance of Apollonian (or rationalist-linear living) over Dionysian (or non-rationalist-spontaneous) living. Although these strains were in tension—in Nietzsche's time, as in the time of the ancient Greeks who formulated them—Nietzsche foresaw the era when Apollonian technocracy would overshadow and level all in its path. To remedy this situation, and to restore the Dionysian spirit, Nietzsche (1889/1982) called for a Dionysian–Apollonian rapprochement. This rapprochement would "afford" people "the whole range and wealth of being natural" but also, and in concert with the latter, the capacity for being "strong, highly educated," and "self-controlled" (p. 554).

The next major revolution in existential–humanistic (E-H) psychology occurred in the early 20th century, with the advent of behaviorism and psychoanalysis. Behaviorism, championed by such advocates as John Watson, stressed the mechanistic and overt aspects of human functioning, whereas psychoanalysis, spearheaded by Freud and his followers, promoted a covert intapsychic determinism. In neither case, existential humanists contended, was the human psyche illuminated in its radiant and enigmatic fullness—its liberating and yet vulnerable starkness—and so they rebelled. Among these rebellions were the rich and far-ranging meditations of William James (1902/1936), Otto Rank (1936), C.G. Jung (1966), and Henry Murray (Murray et al., 1938). But while this group drew tangentially from existential–humanistic philosophy, another group of mainly former Freudians drew directly on the existential–humanistic lineage. Ludwig Binswanger (1958) and Medard Boss (1963), for example, based their psychiatric practices on the existential and phenomenological philosophy of Martin Heidegger (1962) and Edmund Husserl (1913/1962). Expanding on Kierkegaard's emphasis on the subjective, Heidegger developed a philosophy of being. By being, Heidegger meant neither self-enclosed individualism nor deterministic realism but a "lived" amalgam of the two he termed "being-in-the-world." Being-in-the-world" is Heidegger's attempt to illustrate that our Western tradition of separating inner from outer, or subjective from objective, is misleading and that, from the standpoint of experience, there is no clear way to separate them. In a phrase, we are both separate subjective selves *and* related to the external world, according to Heidegger. To develop

his thesis, Heidegger drew on the method and practices of phenomenology, originated by his mentor, Edmund Husserl. According to Husserl (1913/1962), the chief task of phenomenology is to apprehend human experience in its living reality; that is, in its full subjective and intersubjective context (see also Churchill & Wertz, 2001; Giorgi, 1970).

By the 1960s, E-H psychotherapy evolved into a mature and recognized movement, but it was also a diverse movement. Whereas most existential–humanistic practitioners stressed freedom, experiential reflection, and responsibility, they did so with varying degrees of intensity. There were times, for example, such as in the aftermath of World War II, and during the flowering of the human potential movement of the 1960s, when existential freedom may have been stressed to the neglect of responsibility (e.g., see May, 1969, 1981; Merleau-Ponty, 1962; Yalom, 1980), or other times when responsibility was accented to the detriment of freedom (Rowan, 2001) or experiential reflection to the neglect of responsibility (Spinelli, 2001), and so on. These controversies persist today.

However, today's E-H practitioners have an advantage over those of their predecessors—hindsight. With such hindsight, many contemporary E-H therapists are wary of one-sided formulations, be they of the existential–humanistic variety or those with which E-H practitioners traditionally differ. Contemporary E-H practitioners, moreover, tend to value holism, integration, and complementarity. They tend to see the intrapsychic aspects of therapy on a par with those of intersubjectivity; the social and cultural implications of their work on a level with individual transformation and the intellectual and philosophical bases of practice on a plane with those of emotion and spirit; and the contemporary E-H practitioner does not shy away from programmatic or even biological interventions, as those may be appropriate (Schneider, 1995).

This breadth of outlook has widened the existential–humanistic client base. Less and less is E-H practice confined to the rarified environs of its psychoanalytic forebears, or to upper-class elites, but is opening out to the world within which most of us dwell (O'Hara, 2001; Pierson & Sharp, 2001). Put another way, the E-H *attitude* can be seen in a variety of practice setttings, from drug counseling (Ballinger, Matano, & Amantea, 1995) to therapy with minorities (Alsup, 1995; Rice, 1995; Vontress & Epp, 2001) to gay and lesbian counseling (Monheit, 1995) to therapy with psychotic clientele (Mosher, 2001, Thompson, 1995) to emancipatory practices with groups (Lerner, 2000; Lyons, 2001; Montuori & Purser, 2001; O'Hara, 2001).

Yet in spite of their expanded vision, contemporary E-H practitioners still share a core value with their predecessors: the personal or intimate search process that is at the crux of depth practice. As we shall see, this process entails four basic stances or conditions—the cultivation of therapeutic presence, the activation of presence through struggle, the working through of resistance, and the consolidation of meaning.

In the next section we describe the theory of personality that underlies this core value and the practical consequences that follow. (For additional references to the existential–humanistic philosophical heritage, see also Barrett, 1958; Becker, 1973; Buber, 1937/1970; Camus, 1955; deBeauvior, 1948; Friedman, 1991b; Marcel, 1956; Sartre, 1956; Tillich, 1952. For additional references to the psychological heritage of existential humanism, see Bugental, 1965; Frankl, 1963; May, 1983; Moustakas, 1972; Rogers, 1951; Wheelis, 1958; Yalom, 1980.)

THE CONCEPT OF PERSONALITY, PSYCHOLOGICAL HEALTH, AND PATHOLOGY

The concept of personality is useful but, for our purposes, limited. From the standpoint of E-H psychology, one does not experi-

ence a personality; one lives an experience. Similarly, the notions of psychological health and pathology can have static, culturally normative qualities that may not reflect the lived experience of distinctive individuals (see Becker, 1973, Fromm, 1941; Laing, 1967). Nevertheless, there are *patterns* within these lived experiences—characterological structures—which existential humanists have carefully described phenomenologically. Let us consider a sampling of these.

As suggested earlier, the E-H understanding of functionality rests on three interdependent dimensions—freedom, experiential reflection, and responsibility. Although E-H theorists almost invariably highlight all three of these dimensions, they do so in unique and variegated ways. For example, Rollo May (1981) gives primary attention to freedom and that which he terms "destiny." By freedom, May means the capacity to choose within the natural and self-imposed (e.g., cultural) limits of living. Freedom also implies responsibility, for, as he suggests, if we are conferred the power to choose, is it not incumbent upon us to exercise that power?

May defines destiny in terms of the consciousness of our limits. He then goes on to define four basic limits or forms of destiny—the cosmic, the genetic, the cultural, and the circumstantial. Cosmic destiny embraces the limitations of nature (e.g., earthquakes and storms), genetic destiny addresses the limits of physiology (e.g., lifespan and temperament), cultural destiny entails preset social patterns (e.g., language and class), and circumstantial destiny pertains to sudden situational developments (e.g., war and recession).

How then, do we deal with these contending forces according to May, and what happens when we do not? Let us consider the latter first. The failure to acknowledge our freedom, according to May (1981) leads to a dysfunctional identification with destiny or limits, whereas the failure to acknowledge our limits leads to a dysfunctional identification with our possibilities. Hence, the failure to acknowledge freedom can be seen in the forfeit of the capacity for wonder, experimentation, and boldness. Among those who embody those imbalances are the reticent wallflower, the rigid bureaucrat, and the robotic conformist. The failure to acknowledge limits, on the other hand, can be detected in the sacrifice of the ability to discern, discipline, and prioritize one's life. Among those who illustrate this polarity are the aimless dabbler, the impulsive philanderer, and the arrogant abuser.

The great question of course, is how to help people redress these imprisoning dispositions—how to help them broaden and thereby mobilize their range of behavioral, cognitive, and affective resources. Although there is no simple answer to this query, May finds that intra- and interpersonal struggles (or encounter) are key ameliorative dimensions. It is only through struggle, according to May (1981), that freedom and destiny—capabilities and limits—can be illuminated in their fullness, substantively explored, and meaningfully transformed.

The polarities of freedom and destiny or limitation, and the challenge to respond to these polarities, are central to leading E-H conceptions of psychological health. James Bugental (Bugental & Sterling, 1995), for example, draws on a similar dialectic with his emphasis on the self as embodied yet changing; choiceful yet finite; isolated yet related. We are ever in the process of change according to Bugental (see also the ancient Greek philosopher Heraclitus), no matter how we choose to conceive it. Our challenge, Bugental elaborates, is to face that change, sort through its manifold features, and etch out of it a meaningful and action-oriented response.

Irvin Yalom (1980) conceives of four "givens" of human existence—death, freedom, isolation, and meaninglessness. Depending on how we confront these givens, Yalom elaborates, we confront the design and quality of our lives. To the extent that we confront death, for example, we also en-

counter the urgency, intensity, and seriousness that death arouses. To the extent that we confront isolation, we also contact and become aware of our need for relation, or its opposite, solitude. For Yalom, the composition of a life is directly proportional to the composition and array of one's relationship to givens, and the priorities one sets to integrate, explore, or coexist with those givens.

I have elaborated a constrictive/expansive continuum of conscious and subconscious personality functioning (Schneider, 1995, 1999b). This continuum is identified as a capacity that is both freeing and yet limited. We have a vast capacity to "draw back" and constrict thoughts, feelings, and sensations, as well as an equivalent capacity to "burst forth" and expand thoughts, feelings, and sensations. At the same time, each of these capacities is delimited. We can only constrict (e.g., focus and accommodate) and expand (e.g., enlarge and assimilate) so far, before the givens of existence (e.g., death, genes, and culture) deter and curtail us. For me, it is the interplay among constrictive and expansive capacities, the ability to *respond* to those capacities, and the ability to integrate those responses into a meaningful whole that constitute optimal personal and interpersonal dynamics.

Maurice Friedman (1995, 2001) echoes the philosophy of Martin Buber with his "dialogical" approach to psychological functioning. The dialogical approach, based on Buber's philosophy of "I–thou" relationships, emphasizes the interpersonal and interdependent dimension of personality. For Friedman, psychological growth and development proceed, not merely or mainly through the encounter with self but through the encounter with another. This "healing through meeting," as Friedman puts it, is characterized by the ability to be present to and confirming of oneself, at the same time being open to and confirming of another. The freedom and limits of such a relationship then become transferred to the freedom and limits experienced within one's self, and the trust developed to risk affirmation of the self.

THE PROCESS OF CLINICAL ASSESSMENT

The question of assessment is essentially the question of understanding: On what basis do E-H therapists understand an individual's pattern of interaction, symptomatology, and adaptive resources? E-H therapists employ a variety of means to understand lives. Among these means can be paper-and-pencil tests, ratings of symptomatology, and history taking. However, these modalities tend to be implemented sparingly rather than as a staple of practice. The reason for this caveat is that, as a rule, assessment—like therapy—is an ongoing process for E-H practitioners and not a linear or mechanistic procedure. Appraisal is holistic, in other words, and should not be mistaken for a global or rigid declaration (Bugental & Sterling, 1995). Client X may be a "depressive" for an E-H practitioner, but he is also a living, dynamic human being, and this is pivotal information—both for client and therapist.

E-H practitioners are concerned with depth and breadth of context as much as or more than they are with specific overt behaviors. Ideally, nothing is spared in E-H therapeutic assessment—the unfolding moment, the client's explicit and implicit intentions in the moment, the horizons of the past, and the full person-to-person field that is evoked each moment are of equal and abiding import (Fischer, 1994; Schneider, 1995).

Generally speaking, contemporary E-H practice is an integrative practice (Schneider & May, 1995; Watson & Bohart, 2001). E-H practitioners value the whole human being—conscious and nonconscious, past, present, and evolving—in the therapeutic encounter. As such, E-H practitioners are concerned with how best to understand clients in their moment-to-moment un-folding, and their given level of relation and experience. *Presence* is the chief tool of E-H assessment. Through presence, the holding and illuminating of clients' moment-to-moment experience, E-H therapists are able to become attuned to the subtlest nuances of clients' concerns, from the cognitive and behavioral to the affective and spiritual.

Although E-H therapists value the *content* (or explicit features) of clients' experiences, they are acutely and simultaneously attuned to the *process* or implicit aspects of those experiences. For example, whereas the content of a client's report (e.g., binge eating) may be physiological in nature, the process or implicit aspects may be intensely spiritual, ontological, or interpersonal in nature. E-H assessment, therefore, is predicated not only on a client's presenting problem (or complaint) but also on the entire atmosphere of a client's predicament. Everything and anything is open to investigation within the E-H framework, from the initial manner in which the client greets the therapist to the position of the client's hands while elaborating her concern. Put another way, every E-H assessment is holographic. Every moment is believed to be a microcosm and in some sense dovetails with every other moment, and no moment stands in isolation.

For example, one of the first areas of focus within E-H therapy—even before any words are exchanged—is "What is my client expressing in his body?" The E-H therapist is particularly attuned to the manner in which these expressions resonate within him- or herself—their shape, texture, and future intimations. In effect, the E-H therapist uses his or her body as a barometer or register of clients' tacit and overt struggles. Here is a sample of my own thoughts upon greeting a given client:

What kind of world is this man trying to hold together? What kind of life-design do his muscles, gestures, and breathing betray? Is he stiff and waxy or limber and fluid? Is he caved in and hunched over or stout and thrust forward? Does he curl up in a remote corner of the room or does he "plant himself in my face"? What does he bring up in *my* body? Does he make me feel light and buoyant or heavy and stuck? Do my stomach muscles tighten, or do my legs become jumpy? Do my eyes relax, or do they become "hard," or guarded? What can I sense from what he wears? Is he frumpy and inconspicuous or loud and outrageous? What can be gleaned from his face? Is it tense and weather-beaten or soft and innocent? (Schneider, 1995, p. 154)

Each of these observations begins to coalesce with others, cumulatively, to disclose a world. Each oscillates with others to form a shape, sense, and overarching Gestalt of this particular man's strife.

Presence, then is the *sine qua non* of E-H assessment. Through the illumination of presence, E-H therapists open to and begin to discover clients' overt and covert scripts, ostensible and tacit agendas, and unfolding rivalries within the battleground of self. Further, they begin to sense the shape of their own responses to these revelations and how best to "meet" or facilitate them. For example, an E-H therapist might ask (silently to herself), what are the resources, difficulties, and potential tools necessitated to address an acutely fragile client? What about a combative client, or a client who resists exploration? These are issues that challenge any serious-minded therapist but are especially trying to E-H practitioners who prize depth of connection over symptom relief. The question for the E-H therapist is, How can I best meet this client "where he lives," within the abilities and constraints of where he or she lives, and yet hold out the possibility for a fuller and deeper connection? This holding out of the possibility for an enlarged and deepened contact is one of the primary distinctions between prevailing and E-H visions of healing. Whereas conventional practitioners may tend to calibrate their actions to given parts of the therapeutic concern (e.g., those that pertain to behavior or cognition or childhood), E-H practitioners endeavor to be available to

clients across the range of their difficulties, from the measurable and overt to the felt and unformed. It is in this sense that diagnosis is a part of the ongoing contact in E-H therapy, and that formulations must fit people and not the other way around (Fischer, 1994; May, 1983).

Given its evolving and holistic approach, then, E-H assessment must be artfully and mindfully engaged. While psychiatric diagnoses may be useful to E-H practitioners at given stages of therapy, the assessment overall is based on therapist attunement, experience, and clinical judgment. As a rule, the client's desire and capacity for change and the therapist's mindful and sensitive alertness to these criteria guide the ensuing work.

THE PRACTICE OF THERAPY

The aim of E-H therapy is to "set clients free" (May, 1981, p. 19). By freedom, E-H therapists do not at all mean caprice or licentiousness, or even truth in the unqualified sense. What they do mean, however, is the cultivation of the capacity for choice; and choice, as is well established in the existential literature, implies limits, ambiguities, and risk (May, 1981; Tillich, 1952).

Freedom is limited because it arises in a sociobiological–spiritual context, only degrees of which are accessible, changeable, and clear. It is ambiguous because for every choice there is a choice not taken, and for every gain there is a commensurate relinquishment. If I devote myself to sports, for example, my ability to perform intellectually is likely to suffer. If I affirm social visibility, I relinquish my capacity to withdraw, and so on. Finally, freedom is risk because it is ever set against uncertainty and the potential for collapse. But freedom is also vibrant, poignant, and energizing; and for many, it is the point of being alive, in spite of and perhaps even in light of its many challenges.

As suggested earlier, contemporary E-H therapy is both integrative and incremental in its approach to freedom. The client's desire and capacity for change (Schneider, 1995), the alliance and context of the therapy (Bugental, 1987), and practical elements (Yalom, 1989) all figure in. Hence, for some E-H clients, at some stages of therapy, choice can mean drug-induced stability or nutrition-based evenness of mood or reasoned-based empowerment, and so on. However, that which distinguishes E-H facilitation is its ability to address, not merely programmatic (i.e., externally based) adjustments but internally sparked commitments. Commitment, for E-H therapists, refers to a sense "I-ness," agency, or profound caring about a given direction. It implies a sense that the life one chooses really matters to oneself and is worth one's whole (embodied) investment. This ontological or experiential level of commitment manifests clinically as a sense of immediacy (aliveness), affectivity (passion), and kinesthesia (embodiment) and is typified in the deepest and most pivotal stages of therapy. In short, E-H therapists endeavor to meet clients "where they are at" but also to be available to the fullest potential of those clients to "own" or claim the life that is presented to them.

In light of this background, E-H therapy can vary in both length and intensity. It can proceed, on rare occasions, within one or two sessions (e.g., see Galvin, 1995; Laing, 1985); or it can occur in a limited way within a short-term focused format (e.g., Bugental, 1995). Typically, however, E-H engagements are intimate (e.g., trust building), long term (e.g., 3–5 years), and intensive (e.g., weekly to twice weekly). Furthermore, E-H therapy can be of benefit to a more diverse range of clientele than is generally presumed (e.g., see May, 1972; Vontress & Epp, 2001), although those who tend to be introspective, emotionally tolerant, and exploratory are likely to derive maximal benefits.

To summarize then, the chief question for the E-H therapist is how does one help this person (client) find choice—meaning, clarity, and direction—in his or her life, in spite of (and sometimes, in light of) all the threats to these possibilities? Clearly, there are no easy answers to this question, yet it is precisely its difficulty, its *struggle,* that for E-H therapists is key to its unfolding. In other words, E-H therapists challenge clients to grapple with their concerns, and not just intellectually, behaviorally, or programmatically, but experientially, in order to maximize their capacities to transform themselves.

Existential Stances or Conditions

To achieve the aforementioned aims, E-H therapists use a variety of means. These means, however, are not techniques in the classical sense; they are stances or conditions through which experiential liberation, or profound experiential transformation, can take root. Among the core (intertwining and overlapping) E-H stances are the following: *the cultivation of therapeutic presence (presence as ground); the activation of therapeutic presence through struggle (presence as goal); the encounter with the resistance to therapeutic struggle; and the consolidation of the meaning, intentionality, and commitment that result from the struggle.* We now proceed to elaborate on these dimensions.

The Cultivation of Therapeutic Presence: Presence as Ground

As suggested earlier, presence is the *sine qua non* of E-H practice. There is a moving story about the travails of the distinguished existential philosopher, Martin Buber, that vividly illustrates the life-and-death significance of therapeutic presence. As conveyed by Friedman (1991a), Buber was in the throes of a mystical rapture when a curious caller appeared at his door. The caller was a dour and anxious young man who had come to seek Buber's advice: Should he (the caller) volunteer to go to the front of a major battle (during World War I), or should he resist and find refuge as a noncombatant? While Buber greeted this young man with his customary graciousness, his customary attunement was wanting. In short, in the midst of his spiritual distractions, Buber failed to "meet" this young man, and tragedy followed. Some time later, we are told, the young man enlisted in the army and died precipitously on the front. Although multiple in its potential meanings, Buber took this situation as a dire warning to himself and others to never underestimate the gravity of presence, and subsequently, according to Friedman, he never did.

The gravity of presence is further illustrated by Rollo May's (1987) incisive declaration that in dedicated E-H therapy, it is "the client's life that is at stake," and that is how the therapist should view it.

There is a vivid distinction, in my view, between a therapist who approaches a client as a problem-solving "doctor" and a healer who is available for inter- and intrapersonal connection. The former offers a specific set of remedies for an isolated and definable malady; the latter offers a relationship, an invitation and an accompaniment on a journey. And although the former is likely to appeal to a client's immediate needs for relief, the latter is likely to appeal to a client's underlying urges for discovery, self-sustainment, and vitality. To be sure, *both* modalities are often relevant over the course of a given therapy, and both are useful. But in today's market-driven, standardizing atmosphere, rarely are both made available.

Through the dimension of presence, however (including a willingness to negotiate fees!), both the problem-solving and journey-accompanying modalities can be made available to clients. And clients, in turn, can substantively benefit from these resources. Without the latter (journey-accompanying) mode, however, clients are likely to feel short-changed, and, arguably, like Buber's caller, short-circuited.

Presence is the "soup," the seedbed of substantive E-H work. Yalom (1980) draws an intriguing parallel between the masterful preparation of a meal and E-H therapy.

Whereas the average cook prepares a meal in accordance with a standardized menu, the masterful cook, while not ignoring the latter guidelines, attunes to the evolving, emerging, and subjectively engaging in her preparation. The masterful cook, in other words, has a good sense of how to prepare a basic meal but can also throw in spices, seasonings, and flavorful mixtures that can radically enhance and transform it. For Yalom, it is precisely these nonprescriptions, these "throw-ins" (p. 3), as he puts it, that matter most.

Analogously, it is precisely the present and attuned therapist who is prepared to help his or her client most, according to E-H practice philosophy. Such a therapist is optimally prepared to provide the atmosphere, personality, and moment-to-moment adjustments that can mobilize client change (Bugental, 1987). Interestingly, even standardized psychotherapy research upholds the latter postulate: Wampold (2001), for example, found that "common factors," such as therapist–client alliance and personality variables, account for about nine times the variance in outcomes over specific therapeutic techniques. Yalom (1989) puts it this way:

> The capacity to tolerate uncertainty is a prerequisite for the profession. Though the public may believe that therapists guide patients systematically and sure-handedly through predictable stages of therapy to a foreknown goal, such is rarely the case. . . . The powerful temptation to achieve certainty through embracing an ideological school . . . is treacherous: such belief may block the uncertain and spontaneous encounter necessary for effective therapy. (p. 13)

"This encounter," Yalom concludes, is "the heart of psychotherapy, . . . a caring, deeply human meeting between two people, one (generally, but not always, the patient) more troubled than the other" (p. 13).

Finally, the value of being present as a vulnerable and yet distinctive *person,* is illustrated by Friedman (1995) in the following client-authored vignette. Following a 4-year therapy with Friedman, his client, "Dawn," reports the following:

> When I think about our therapeutic relationship, it is the *process* that stands out in my memory, not the content.
>
> Up until the time I met Maurice, I had always "picked out" a male authority figure (usually a teacher or psychologist), put him on a pedestal, and obsessed about him a lot—not usually in a romantic or sexual way, although there was an erotic element. I just wanted him to like me and approve of me and to think I was smart and interesting. A real relationship, though, was terrifying to me—I kept my distance and rarely ever talked to them. The greater the attraction, the greater the fear.
>
> When I first met Maurice, I could feel myself wanting to fall into this same pattern with him. However, I could never quite feel intimidated by him—although I think I really wanted to. He was too human for that. I never felt that I had to be interesting or smart, good, bad, happy, or sad—it just wasn't something I had to be concerned with. If the therapist can be human and fallible, that gives me permission to be human and fallible, too. (p. 313)

For Friedman, as with most E-H therapists, then, presence is the foundation, which both holds and illuminates. It holds by supporting, embracing, and opening to clients' travails, and it illuminates by witnessing, disclosing, and engaging with those travails. In short, presence holds and illuminates that which is palpably (immediately, affectively, kinesthetically, and profoundly) relevant within the client and between the client and therapist, and it is the ground and goal of substantive E-H transformation.

The Activation of Therapeutic Presence through Inner Struggle: Presence as Goal

As suggested earlier, presence not only forms the ground for E-H encounter, it also culminates in its goal. To the extent that clients can attune, at the most embodied

levels, to their severest conflicts, healing in the E-H framework is likely to ensue. This healing is a kind of reoccupation of oneself—an immersion in the parts of oneself that one has designed a lifetime to avoid, and it is an integration thereby of the potential or openings that become manifest through that reoccupation. The question for this particular phase of the therapeutic process is: What are the ways and means to activate presence in the client? Or, how can therapists help to *mobilize* clients' presence? (Bugental, 1987).

As we shall see, the activation of client presence within E-H therapy is characterized by two basic modes or access points—the intrapsychic and the interpersonal. Although these modalities overlap, and indeed intertwine (Merleau-Ponty, 1962), they nevertheless reflect two basic E-H practice styles that are gradually, and for many, refreshingly, beginning to merge (Portnoy, 1999).

Bugental (1987), for example, is more representative of the intrapsychic or individualist tradition, although this characterization is far from discrete and much about his approach can be considered interpersonal as well. Within the former tradition, then, Bugental (1987) outlines four basic practice strategies, or that which he terms "octaves" for activating clients' presence. These are listening, guiding, instructing, and requiring.

The first octave, *listening,* draws clients out, encourages them to keep talking, and obtains their story without "contamination" by the therapist. Examples of listening include, "getting the details" of clients' experiences, "listening to emotional catharsis, learning [clients' views of their] own life or . . . projected objectives" (Bugental, 1987, p. 71). The second octave, *guiding,* gives direction and support to clients' speech, keeps it on track, and brings out other aspects. Examples of guiding include, exploration of clients' "understanding of a situation, relation, or problem; developing readiness to learn new aspects or get feedback" (p. 71).

The third octave is *instructing*. Instructing transmits "information or directions having rational and/or objective support." Examples include "assignments, advising, coaching, describing a scenario of changed living," or reframing (Bugental, 1987, p. 71). Finally, the fourth octave is *requiring*. Requiring brings a "therapist's personal and emotional resources to bear" to cause clients to change in some way. Examples of requiring include, "subjective feedback, praising, punishing [e.g., admonishing], rewarding," and "strong selling of [a] therapist's views" (p. 71).

Listening and guiding comprise the lion's share of E-H activation of presence. Whereas instructing and requiring can certainly be useful from the E-H point of view, they are implemented in highly selective circumstances. For example, instructing may be helpful to clients at early stages of therapy, or for those who have fragile emotional constitutions, such as victims of chronic abuse, or for clients from authority-dependent cultures. Requiring, similarly, may be useful in the foregoing situations, but also in the case of therapeutic impasses or entrenched client patterns, as we shall see. For the majority of E-H practice situations, however, listening and guiding are pivotal to the deepening, expanding, and consolidating of substantive client transformation.

May (1981) illustrates the value of listening with his notion of the pause. "It is in the pause," he writes,

> that people learn to listen to silence. We can hear the infinite number of sounds that we normally never hear at all—the unending hum and buzz of insects in a quiet summer field, a breeze blowing lightly through the golden hay. . . . And suddenly we realize that this is *something*—the world of "silence" is populated by a myriad of creatures and a myriad of sounds. (p. 165)

The client, similarly, is almost invariably enlivened in the pause. As Bugental (1987, p. 70) suggests, it is in the therapist's silence at given junctures, that abiding change can take root.

The provision of a working "space," a therapeutic pause, not only helps the therapist to understand, but most importantly, assists the client to vivify him or herself. Vivification of a client's world is one of the cardinal tasks of E-H therapy. To the extent that clients can "see" the worlds in which they have lived, the obstacles they have created, and the strengths or resources they possess to overcome those obstacles, they can proceed to a foundational healing. Listening promotes one of the most crucial realizations of that vivification—the contours of a client's battle.

The client's battle—and virtually every client has one—becomes evident at the earliest stages of therapy. For some this battle takes the form of an interpersonal conflict, for others an intrapsychic split; for some it may encompass the compulsion for and rejection of binge eating; for others it may relate to a conflict with one's boss; for still others it may be a struggle between squelched vocational potential and evolving aspirations, and so on. Regardless of the content of clients' battles, however, their form can be understood in terms of two basic valences—the part of themselves that endeavors to emerge, and the part of themselves that endeavors to resist, oppose, or block themselves from emerging (Schneider, 1998a).

Whereas therapeutic listening acquaints and sometimes immerses clients in their battle, therapeutic guiding intensifies that contact. Therapeutic guiding can be further illustrated by encouragements to clients to personalize their dialogue (e.g., to give concrete examples of their difficulties, to speak in the first person, and to "own" or take responsibility for their remarks about others). Guiding is also illustrated by invitations to expand or embellish on given topics, such as in the suggestion "Can you say more?" or "How does it feel to make that statement?" or "What really matters about what you've conveyed?" Finally, guiding is exemplified by the notation of content/process discrepancies, such as "you smile as you vent your anger at him," or "notice how shallow your breathing is right now" (Bugental, 1987; Schneider, 1995).

I have formulated a mode of guiding that I call guided or *embodied meditation* (Schneider, 1995, 1998a). Embodied meditation begins with a simple grounding exercise, such as breathing awareness or progressive relaxation (usually assisted by the closing of the eyes). From there, it proceeds to an invitation to the client to become aware of his or her body. The therapist may then ask what, if any, tension areas are evident in the client's body. If the client identifies such an area, which often occurs, the therapist asks the client to describe, as richly and fully as possible, where the tension area is and what it feels like. Following this and assuming the client is able to proceed with the immersion, he or she is invited to place his or her hand on the affected area (I find that this somatic element can often be, although not necessarily, experientially critical). Next, the client is encouraged to experientially associate to this contact. Prompts such as, "What if any feelings, sensations, or images emerge as you make contact with this area?" can be of notable therapeutic value. I have seen clients open emotional "floodgates" through this work, but I have also seen clients who feel overpowered by it. It is of utmost importance, again, for the therapist to be acutely attuned while practicing this and other awareness-intensive modes.

Guidance is also illustrated by a variety of experimental formats that can be offered in E-H therapy. These experiments, including role-play, rehearsal, visualization, and experiential enactment (e.g., pillow hitting and kinesthetic exercises), serve to liven emergent material and vivify or deepen the understanding of that material (Mahrer, 1996; May, 1972; Schneider, 1995; Serlin, 1996). The phrase, "truth exists only as it is produced in action" (Kierkegaard, cited in May, 1958, p. 12), has much cache in this context. When clients can enact (as appropriate) their anxieties, engage their aspirations, and

simulate their encounters, they bring their battles "out on the table," so to speak—in "living color"—for close and personal inspection.

While experimentation within the therapeutic setting is invaluable, experimentation outside the setting can be of equivalent or even superior benefit. After all, it is the life outside therapy that counts most for clients, and it is in the service of this life that therapy proceeds. Experimentation outside therapy, then, has two basic aims: (1) it reinforces intratherapy work and (2) it implements that work in the most relevant setting possible—the lived experience. Accordingly, E-H therapists encourage clients to practice being aware and present in their outside lives. They may gently challenge clients to reflect on or write about problematic events, or they may propose an activity or therapeutic commitment (e.g., Alcoholics Anonymous or assigned readings). They may also challenge clients to do *without* a given activity or pattern. For example, Yalom (1980) challenged his promiscuous client Bruce to try living without a sexual partner for an extended period. This was a highly demanding exercise for Bruce, whose sexual compulsions were formidable and afforded no pause. Yet after the exercise, Bruce reported rich therapeutic realizations, like the degree to which he felt empty in his life and the blind and compulsive measures he took to fill that emptiness. Emptiness, Yalom reported, subsequently became the next productive focus.

Prompts to clients to "slow down," or "stay with" charged or disturbing experience can also facilitate intensified self-awareness. I have known many a supervisee (and even seasoned colleague) who has had difficulties with this latter facilitation. They are superb at helping clients to reconnect with the parts of themselves they have shunted away, and they inspire deep somatic immersion in expressiveness, but they are left with one gaping question: "What do I do after the client is immersed?" The exasperation in this puzzlement is understandable. E-H work can seem tormenting. It can instigate profound moments of unalloyed pain. The last thing a therapist wishes to do in such a situation is to enable increased suffering, or to hover in continued despair. And yet, given the client's desire and capacity for change, these are precisely the allowances that E-H therapists must provide; precisely the groundworks they must pursue. They must develop trust, and a sense that the work will unfold (Welwood, 2001). Hence, what do I advise my supervisees and colleagues? I suggest that it is in their interest to trust; in particular, to trust that gentle prompts to "stay with" or "allow" intensive material will almost invariably lead to changes in that material. Although these changes may not feel immediately welcome or gratifying—indeed, they may even feel regressive for a time—they do represent evolution, the "more" that every person is capable of experiencing.

Much of the therapist's task within E-H therapy is to facilitate this "more." In time, and as clients become aware of their wounds, they also tend to feel less daunted by those wounds, less imprisoned; they begin to realize, in other words, that they are *more* than their wounds, and through this process, that they are more than their "disorder." For example, client X felt sure that he was despicable, plague-like, and demonic. His parents had convinced him so over a period of 18 years, and not through the usual route of abuse and punishment but exactly the opposite, through indulgence. Client X was led to believe he was a king, a seer, and a god. He was given "everything," and praised for virtually every routine move. The result: As soon as client X hit adulthood, the trials and pressures of college, dating, and vocation, his bubble burst. No longer could he live under his former illusions but now had to face his incompetencies, inabilities to compete, and his far from developed will. The convergence of these factors sent client X into a tailspin.

His view of himself completely reversed—such that he now (in his 30s) repudiated himself whereas he had earlier glorified himself; and where he once saw a titan for whom every whim was fulfilled, he now saw an outcast for whom every desire was unreachable.

The work with client X is highly illustrative of the trust dimension in the activation of presence. Although his self-hatred was formidable, it was not irrevocable. We spent many sessions on his anguish, self-pity, and searing guilt. There were many times when he could go only so far with these feelings, and had to warp back into the semblance of self and self-image that he had constructed as a defense. But there were times, increasingly productive times, when he could glimpse a counterpart. For example, in the midst of his self-devaluing, he might suddenly become frustrated and realize moments of self-affirmation; that is, times when he actually liked himself, and liked being alive, regardless of the strokes he would receive from doting associates. At first this realization was fleeting but eventually, as he stayed with it, it became the major counterpoint to his despairing self-reproach. Back and forth he would swing, between burning self-debasement and gleaming self-validation—including compassion, appreciation, and even exultation at being alive. This latter quality was also connected to his growing sense of outrage, not only at his outdated sense of self but at his upbringing and his well-intentioned but clueless parents. He began to realize that his lowliness was far from an inherent defect but a product of environment, circumstance, and, in part, choice.

To summarize, despite client X's repeated resistance and readiness to give up, the therapist's empathic invitations to "give his hurt a few moments," or to "see what unfolds," were crucial to his reengagement with his larger self. And through this reengagement he began to discover that he was so much vaster than his stuck sense of unworthiness; he began to see that he was sensitive, alive, and resiliently mortal—and that these were enough.

The Interpersonal Activation of Presence

The activation of presence can also occur through the interpersonal route, or that which E-H therapists term the "encounter" (Phillips, 1980–1981). The *encounter* is illustrated by E-H therapists in myriad and diverse forms. For example, the calling of attention to disturbances or undercurrents in the immediate relationship exemplifies the E-H concern with encounter, as does the recognition of transference and countertransference projections, as does the encouragement to explore the status of the therapeutic bond at given junctures. As a whole, E-H encounter is characterized by the following three criteria: (1) the real or present relationship between therapist and client (which can include past projections but chiefly as they are experienced now rather than in the remoteness of reminiscences, e.g., the difference between reporting about and "living" transferential material); (2) the future and what is potential in the relationship (vs. strictly the past and what has already been scripted); and (3) the enactment or experiencing, to the degree possible, of relational material.

Attention to the encounter or "intersubjective," as an emerging cadre of psychoanalysts are calling it (Stolorow, Brandchaft, & Atwood, 1987) is a vital part of E-H facilitation. The reason for this is that interpersonal contact has a uniquely intensive quality that both accentuates and mobilizes clients' presence. The encounter accentuates presence by awakening it to what is real, immediate, and directly personal, and it mobilizes presence by demanding of it a response, engagement, and address. There is something profoundly naked about the turn to an immediate interaction. It takes the parties out of their inward routine (assuming that is there) and focuses the spotlight on a new and utterly alternative reality—themselves. In short, there is something un-

deniably "living" about face-to-face interactions; they peel away the layers of pretense and expose the inflamed truth of embattled humanity. There are no easy exits from such interactions, and there are fewer "patch-up jobs" as a result.

Take the case of Elva. A thorny and self-aggrandizing widow, Elva spared few with her humor-laced vitriol. Yet Elva's battle was the profound sense of helplessness that underlay her bravado. Since the death of her husband, and despite her bouts with loneliness, Elva had been making a comeback through therapy. She was just beginning to reclaim her self-worth, and her jokes were becoming less caustic, when the bubble burst and she was mugged. The period following this attack, a callous purse snatching, was a trying one for Elva. She was retraumatized, and even her attempts at false bravado fell short.

Yet Elva's battle was clear—she was face to face with her worst fears of helplessness, and her wounds were exposed raw. It was at this critical juncture that Elva's therapist and author of this case, Yalom (1989), took a risk. Instead of encouraging her to report *about* her terrors, which might have alleviated some of her internal pressure but not genuinely confronted her wound, he invited her to experience her terrors directly with him. But instead of making it a one-sided exercise, he encouraged her disclosure with some disclosures of his own: "When you say you thought [the purse-snatching] would never happen to you," Yalom confided to Elva, "I know just what you mean," he elaborated. "It's so hard for me, too, to accept that all these afflictions—aging, loss, death—are going to happen to me, too" (p. 150).

He went on: "You must feel that if Albert [her deceased husband] were alive, this would never have happened to you. . . . So the robbery brings home the fact that he's really gone" (p. 150). "Elva was really crying now," Yalom (1989) continued, "and her stubby frame heaved with sobs for several minutes. She had never done that before with me. I sat there and wondered, 'Now what do I do?'" But he sensed "instinctually," just what to do. He took one look at her purse—"that same ripped-off, much abused purse" (p. 150), and challenged—"Bad luck is one thing, but aren't you asking for it carrying around something that large" (p. 150)?

This sardonic quip, which was also an offering to dialogue, set off a whole new direction for Elva and Yalom. Not only did she proceed to open up her purse to him, they shared intimately the discussion of its contents. Finally, "when the great bag had . . . yielded all," Yalom elaborated, "Elva and I stared in wonderment at the contents. . . . We were sorry the bag was empty and that the emptying was over" (1989, p. 150). But what struck Yalom most of all was how "transforming" that engagement had been, for Elva, in his view, had "moved from a position of forsakenness to one of trust" (p. 150). That was "the best hour of therapy I ever gave" (p. 150), Yalom concluded.

Through sharing that bag, Elva accessed more vulnerability, more anxieties about trust, and more possibilities for risking, healing, and bridging than she would likely ever have, had she simply reflected on its contents.

The interpersonal encounter for E-H therapists is rife with responsibility, the ability to respond to the injured other (i.e., client) such that he or she can respond to and reconnect with the parts of him- or herself that have been damaged. According to Buber, and following him, Friedman (2001), such responsibility entails "hearing the unreduced claim of each hour in all its crudeness and disharmony and answering it out of the depths of one's being. . . . [It entails] the great character who can awaken responsibility in others . . . [and] who acts from the whole of his or her substance and reacts in accordance with the uniqueness of every situation" (p. 343).

Mutual confirmation, or what Buber calls an "I–Thou" relationship, "a relationship of openness, presence, directness, and immediacy," is essential to the therapist's re-

sponsibility according to Friedman (2001, p. 344). Although there is a place, of course, for modulating this confirmation, and no professional relationship can be mutual in the sense of a friendship, such a notion is nevertheless a bellwether, a palpable and reliable indicator, of intensive therapeutic transformation. Why is this so? Because the further that one can be present to and work out differences with another, the more one can generally engage in the same relational dynamics toward oneself.

In her discussion of Sylvia, Molly Sterling (2001) articulates both sides of the responsibility question, and she does so poignantly and incisively. "My client leaned forward," Sterling begins her case presentation, "eyes intently on me, voice passionately intense, and said to me, 'I just want to be in your kitchen while you cook.' "Inwardly," Sterling goes on, "I froze.

> Not one therapist sinew, not one trained muscle of years of practice, flexed into action. Nowhere in me was there a standard response, and I parody our standard psychotherapeutic repertoire a bit here: "Tell me how that would be" or "You would like to be closer to me" or "Our meetings aren't enough for you" or just a genuinely open and quiet waiting for my client to continue. "Instead I reacted viscerally," elaborated Sterling. "In my frozen moment, I saw the dishes left as I hurried out early that morning. I felt my pleasure in my own rhythm of my pottering about. I wondered how my family would take to this new person slipped into their lives. These images supplanted my unawareness that I could not sustain my client's intense pressure. I felt, in short, inadequate to her proposition. (p. 349)

Sterling (2001) took Sylvia's request as a "concrete proposition to which [Sterling] was called to give a concrete answer. . . . And so, the gist of [Sterling's] reply carried all of these [above] feelings and many more to which [she] was then blind: 'Oh, you might not like me so much if you were around me more.'" And "in one blind stroke," Sterling conceded, "I had cleaved open a chasm of distance, betrayal, shame, fury, and misconstrual" (p. 349).

Sylvia was a "successful . . . kind, intelligent, and savvy" therapy client, according to Sterling (2001, p. 349). She took "care of herself and her life everywhere but in her most private heart, where she [hid] shame, guilt, and grief," and where she "neither is loved nor loves (she believes)" (p. 349). To Sterling, her "blind remark" to Sylvia rejected Sylvia's "plea for abiding acceptance," and "violently broke open her heart" (p. 349). Sylvia "wanted something" from Sterling, according to Sterling, and she (Sterling) failed to provide it. Caught up in her own discomfiting anxieties about being wanted, needed, and accompanied, Sterling reacted—as would many therapists in similar situations—with modified, low-grade panic.

But, and this is where the existential, I–thou notions of encounter become so relevant, Sterling (2001) did not *desist* at the point of her anxiety. She did not "fold up" and revert to some stilted or rehearsed professionalism; nor did she abandon Sylvia, either physically or emotionally. To the contrary, she stayed profoundly with her evolving distress, immersed in it, took time to study it, explored it with Sylvia, and gradually, charily, fashioned a response to it.

The response that Sterling fashioned recognized both her own and Sylvia's shortcomings but also their humanity. Sterling *was* overwhelmed by Sylvia's neediness in her request, and she had a right to experience this sensibility; at the same time, Sylvia had a right to expect something more from Sterling, something that acknowledged her plea. Sterling took inspiration from the existential–phenomenological philosopher Levinas:

The ability to respond is the primary meaning of responsibility. Levinas took this further to show that responsibility also carries the experience of being beholden to the other person. . . . Responsibility, for Levinas, meant that simply by the fact of the face of the other person, one is "taken hostage"—before

thought, choice, or action. . . . It is this level of our human condition, brought into presence by our naked encounter, that Sylvia and I . . . had to reckon with. (2001, p. 351)

Although Sterling "failed" to meet the "obligation" of human encounter, in her very failure, she realized, were the seeds of her success. For as Sterling put it about her discouraging remark to Sylvia, "Sylvia *was* [nevertheless] in my kitchen with me—conflicts, mess, hurry, and all. At that moment, [Sylvia] had what she would get in my kitchen in actuality, if not what she wanted in feeling. I was as naked as she was, if only she (and I) could see it" (2001, p. 352).

But Sterling did see it. In time, she acknowledged how overwhelmed she was by Sylvia's fantasy. She opened up some about her own weaknesses, fears, and misgivings, and this, as Sterling put it, "altered" (2001, p. 352) their relationship. From that point on, Sylvia was freed to respond as a person to Sterling, because Sterling, in turn, had responded as a person with Sylvia. But by acknowledging her limits with Sylvia, both as person and professional, Sterling helped free Sylvia to respond to something else—her nurture of herself—and the challenge thereby to actualize that relationship.

To summarize, E-H encounter is a complex and dynamic process whereby the entire therapeutic context is taken into consideration; among the salient factors within this context are the client's desire and capacity for change, the therapeutic alliance, and practical considerations. The guiding therapeutic question is, To what extent does encounter further the cause of immersion in, engagement with, and integration of clients' intensive struggles; or, on the other hand, to what extent does encounter do the opposite and defeat or stifle facilitative processes?

The Encounter with Resistance

When the invitation to explore, immerse, and interrelate, is abruptly or repeatedly declined by clients, then the perplexing problem of resistance must be considered. Resistance is the *blockage* to that which is palpably (immediately, affectively, kinesthetically) relevant within the client and between client and therapist. Several caveats must be borne in mind when considering client resistance. First, therapists can be mistaken about resistance. What therapist A, for example, labels resistance may in 'fact be a refusal on the part of client B to accept therapist A's agenda for him or her. Resistance may also be a safety issue for a given client, or an issue of cultural or psychological misunderstanding. From an E–H perspective then, it is of utmost importance that therapists suspend their attributions of resistance and discern their relevant contexts.

Second, it is crucial to respect resistance, from an E–H point of view. Resistance is a lifeline to many clients and as miserable as their patterns may be, this lifeline represents the ground or scaffolding of an assured or familiar path. Although this path may seem crude or even suicidal, to clients who experience it, it is starkly preferable to the alternatives (May, 1983, p. 28). Accordingly, it is important for E–H therapists to tread mindfully when it comes to resistance; acknowledging *both* its life-giving *and* life-taking qualities. It is also important to be cognizant of challenging clients' resistance prematurely, lest such challenges exacerbate rather than alleviate defensive needs.

From an E–H point of view, resistance work is mirroring work. By mirroring work, I mean the feeding back and elucidation of clients' monumental experiential battle. As suggested earlier, this battle consists of two basic factions: the side of the client that struggles to emerge (e.g., to liberate from, transcend, or enlarge his or her impoverished world), and the side that vies to suppress that emergence and revert. Whereas the activation of presence (e.g., the calling of attention to what is alive) mirrors clients' struggles to emerge, resistance work, as previously noted, elucidates clients' barriers to that emergence, and the ways and means they immobilize.

In sum, resistance work must be artfully engaged. The more that therapists invest in changing clients, the less they enable clients to struggle with change. By contrast, the more that therapists enable clients to clarify how they are willing to live, the more they fuel the impetus (and often frustration!) required for lasting change (Schneider, 1998a).

There are two basic forms of resistance work: vivification and confrontation. *Vivification of resistance* is the intensification of clients' awareness of how they block or limit themselves. Specifically, vivification serves three basic functions: (1) it alerts clients to their defensive worlds, (2) it apprises them of the consequences of those worlds, and (3) it reflects back the counterforces (or counterwill, as Otto Rank, 1936, put it) aimed at overcoming those worlds. There are two basic approaches linked to vivifying resistance—noting and tagging. *Noting* apprises clients of initial experiences of resistance. Here is an illustration: "you suddenly get quiet when the subject of your brother arises"; or "you laugh when speaking of your pain"; or "we were just speaking about your anxieties working with me and you suddenly switched topics"; or "I sense that you're holding down your anger right now."

In a distinctly dramatic illustration of noting resistance, Bugental (1976) reported a highly stilted initial interview with a client in which decorum rather than genuine feeling permeated. Laurence (Bugental's client) took extensive pains to show how competent he was, how many accolades he had won, and how important his life was. But after some period of this self-puffery, Bugental "took a calculated risk" (p. 16). Instead of placating his new client or emulating the standard intake role of detached observer, Bugental turned to Laurence, faced him directly and averred: "You're scared shitless"—and at that, Laurence shed his mask of bravado, and began a genuine interchange with Bugental.

Sometimes noting resistance takes the form of nonverbal feedback. For example, just sitting with clients in their uncertainty at a given moment, can feed back to them the realization that a change or mobilization of some sort is necessary in their life. Or through the therapist's mirroring of clients' crossed arms or furrowed brow, clients may begin to become clearer about how closed they have been, or how tensely they hold themselves.

Tagging alerts clients to the repetition of their resistance. Examples of tagging include, "So here we are again; at that same bitter place"; or "Every time you note a victory, you go on and beat yourself up"; or "You repeatedly insist on the culpability of others"; or "What is it like to feel helpless again?" Like noting, tagging implies a subtle challenge, a subtle invitation to reassess one's stance. Implicitly, it enjoins clients to take responsibility for their self-constructions and to revisit their capacities to transform.

Revisitation is a key therapeutic dimension. Every time clients become aware of how they stop (or deter) themselves from fuller personal and interpersonal access, they learn more about their willingness to approach such situations in the future. Frequently, there are many revisitations required before "stuck" experiences can be accessed; clients must revisit many frustrations and wounds before they are ready to substantively reapproach those conditions. Yet, as entrenched as their miseries may be, each time clients face them, they face remarkable opportunities for change; and each incremental change can become monumental—a momentum shift of life-changing proportions.

Another form of vivifying resistance is "tracing out." *Tracing out* entails encouraging clients to explore the fantasized consequences of their resistance. For example, I have encouraged obese clients who fear weight loss to review and grapple with the expectations of that weight loss, and not just intellectually but experientially, through dramatizing an anticipated scene; identifying the feelings, body sensations, and images associated with the scene; and encountering the fears, fantasies, and anticipated consequences of following the scene to its ultimate conclusion. Although clients often find such tracing out disconcerting, they also often find it illuminating, as it animates their overinflated fears, unexpected resources, and resolve, in addition to their harrowing frailties. The tracing out of *capitulating* to a behavior or experience is also highly illuminating. Such tracing out, for example, might take the form of foregoing weight loss and the anticipated fears, fantasies, and implications of maintaining the status quo. The question "Where does this (reluctance to lose weight) leave you?" or "How are you willing to respond (to such intransigence)?" can help elaborate these exercises.

When clients' stuckness becomes intractable but with a potential for substantive change, a confrontation may be called for. *Confrontation* with resistance is a direct and amplified form of vivification. However, instead of *alerting* clients to their self-destructive refuges, confrontation *alarms* them, and in lieu of *nurturing* transformation, confrontation *presses* for and *demands* (or "requires," to use Bugental's [1987] phrase) such transformation (Schneider, 1995). There are several caveats, however, about confrontation that bear consideration. First, confrontation may risk an argument or power struggle between client and therapist, versus a deepening or facilitative grappling. Second, confrontation risks the surrender of clients' decision-making power to therapists with the resultant withdrawal of that decision-making power from clients' own lives. Third, confrontation risks alienating clients—not merely from an individual therapist but from therapy as a whole.

As unfortunate as these potentially calamitous outcomes may be, they are not, by any means foreordained. Engaged optimally, confrontation requires careful and artful encouragements to clients to change, but also, and equally important, a full appreciation for the consequences of such encouragements. Prior to decisions to confront, therefore, therapists must carefully weigh the stakes—such as their intervention's timeliness, their degree of alliance with clients, and their own personal and professional preparedness.

Bugental (1976) provides a keen illustration of confrontation with his case of Frank. Frank was an obstinate and reproachful young man. He repeatedly scorned life and yet refused to entertain its possibilities for betterment as well. At one peculiarly frustrating juncture, Frank chastises Bugental: "Whenever you guys want to make a point but can't do it directly, you tell the sucker he's got some unconscious motivation. That way. . . ."

> [Bugental responds:] "Oh shee-it, Frank. You're doing it right now. I answer one question for you and get sandbagged from another direction. You just want to fight about everything that comes along."
> [Frank:] "It's always something I'm doing. Well, if you had to eat as much crap everyday as I do, you'd . . ."
> [Bugental:] "Frank, you'd rather bellyache about life than do something about it."
> [Frank's "pouting tone" changes.]
> [Bugental continues:] "Frank, I don't want all this to get dismissed as just my tiredness or your sad, repetitive life. I am tired, and maybe that makes me bitch at you more. I'll take responsibility for that. But it is also true that somehow you have become so invested in telling your story of how badly life treats you that you do it routinely and with a griping manner that turns people off or makes them angry. You don't like to look at that, but it's so, and I think some part of you knows it." (p. 109)

This vignette illustrates several important points. First, by intensifying his description of Frank's behavior, Bugental stuns or gently shocks Frank into a potentially new view of himself—that of a responsible agent rather than passive victim. By accenting Frank's "investment" in complaining, he tacitly asks Frank to reassess that investment, and his entire stance, in fact, of treating himself as a victim. Second, the vignette illustrates how a therapeutic interaction can reflect a more general reality in a client's day-to-day world. As Bugental's comment makes plain, Frank's "griping" must turn off a lot of people, and, as in the case with Bugental, this reaction can only complicate, if not exacerbate, Frank's intransigent bitterness. Third, and by way of summary, Bugental's remarks challenge Frank to reassess his whole stance, the issues leading up to that stance, and the necessity of maintaining that stance. In effect, Bugental beseeches, "What is the pay-off of staying bitter, and is it worth the price"?

On the other hand, there are notable times when such imploring (or even gentle inquiring) with clients is futile, if not outright hazardous. At such times, clients may feel sapped, "spent," or defiantly entrenched, and instead of confronting or challenging those states (which may have the unintended effect of threatening and thereby hardening intractable defenses) the best strategy, from the E-H view, may simply be to enable or allow those devitalizing realities (e.g., see Schneider, 1999b). Frequently, for example, I have found that clients' investments in their resistance directly parallel my own investment in their overcoming of that resistance. Furthermore, when I have pulled back some from my own intransigence, clients' too have seemingly loosened up and pulled back. This dynamic makes sense; for what is being asked of clients, in effect, is to leap headlong into the doom that they have designed a lifetime to avoid. However, to the extent that such clients feel that they have room, can take their own pace, and can shift in their own time-tested fashion, they are often more pliable, flexible, and inclined toward change.

To summarize, resistance work is mirror work and must be skillfully facilitated. Vivification (noting and tagging) of resistance alerts whereas confrontation alarms clients about their self-constructed plights. Presumptuousness, however, must be minimized in this work. Whereas some clients are amenable to the accentuation and vivification of their life patterns, others are more reticent, and such reticence should not be undervalued. It too can be informative and eventually facilitate a fuller and deeper stance.

The Consolidation of Meaning, Intentionality, and Commitment

As clients are able to face and overcome the blocks to their aliveness, as they begin to *choose* rather than succumb to the paths that beckon them, they develop a sense of life meaning. This meaning is wrought out of struggle, deep presence to the rivaling sides of oneself, and embodied choice about the aspect of oneself that one intends to live out. The overcoming of resistance, in other words, is preparatory to the unfolding of meaning, and the unfolding of meaning is preparatory to revitalization.

Such revitalization, or what Rollo May (1969) terms, "intentionality," is the full-bodied orientation to a given goal or direction. It is different from intellectual or behavioral change because its impetus derives from one's entire being, one's entire sense of import and one's entire sense of priority (see also the "I am" experience in May, 1983).

The consolidation of meaning, intentionality, and commitment takes many forms. Sometimes clients find it on the job site, in the home, with friends, or with community. At times it takes the form of a sport or a class or a trip, and sometimes it is without form. The pivotal issue here is attitude. To what extent does a client's life meaning align with his or her inmost aspirations, sensibilities, and values, and how much is the client willing to risk (take responsibility for) the consequences of those alignments?

The task of the therapist at this stage is to assist clients in their quest to *actualize their life meanings*. This assistance may take the form of a Socratic dialogue about possible ways to change one's lifestyle, or relate to a partner, or begin a new project. It may be manifest as an invitation to visualize or role-play new scenarios, inner resources, or concerted actions. It may develop as a reflection on one's dream life and the symbols, patterns, and affects associated with the dream's message. It may take the shape of a challenge to try out newfound capacities in real-life circumstances—a desired encounter, a wished for avocation, a contemplated journey. Following each of these explorations, meaning is further consolidated by encouraging clients to sort through their experiential discoveries. For example, by attuning to the feelings, sensations, and general life impact of risking a new relationship, clients are in an enhanced position to evaluate the significance of that relationship.

A Note about the Social and Spiritual Dimensions of E-H Transformation

In recent years, psychotherapy has received a glut of criticism. This criticism centers on three main points: (1) that psychotherapy is overly individualized; (2) that it feeds a materialist, consumerist mind-set; and (3) that it is politically naïve or regressive (Cushman, 1995; Hillman & Ventura, 1992). "We have had 100 years of psychotherapy," Hillman and Ventura (1992) inveigh, "and the world's getting worse."

The question, however, is which *form* of psychotherapy are the detractors focusing on, and whose particular world is "getting worse"? Although Hillman and Ventura appear to include E-H therapy in their generalized indictment, is this inclusion warranted? From an E-H point of view, for example, there is certainly merit to the problem of a worsening world. In many quarters of the globe, class divisiveness and materialist ambition appear to be on the rise, whereas, at the same time, conviviality, interethnic understanding, and magnanimity appear to be on the descent. But is E-H practice among the instigators of these developments? I would say both yes and no. "Yes" in the sense that it is sometimes overly individualistic, but "no" in the sense that it has consistently opposed the simplistic, cosmetic, and mechanical in therapeutic conduct, which are the primary corrosive influences in my view (e.g., see Laing, 1967; May, 1983).

In any case, one point has become increasingly clear: One cannot simply heal individuals to the neglect of the social context within which they are thrust. To be a responsible practitioner, one must develop a vision of responsible social change, alongside of and in coordination with one's vision of individual transformation—and increasingly, E-H practitioners are becoming conscious of this interdependence (Mendelowitz, 2001; O'Hara, 2001; Pierson & Sharp, 2001; Wadlington, 2001).

The question is one of social advocacy; on whose behalf does a therapist function—the culture, the institutional norm, the conventions of the health care industry, or the client him- or herself? Although none of these can be neglected from an E-H point of view, it is emphatically the client, and the profound subjective and intersubjective realizations of depth-experiential inquiry, that reflect E-H therapy's chief priority. This person-centered priority, moreover, is not just for the revitalization of individuals; it is for the revitalization of their (our) community, culture, and indeed, world (e.g., see Buber, 1937/1970; Bugental & Bracke, 1992; Friedman, 2001; Hanna, Giordano, Dupuy, & Puhakka, 1995; May, 1981). To put it another way, E-H therapy promotes depth inquiry, and depth inquiry promotes a sense of what deeply matters. Although such a sense does not always lead to social and spiritual consciousness, in my experience—and that of many E-H practitioners—this is predominantly what results.

CURATIVE FACTORS OR MECHANISMS OF CHANGE

As previously indicated, the core of E-H change processes is presence. Without presence, there may well be intellectual or behavioral or physiological change but not necessarily the sense of agency or personal involvement that core change requires. To put it another way, E-H therapy stresses presence to *what really matters,* both within the self and between the self and the therapist. This presence has two basic functions: (1) it reconnects people to their pain (e.g., blocks, fears, and anxieties), and (2) it attunes people to the opportunities to transform or transcend that pain.

Presence, then, is both the ground (condition, atmosphere) and the goal for E-H facilitation. As ground, presence holds and illuminates that which is palpably (immediately, affectively, and kinesthetically) relevant within the client and between the client and therapist. Presence in this sense provides the holding environment whereby deeper and more intensified presence can take root. As goal, presence mobilizes clients. It accompanies them during their deepest struggles, their search to redress those struggles, and their day-to-day integration of those struggles (Bugental, 1987; Frankl, 1963; May, 1969).

In addition to facilitating experiential forms of change, such as those previously mentioned, presence also guides and provides a container where appropriate, for more behavioral or programmatic levels of change. The question that presence illuminates is, "What is really going on with this client, and how can I optimize my assistance to her?"; or, to put it another way, What is this client's desire and capacity for change?" (Schneider, 1995).

Insight in E-H therapy is more like "inner vision," as Bugental (1978) frames the term. Inner vision facilitates an *experience* of past, present, or future issues rather than an explanation or formulation *about* them. The end goal of inner vision is not so much to "figure issues out" as to stay with them, attend to their affective and kinesthetic features, and sort out how or whether one is willing to *respond* to them. To the degree that one can follow this process through, one can become more intentional (i.e., concerted, purposeful) in one's life, but also, and paradoxically, more flexible, tolerant, and capable of change.

Interpretations are provided in E-H therapy to facilitate a deepening of experience more than a strengthening of analytical skills. Although a strengthening of analytical skills can certainly be of benefit over the course of an E-H regimen, the thrust of the work is toward empowering *clients* to find their logical or adaptive paths. In this sense, interpretations tend to take the form of mirroring responses in E-H therapy, reflecting and amplifying clients' rivaling impulses.

E-H change processes comprise both an intra- and interpersonal dimension. The intrapersonal aspect is facilitated through concerted efforts to survey the self, whereas the interpersonal dimension is facilitated through the naturally evolving "I–thou" dynamic of relationship. Although E-H practitioners tend to emphasize different aspects of intra- and interpersonal exploration, there is essential unanimity when it comes to the core of these emphases—immediacy and presence.

To summarize, E-H therapy has two essential aims: (1) to cultivate presence (i.e., attention, choice, and freedom), and (2) to cultivate responsibility (i.e., ability to respond) to that presence. These aims are fulfilled by therapists through their capacity to attune, tolerate struggle, and vivify emergent patterns, and by clients through their commitment and desire and capacity for change. Although E-H therapy parallels, and indeed grounds, many other intensive therapies (see the section "Research Support"), its emphasis on presence, struggle, and whole-bodied responsiveness renders it unique.

TREATMENT APPLICABILITY AND ETHICAL CONSIDERATIONS

As suggested earlier, E-H therapy applies to a diverse population of clients. Despite its high-brow image, E-H practice has been applied to substance abusers, ethnic and racial minorities, gay and lesbian clientele, psychiatric inpatients, and business personnel (Schneider & May, 1995; Schneider, Bugental, & Pierson, 2001). Furthermore, E-H principles of presence, I–thou relationship, and courage have been adopted by a plethora of practice orientations (see, e.g., Stolorow et al., 1987). That said, however, the expansion and diversification of E-H therapy is a relatively recent phenomenon; most E-H practice still tends to take place in white middle- to upper-class neighborhoods with white middle- to upper-class clientele. And yet there is no necessary link between such clientele and successful E-H therapy; as E-H practitioners are discovering, the benefits of presence, I–thou encounter, and responsibility are cross-cultural as well as cross-disciplinary (Vontress & Epp, 2001).

While E-H therapists realize that they cannot be "all things to all people," and that certain problems (e.g., circumscribed phobias and brain pathology) are best handled by specialists, there is a definite ecumenism impacting contemporary E-H practice. This ecumenism is correlating with cross-disciplinary openness, adaptations for diverse populations, and sliding-fee scales.

In the end, however, there is no formulaic guideline that determines the course of E-H practice. Each client and therapist pair, each humanity, must have his or her say.

RESEARCH SUPPORT

E-H practice has produced some of the most eloquent case studies in the case literature (e.g., Binswanger, 1958; Boss, 1963; Bugental, 1976; May, 1983; Schneider & May, 1995; Spinelli, 1997; Yalom, 1980). At the same time, however, the systematic, corroborative evidence for E-H therapy is relatively limited (Walsh & McElwain, 2002; Yalom, 1980). There are two major reasons for this situation. First, the E-H theoretical

outlook has tended to attract philosophically and artistically oriented clinicians who
are more at home with clinical practice or
case study narratives than they are with laboratory procedures or controlled investigations (DeCarvalho, 1991). Second, when E-
H therapists or theorists have attempted to
conduct research, they have found themselves facing an array of theoretical, practical, and political barriers. Among these barriers are the difficulties of translating
long-term, exploratory therapeutic processes and outcomes into controlled experimental designs and requirements (Schneider, 1998b; Seligman, 1996), the problems
of quantifying complex life issues (Miller,
1996a), and the hardships of obtaining research funds for "alternative" therapeutic
practices (Miller, 1996b). Furthermore, the
obstacles are even more daunting for those
in the E-H therapy community who have
called for qualitative (e.g., phenomenological) assessment of their practices. Although
many consider such assessments more appropriate than their conventional counterparts to evaluate E-H subject matter, there
are substantial costs associated with their
implementation (Wertz, 2001). Among
them are perplexing theoretical and practical challenges but also, and no less con-
founding, estrangement from a quantifying,
medicalizing research community (Elliott,
2001; Wertz, 2001).

This state of affairs, however, appears to
be changing. In the past decade, mainstream
conceptions of therapeutic process and outcome research have undergone notable
reevaluations, and models, once considered
invulnerable are now being revised. The
randomized controlled trial, for example,
once considered the "gold standard" of
therapeutic evaluation research, has been
criticized as well (see Bohart, O'Hara, &
Leitner, 1998; Goldfried & Wolfe, 1996;
Schneider, 2001). Conversely, qualitative research, once considered practically and scientifically untenable, has attained professional legitimacy (Elliott, 2002; Wertz,
2001).

In light of these changes, E-H therapy
has been accumulating a considerable base
of empirical support. Although still comparatively small, this base is both rigorous and
promising (Elliott, 2002; Walsh & McElwain, 2002). In the domain of systematic
quantitative inquiry, for example, there is
growing support for key E-H principles of
practice. This support is reflected in the
"common factors" research which consistently upholds the relationship as opposed
to technical factors as the core facilitative
condition (Wampold, 2001). It is echoed in
the research on therapeutic alliance (Hovarth, 1995), empathy (Bohart & Greenberg,
1997), genuineness and positive regard (Orlinsky, Grawe, & Parks, 1994), and clients'
capacity for self-healing (Bohart & Tallman,
1999), and it is mirrored in the burgeoning
research on expressed emotion (e.g.,
Gendlin, 1996; Greenberg, Rice, & Elliott,
1993). Greenberg and colleagues (1993), for
example, demonstrated that such E-H compatible facilitations as evocative unfolding
(or vivifying a problematic scene), empty-
chair technique (role play with an imagined
other), and experiential processing (which
includes evoking awareness of experience,
attendance to unclear or emergent experience, ownership of emotional reactions, interpersonal contact, development of a
meaning perspective, and translation of
emerging awareness into daily life) all correlated with positive outcome (see also Elliott & Greenberg, 2002).

Finally, in a little known but provocative
study of E-H therapy with patients diagnosed as schizophrenic and treated in an alternative, minimally medicating psychiatric
facility, Mosher (2001), reported the following: At 2-year follow-up, the experimental
(E-H treated) population ($n = 68$) "had significantly better outcomes . . . representing
the dimensions of rehospitalization, psychopathology, independent living, and social and occupational functioning" than
their conventionally treated (medicated)
counterparts ($n = 61$) over the same investigative period (p. 392).

On the qualitative side of the equation, Bohart and Tallman (1999), Rennie (1994), and Watson and Rennie (1994) have demonstrated the value of such E-H stalwarts as presence and expanding the capacity for choice in effective facilitation. Specifically they showed that successful therapy as understood by clients necessitates "a process of self-reflection," consideration of "alternative courses of action, and making choices" (Walsh & McElwain, 2002, p. 261). In a related study, Hanna and colleagues (1995) investigated what they termed "second order," or deep and sweeping change processes in therapy. Compatible with existential emphases on liberation, they found that "transcendence," or moving beyond limitations, was the essential structure of change. Furthermore, they found that transcendence consisted of "penetrating, pervasive, global and enduringly stable" insight, accompanied by "a new perspective on the self, world, or problem" (p. 148).

Finally, in a study of clients' perceptions of their E-H oriented therapists, Schneider (1985) reported that although techniques were important to the success of long-term (i.e., 2-year-plus) therapeutic outcomes, the "personal involvement" of the therapist—which comprised his or her genuineness, support, acceptance, and deep understanding—was by far the most critical factor identified. Such involvement, moreover, inspired clients to become more self-involved, and to experience themselves as more capable, responsible, and self-accepting. (For a comprehensive review of these and other E-H therapeutic investigations, see Elliott, 2002; Rennie, 2002; Walsh & McElwain, 2002; Watson & Bohart, 2001.)

To summarize, empirical investigation of E-H therapy is in a nascent but flowering stage. Many conceptual dimensions of E-H practice have been confirmed by both quantitative and qualitative investigation, and many remain to be more fully illuminated. Yet if the trends in therapy research continue, E-H practice may become a model, evidence-based modality which stresses three critical variables: (1) the therapeutic relationship, (2) the therapist's presence or personality, and (3) the active self-healing of clients. By implication, on the other hand, statistically driven manuals, programs, and techniques may become increasingly adjunctive, if not peripheral, in their facilitative role (Bohart & Tallman, 1999; Messer & Wampold, 2002; Westen & Morrison, 2001).

CASE ILLUSTRATION

Mary was a self-referred, 240-pound, single, Caucasian sales clerk. She had a minimal, 3-month history of "mental health" counseling (as a young adolescent), and no history of psychiatric medication. From the moment Mary stepped into my office, I could sense a deep connection with her, and yet at the same time, a curious reluctance on her part to engage.

Seduced and teased as a child, Mary had negligible trust in men, little trust in herself in the presence of men, and minute trust in the culture that tacitly assented to these calamities. Yet here she was, at 30 years old, declaring her commitment to reenvision and reassemble her life. Here she was—partly with my encouragement—spending hours of the evening dashing off reams of pages about the pain, injustice, and outrages of her life but at the same time, the dreams, desires, and possibilities that could be her life. She would read from, and we would share reflections about, her entries, and she would scrap tirelessly with them. Back and forth, she would swing—between searing self-abasement and rising self-attunement; between depleting worry and replenishing confidence. Her struggle displayed all the earmarks of the depth excursion, the depth entanglement, that precedes restoration. She, like so many therapy clients, had to straddle contending life paths, to sift out the intimations of those life paths, and to consolidate a plan, direction, and vision that were based on those intimations. Following

3 years of such wrangling and deep experiential immersions, she gradually and doggedly reemerged. She found that capitulating to her father, the culture, and the taboo of asserting herself were no longer tolerable and that changes had to occur.

Her first step, which I encouraged, was to allow herself to be angry enough and indignant enough to halt her automatic bingeing and to peer into the void it replaced. Instead of instantly seeking food as a refuge, therefore, and based on my recommendation, she instituted a pause in her experience; she allowed the fears and hurts to percolate. Yet, in this percolation were much more than fears and hurts. She realized, for example, that she did not have to be so readily panicked over being seen by others, that she would not inexorably be attacked by the person she feared, and that greatest of all, she had a value and truth that she could not squander. Regardless of her obesity, she realized, *she* had worth; a tender, loving essence inside her, yearning to be felt, heard, and held.

Her second step, which we coordinated with a local weight loss clinic, was the long and arduous process of losing her excess girth, and of confronting the barriers to this toilsome process. It is not that she felt an *obligation* to lose pounds or even that this ordeal was mandatory for her physical health. All these "supposed to's" were increasingly peripheral to her. By contrast, that which was mandatory for her was an internal rightness about losing her weight. She did not want to go into a program until she felt clear that health, attractiveness, and integrity were necessary for *her*—not for some imagined other.

Following this clarification, she embarked on an 8-month trial with a powder diet as a replacement for meals. This course had its own thorny challenges, but she met them well. On the one hand, the powder was "easy," because it was readily available, habit forming, and required little forethought. On the other hand, precisely because it was *not* food, the powder presented

Mary with opportunities to reassess her associations to food. Among these associations were the comfort value of food, the special linkages to sweets, and the pleasure of cooking. But chief among Mary's discoveries was that behind all these compelling features of food was the daunting capacity of food to protect. From the standpoint of protection, Mary realized, food was not simply a distraction or a pleasurable obsession; it was a refuge from perceived annihilation. By eating the powder, and particularly, by attending to the feelings, sensations, and images conjured up by her abstinence from food, Mary began to confront death, the "death" (or brutality) she associated with her nakedness, beauty, and rawness, removed of her culinary refuge. As a result, she began to cope better with that death anxiety. She became less anxious and acquired new patterns of self-support—such as speaking up for herself, or associating with caring company. She also found freedom in her newfound visibility, particularly the freedom to play. She indulged in play like a kid on her first visit to a beach. She ran, worked out, and hiked and simply reveled in her newfound (130-pound) mobility. She also reveled in her newfound attractiveness to men.

Despite these Herculean developments, however, and like so many who embark on the dieting path (see, e.g., Wadden & Stunkard, 1986), Mary emphatically relapsed. After 8 energizing months, and upon transitioning to real food, Mary discovered yet another layer to her ordeal: she had yet to confront her rage. Oh, Mary could get angry. She could rail at the indignities of life, the injustices of culture, the cruelty of her narrow-minded peers, and so on. Yet what she could not do earlier, in the ease and comfort of her powdered diet, was to rail at the chief source for her oppression— her incest-mongering father.

The reexposure to food then brought back a torrent of memories, hurts, and defenses for Mary. She conveyed a dream— early on in this transition—that coupled a hovering, heavily breathing face, with a tiny, prenatal body. I asked her to focus on the feeling tone of this dream and to explore the affective and kinesthetic associations to this feeling tone. Although reluctant at first, she soon was able to "live out" the sequences of the dream, and to "speak" from its urgent depths. The voice that stood out consequently was the prenatal voice, which was her voice, of course, struggling for its survival. But suddenly, a shift occurred: the ostensibly fragile, prenatal cry, became a blood-curdling scream; and the scream became an attacking fist. But this sequence only lasted a few seconds. In moments, she would revert back again to a cry. Mary spent many subsequent months unpacking the above sequence, delving ever closer to her core battle. Repeatedly, we would call attention to her swings between abject timidity, helplessness, and vulnerability and flagrant rebellion, vengefulness, and fury; then her fear and guilt would set in, the whole cycle would be repeated.

The instantiation of this pattern was evident in Mary's daily life. Consistently she would oscillate between holing herself up in her house with bags of candy to bulldozing her coworkers to bloating and flagellating herself again with food. After 6 months of her transition back to food, Mary regained 60% of her postdietary weight.

There were, of course, livelier times for Mary, but at this juncture, they were mercilessly under siege. The encrusted layers of pain, dormant just 6 months ago (in association with her powder diet), now broke open into raw, exposed gashes; and although Mary empathized with these gashes, their intensity sometimes overwhelmed her. Binge eating, as noted previously, was one avenue of defense against this intensity, but so were vain efforts to gain control, such as bulimic purging and even mild cutting.

At one point I mirrored these patterns back to Mary. I echoed back to her what I experienced as her slow "suicide," her pull to "give up," and her readiness to defer her power. In turn, Mary bristled at my charac-

terizations, denied that she was in crisis, and simmered in defiance. Yet, at the same time, Mary and I both knew that I had touched a chord at some level, that death was at her doorstep, and that time was slipping fast. It is during just such periods that clients stand before a crossroad in E-H therapy—the crossroad of life or death, possibility or foreclosure, and it is precisely the handling of that crossroad (by both therapist and client) that has an indelible impact on recovery. In light of these contexts, I concertedly invited Mary to stay present to herself, to reverberate to her agonizing dilemma, and to open to the possibilities, the "more" that her dilemma foretold. A part of this "more" encompassed Mary's relationship with me. To the degree that Mary and I could tussle with one another—could face one another's ire and awkwardness and discomfort—to that extent could we also begin to appreciate one another, and the "truth" that we separately offered to one another. Mary's truth, as I grew to appreciate it, was the stark terror of confronting and overcoming her father's wrath. It was the dread of change, and of becoming the "new" person who has to embody that change. The truth that I held for Mary, on the other hand, which she grew to appreciate, was the anguish, self-deprecation, and disability she countenanced by remaining in her father's thrall, and, conversely, the freedom, mobility, and life that awaited her on the other side of that thrall.

This I–thou meeting afforded Mary a chance to reappraise her relationship to herself, her father, and me. It helped her see—in vivid and experiential immediacy—that she was more than her paralyzing fragility, more than a rape victim, and even more than a victim of women-hating men but a person who could struggle and be vulnerable with another person and yet emerge with renewed vigor.

Gradually then, and with mounting force, the side of Mary that aspired to feel, deepen, and live began to predominate; whereas the regressive side, the side that pulled to hide, waned. (Although this was not a permanent state of affairs, it definitely set the tone for the future.)

These changes afforded Mary and me a chance to revisit the question of her transformation. The first step in our reassessment was to institute a stopgap measure; in order for Mary to reemerge, the "blood-letting" had to be stanched. Accordingly, Mary limited her bingeing, stopped her cutting, and ceased her purging. With my encouragement, furthermore, she enrolled in an intensive, year-long rehabilitation program. This program—which comprised nutritional counseling, group therapy, and behavioral modification training—was aimed at curtailing her bingeing, bolstering her life-management skills, and strengthening her capacity to communicate.

Once Mary began stabilizing—which was about 8 months after her transition to food—and could learn to exercise some control over her external patterns, the long and continuing inner work could be engaged more fully. Her behavioral skill building, in other words, paved the way for the next and more pivotal phase of internal skill building; which illustrates the integrative dimension of E-H therapy.

In the final phase of our work, Mary focused on living while dieting rather than dieting to live. Over the course of her many ordeals, Mary had learned to grab into the life that awaits her *now* rather than postponing it for some unreachable ideal. In accord with this philosophy and in the midst of her ongoing weight management, she began dating again, went on trips that she had deferred, and resumed her "working through" with her father. For example, to facilitate Mary's rising self-confidence in relation to her father, we worked with a variety of exploratory outlets—from role plays to drawings to rituals with effigies.

Yet, whereas these initial encounters with her father were imaginary, she soon began to shift her tack and contemplate an actual confrontation. She spent many weeks exploring the necessity of such a confrontation, but by closely attending to her experience—immediately, affectively, and kinesthetically—she emphatically arrived at a decision: She would write him a letter, spelling out her entire experience of him—decimating as well as ambivalent and loving—and she would offer to personally discuss that letter at a location of her choosing.

This decision on Mary's part was a turning point of therapy. Regardless of how her father would have responded, in my view Mary had turned the tide with this decision, from floundering panic to concerted choice, and from impotence to agency. As it turned out, Mary fulfilled her plan and met with her father. Although he was reportedly "shaken" by the ordeal, it did bring a renewed life to their relationship, and most important, it helped to restore Mary's life, the "life" that she could give to herself.

By the end of our work together—about 3½ years of therapy—Mary acquired a revivified sense of self. Although she continued to contend with weight issues (e.g., she was now about 30% overweight), and harbored residual anxieties, these no longer stifled her or prevented her from *concertedly* living. She enjoyed most of her food, ate healthfully, and began a promising romantic relationship. She also experienced a great deal more freedom in her life, and that sensibility paid off in her deepened friendships, expanded physical activities, and enhanced service to the community.

Finally, although Mary was "liberated," she did not completely eradicate her symptoms. What she did eradicate, on the other hand, was a corrosive view of life, which was a partial view that stressed helplessness over possibility and anxiety over courage. Like many E-H therapy clients, Mary formed a new relationship with her symptoms; she learned that she could expand beyond them and through that expansion, discover new relationships to food, to her father, and even to existence itself.

Mary was not unlike another weight-loss survivor, Karen, who after about 3 years of her own therapy declared:

I wish I could tell you that being a size twelve is all wonderful but I'm finding out that being awake and alive is a package deal. I don't get to go through the line and pick only goodies. On one side is wonder, awe, excitement and laughter—and on the other side is tears, disappointment, aching sadness. Wholeness is coming to me by being willing to explore ALL the feelings.

So . . . 275 pounds later, my life is a mixture of pain and bliss. It hurts a lot these days but it's real. It's my life being lived by me and not vicariously through a soap opera. . . . I don't know where it's all heading, but one thing I know for sure, I'm definitely going. (Roth, 1991, pp. 183–184)

Mary was a deeply troubled but extraordinarily dedicated E-H therapy client. She grappled with some of the most trying personal and social barriers with which humans must contend—incest, obesity, depersonalization—and yet she comparatively and realistically triumphed. Beginning with her furious journal writing; our introductory struggles; and her fitful alignment with fears, desires, and outrages, Mary gradually reconstructed her life. Through my presence and our presence to each other, Mary was able to experience the safety to do more than merely report about her life but to "work out" that life amid torments of the past, promptings of the present, and callings of the future. Through invitations to stay present to herself—particularly the feelings, sensations, and images evoked within herself—she began to illuminate what she profoundly desired in her life (e.g., freedom, mobility, and intimacy) but also, and equally important, what separated her from those profound desires (e.g., terror of annihilation [her father, men], suppressed rage, and entrenched habits).

In the meantime, adjunctive therapies were employed at key stages throughout the E-H therapy process. These therapies, such as nutritional counseling and behavioral skills training, provided a key confidence-building component to the E-H work. At the same time that they helped Mary to stabilize, they also helped empower her, and this empowerment translated into her willingness to take risks in depth therapy.

In short, E-H therapy provided a forum whereby presence and its activation through inner struggle, resistance work, and meaning creation, along with an adjunctive program of rehabilitation, could converge to reassemble a life. To the extent that such opportunities for meaningful convergence are being economically hampered today, there are dwindling opportunities to reassemble lives, and this, lamentably, may be the direst legacy of market-driven mental health.

CURRENT AND FUTURE TRENDS

The outlook for E-H therapy is both guarded and promising. It is guarded to the extent that all depth therapies are guarded and under threat today—by an encroaching medicalized ethos. Moreover, as students, instructors, and professional organizations acquiesce to, and in some cases encourage, the foregoing ethos, there is a decreasing incentive to teach let alone apply E-H alternatives (Bohart et al., 1997; Schneider, 1998b, 1999a).

On the other hand, the outlook for the future is not so one-sided as it may seem. As previously suggested, there are trends, such as the embrace of experientially informed practice, that run directly counter to the aforementioned scenario. These trends suggest that a backlash is building, and that E-H therapy is on its cutting edge—as is holistic and integrative medicine, comprehensive health care, and social and spiritual activism (see, e.g., Criswell, 2001; Elkins, 2001; Lyons, 2001; Montouri & Purser, 2001; Schneider, 1998b).

As E-H therapy evolves, moreover, it is converging with other "liberation-based" therapies. These therapies are influencing the culture, beyond the traditional two-person context. Drawing on E-H practice principles, for example, Holzman and New-man have formulated "performative social therapy" (Waddlington, 2001). This therapy is present-centered, improvisational, and egalitarian and addresses through an "edu-cational community, a theater space, and a therapy environment," challenging cultural predicaments, as well as those that afflict in-dividuals (Waddlington, 2001, p. 496). Re-ferring to that which she terms "emancipa-tory therapy," O'Hara (2001) has elaborated an ever-widening E-H application. She documents the use of E-H approaches in the schools, business community, and hu-man service fields, and pleads for a society-wide E-H reformation.

Finally, what I (Schneider, 1998b) have termed the "romantic" in psychology ties together existential, emancipatory, psycho-dynamic–relational, and spiritual spheres of inquiry. This perspective is defined by three overarching emphases: (1) the interrelated wholeness of experience; (2) access to such wholeness by means of tacit processes—affect, intuition, kinesthesia, and imagina-tion; and (3) qualitative or descriptive ac-counts of such processes (p. 278).

To the extent that the aforementioned trends grow—and there is reason for opti-mism that they will (e.g., Ray, 1996)—then correlative trends should also grow, such as funding for E-H practices, support for E-H training, and investment in EH theory building.

On the other hand, I do not want to sound glib about the difficulties E-H and related practice modalities face in the com-ing years. Managed care, programmatic mental health practices, and medicalization are here to stay, and there are sound bases for their existence (e.g., Schneider, 1995). But what I do wish to emphasize is that with discernment, focus, and passion, a ma-jor transformation can be staged in psychol-ogy. This change will not be exclusivist—it will not reject conventional modalities, but it will widen, deepen, and integrate these modalities, and it will weave them into a liberating whole.

SUGGESTIONS FOR FURTHER READING

Case Reports

Bugental, J. F. T. (1976). *The search for existential identity: Patient-therapist dialogues in humanis-tic psychotherapy*. San Francisco: Jossey-Bass.—This book is a classic of the E-H case literature. In addition to lively and in-structive case synopses, Bugental provides a rare glimpse of himself, as he grapples per-sonally with each of his encounters. Unfor-tunately, *Search* is out of print, but was up-dated in a later work titled, *Intimate Journeys* (San Francisco: Jossey-Bass, 1990).

Schneider, K. J., & May, R. (Eds.). (1995). *The psychology of existence: An integrative, clinical perspective*. New York: McGraw-Hill.—This edited volume extends E-H therapy to a new, more diverse generation of practition-ers. In addition to providing an integrative framework for existential–humanistic prac-tice, it also features 16 ethnically and diag-nostically diverse case studies, including Rollo May's germinal, "Black and Impo-tent: The Case of Mercedes."

Yalom, I. (1989). *Love's executioner*. New York: Basic Books.—This is an enlightening, earthy, and superbly written volume, fea-turing many memorable vignettes. Yalom's observations are not always comfortable, but they are pithy, candid, and true to life.

Research

Cain, D. J., & Seeman, J. (Eds.). (2002). *Humanis-tic psychotherapies: Handbook of research and practice*. Washington, DC: American Psy-chological Association.—This is an excel-lent compendium, featuring top-notch in-vestigations of E-H practices. Although these investigations tend to be quantitative, they are highly illuminating to mainstream clinicians and researchers who are skeptical of E-H offerings.

Schneider, K. J., Bugental, J. F. T., & Pierson, J. F. (Eds.). (2001). *The handbook of humanistic psychology: Leading edges in theory, research, and practice*. Thousand Oaks, CA: Sage.—This edited volume comprises an unprece-dented qualitative research section, which explores both active and hypothetical E-H case material. The section features phenomenological, heuristic, narrative, multi-ple-case, and hermeneutic modes of inves-tigation.

Yalom, I. (1980). *Existential psychotherapy.* New York: Basic Books.—Yalom's classic features an important section on E-H process and outcome research, with the dimension of death as a prominent investigative focus.

Further Reading

Cooper, M. (2003). *Existential therapies.* London: Sage.—A clear and comprehensive survey of the latest E-H (American) and existential–analytic (European) practice philosophies. Although the European perspectives are highlighted, there is a lively, if somewhat controversial, consideration of the American position.

Frie, R. (Guest Ed.). (1999). Understanding existence: Perspectives in existential analysis. *The Humanistic Psychologist, 27*(1).—This special issue provides a timely and absorbing overview of recent trends in existential-analytic, existential-humanistic, and existential-postmodern therapeutic perspectives. The therapeutic relationship and social context are of particular focus.

Laing, R. D. (1969). *The divided self: An existential study in sanity and madness.* Middlesex, UK: Penguin.—This is a stunning illustration of the E-H perspective on psychosis; it is a standard reference, moreover, for all those interested in minimally medicating psychiatric alternatives.

May, R., Angel, E., & Ellenberger, H. (Eds.). (1958). *Existence.* New York: Basic Books.—This is the volume that began it all—the importation of E-H therapy to the United States. May's opening chapters in particular, are foundational to the E-H theoretical base.

REFERENCES

Alsup, R. (1995). Existentialism of personalism: A Native American perspective. In K. J. Schneider & R. May (Eds.), *The psychology of existence: An integrative, clinical perspective* (pp. 247–253). New York: McGraw-Hill.

Ballinger, B., Matano, R., & Amantea, M. (1995). A perspective on alcoholism: The case of Mr. P. In K. J. Schneider & R. May (Eds.), *The psychology of existence: An integrative, clinical perspective* (pp. 264–270). New York: McGraw-Hill.

Barrett, W. H. (1958). *Irrational man: A study in existential philosophy.* New York: Doubleday.

Becker, E. (1973). *Denial of death.* New York: Free Press.

Binswanger, L. (1958). The case of Ellen West. In R. May, E. Angel, & H. Ellenberger (Eds.), *Existence* (pp. 237–364). New York: Basic Books.

Bohart, A. C., & Greenberg, L. S. (Eds.). (1997). *Empathy reconsidered.* Washington, DC: American Psychological Association.

Bohart, A. C., O'Hara, M., & Leitner, L. M. (1998). Empirically violated treatments: Disenfranchisement of humanistic and other psychotherapies. *Psychotherapy Research, 8,* 141–157.

Bohart, A. C., O'Hara, M., Leitner, L. M., Wertz, F. J., Stern, E. M., Schneider, K. J., Serlin, I. A., & Greening, T. C. (1997). Guidelines for the provision of humanistic psychosocial services. *Humanistic Psychologist, 24,* 64–107.

Bohart, A. C., & Tallman, K. (1999). *How clients make therapy work: The process of active self-healing.* Washington, DC: American Psychological Association.

Boss, M. (1963). *Psychoanalysis and daseinsanalysis* (L. B. Lefebre, Trans.). New York: Basic Books.

Buber, M. (1970). *I and thou.* (W. Kaufmann, Trans.). New York: Scribner's. (Originally published 1937)

Bugental, J. F. T. (1965). *The search for authenticity: An existential–analytic approach to psychotherapy.* New York: Holt, Rinehart, & Winston.

Bugental, J. F. T. (1976). *The search for existential identity: Patient–therapist dialogues in humanistic psychotherapy.* San Francisco: Jossey-Bass.

Bugental, J. F. T. (1978). *Psychotherapy and process: The fundamentals of an existential–humanistic approach.* New York: McGraw-Hill.

Bugental, J. F. T. (1987). *The art of the psychotherapist.* New York: Norton.

Bugental, J. F. T. (1995). Preliminary sketches for a short-term existential therapy. In K. J. Schneider & R. May (Eds.), *The psychology of existence: An integrative, clinical perspective* (pp. 261–264). New York: McGraw-Hill.

Bugental, J. F. T., & Bracke, P. (1992). The future of existential–humanistic psychotherapy. *Psychotherapy, 29,* 28–33.

Bugental, J. F. T., & Sterling, M. (1995). Existential psychotherapy. In A. S. Gurman & S. B. Messer (Eds.), *Essential psychotherapies* (pp. 226–260) New York: Guilford Press.

Camus, A. (1955). *The myth of Sisyphus and other essays.* (J. O'Brien, Trans.). New York: Knopf.

Churchill, S., & Wertz, F. J. (2001). An introduction to phenomenological research in psychology: Historical, conceptual, and methodological foundations. In K. J. Schneider, J. F. T. Bugental, & J. F. Pierson (Eds.), *The handbook of humanistic psychology: Leading edges in theory, practice, and research* (pp. 247–262). Thousand Oaks, CA: Sage.

Criswell, E. (2001). Humanistic psychology and mind/body medicine. In K. J. Schneider, J. F. T. Bugental, & J. F. Pierson (Eds.), *The handbook of humanistic psychology: Leading edges in theory, practice, and research* (pp. 581–591). Thousand Oaks, CA: Sage.

Cushman, P. (1995). *Constructing the self, constructing America: A cultural history of psychotherapy.* Reading, MA: Addison-Wesley.

deBeauvoir, S. (1948). *The ethics of ambiguity.* New York: Citadel.

DeCarvalho, R. (1991). *The founders of humanistic psychology.* New York: Praeger.

Elkins, D. N. (2001). Beyond religion: Toward a humanistic spirituality. In K. J. Schneider, J. F. T. Bugental, & J. F. Pierson (Eds.), *The handbook of humanistic psychology: Leading edges in theory, practice, and research* (pp. 201–212). Thousand Oaks, CA: Sage.

Elliott, R. (2001). Hermeneutic single-case efficacy design: An overview. In K. J. Schneider, J. F. T. Bugental, & J. F. Pierson (Eds.), *The handbook of humanistic psychology: Leading edges in theory, practice, and research* (pp. 315–324). Thousand Oaks, CA: Sage.

Elliott, R. (2002). The effectiveness of humanistic therapies: A meta-analysis. In D. J. Cain, & J. Seeman (Eds.), *Humanistic psychotherapies: Handbook of research and practice* (pp. 57–81). Washington, DC: American Psychological Association.

Elliott, R., & Greenberg, L. S. (2002). Process–experiential psychotherapy. In D. J. Cain, & J. Seeman (Eds.), *Humanistic psychotherapies: Handbook of research and practice*

(pp. 279–306). Washington, DC: American Psychological Association.

Fischer, C. T. (1994). *Individualizing psychological assessment.* Hillsdale, NJ: Erlbaum. (Original work published 1985)

Frankl, V. E. (1963). *Man's search for meaning: An introduction to logotherapy.* New York: Pocket Books.

Friedman, M. (1991a). *Encounter on the narrow ridge: A life of Martin Buber.* New York: Paragon House.

Friedman, M. (1991b). *The worlds of existentialism: A critical reader.* New York: Humanities Press.

Friedman, M. (1995). The case of Dawn. In K. J. Schneider & R. May (Eds.), *The psychology of existence: An integrative, clinical perspective* (pp. 308–315). New York: McGraw-Hill.

Friedman, M. (2001). Expanding the boundaries of theory. In K. J. Schneider, J. F. T. Bugental, & J. F. Pierson (Eds.), *The handbook of humanistic psychology: Leading edges in theory, practice, and research* (pp. 343–348). Thousand Oaks, CA: Sage.

Fromm, E. (1941). *Escape from freedom.* New York: Holt, Rinehart, & Winston.

Galvin, J. (1995). Brief encounters with Chinese clients: The case of Peter. In K. J. Schneider & R. May (Eds.), *The psychology of existence: An integrative, clinical perspective* (pp. 254–261). New York: McGraw-Hill.

Gendlin, E. T. (1996). *Focusing-oriented psychotherapy.* New York: Guilford Press.

Giorgi, A. (1970). *Psychology as a human science: A phenomenologically based approach.* New York: Harper & Row.

Goldfried, M. R., & Wolfe, B. E. (1996). Psychotherapy practice and research: Repairing a strained alliance. *American Psychologist, 51,* 1007–1016.

Greenberg, L. S., Rice, L. N., & Elliott, R. (1993). *Facilitating emotional change: The moment-by-moment process.* New York: Guilford Press.

Grondin, J. (1995). *Sources of hermeneutics.* Albany: State University of New York Press.

Hanna, F. J., Giordano, F., Dupuy, P., & Puhakka, K. (1995). Agency and transcendence: The experience of therapeutic change. *Humanistic Psychologist, 23,* 139–160.

Heidegger, M. (1962). *Being and time* (J. Macquarrie & E. Robinson, Trans.). New York: Basic Books.

Hillman, J., & Ventura, M. (1992). *We've had a hundred years of psychotherapy and the world's getting worse.* San Francisco: HarperSan-Francisco.

Hovarth, A. O. (1995). The therapeutic relationship: From transference to alliance. *In Session, 1,* 7–17.

Husserl, E. (1962). *Ideas: General introduction to pure pheneomenology* (W. R. Boyce Gibson, Trans.). New York: Collier. (Original work published 1913)

James, W. (1936). *The varieties of religious experience.* New York: Modern Library. (Original work published 1902)

Jung, C. G. (1966). *Two essays on analytical psychology* (R. F. C. Hull, Trans.). Princeton, NJ: Princeton University Press.

Kierkegaard, S. (1944). *The concept of dread* (W. Lowrie, Trans.). Princeton, NJ: Princeton University Press. (Original work published 1844)

Laing, R. D. (1967). *The politics of experience.* New York: Ballantine.

Laing, R. D. (Speaker). (1985). Theoretical and practical aspects of existential therapy (Cassette Recording No. L330-W1A). Phoenix, AZ: The Evolution of Psychotherapy Conference, sponsored by the Erickson Institute.

Lerner, M. (2000). *Spirit matters.* Charlottesville, VA: Hampton Roads.

Lyons, A. (2001). Humanistic psychology and social action. In K. J. Schneider, J. F. T. Bugental, & J. F. Pierson (Eds.), *The handbook of humanistic psychology: Leading edges in theory, practice, and research* (pp. 625–634). Thousand Oaks, CA: Sage.

Marcel, G. (1956). *The philosophy of existentialism.* New York: Philosophical Library.

Mahrer, A. R. (1996). *The complete guide to experiential psychotherapy.* New York: Wiley.

May, R. (1958). The origins and significance of the existential movement in psychology. In R. May, E. Angel, & H. Ellenberger (Eds.), *Existence* (pp. 3–36). New York: Basic Books.

May, R. (1969). *Love and will.* New York: Norton.

May, R. (1972). *Power and innocence.* New York: Norton.

May, R. (1981). *Freedom and destiny.* New York: Norton.

May, R. (1983). *The discovery of being.* New York: Norton.

May, R. (1987). (Speaker). *The relevance of existential therapy to today's world* [Videotape]. (Available on a limited basis from the author, c/o Saybrook Graduate School, 450 Pacific Street, San Francisco, CA 94133)

Mendelowitz, E. (2001). Fellini, Fred, and Ginger: Imagology in a postmodern world. In K. J. Schneider, J. F. T. Bugental, & J. F. Pierson (Eds.), *The handbook of humanistic psychology: Leading edges in theory, practice, and research* (pp. 153–159). Thousand Oaks, CA: Sage.

Merleau-Ponty, M. (1962). *The phenomenology of perception* (C. Smith, Trans.). London: Routledge & Kegan Paul.

Messer, S. B., & Wampold, B. E. (2002). Let's face facts, common factors are more potent than specific therapy ingredients. *Clinical Psychology: Science and Practice, 9*(1), 21–25.

Miller, I. J. (1996a). Managed care is harmful to outpatient mental health services: A call for accountability. *Professional Psychology: Research and Practice, 27,* 349–363.

Miller, I. J. (1996b). Time-limited brief therapy has gone too far: The result is invisible rationing. *Professional Psychology: Research and Practice, 27,* 567–576.

Monheit, J. (1995). A gay and lesbian perspective: The case of Marcia. In K. J. Schneider & R. May (Eds.), *The psychology of existence: An integrative, clinical perspective* (pp. 226–232). New York: McGraw-Hill.

Montuori, M., & Purser, R. (2001). Humanistic psychology and the workplace. In K. J. Schneider, J. F. T. Bugental, & J. F. Pierson (Eds.), *The handbook of humanistic psychology: Leading edges in theory, practice, and research* (pp. 635–644). Thousand Oaks, CA: Sage.

Mosher, L. (2001). Treating madness without hospitals: Soteria and its successors. In K. J. Schneider, J. F. T. Bugental, & J. F. Pierson (Eds.), *The handbook of humanistic psychology: Leading edges in theory, practice, and research* (pp. 389–402). Thousand Oaks, CA: Sage.

Moss, D. (Ed.). (1999). *Humanistic and transpersonal psychology: A historical and biographical sourcebook.* Wesport, CT: Greenwood Press.

Moustakas, C. (1972). *Loneliness and love.* Englewood Cliffs, NJ: Prentice Hall.

Murray, H. A., Barret, W. G., Homburger, E., et al. (1938). *Explorations in personality.* New York: Oxford University Press.

Nietzsche, F. (1982). Twilight of the idols. In W. Kaufmann (Ed.), *The portable Nietzche* (pp. 465–563). New York: Penguin. (Originally published 1889)

O'Hara, M. (2001). Emancipatory therapeutic practice for a new era: A work of retrieval. In K. J. Schneider, J. F. T. Bugental, & J. F. Pierson (Eds.), *The handbook of humanistic psychology: Leading edges in theory, practice, and research* (pp. 473–489). Thousand Oaks, CA: Sage.

Orlinsky, D. E., Grawe, K., & Parks, B. K. (1994). Process and outcome in psychotherapy—noch einmal. In A. E. Bergin & S. L. Garfield (Eds), *Handbook of psychotherapy and behavior change* (pp. 270–378). New York: Wiley.

Phillips, J. (1980–1981). Transference and encounter: The therapeutic relationship in psychoanalytic and existential therapy. *Review of Existential Psychology and Psychiatry, 17*(2 &3), 135–152.

Pierson, J. F., & Sharp, J. (2001). Cultivating psychotherapist artistry: A model existential-humanistic training program. In K. J. Schneider, J. F. T. Bugental, & J. F. Pierson (Eds.), *The handbook of humanistic psychology: Leading edges in theory, practice, and research* (pp. 539–554). Thousand Oaks, CA: Sage.

Portnoy, D. (1999). Relatedness: Where humanistic and psychoanalytic psychotherapy converge. *Journal of Humanistic Psychology, 39*(1), 19–34.

Rank, O. (1936). *Will therapy* (J. Taft, Trans.). New York: Knopf.

Ray, P. (1996). The rise of integral culture. *Noetic Sciences Review*, pp. 4–15.

Rennie, D. L. (1994). Storytelling in psychotherapy: The client's subjective experience. *Psychotherapy, 31,* 234–243.

Rennie, D. L. (2002). Experiencing psychotherapy: Grounded theory studies. In D. J. Cain, & J. Seeman (Eds.), *Humanistic psychotherapies: Handbook of research and practice* (pp. 117–144). Washington, DC: American Psychological Association.

Rice, D. (1995). An African American perspective: The case of Darrin. In K. J. Schneider & R. May (Eds.), *The psychology of existence: An integrative, clinical perspective* (pp. 204–214). New York: McGraw-Hill.

Rogers, C. R. (1951). *Client-centered therapy: It's current practice, implications, & theory.* Boston: Houghton Mifflin.

Roth, G. (1991). *When food is love.* New York: Plume.

Rowan, J. (2001). Existential analysis and humanistic psychotherapy. In K. J. Schneider, J. F. T. Bugental, & J. F. Pierson (Eds.), *The handbook of humanistic psychology: Leading edges in theory, practice, and research* (pp. 447–464). Thousand Oaks, CA: Sage.

Sartre, J. P. (1956). *Being and nothingness* (H. Barnes, Trans.). New York: Philosophical Library.

Schneider, K. J. (1985). Clients' perceptions of the positive and negative characteristics of their counselors. *Dissertation Abstracts International, 45*(10), 3345b.

Schneider, K. J. (1995). Guidelines for an existential–integrative (EI) approach. In K. J. Schneider & R. May (Eds.), *The psychology of existence: An integrative, clinical perspective* (pp. 135–184). New York: McGraw-Hill.

Schneider, K. J. (1998a). Existential processes. In L. S. Greenberg, J. C. Watson, & G Lietaer (Eds.), *Handbook of experiential psychotherapy* (pp. 103–120). New York: Guilford Press.

Schneider, K. J. (1998b). Toward a science of the heart: Romanticism and the revival of psychology. *American Psychologist, 53,* 277–289.

Schneider, K. J. (1999a). Clients deserve relationships, not merely "treatments." *American Psychologist, 54,* 206–207.

Schneider, K. J. (1999b). *The paradoxical self: Toward an understanding of our contradictory nature* (2nd ed.). Amherst, NY: Humanity Books.

Schneider, K. J. (2001). Closing statement. In K. J. Schneider, J. F. T. Bugental, & J. F. Pierson (Eds.), *The handbook of humanistic psychology: Leading edges in theory, practice, and research* (pp. 672–675). Thousand Oaks, CA: Sage.

Schneider, K. J., Bugental, J. F. T., & Pierson, J. F. (Eds.). (2001). *The handbook of humanistic psychology: Leading edges in theory, research, and practice.* Thousand Oaks, CA: Sage.

Schneider, K. J., & May, R. (Eds.). (1995). *The psychology of existence: An integrative, clinical perspective.* New York: McGraw-Hill.

Seligman, M. E. P. (1996). Science as an ally of practice. *American Psychologist, 51,* 1072–1079.

Serlin, I. A. (1996). Kinesthetic imagining. *Journal of Humanistic Psychology, 36*(2), 25–34.

Spinelli, E. (1997). *Tales of unknowing: Therapeutic*

encounters from an existential perspective. London: Duckworth.

Spinelli, E. (2001). A reply to John Rowan. In K. J. Schneider, J. F. T. Bugental, & J. F. Pierson (Eds.), *The handbook of humanistic psychology: Leading edges in theory, practice, and research* (pp. 465–471). Thousand Oaks, CA: Sage.

Sterling, M. (2001). Expanding the boundaries of practice. In K. J. Schneider, J. F. T. Bugental, & J. F. Pierson (Eds.), *The handbook of humanistic psychology: Leading edges in theory, practice, and research* (pp. 349–353). Thousand Oaks, CA: Sage.

Stolorow, R. D., Brandschaft, B., & Atwood, G. E. (1987). *Psychoanalytic treatment: An intersubjective approach.* Hillsdale, NJ: Analytic Press.

Taylor, E. T. (1999). An intellectual renaissance in humanistic psychology? *Journal of Humanistic Psychology, 39*(2), 7–25.

Tillich, P. (1952). *The courage to be.* New Haven, CT: Yale University Press.

Thompson, M. G. (1995). Psychotic clients, Laing's treatment philosophy, and the fidelity to experience in existential psychoanalysis. In K. J. Schneider & R. May (Eds.), *The psychology of existence: An integrative, clinical perspective* (pp. 233–247). New York: McGraw-Hill.

Vontress, C. E., & Epp, L. R. (2001). Existential cross-cultural counseling: When hearts and cultures share. In K. J. Schneider, J. F. T. Bugental, & J. F. Pierson (Eds.), *The handbook of humanistic psychology: Leading edges in theory, practice, and research* (pp. 371–387). Thousand Oaks, CA: Sage.

Wadden, T. A., & Stunkard, A. J. (1986). Controlled trial of very low calorie diet, behavior therapy, and theier combination in the treatment of obesity. *Journal of Consulting and Clinical Psychology, 54*(4), 482–488.

Wadlington, W. (2001). Performative therapy: Postmodernizing humanistic psychology. In K. J. Schneider, J. F. T. Bugental, & J. F. Pierson (Eds.), *The handbook of humanistic psychology: Leading edges in theory, practice, and research* (pp. 491–501). Thousand Oaks, CA: Sage.

Walsh, R. A., & McElwain, B. (2002). Existential psychotherapies. In D. J. Cain & J. Seeman (Eds.), *Humanistic psychotherapies: Handbook of research and practice* (pp. 253–278). Washington, DC: American Psychological Association.

Wampold, B. E. (2001). *The great psychotherapy debate: Models, methods, findings.* Mahwah, NJ: Erlbaum.

Watson, J. C., & Bohart, A. C. (2001). Humanistic–experiential therapies in the era of managed care. In K. J. Schneider, J. F. T. Bugental, & J. F. Pierson (Eds.), *The handbook of humanistic psychology: Leading edges in theory, practice, and research* (pp. 503–517). Thousand Oaks, CA: Sage.

Watson, J. C., & Rennie, D. L. (1994). Qualitative analysis of clients' subjective experience of significant moments during the exploration of problematic experiences. *Journal of Counseling Psychology, 41,* 500–509.

Welwood, J. (2001). The unfolding of experience: Psychotherapy and beyond. In K. J. Schneider, J. F. T. Bugental, & J. F. Pierson (Eds.), *The handbook of humanistic psychology: Leading edges in theory, practice, and research* (pp. 333–341). Thousand Oaks, CA: Sage.

Wertz, F. J. (2001). Humanistic psychology and the qualitative research tradition. In K. J. Schneider, J. F. T. Bugental, & J. F. Pierson (Eds.), *The handbook of humanistic psychology: Leading edges in theory, practice, and research* (pp. 231–245). Thousand Oaks, CA: Sage.

Weston, D., & Morrison, K. (2001). A multidimensional meta-analysis of treatments for depression, panic, and generalized anxiety disorder: An empirical examination of the status of empirically supported theories. *Journal of Consulting and Clinical Psychology, 69,* 875–899.

Wheelis, A. (1958). *The quest for existential identity.* New York: Norton.

Yalom, I. (1980). *Existential psychotherapy.* New York: Basic Books.

Yalom, I. (1989). *Love's executioner.* New York: Basic Books.

6

Behavior Therapy

MARTIN M. ANTONY
LIZABETH ROEMER

Behavior therapy is not a unified approach to psychotherapy. In fact, in their *Dictionary of Behavior Therapy Techniques,* Bellack and Hersen (1985) list more than 150 different behavioral strategies for treating psychological problems. Behavior therapy includes a wide range of techniques, including exposure-based therapies for anxiety disorders, relaxation training, biofeedback, reinforcement-based treatments, assertiveness training, sensate focus for sexual dysfunction, "bell and pad conditioning" to prevent bed wetting, and many others. In addition, modern behavioral treatments often include components of other therapies, including cognitive therapy and, more recently, meditation-based treatments. Finally, the theoretical assumptions of modern behavior therapy are also quite diverse in a number of ways. Behavior therapists differ with respect to the relative importance placed on factors such as environmental contingencies and the role of cognitions in understanding behavior. There is also disagreement regarding the importance of developing a unique, individualized, evidence-based treatment plan for each client versus relying only on standardized, session-by-session, treatment protocols that have been subjected to random-

ized, controlled outcome studies (Addis, 1997; Addis, Wade, & Hatgis, 1999; Wilson, 1996, 1998).

Despite the differences among different behavioral treatments, there are also a number of shared characteristics that distinguish behavioral treatments from other forms of psychotherapy. First, behavior therapy is a form of psychotherapy in which the emphasis is on directly changing those relatively immediate factors that are thought to predispose, trigger, strengthen, or maintain problematic behaviors. Unlike some other forms of psychotherapy, wherein the goal may be to help an individual to develop insight into the early developmental factors that may have initially contributed to a problem, behavior therapists work directly on problematic patterns of behavior, by helping their clients to make changes such as decreasing avoidance of feared situations (e.g., in phobias), eliminating compulsive rituals (e.g., in obsessive–compulsive disorder [OCD]), improving social skills (e.g., in schizophrenia), or changing unhealthy eating patterns (e.g., in anorexia nervosa or obesity). Behavioral treatments may also involve changing aspects of the environment that *reinforce* a particular problem. For example, if a child's behavioral problems appear to be reinforced by the parents' giving in to their son's or daughter's unreasonable demands whenever he or she has a tantrum, the parents may be taught alternative ways of responding to the child's screaming and crying. Similarly, someone who has withdrawn from almost all activities as a result of severe depression might be encouraged to begin to reintroduce various activities into his or her daily routine as a way of increasing the rewards that occur when a person is actively engaged in life.

Second, whereas therapists in traditional psychodynamic psychotherapy and person-centered psychotherapy tend to be relatively nondirective, behavior therapists tend to be quite directive, modeling or demonstrating alternative behaviors, encouraging the client to try particular exercises, and assigning homework at the end of each session. Behavioral treatments tend to emphasize the importance of learning new skills and unlearning old behaviors that contribute to the individual's problems. In fact, clients sometimes point out the similarities between being in behavior therapy and being in school. Like formal education, behavior therapy tends to be focused on achieving particular goals, may include instruction and education, involves the completion of homework between sessions, and is associated with repeated assessments to measure the extent to which goals are being met.

The duration and setting of treatment can sometimes be quite different in behavior therapy than in other forms of therapy. First, behavior therapy is often brief, particularly when standard evidence-based protocols are followed. For example, in typical research studies on behavior therapy, treatment for anxiety disorders is often completed in as little as one session for a specific phobia of spiders (Öst, 1997) or 10–15 sessions for other anxiety disorders such as panic disorder and social anxiety disorder (Antony & Swinson, 2000a). In addition, whereas most psychotherapies take place in the therapist's office, during a 50-minute

hour, behavior therapy sessions may last longer and may occur outside the therapist's office.

For example, a client who fears elevators might have entire treatment sessions on elevators. Similarly, an individual with an eating disorder might have some sessions in restaurants, where it is often easier to work on problem eating behaviors. Long sessions (e.g., 90 minutes to 2 hours) are often used during the course of exposure-based treatments for anxiety disorders, where it is recommended that exposure sessions last long enough for the client's fear to decrease.

Finally, behavioral treatments are strongly rooted in empirical research, more than many other forms of psychotherapy. As a result, the techniques used by behavior therapists change over time, as new information is learned about which techniques are most helpful and which are unnecessary. For example, one of the earliest behavioral treatments for phobias was systematic desensitization (Wolpe, 1958). This approach involved overcoming a fear using a combination of progressive muscle relaxation and gradual exposure (in imagination) to the feared situation or object. Although systematic desensitization is still sometimes used in clinical practice, it is no longer considered to be the treatment of choice for phobias (Antony & Swinson, 2000a). First, it is now established that live (*in vivo*) exposure is more effective than exposure in imagination for treating phobias (Emmelkamp & Wessels, 1975; Stern & Marks, 1973). Second, relaxation training does not seem to add much to exposure-based treatments for phobias; exposure works just as well with or without adding relaxation (e.g., Öst, Lindahl, Sterner, & Jerremalm, 1984). Therefore, as a result of numerous carefully controlled trials, the treatment of choice for specific phobias is now considered to be *in vivo* exposure without the addition of relaxation training.

The purpose of this chapter is to provide the reader with an understanding of the theory and practice of behavior therapy. We begin with a discussion of the historical and conceptual foundations of behavior therapy, followed by a review of behavioral assessment strategies. Much of this chapter describes standard behavioral techniques and provides sample behavior therapy protocols and case examples for particular conditions. Other topics covered include therapist factors and their effect on treatment, theoretical perspectives on change, ethical considerations, and future directions in behavior therapy.

Although modern behavior therapy is usually delivered as part of a comprehensive treatment package that also includes cognitive strategies, this chapter does not describe the cognitive aspects of treatment in detail. Instead, the reader is encouraged to refer to Chapter 7 (Reinecke and Freeman, in this volume) on cognitive therapy. However, it should be noted that despite the fact that they have been divided into separate chapters in this book, cognitive and behavioral treatments are often used in combination.

HISTORICAL BACKGROUND

Despite a few early papers describing exposure-based treatments for fear (e.g., Jones, 1924a, 1924b; Terhune, 1948), it was not until the 1950s and 1960s that interest in behavior therapy started to blossom thanks to several researchers (e.g., Hans Eysenck, Cyril Franks, Arnold Lazarus, Isaac Marks, S. Rachman, G. Terence Wilson, and Joseph Wolpe) working in South Africa, England, and the United States. According to Margraf (1998), two conditions set the stage for the early popularity of behavior therapy. First, in the 1950s, basic research on learning theory-based explanations for clinical phenomena was becoming popular. For example, researchers with an interest in phobias were influenced by Mowrer's (1939) two-factor model, which explained phobias as being initially triggered by a traumatic *classical conditioning* experience (e.g., developing a fear of dogs after being bitten by a

dog) and later maintained by *operant conditioning* or reinforcement for avoiding the feared stimulus (e.g., experiencing relief by avoiding dogs). Second, a number of clinical researchers (e.g., Eysenck, 1952) were becoming increasingly disenchanted with psychoanalysis, the dominant form of psychotherapy at the time. Eysenck and others criticized psychoanalysis for lacking empirical support and for being an ineffective treatment in many cases. The growing dissatisfaction with psychoanalysis, combined with the increasing interest in learning theory, set the stage for the birth of behavior therapy.

According to O'Donohue and Krasner, the first professional publication that used the term "behavior therapy" was a report published by Lindsley, Skinner, and Solomon in 1953, in which the term referred to the application of an operant conditioning model to change problem behaviors in psychotic patients. Arnold Lazarus (1958) subsequently used the term to refer to Joseph Wolpe's procedures for treating neurotic clients by reciprocal inhibition (Wolpe, 1958), and shortly thereafter, other influential writers (e.g., Eysenck, 1959, 1960) had begun to employ the term more broadly to refer to any treatment procedures based on learning theory, and especially the principles of classical and operant conditioning. Beginning in the 1960s, the term "behavior modification" began to be used as well (Bandura, 1969; Krasner & Ullmann, 1965; Ullmann & Krasner, 1965). Although the terms "behavior modification" and "behavior therapy" are sometimes used interchangeably, the term "behavior modification" has also been called on to describe treatment procedures that are specifically based on operant conditioning (e.g., token economy and aversive conditioning) (O'Donohue & Krasner, 1995), and the term "behavior therapy" is more often used in discussions of the outpatient clinic-based practice of behavioral approaches.

By the 1960s, behavior therapy was quickly being established as a bona fide approach to treating psychopathology. In 1963, the first major journal devoted to behavior therapy, *Behaviour Research and Therapy,* was founded by Hans Eysenck (later to be edited by S. Rachman, and now G.T. Wilson), and 3 years later, the Association for Advancement of Behavior Therapy (AABT) was formed, with Cyril Franks as the founding president. Today, a much larger number of journals are devoted to behavior therapy (e.g., *Behavior Modification, Behavior Therapy, Behavioural and Cognitive Psychotherapy, Cognitive and Behavioral Practice, Cognitive Behaviour Therapy, Journal of Applied Behavior Analysis, Journal of Behavior Therapy and Experimental Psychiatry*), and AABT remains the largest professional association in North America devoted to the study and practice of behavioral and cognitive therapy.

The domain of behavior therapy is no longer limited to treatments based on traditional learning theory. Many behaviorally oriented clinicians now include a wide range of evidence-based techniques in their practices, including cognitive therapy, relaxation training, biofeedback, social skills training, and meditation. In addition, almost all the journals that specialize in behavior therapy publish papers on a broad range of empirically supported psychological treatments. Although the variety of behavioral treatments has expanded over the years, the importance of using treatments that are supported by rigorous scientific study remains a hallmark of behavior therapy.

THE CONCEPT OF PERSONALITY

The notion of personality is based on the idea that individuals have characteristic patterns of feeling, thinking, and acting. Trait theories of personality suggest that given a particular situation, different individuals will respond in different ways, depending on the unique combination of personality traits we each possess. For example, some people (i.e., those with greater *trait anxiety*) are more likely than others to react with anxiety in a potentially threatening situation. In its most extreme form, trait theory places the cause of an individual's behavior in the person. That is, it is presumed that the individual's personality causes his or her behavior.

In contrast, behavioral theorists have tended to emphasize the role of context or situational factors in determining a particular individual's behavior. Walter Mischel (1968, 1984) is perhaps best known for demonstrating that people do not act consistently across situations, and that it is, in fact, difficult to accurately predict behavior based on measures of personality. For example, most people who report high levels of trait anger on personality measures are not angry in *all* situations. A person may be angry in one situation (e.g., being cut off while driving) and calm in other challenging situations (e.g., when a child spills his or her soup). From a behavioral perspective, as described here, it is the situation that determines behavior—not the presence or absence of particular personality traits.

On the surface, behavioral theory may seem to be at odds with a trait-based approach to understanding personality. However, the apparent differences probably have more to do with common misunderstandings about both approaches rather than actual differences. In fact, the two approaches are quite compatible. Most trait theorists acknowledge the role of context and situational factors in determining behavior. However, all other factors being equal, a trait approach would predict two different individuals to behave in characteristically different ways given the same situation. For example, an individual who is extroverted would be expected to be more social at a party than would an individual who is relatively introverted, assuming that all other factors (the person's mood, life stresses, the number of familiar people at the party, etc.) are equal for both individuals.

Similarly, most behaviorists would acknowledge that there are predisposing factors that affect how an individual responds to particular situations and that, in some cases, individuals respond similarly to a broad range of situations. However, behaviorists differ from other theorists in the way they define and explain these stable tendencies to respond to a wide range of situations in similar ways (i.e., personality). From a behavioral perspective, personality is defined in terms of an individual's behaviors, and behaviors are assumed to occur primarily as a result of an individual's learning history. So, to a behaviorist, an individual who is particularly introverted across a wide range of social situations might be introverted because he or she never learned any alternative ways to behave in these situations, or because being in social situations is not reinforcing for the individual.

Most behaviorists would also acknowledge the role of biological constraints on learning. In other words, one's unique genetic composition, temperament, and other biologically determined factors are thought to influence the ways in which one learns, thereby influencing one's personality.

When behavior therapists refer to an individual's learning history, they are typically including a broad range of experiences. For example, a number of repeated assaults in various public places could lead a person to fear being alone in public through a process of *classical conditioning* (i.e., the pairing of a neutral stimulus, such as being outside, with a motivationally relevant event, such as an assault). Through *stimulus generalization* (i.e., the spreading of the conditioned response to new situations that are similar to the situation where the trauma occurred), the individual might begin to feel unsafe in a wider range of situations, developing what one might consider an "anxious personality."

Although classical conditioning may contribute to the development of personality, operant conditioning is often thought to play an even larger role. B. F. Skinner and other *radical behaviorists* suggested that behaviors, including those behaviors that make up a person's personality, are deter-

mined by patterns of reinforcement and punishment from the environment (Skinner, 1974). For example, from a radical behavioral perspective, someone who is generally dishonest, manipulative, and antisocial might have been reinforced for these behaviors in the past (e.g., spending time with friends who also engaged in these behaviors), whereas someone who does not display these traits would likely not have been reinforced for these behaviors, and might even have been punished for behaving dishonestly.

In addition to classical and operant conditioning, other forms of learning are also thought to contribute to personality, according to a behavioral perspective. For example, social learning theorists such as Albert Bandura discuss the role of *modeling* (observing others who exhibit a particular type of behavior) and its influence on behavior. Cognitive-behavioral theorists emphasize the role of an individual's beliefs and assumptions in determining behavior, as do social learning theorists. Our beliefs are thought to arise from various types of learning experiences, including classical conditioning events, operant conditioning, watching others behave in particular ways, or being exposed to various forms of information or misinformation from things that we hear, see, or read. According to cognitive-behavioral theory, one's cognitions mediate the relationship between one's learning history and one's behavior. In contrast, radical behaviorists see cognitions as just another form of behavior, influenced by one's learning history, just like any other behavior. For radical behaviorists, cognitions are not thought to *cause* behavior. Rather, cognitions are thought to be just a particular form of behavior.

To summarize, a behavioral perspective views personality as nothing more than *behaviors* that are consistent across a range of situations. These behaviors are responses to environmental events and other learning experiences. Because an individual's learning history is constantly evolving, personality is also viewed to be something that develops and changes throughout an individual's life. Behaviorally oriented theorists disagree about the relative role of cognition in determining these behaviors, but most behaviorists acknowledge the role of biological factors such as genetics as having effects on the ways in which individuals learn and behave.

PSYCHOLOGICAL HEALTH AND PATHOLOGY

Theoretically speaking, a behavioral approach to psychopathology does not judge behaviors as healthy or unhealthy, separate from their context and their consequences. Instead, behaviors, whether deficient or excessive, are usually discussed with respect to whether they are *adaptive* or *maladaptive* in a particular cultural or social context. In this way, the definition of mental disorder from a behavioral perspective is consistent with the definition published in the text revision of the fourth edition of the *Diagnostic and Statistical Manual of Mental Disorders* (DSM-IV-TR; American Psychiatric Association, 2000). DSM-IV-TR defines a mental disorder as "a clinically significant behavioral or psychological syndrome or pattern that occurs in the individual and that is associated with present distress (e.g., a painful symptom), disability (impairment in one or more important areas of functioning) or with a significantly increased risk of suffering death, pain, disability, or an important loss of freedom" (p. xxxi). In other words, whether a pattern of behavior is considered pathological depends on the consequences of the behavior and not on the content or form of the behavior. This definition allows for appreciating differences between cultures and other groups. For example, a behavior that is considered normal in one culture or social group may be considered deviant in another culture or group. A behavior would not be considered unhealthy if it were normal and adaptive in the context in which it occurs.

Also, according to behavioral theory, adaptive and maladaptive behaviors are caused by the same basic learning processes. Differences between nonclinical manifestations of a problem and clinically relevant symptoms (e.g., normal sad moods vs. depression and occasional worry vs. generalized anxiety disorder) are typically thought to be quantitative differences. In other words, the most important differences between an individual with clinical depression and a healthy individual who occasionally experiences sad mood are in the frequency, intensity, and consequences of the depression, not in the quality of the mood state.

THE PROCESS OF CLINICAL ASSESSMENT

Conceptual Issues in Behavioral Assessment

There are three general purposes of assessment in the context of behavior therapy—to understand an individual's problem, to plan treatment, and to measure change. In traditional behavior therapy, understanding a problem typically includes a comprehensive *functional analysis*. The process of functional analysis involves considering four different areas that can be summarized by the acronym SORC (Stimulus–Organism–Response–Consequence; Nelson & Hayes, 1986). The term "stimulus" refers to the antecedents of a problem behavior, including the controlling variables that trigger or cause the behavior. For example, antecedents of problem drinking for a particular person may include such factors as being around drinking cues (e.g., friends who drink, places that serve alcohol, and smoking), life stresses (e.g., a hard day at the office), and having extra money to spend (e.g., payday). Variables having to do with the *organism* are those that are unique to the individual, including such things as physiological factors, temperament, learning history, expectancies, and other cognitive factors.

Describing the person's *responses* involves conducting a detailed analysis of the individual's behavior. For example, in the case of the individual who drinks excessively, the behavior therapist would likely want to know how frequently the person is drinking, how much the person drinks, and what the person is drinking. The assessment should identify problem *target behaviors* (e.g., behavioral *excesses* and *deficits* that will be the focus of change) as well as *alternative behaviors* (i.e., behaviors that can replace the problem behaviors). Finally, functional analysis involves examining the *consequences* of the behavior in order to understand the patterns of reinforcement and punishment from the environment that may be influencing the problem. For example, consequences of problem drinking may include positive effects such as intoxication, reduced anxiety, and social support from one's drinking buddies and negative effects such as being late for work, relationship problems, and withdrawal symptoms the next morning. The results of a functional analysis may be used to develop an individualized treatment plan that will involve changing the triggers and reinforcing consequences for the problem behavior.

In practice, behavior therapists differ in the extent to which to which they rely on idiographic or individualized assessments, such as functional analysis, versus using standardized assessment tools such as symptom questionnaires or structured diagnostic interviews. In recent years, many behavior therapists have shifted away from traditional functional analysis toward a more symptom-focused assessment, with the goal of measuring the presence, absence, and severity of particular symptoms (panic attacks, depressed mood, drinking, binge eating, etc.), understanding the triggers for these symptoms, and establishing a diagnosis, based on DSM-IV criteria. Over the past few decades, effective behavioral treatments have been developed for a number of psychological disorders, and many of these have been empirically validated in the context of particular DSM-IV diagnoses. Thus, knowing whether a particular person suffers from panic disorder or social anxiety disorder can inform decisions regarding the best treatment for the problem. In addition, insurance companies typically require a diagnosis in order to reimburse clients for psychological treatments—a practical reason why behavior therapists may have become more interested in diagnosis in recent years. Ideally, a comprehensive behavioral assessment should include aspects of both approaches, obtaining information about the types of symptoms a person is experiencing as well as learning about any individual characteristics (patterns of reinforcement in the client's environment, cultural factors, etc.) that may have an impact on treatment.

From a behavioral perspective, a thorough assessment is thought to be essential for treatment planning. For example, the information obtained during the assessment is often used to establish the goals for treatment. A client with OCD who reports washing her hands several hundred times per day might have a goal of reducing her hand washing to no more than 10 times daily. Information from the assessment is also used to select appropriate treatment strategies. In this case example, the assessment would involve making a list of situations that trigger a feeling of contamination and subsequent hand washing, and this list of situations would then be used to generate possible exposure practices (e.g., having the client touch various "contaminated" objects).

One way in which behavior therapy is different from most other forms of therapy is the importance placed on measuring outcome. A hallmark of behavior therapy is the use of empirically supported treatments and the measurement of treatment outcome for each client, using empirically supported assessment tools. Before treatment begins, measures are taken during a baseline period to establish the pretreatment level of symptoms. Ideally, measurement of the problem behaviors continues throughout treatment, followed by a thorough posttreatment assessment and occasional repeated assessments during follow-up.

Assessment Strategies Used in Behavior Therapy

Behavior therapists usually recognize that information obtained during an assessment is often inconsistent, depending on the way in which the information is collected. Therefore, a *multimodal* approach to assessment is typically recommended, in which a number of different sources of information (e.g., client, family members, and teachers) and methods of collecting information are used in combination. Assessment tools used by behavior therapists may include such methods as behavioral observation, diaries, clinical interviews, self-report scales, and psychophysiological measures. Each of these approaches is discussed in this section.

Direct Behavioral Observation

Behavior therapists often use observation to assess their client's symptoms directly. For example, a therapist who is interested in measuring the frequency of a young boy's disruptive behaviors in the classroom might ask the child's teachers to observe the child and to record each time he engages in particular target behaviors. Similarly, therapists who treat phobias behaviorally often use *behavioral approach tests* (BATs) to assess their clients' symptoms directly. A BAT involves instructing a client to enter a feared situation and measuring his or her responses, including subjective fear ratings (e.g., based on a scale ranging from 0–100, called a *subjective units of discomfort scale,* or SUDS), physical symptoms, overt behaviors, and anxious thoughts. Sometimes, videotaping clients can be a useful way of assessing behavior. For example, during social skills training, behavior therapists often use videotapes to record a client's performance and may play the tapes for the client as a tool for facilitating change in particular social behaviors.

Unobtrusive observation (i.e., observation in which the client is unaware that he or she is being observed) is often most likely to provide a more typical sample of the client's behavior, as people tend to behave differently when they know they are being observed. However, in many situations unobtrusive observation is either impractical or unethical. The effect on behavior of knowing that one is being observed can be minimized by observing the client for long periods (allowing time for the client to habituate to the presence of the observer), or by ensuring that the client is unaware of which specific behaviors are being measured during the observation period.

Monitoring Forms and Behavioral Diaries

Almost all behavioral treatments involve the monitoring of symptoms using a variety of diaries and other monitoring forms. For example, in the behavioral treatment of panic disorder, clients are asked to complete a Panic Attack Record each time they experience a panic attack (Barlow & Craske, 2000; see Figure 6.1). On this diary, clients record the time and date of the attack, whether the attack was expected or unexpected, the triggers for the attack, and the specific symptoms experienced during the attack. Similarly, behavioral diaries are used to measure food intake in clients with eating disorders, depressed mood in clients with depression, and the frequency and content of worry in clients with generalized anxiety disorder. Diaries are also a helpful tool for facilitating compliance with homework during behavior therapy. For example, an individual being treated for a phobia of driving might be encouraged to complete a behavioral diary each time he or she practices driving. The diary can provide information about the location and duration of the practice, the fear level experienced (based on the SUDS), any anxious behaviors or thoughts that were experienced, and the outcome of the practice.

Perhaps the biggest advantage of having clients complete behavioral diaries is that

Panic Attack Record

Date _____ Time Began _____ AM/PM

☐ Expected   Triggers _____
☐ Unexpected   _____
                _____

Maximum Fear *(circle)*

0	1	2	3	4	5	6	7	8
None		Mild		Moderate		Strong		Extreme

Symptoms
(Check all symptoms present to at least a mild degree.)

☐ Difficulty Breathing   ☐ Nausea/Abdominal Distress   ☐ Unsteadiness/Dizziness/ Faintness

☐ Racing/Pounding Heart   ☐ Chest Pain/Discomfort   ☐ Fear of Dying

☐ Choking   ☐ Hot/Cold Flashes   ☐ Fear of Losing Control/ Going Crazy

☐ Numbness/Tingling   ☐ Sweating

☐ Trembling/Shaking   ☐ Feelings of Unreality

FIGURE 6.1. Panic attack record. From Barlow and Craske (2000). Copyright 2000 by Graywind Publications. Adapted and reproduced by permission of the Publisher, Graywind Publications Incorporated. All rights reserved.

they circumvent the problem of clients not recalling the details of their symptoms and experiences from the previous week. Having individuals record their experiences as they occur increases the likelihood that the information will be accurate. However, from a measurement standpoint, one disadvantage of behavioral diaries is the problem of *reactivity*. There is a considerable literature demonstrating that monitoring one's own behavior can lead to changes in behavior, particularly when the client first starts completing the diaries. For example, counting cigarettes smoked can lead to a reduction in smoking (McFall, 1970) and monitoring food intake in obese individuals can lead to a reduction in eating (Green, 1978), even before the actual treatment begins. Therefore, therapists should be aware that baseline symptoms and behaviors measured by diaries may not reflect the true baseline levels of these symptoms and behaviors.

Clinical Interviews

Like professionals who practice other forms of psychotherapy, behavior therapists typi-cally use clinical interviews to collect important information about their clients, including information about such things as the types of problems the individual is experiencing, relevant symptoms, behavioral manifestations of the problem (e.g., avoidance behaviors and binge eating), cognitive manifestations of the problem (e.g., dysfunctional beliefs), contributing factors and triggers, consequences of the problem, and treatment history. For much of the information collected, therapists must rely on unstructured clinical interviews, in which the clinician is entirely responsible for determining what questions to ask and how the resulting information is to be used. The specific questions asked are of course determined by the types of information that the client provides.

Although they provide maximum flexibility, unstructured interviews are generally thought to be unreliable, leading different interviewers to obtain considerably different information. Therefore, whenever possible, behavior therapists prefer to use structured or semistructured interviews to supplement the information obtained during their unstructured clinical interviews. Structured and semistructured interviews address the issue of unreliability by standardizing the content, format, and order of questions, and the psychometric properties of these instruments are often well established. Generally, for the purpose of establishing a diagnosis, semistructured interviews are preferable to fully structured interviews, because they permit the interviewer to ask follow-up questions (after the standardized question has been asked) to clarify an incomplete response or a response that suggests the client has not understood the question. In contrast, fully structured diagnostic interviews do not allow for any deviation from the interview script, even to clarify information given by the client. Recently the utility of fully structured diagnostic interviews for establishing a valid diagnosis has been challenged (e.g., Antony, Downie, & Swinson, 1998; Antony & Swinson, 2000a). In contrast, semistructured interviews are often considered the gold standard for diagnostic assessment in that they combine the strengths of a structured interview with the flexibility of an unstructured interview.

Structured and semistructured interviews are typically each designed for a specific purpose. For example, the Structured Clinical Interview for DSM-IV (SCID-IV; First, Spitzer, Gibbon, & Williams, 1996) is a popular semistructured interview that takes about 2 hours to administer and assesses the diagnostic criteria for a large number of DSM-IV disorders (see Summerfeldt & Antony, 2002, for a review of the SCID-IV and other diagnostic interviews). The Yale–Brown Obsessive–Compulsive Scale (Y-BOCS) is another example of a popular semistructured interview, designed to assess the range and severity of symptoms in OCD. Because most structured and semistructured interviews are quite narrow in their focus, they cannot possibly cover all relevant areas in a clinical interview. Therefore, most behavior therapists who use these interviews also rely on unstructured interviews to gather certain types of information.

Self-Report Scales

Literally thousands of self-report questionnaires and tests exist for measuring a wide range of problems. For example, Antony, Orsillo, and Roemer (2001) recently reviewed more than 200 evidence-based measures related to anxiety disorders alone. Ideally, a comprehensive behavioral assessment should include some client-administered measures to balance information obtained from clinician-administered scales, which can be influenced to a greater extent by interviewer biases. In addition, self-report scales have the advantage of being relatively cost-effective in that they are typically easy to score and do not require any clinician time to administer.

An example of a popular self-report scale is the second edition of the Beck Depression Inventory (BDI-II; Beck, Steer, & Brown, 1996). This scale contains 21 items, takes a few minutes to complete, and provides a reliable and valid measure of depression severity. In addition, it includes questions that assess most of the official DSM-IV symptoms of depression (changes in appetite, loss of interest, suicidal thoughts, etc.); thus it can be a useful way of confirming the results of a thorough diagnostic interview. In the behavioral treatment of depression, the BDI-II is often completed at each session, so the severity of depression can be tracked over the course of treatment.

Psychophysiological Assessment

Psychophysiological assessment involves measuring aspects of an individual's physiological functioning. This form of assessment is typically not used in routine clinical practice, but there are a number of situations in which it can be useful. For example, therapists and researchers who work with anxious clients will sometimes measure the individual's heart rate as a physiological indication of fear (Yartz & Hawk, 2001). Changes in heart rate can be used to measure improvements over the course of treatment, along with more subjective measures such as self-report scales, behavioral approach tests, and clinical interview data. Similarly, individuals suffering from sleep disorders (e.g., insomnia) will often undergo all-night electrophysiological monitoring of sleep as measured by electroencephalography (EEG; measurement of brain activity), electrooculography (EOG; measurement of eye movements), and electromyography (EMG; measurement of muscle activity) (Savard & Morin, 2002). These measures are useful for the purpose of diagnosis in that they may help to distinguish among different sleep-related disorders

PRINCIPLES OF BEHAVIORAL TREATMENT

Many of the most important defining features of behavior therapy are described elsewhere in this chapter; thus in this section we provide only a brief summary of the key principles underlying behavioral treatment.

- Behavior therapy is evidence-based. Treatments are selected based on available research regarding what works and what does not. In addition, behaviorally oriented therapists collect data from each and every client to assess the impact of the treatment. When possible, therapists may conduct single case "experiments" to assess whether treatment (vs. the passage of time, for example) is actually causing the changes observed (Hersen & Barlow, 1984). An example of such an experiment might be to withdraw treatment for a brief time and to see whether the improvements continue.
- Behavior therapy focuses on changing those variables that are thought to be currently maintaining a problem rather than on discussing experiences earlier in a person's development that may have contributed to the creation of a problem.

- Behavior therapy is problem-oriented. Behavioral assessment focuses on identifying key problems and realistic goals, and treatment strategies are selected to facilitate alleviating problems and meeting goals.
- Behavior therapy is transparent. In other words, clients are provided with a behavioral model for understanding their problems as well as a full rationale for each strategy that is used. In addition, clients are often provided with readings that include information about the treatment, as well as the research supporting it. By the end of treatment, most clients have a good understanding of the nature and theoretical underpinnings of the treatment they have received.
- Behavior therapy is action-oriented. Treatment involves taking active steps such as confronting feared situations, changing eating habits, recording information on diaries, and changing other behaviors. In addition, treatment is not limited to the traditional therapy session. Much of the change is thought to occur during homework practices between sessions. In fact, homework compliance in behavior therapy appears to be directly related to the outcome of treatment (e.g., Edelman & Chambless, 1993, 1995; Leung & Heimberg, 1996).
- The format of behavior therapy is flexible. The location and duration of sessions varies depending on the problem, as does the number of sessions.
- Traditional behavior therapy emphasizes an idiographic approach to changing behavior. In other words, each client receives an individually tailored treatment, depending on the specific symptoms that he or she reports and the particular variables that appear to be maintaining those symptoms.
- More recently, there has been a move toward the development of standardized treatment packages that are designed to treat particular diagnostic categories, that contain particular behavioral and cognitive techniques, and that have been validated in controlled clinical trials. Several of these

protocols are described later in this chapter. Although the movement toward using standardized treatments in clinical practice has been controversial (Addis, 1997; Addis et al., 1999; Wilson, 1996, 1998), this development has arisen for several reasons. First, the identification and validation of empirically based treatments has helped to distinguish behavioral treatments from the numerous other forms of psychotherapy that often have little evidence supporting their use. In addition, the development of treatment manuals has facilitated the dissemination of effective psychological treatments, despite competition from psychotherapies with less empirical support, and pharmacological treatments, which are also marketed for particular diagnostic syndromes. Finally, the move toward managed care in the United States has demanded that clinicians deliver short-term treatments that work and evidence-based psychological treatments have met those demands fairly well. The Society of Clinical Psychology (Division 12 of the American Psychological Association) has identified a list of empirically supported treatments, most of which come from cognitive-behavioral approaches (Woody & Sanderson, 1998). More information on empirically supported psychological treatments is available on the Society's website: *www.apa.org/divisions/div12/rev_est/index. shtml,* as well as in several recent books (e.g., Barlow, 2001; Nathan & Gorman, 2002).

• In practice, differences between traditional ideographic approaches to treatment and a more protocol-driven, symptom-focused approaches are often relatively small, especially when used by experienced behavior therapists. Most individualized treatment plans rely on strategies that are similar to those described in standard protocols. In addition, many standard protocols allow therapists to be flexible with respect to the strategies that are selected for particular clients. Finally, despite the emphasis among behaviorally oriented therapists on empirically supported *techniques,* there is now increasing awareness of the importance of other factors, such as empirically supported *therapeutic relationships,* in affecting the outcome of treatment (Norcross, 2002).

THE PRACTICE OF THERAPY

Psychoeducation

Most behavioral treatments include some form of psychoeducation. In fact, the first session or two are often devoted exclusively to psychoeducation. This aspect of treatment is consistent with the notion that behavior therapy is transparent, as discussed earlier. Some of the topics covered during the initial psychoeducation sessions include discussion of a behavioral model for the problem being treated, a description of the treatment process, and an overview of the ways in which the treatment procedures are likely to have an impact on the problem. Ideally, psychoeducation should not involve lecturing to the client. Instead, it should involve a two-way discussion, in which the client is presented with new information and is also asked to provide feedback about the ways in which his or her symptoms are consistent (or inconsistent) with the model. Psychoeducation may also involve correcting misinformation that the client has picked up along the way and suggesting recommended readings about the target problem or about effective methods for treating it.

For example, the initial session for a client being treated for a phobia of heights would typically emphasize psychoeducation, with the goal of making several important points (Antony & Swinson, 2000a). First, the session might begin with a general discussion of the nature of fear and phobias. The therapist would discuss the notion that fear is a normal and healthy emotion that everyone experiences from time to time. The function of fear (to protect the individual from perceived danger) would also be discussed. The client would be reminded that the goal of treatment is not to remove all fear of heights (e.g., it is helpful to be apprehensive in high situations that are truly dangerous, such as standing on the edge of a cliff) but, rather, to bring the fear to a realistic level that no longer creates significant distress or impairment.

Some portion of the initial session might also be spent discussing fear in terms of its three components (i.e., physical feelings, cognitions, and behaviors) and the role of that each of these components plays in maintaining the fear. People with height phobias are often anxious about the feelings they experience in high places, such as dizziness and unsteady legs, which in turn can increase levels of fear when these sensations occur. The beliefs that people hold ("I will fall, be pushed, or jump from the high place; the structure of the building will collapse," etc.) are also thought to maintain the fear. Perhaps the most important factor in maintaining a fear of heights is the avoidance of high places, including overt avoidance (i.e., not going into high places) and more subtle forms of avoidance (e.g., standing away from the ledge and holding on to a railing). Avoidance behavior reinforces the phobic reaction and prevents the individual from ever learning that the situation is safer than he or she thinks.

An in-depth description of the treatment would also be included in the first session. In the case of height phobia, the treatment of choice almost always includes *in vivo* exposure to high places. Therefore, the therapist would likely spend some time in the initial session describing the content of exposure-based treatment and the guidelines for maximizing the effectiveness of exposure (as described in the next section). Reasons for the effectiveness of exposure are explored as well. The session might end with assigning readings on the treatment of specific phobias (e.g., Antony, Craske, & Barlow, 1995) as homework.

Although psychoeducation is an important feature during the initial phases of treatment, it continues to be used throughout treatment as well. For example, whenever a new therapy technique or assessment tool is introduced, some time needs to be spent discussing how it is to be used. In addition, toward the end of treatment, the therapist will likely spend some time reviewing with the client strategies for maintaining improvements after treatment has ended.

Exposure-Based Treatments

Some of the earliest behavioral treatments to be studied were based on the notion that exposure to feared objects and situations leads to a reduction in fear. Today, exposure is usually considered to be a necessary component of treatment for phobias, OCD, and other fear-based problems. In fact, in the case of certain specific phobias, a single session of *in vivo* exposure is enough for the majority of sufferers to overcome their fear (for a review, see Antony & Barlow, 2002; Antony & McCabe, in press). For other anxiety disorders, such as panic disorder and social phobia, exposure is an important component of a treatment package that typically includes a number of different strategies and typically occurs over a period of months.

Exposure Modalities

Exposure can be delivered in a number of different ways. In most cases, the method of choice is *in vivo exposure,* which involves exposing a person to his or her feared object or situation in real life. For example, an individual who fears driving is encouraged to drive; an individual who fears dogs is encouraged to be near, and eventually handle, dogs; an individual with OCD who fears contamination is encouraged to touch things that he or she perceives as contaminated. In the case of social phobia, exposure practices may include role plays or simulated exposures as part of the treatment and are often combined with cognitive therapy and sometimes social skills training.

A second manner by which exposure can be administered is in imagination. *Imaginal exposure* involves having a client imagine being in a feared situation. Although imaginal exposure can lead to a reduction in fear, it is typically not used for treating phobias because it is not considered to be as powerful a method as *in vivo* exposure. However, there are two situations in which imaginal exposure is considered appropriate: (1) for clients who are afraid of thoughts, images, or memories and (2) for clients who are unable or unwilling to do *in vivo* exposure.

A number of anxiety disorders are associated with a fear of thoughts, images, or memories. For example, individuals with OCD who have violent, religious, or sexual obsessions are often terrified of having thoughts that they perceive as inappropriate or dangerous, and in these cases the suppression of such thoughts is often thought to help maintain the OCD symptoms over time (Salkovskis, 1998). In such cases, teaching clients to purposely bring on the frightening thoughts and images until they are no longer distressing can be a useful way of decreasing OCD symptoms and may add to the effectiveness of *in vivo* exposure alone (Abramowitz, 1996). Another anxiety disorder that is associated with a fear of memories is posttraumatic stress disorder (PTSD). As with exposure to feared thoughts in OCD, systematic imaginal exposure to the memories of a trauma can lead to a reduction in PTSD symptoms (Foa & Rothbaum, 1998; Tarrier et al., 1999).

As mentioned earlier, imaginal exposure may also be appropriate for clients who are unwilling or unable to do *in vivo* exposure. For example, for individuals who suffer from a phobia of storms, imaginal exposure may be a useful tool to use between thunderstorms. Similarly, an individual who fears snakes but is unwilling to be anywhere near a live snake may benefit from exposure to snakes in imagination until reaching a point at which exposure to live snakes is possible. Using videotaped snakes or photos of snakes may also be helpful as the client progresses to the point of being willing to try exposure *in vivo*.

A third form of exposure, *interoceptive exposure,* essentially involves exposure to feared sensations. This method of exposure is used particularly when treating panic disorder, a problem in which individuals are usually frightened of the sensations associated with physical arousal and panic attacks (e.g., racing heart, dizziness, and breathlessness). Interoceptive exposure involves repeatedly exposing oneself to feared sensations using a series of exercises such as hyperventilation (to induced lightheadedness and other symptoms), aerobic exercise (to induce racing heart and breathlessness), and spinning around (to induce dizziness). Over time, exposure to these and other exercises decreases the fear of panic symptoms that contributes to the occurrence of panic attacks and related symptoms by the process of *extinction* (Antony & Swinson, 2000a).

A fourth modality by which exposure can be delivered is a more recent development. In the past few years, virtual reality has been used as a method of exposing individuals to the situations they fear. *Virtual reality exposure* involves using three-dimensional computer-generated images projected on the inside of a visor worn in front of the eyes. As reviewed elsewhere (Antony & Barlow, 2002), published case studies and a few controlled studies have used virtual reality exposure to treat a range of specific phobias, including fears of heights, flying, driving, and spiders. In addition, recent studies have found virtual reality to be as effective as *in vivo* exposure for treating flying phobia (Emmelkamp et al., 2002) and height phobia (Emmelkamp, Bruynzeel, Drost, & van der Mast, 2001). Exposure-based treatments with virtual reality have also been used successfully used with people suffering from body image disturbances (Perpina et al., 1999) and PTSD (Rothbaum, Hodges, Ready, Graap, & Alarcon, 2001).

Guidelines for Effective Exposure

How exposure is conducted appears to have a significant impact on the outcome of treatment. Antony and Swinson (2000a) recently summarized the relevant research on this topic with the following conclusions:

- Exposure works best when it is *predictable* (i.e., the client knows what the exposure will involve and when it will occur) and under the client's *control* (i.e., the client is able to control the intensity and duration of the exposure) (see Antony & Swinson, 2000a). Therefore, behavior therapists should never surprise their clients during an exposure practice, or force their clients to do anything they have not agreed to try.
- Longer exposures (e.g., 2 hours) lead to greater reduction in fear than shorter exposures (e.g., 30 minutes) (e.g., Stern & Marks, 1973). It is generally recommended that exposure practices last long enough for the client's fear to decrease. If a practice is inherently brief (e.g., driving over a bridge), clients are encouraged to repeat the practice over and over, until their fear has decreased.
- For exposure to be useful, it should be intense enough to trigger a fear response, but it is not necessary (or probably even helpful) for the fear to be overwhelming (Foa, Blau, Prout, & Latimer, 1977).
- Exposure sessions should be spaced close together. Foa, Jameson, Turner, and Payne (1980) found that 10 daily exposure sessions led to a greater reduction in agoraphobic fear than did 10 weekly sessions. Because therapists typically cannot see their clients every day, completion of exposure homework is particularly important in light of these findings.
- Varying the stimulus across exposure practices appears to improve long-term outcome following exposure-based treatment (Rowe & Craske, 1998). For example, an individual being treated for a bridge phobia should practice driving over a number of bridges to facilitate generalization of the fear reduction across situations.
- Conducting exposure practices in multiple contexts appears to protect clients against experiencing a return of fear, compared to conducting exposure in only one context (Gunther, Denniston, & Miller, 1998). For example, an individual who is fearful of spiders should practice exposure to harmless spiders in various places (therapist's office, bedroom, basement, garden, etc.).
- Although findings have been mixed (e.g., Antony, McCabe, Leeuw, Sano, & Swinson, 2001), some studies have found that distraction during exposure practices can interfere with a successful treatment outcome, particularly over the long term (e.g., Craske, Street, & Barlow, 1989; Haw & Dickerson, 1998). Therefore, it is generally recommended that clients focus on the feared stimulus during exposure practices rather than distracting themselves, and thus avoiding. In addition, other forms of subtle avoidance, such as relying on safety cues, should be eliminated during exposure (Morgan & Raffle, 1999).

Exposure Hierarchies

To help facilitate the process of exposure, therapists typically work with their clients to generate an exposure hierarchy. Table 6.1 provides an example of such a hierarchy for an individual suffering from PTSD following a sexual assault. Essentially, a hierarchy is a list of situations (usually 10 to 15) that an individual fears and avoids, rank-ordered from most difficult (at the top) to less difficult (at the bottom). The hierarchy can then be used as a road map to guide the content of future exposure practices. Typically, the client starts with items near the bottom of the hierarchy and, as these are dealt with successfully, progresses to more and more difficult items until he or she is able to ad-

TABLE 6.1. Exposure Hierarchy for a Sexual Assault Victim with Posttraumatic Stress Disorder

Item	Fear	Avoidance
1. Have sexual relations with partner	100	100
2. Go out for dinner at night with friends	85	90
3. Park in an underground parking lot during the day	85	85
4. Drive by the park where I was assaulted	60	75
5. Hug my partner	50	50
6. Sit in my car, in my driveway, at night with the doors locked	45	45
7. Ask a man at a bus stop for directions	40	40
8. Walk through a crowded mall	30	40
9. Stay home alone at night	30	20
10. Walk down a busy street during the day	25	25

Note. Fear and Avoidance are rated on scales ranging from 0 to 100.

dress the items near the top of the hierarchy with little fear. The hierarchy can also be used as an outcome measure by having the client rate his or her fear and avoidance levels for each item and repeating the ratings at each session.

Response Prevention

Response prevention involves preventing behaviors that are designed to decrease anxiety, fear, or tension, until the urge to perform these overprotective behaviors subsides. Conceptually, response prevention is a means of providing exposure experiences, and in practice, these two strategies are often used together. Perhaps the most common use of response prevention is in the treatment of OCD, where this method is also referred to as *ritual prevention* (Foa, Franklin, & Kozak, 1998). In fact, the gold standard psychological treatment for OCD is the combination of exposure to OCD triggers (e.g., contamination and frightening thoughts) and prevention of OCD rituals (e.g., checking, washing, and counting). Clients are encouraged to do whatever they can to prevent their rituals, until the urge to perform the ritual decreases. If a person feels unable to completely prevent a ritual, he or she might be asked to delay the ritual for progressively longer periods. Over the

course of treatment, the urge to perform rituals usually decreases considerably and may be eliminated completely, in some cases. Exposure and response prevention are supported by numerous studies for the treatment of OCD, and response prevention seems to contribute to successful treatment outcome over and above the effects of exposure alone (for a review, see Franklin & Foa, 2002).

In addition to OCD, response prevention has been used successfully in a number of other psychological disorders, including bulimia nervosa (Bulik, Sullivan, Carter, McIntosh, & Joyce, 1998; Leitenberg, Rosen, Gross, Nudelman, & Vara, 1988), body dysmorphic disorder (McKay, Todaro, Neziroglu, & Campisi, 1997), alcohol use disorders (Rankin, Hodgson, & Stockwell, 1983), and hypochondriasis (Visser & Bouman, 2001).

Operant Strategies

A basic tenet of behavioral theory is that behavior is functional; that is, behaviors that have been followed by desirable consequences (*reinforcers*) will become more likely and behaviors that have been followed by undesirable consequences (*punishment*) will become less likely. Reinforcement can be either *positive* (i.e., receiving a reward, such as a promotion at work or a gift, in response to a particular behavior) or *negative* (i.e., removing an aversive consequence in response to a particular behavior). An example of negative reinforcement is the reduction in distress that people experience after escaping from a feared situation. Punishment can also be defined as either *positive* or *negative*. Positive punishment involves receiving an aversive consequence (e.g., electrical shock) in response to a particular behavior, whereas negative punishment involves the removal of something desirable (e.g., permission to borrow the family car) in response to a particular behavior.

Behavior is thus determined by environmental cues (signals technically known as *discriminative stimuli*) that indicate whether a behavior is likely to be rewarded or punished and by previous history of reward or punishment for a given behavior in a given context. This model helps clients and therapists understand seemingly incomprehensible behavior (e.g., a heroin addict is responding to the strong negatively reinforcing contingency of removal of distress that follows heroin use, not purposely creating havoc in his or her family life). In addition, this model provides clear targets for clinical intervention through contingency management (i.e., arranging for different consequences to follow a given response). Applied behavior analysis incorporates these principles into comprehensive, individually focused treatment plans (see Nemeroff & Karoly, 1991, for a review). These interventions have demonstrated efficacy across a wide range of presenting problems and settings (see Miltenberger, 1997, for a review)

Space does not permit detailed description of operant interventions; however, a brief overview of the procedures described by Nemeroff and Karoly (1991) will be provided. An essential first step is careful assessment of the stimuli and consequences associated with target behaviors (including behaviors for which reduced frequency is desired and those for which increased fre-

quency is desired). It is particularly important to identify the contingencies that are maintaining problematic behaviors. Efforts can then be made to eliminate *reinforcement* of problematic behavior and to introduce reinforcement of less frequent, desired behavior. For instance, a parent might be encouraged to ignore a child when he or she is yelling but then attend to the child when he or she begins speaking more quietly. When a desired behavior does not occur at all, *shaping* can be used to reinforce successive approximations of the desired behavior. It is important to keep in mind that what constitutes reinforcement is not determined subjectively. A consequence is "reinforcing" only if it increases the likelihood of an individual's previous response. Consequences have different effects on different individuals; successful operant interventions must take into account what is reinforcing for the given individual.

Extinction (withdrawal of reinforcers) often helps reduce the frequency of problematic behaviors, but in some cases punishment may also be used. Most commonly, *negative punishment* (or *response cost* procedures) are implemented. These involve removal of available rewards contingent upon an undesired behavior; the most widely recognized examples are *time-out* procedures. In extreme cases (such as self-injurious behavior), *positive punishment* or *response contingent aversive stimulation* (e.g., applying a negative consequence, such as electrical shock, after a behavior is performed) may be used. However, a wealth of problems associated with these procedures (e.g., modeling of aggression, invoking fear of the situation, failure to provide alternative responses, and short-term efficacy) have made them infrequent. All procedures aimed at reducing behaviors are more efficacious when they are paired with procedures aimed at increasing desirable behaviors. The latter intervention provides clients with a sense of how to get what they want out of life and other people, rather than just teaching them how to avoid what they do not want (Nemeroff & Karoly, 1991).

In addition to altering *consequences* for clinically relevant behaviors, *cues* (i.e., discriminative stimuli) for behaviors can also be the targets of intervention. Individuals learn that responses in a specific context will yield certain consequences; therapy can focus on the stimuli that signal potential reinforcement or punishment. These procedures involve bringing a target behavior under *stimulus control*. For instance, a client with weight problems might be encouraged to eat only in the kitchen, or only in response to hunger cues, thus reducing the stimuli that signal a response of eating. Similarly, individuals with insomnia might be instructed to engage in all nonsleep behaviors in rooms other than the bedroom, in order to increase the strength of the association between bedroom cues and sleeping.

Although contingency management procedures are often applied in controlled environments such as institutions or schools, these same principles can in fact be applied quite flexibly in many contexts. Natural reinforcers, rather than artificial reinforcers, are more likely to lead to maintenance and generalization of behavior change. Natural reinforcers are those that often occur in people's everyday environment and lives. For example, a therapist who responds with empathy and caring when a client shares a painful emotion would likely be more effective than a therapist who responds with a statement such as "thank you for sharing that feeling with me." Even traditional talk therapy likely involves therapists reinforcing certain classes of client behavior (e.g., emotional communication) and extinguishing other classes of behaviors (e.g., superficial conversation). Clients can also use *self-management* or *self-control* procedures to provide contingencies themselves (Kanfer & Gaelick-Buys, 1991). For instance, clients might put aside money not spent on cigarettes each day and then use that money to buy a reward for smoking abstinence. The stimulus control procedures described previously would also be considered self-management procedures—clients choose to engage in behav-

iors in certain contexts in order to strengthen certain habits (e.g., sleep in the bedroom) and weaken others (e.g., eating excessively).

Social and Communication Skills Training

Many, if not all, psychological problems have the potential to affect relationships in negative ways. Deficits in social and communication skills can make it difficult for individuals to deal effectively with relationship problems that arise as a result of their problems. In some cases, social skills deficits can also contribute to the target problem.

Social skills and communication training involves teaching individuals or groups to communicate more effectively. This process may include learning basic skills, such as making eye contact, ordering food in a restaurant, standing at an appropriate distance from others, and allowing others to speak without interrupting. Or, it may involve learning more complex skills, such as being more assertive, becoming a more effective lecturer, developing improved dating skills, or performing more effectively in job interviews. Typically, social skills training includes such strategies as psychoeducation, modeling (e.g., having a teacher, therapist, or other individual demonstrate the behavior), behavioral rehearsal or role plays, and feedback. Clients may also be videotaped while role-playing a particular social interaction so they can later observe their performance.

Social skills training has been used across a large number of psychological and interpersonal problems. It is a standard psychological treatment for schizophrenia (e.g., Bellack, Mueser, Gingerich, & Agresta, 1997; Liberman et al., 1998) and is often included in the treatment of social anxiety (Franklin, Jaycox, & Foa, 1999). It is used in school-based programs (Elias & Clabby, 1992), and for helping children with severe behavior disorders (Durand, 1991). Adults with depression may also be treated with social skills training (Becker, Heimberg, & Bellack, 1987). In fact, interpersonal psychotherapy for depression, an empirically supported treatment that is not normally considered a form of behavior therapy, includes social skills training as a component (Weissman, Markowitz, & Klerman, 2000). Finally, communication training is often included as a component of behavioral treatment for couples (e.g., Lawrence, Eldridge, Christensen, & Jacobson, 1999).

Modeling

As discussed earlier, modeling was first described early in the history of behavior therapy by social learning theorists such as Albert Bandura (1969). Essentially, this procedure involves demonstrating a particular behavior in the presence of a client, usually before asking the client to perform the same behavior. Modeling may also include reinforcement of an appropriate response by the client. This procedure is often used in social skills training (e.g., demonstrating for a client appropriate responses during a job interview) as well as in teaching clients basic skills of living (cooking, dressing, etc.).

Modeling is also often used in the treatment of phobias and other fear-based problems. For example, therapists will often demonstrate exposure to a feared situation before asking the client to try the exposure practice. Although modeling is often thought to be helpful clinically, studies that have examined the impact of adding modeling when treating specific phobias (Bourque & Ladouceur, 1980; Menzies & Clarke, 1993; Öst, Ferebee, & Furmark, 1997) have not found much benefit of adding modeling over and above the effects of exposure alone. The unique effects of modeling have not been examined systematically for the treatment of most other anxiety disorders, although this procedure is often used in clinical practice.

Problem-Solving Training

Problem-solving training is a behavioral strategy for teaching clients to understand their problems and to solve them more effectively, instead of seeing problems as being vague and undefined, becoming overwhelmed by problems, reacting with excessive anxiety and depression, or attempting to solve problems in ways that make the situation worse. The process of problem solving is typically broken down into steps (e.g., D'Zurilla & Goldfried, 1971; Hawton & Kirk, 1989; Mueser, 1998). The first step involves helping the person to assess, define, and understand the problem. The second step involves generating as many solutions to the problem as possible, initially without filtering or judging the solutions listed. The third step involves considering the costs and benefits of each solution, taking into account the likelihood that the solution will be effective and whether the solution is practical. Next, the individual is taught to select the best solution or solutions and to implement them. The final step should involve considering the outcome of the exercise and whether the problem was in fact solved. Problem-solving training has been used successfully (either alone, or as part of a multicomponent treatment package) in the treatment of a variety of conditions, including depression (Nezu, 1986), bipolar disorder (Miklowitz, 2001), and conduct disorder in children (Kazdin, 2002).

Relaxation-Based Treatments

Relaxation training is often used in behavior therapy, either as a stand-alone intervention or integrated into a multicomponent treatment package. The most extensively studied form of this intervention is progressive relaxation training (PRT; Bernstein, Borkovec, & Hazlett-Stevens, 2000; Jacobson, 1938) as well as applied relaxation, in which PRT is taught and clients then learn how to use the relaxation response effectively in their daily lives (Bernstein et al., 2000). As recently reviewed by Bernstein and colleagues (2000), these interventions have demonstrated efficacy for a range of anxiety disorders (generalized anxiety disorder, social phobia, specific phobia and panic disorder with and without agoraphobia) and health-related problems (e.g., hypertension, headache, chronic pain, insomnia, irritable bowel syndrome, and cancer chemotherapy). In addition, relaxation is a component of efficacious treatment packages for these disorders as well as PTSD (e.g., stress inoculation training). However, relaxation training is not an efficacious treatment for OCD, and recent dismantling studies (i.e., those in which the independent effects of multifaceted treatments are separated out) have suggested breathing retraining may not add to (and potentially detracts from) the efficacy of panic control treatment for panic disorder (Schmidt et al., 2000). As noted previously, exposure seems to be the central ingredient than relaxation in the treatment of most anxiety disorders, although relaxation may still be a beneficial component in many cases, particularly among individuals reporting high levels of muscle tension (Bernstein et al., 2000).

PRT was first developed by Jacobson (1938) as a systematic way to help individuals relax muscle fibers, thus removing tension and anxiety. Wolpe (1958) later adopted and shortened this procedure in order to use it to inhibit anxiety in response to cues in systematic desensitization. Bernstein and colleagues (2000) present a comprehensive guide for implementing relaxation training in a procedure that is commonly adopted in treatment outcome trials. A brief review of this procedure is provided next.

Clients are taught that relaxation is a skill, just like any other skill, and therefore requires repeated practice to develop. Relaxation is presented as a process, rather than an outcome, so that any increase in relaxing sensations is seen as progress. PRT involves instructing clients to progressively attend to 16 muscle groups, first briefly tensing them (5–7 seconds) and then releasing them or "letting go" (30- to 60-second cycles). The tension cycles are provided to increase awareness of tense sensations in each muscle group and in order to provide momentum

that enables a deeper level of relaxation. The therapist provides suggestions that facilitate attention to both tense and relaxing sensations across muscle groups. After completing the full cycle with the therapist (tensing each muscle group twice), clients are instructed to practice twice a day between sessions. Again, the importance of practice in developing a new skill (particularly when strong habits of anxious responding exist) is emphasized.

The process of relaxation is gradually shortened over the course of treatment, first to seven, then to four muscle groups, then to relaxation by recall ("remember what it felt like when you released those muscles"), and finally to counting. In addition, differential relaxation (tensing only those muscles needed for an activity and only to the level that is necessary) and conditioned relaxation (pairing relaxation with a cue, such as the word "calm") are introduced as the client becomes more skilled in relaxation. Finally, in applied relaxation, clients are taught to self-monitor and detect anxious cues early and practice invoking relaxation in response to these cues both in session (*in vivo* and imaginally) and between sessions. Practice with multiple forms of relaxation allows for flexibility in response to anxious cues and is thought to increase efficacy of applied relaxation (Bernstein et al., 2000).

Other forms of relaxation training are also incorporated in behavior therapy. In Borkovec's cognitive behavioral treatment for generalized anxiety disorder (Borkovec & Newman, 1998), clients are taught diaphragmatic breathing in the first session and encouraged to practice it during the week. The different autonomic effects of breathing shallowly from one's chest muscles and deeply from one's diaphragm are discussed and demonstrated, with clients typically noting that they habitually breathe shallowly. Clients then practice breathing more deeply from their diaphragm during both times of rest and times of stress throughout the week. Clients often report noticing rapid effects of this relatively brief intervention.

Biofeedback is another technique often incorporated in behavior therapy. Biofeedback provides direct feedback to clients of their biological responses and teaches them how to control these biological responses through repeated feedback and signaling (see Schwartz, 1995, for reviews of these interventions and their efficacy). These interventions are often used in behavioral medicine settings.

Bernstein and colleagues (2000) also note that the metaphor of "letting go" used in PRT can be applied to other anxious symptoms such as intrusive thoughts or images. Similar to the process of noticing muscle tension and then releasing it, clients can notice their distressing thoughts and then gently let go of them. However, it is important to distinguish between this process and suppression or avoidance of thoughts, which may perpetuate anxious meanings.

Acceptance and Mindfulness-Based Treatment Strategies

Over the past decade or so, several behavioral approaches to treating clinical problems have begun to emphasize the importance of acceptance-based strategies, often incorporating mindfulness skills training as one way of encouraging acceptance (see Hayes, Jacobson, Follette, & Dougher, 1994, for an early review of these approaches, and Hayes, Follette, & Linehan, in press). Acceptance is, in a sense, an implicit aspect of traditional exposure-based treatments, which encourage increased contact with rather than avoidance of internal and external stimuli (e.g., accepting rather than avoiding panic-related sensations in panic control treatment; Craske & Barlow, 2001). However, proponents of these newer approaches note that behavior therapy's traditional explicit focus on change may inadvertently overlook the importance of clients learning to give up some of their futile efforts of control (e.g., over their internal experiences, Hayes, Strosahl, & Wilson, 1999; or their partner's behavior, Wheeler, Chris-

tensen, & Jacobson, 2001) and learning to accept and validate their own experience (Linehan, 1993). These clinical scientists have borrowed from Eastern and humanistic/experiential traditions in incorporating acceptance into their behavioral approaches to clinical problems. Acceptance should not be confused with resignation; these therapies all emphasize that an acceptance of things as they are does not preclude efforts to make changes in one's life—it may in fact enable such changes.

Linehan's (1993; Linehan, Cochran, & Kehrer, 2001) dialectical behavior therapy (DBT) for borderline personality disorder (BPD) incorporates both acceptance and change strategies, with each thought to facilitate the other. For instance, therapists provide validation of the client's experience while also using problem-solving strategies to help clients change problematic behaviors. The skills-training component of the treatment similarly balances acceptance and change. Clients are taught mindfulness skills, adapted from Eastern traditions, in which present moment experience is observed, described, and participated in nonjudgmentally. Change-based skills, such as interpersonal effectiveness, are also taught. Dialectical philosophy (in which polar opposites are considered an inherent part of reality) provides a coherent model in which acceptance and change strategies necessarily coexist and complement each other, despite their apparent contradictory nature. Four randomized clinical trials have explored the efficacy of DBT with individuals with BPD and substance use disorders; all trials found significant reductions in target problem behaviors in DBT compared to treatment as usual (Linehan et al., 2001), suggesting this is a promising treatment approach.

Jacobson and Christensen (1998; Wheeler et al., 2001) have similarly integrated acceptance-based strategies into their integrative behavioral couples therapy (IBCT). Based on research that revealed that traditional cognitive-behavioral couples treatments were only efficacious for about half the couples treated and that older, more emotionally disengaged, more distressed couples were less likely to have successful outcomes, Jacobson and Christensen switched the focus of their treatment to an emphasis on *why* distressing behaviors were occurring in order to facilitate each partner's acceptance of the other. Such understanding and acceptance is thought to promote closeness and intimacy, reducing the ongoing conflict regarding "irreconcilable differences." These changes may in fact then lead to changes in the initially targeted behavior more effectively than a direct focus on the target behavior, which may instead increase the conflict between partners. A randomized pilot clinical trial found that couples in ICBT reported greater marital satisfaction and improvement than couples in traditional cognitive-behavioral couple therapy (Wheeler et al., 2001).

Hayes and colleagues (1999) developed acceptance and commitment therapy (ACT) based on extensive basic research in relational frame theory. They note that due to human beings' ability to learn bidirectional relationships between thoughts, feelings, and events, individuals come to respond to negative thoughts and feelings as if they are the actual events with which they are associated. This leads to efforts to control these internal experiences, which are largely not under instrumental control, as well as to *rule-governed* rather than *contingency-based* behavior (i.e., actions based on verbal rules rather than on the contingencies present in the current environment). Treatment focuses on reducing efforts at internal control, reducing clients' literal response to their own thoughts (e.g., recognizing that having the thought, "I'm hopeless," does not mean that the person's life truly is hopeless), and helping clients act in ways that are consistent with how they prefer to live their lives. Thus, a willingness to experience internal events is encouraged and practiced, while control efforts are aimed at actions, which are under instrumental control. An initial study demonstrat-

ed the effectiveness of ACT in an outpatient setting (Strosahl, Hayes, Bergan, & Romano, 1998); more controlled trials are currently under way.

These approaches are only a sample of the ways that acceptance has been integrated into behavioral approaches; the reader is encouraged to read the sources cited here for more examples and more detailed descriptions. Acceptance strategies have also been incorporated into treatments for substance use, depression, and anxiety disorders. Marlatt and Gordon (1985) note that efforts to control urges to drink are likely to have paradoxical effects and, instead, they incorporate "urge surfing," an acceptance-based strategy, in their treatment for substance use disorders. Borkovec's (Borkovec, Alcaine, & Behar, in press) cognitive-behavioral treatment for generalized anxiety disorder includes an emphasis on "letting go" of worries and focusing on present-moment experience rather than trying to predict the future; treatment development in this area has begun to focus more explicitly on mindfulness and acceptance-based strategies, borrowing from the treatments described previously (Roemer & Orsillo, 2002). Within the cognitive area, Segal, Williams, and Teasdale (2002) are using mindfulness meditation techniques in order to reduce depressive relapse; preliminary data suggest that this approach is efficacious. Incorporation of acceptance and mindfulness interventions is an exciting new direction in the behavior therapies. Although initial data are promising, more research is needed to determine active ingredients and mechanisms of change associated with these approaches.

EXAMPLES OF BEHAVIORAL PROTOCOLS FOR PARTICULAR CONDITIONS

Panic Control Treatment for Panic Disorder and Agoraphobia

Panic control treatment (PCT) is a cognitive-behavioral treatment shown to be effective for alleviating symptoms of panic disorder and agoraphobia. The underlying assumption of this approach to treatment is that unexpected panic attacks are caused by a fearful reaction to benign physical symptoms, such as racing heart, dizziness, and breathlessness (see Barlow, 2002; Clark, 1986), and that panic disorder is maintained by anxious apprehension over having more attacks and avoidance of feared situations and symptoms. PCT was developed in the mid- to late-1980s by David Barlow, Michelle Craske, and colleagues (see Craske & Barlow, 2001) and includes a number of components: psychoeducation, breathing retraining, cognitive therapy, interoceptive exposure, and *in vivo* exposure, for clients with agoraphobia. Note that this is not the only "brand" of cognitive-behavioral treatment that has been shown to be effective for panic disorder. For example, Clark and colleagues (1994, 1999) have developed a form of cognitive therapy that combines challenging anxious thoughts with behavioral experiments to test out the validity of catastrophic beliefs about panic-related sensations. In contrast, Isaac Marks (e.g., Marks et al., 1993) has studied a behavioral treatment involving repeated exposure to agoraphobic situations.

PCT typically occurs over 10 to 12 sessions. It is designed to target and prevent the occurrence of panic attacks and to decrease associated symptoms such as worry about panic attacks and agoraphobic avoidance. The initial one or two sessions of PCT include psychoeducation, during which the client is taught that (1) anxiety and fear are normal, (2) panic attacks are time limited, (3) panic symptoms have a survival function (e.g., a racing heart gets blood to the parts of the body that need it, to prepare us for escape from danger), and (4) panic and anxiety can be conceptualized as being comprised of three components (physical symptoms, anxious cognitions, and anxious behaviors, such as phobic avoidance). The ways in which these three components interact are also discussed, and corrective in-

formation is provided to dispel any beliefs that clients may hold (e.g., that panic attacks can cause heart attacks and that panic attacks can cause an individual to "go crazy"). Finally, clients are provided with a description of the treatment, with an emphasis on how each component of treatment targets a particular component of the problem (e.g., breathing retraining targets physical symptoms, cognitive therapy targets anxious thoughts, and exposure targets phobic avoidance).

Breathing retraining is typically introduced at the third PCT session. This strategy involves teaching clients to breath slowly, and from their diaphragm, to reduce symptoms caused by hyperventilation. Although the PCT package includes this particular strategy, researchers have recently shown that breathing retraining does not add to the effectiveness of this treatment (Schmidt et al., 2000), and some authors (Antony & Swinson, 2000a) have argued against including this component of treatment routinely.

The next two sessions focus on cognitive therapy, with the aim of teaching the client to replace anxious thoughts with more realistic ways of thinking about the feared situations. For example, clients may be encouraged to consider a wide range of evidence supporting and contradicting their anxious thoughts before assuming that their racing heart is a sign that they are about to die. They may be asked to recall all the other times that their heart has raced without leading to death, and to consider the implications of their history for the likelihood of having a heart attack the next time they experience a racing heart. Although only two sessions are devoted exclusively to cognitive restructuring, clients are encouraged to use the cognitive techniques throughout the remainder of the treatment, and therapists continue to use some of the time each session to work on changing the client's anxious thoughts.

Interoceptive exposure is introduced next. This intervention involves identifying exercises that bring on panic-like sensations for the client and having the client practice these exercises until the exercieses are no longer frightening. For example, a client who is fearful of experiencing dizziness might practice spinning in a chair for 2 minutes at a time to induce a feeling of dizziness. This exercise would be repeated six or seven times in a row (with a short break between each trial), until the fear decreases, and then the series of six or seven trials would be repeated twice daily for a week or more, until the exercise no longer produces fear. For clients who avoid situations in which panic attacks may occur (i.e., those with agoraphobia), situational or *in vivo* exposure is also included. In fact, clients with severe agoraphobic avoidance may need to spend significant amounts of time on situational exposure to get the most benefit from treatment. The final session of PCT is spent discussing issues related to terminating treatment and strategies for maintaining gains.

Studies on PCT demonstrates that it is among the most effective treatments for anxiety disorders, with gains being maintained over time (Craske, Brown, & Barlow, 1991). PCT works well in both individual (Barlow, Craske, Cerny, & Klosko, 1989) and group (Telch et al., 1993) formats and has been shown to be at least as efficacious as medication treatments, such as imipramine (Barlow, Gorman, Shear, & Woods, 2000) and alprazolam (Klosko, Barlow, Tassinari, & Cerny, 1990). Finally, evidence shows that treating panic disorder using PCT can lead to improvements in comorbid conditions, such as generalized anxiety disorder (Brown, Antony, & Barlow, 1995).

Depression

Jacobson and colleagues (Jacobson, Martell, & Dimidjian, 2001; Martell, Addis, & Jacobson, 2001) have been engaged in developing and empirically investigating behavioral activation (BA) treatment for depression over the past several years. Their interest in this intervention began with a dismantling study that revealed that BA alone had comparable efficacy to cognitive therapy, which includes both behavioral activation techniques and cognitive restructuring (Jacobson et al., 1996). Based on these findings, Jacobson and colleagues began to work on developing BA as a treatment in its own right, aimed at helping depressed individuals increase their contact with positive reinforcers and decrease patterns of avoidance and inactivity.

Jacobson and colleagues base their conceptual model on Ferster's (1973) radical behavioral model of depression. Consistent with a contextualist perspective, they focus on factors external to the individuals (i.e., environmental factors) as potential causal and maintaining factors for depression and aim their intervention at these factors. Consistent with all behavioral models of depression, they note that the inactivity characteristic of depressed individuals leads to decreased contact with potential positive reinforcers, thus reducing opportunities for action to be reinforced. In addition, they note that the inertia and withdrawal typical of depressed individuals serve a negatively reinforcing function, similar to avoidance behaviors characteristic of anxiety disorders. Despite the short-term relief that likely results from inactivity (by reducing experiences with nonreinforcing environments), these avoidance behaviors can lead to secondary problems (such as occupational or relational difficulties) and also limit opportunities for contact with positive reinforcers. Furthermore, these avoidance patterns likely lead to disruptions in routines, which are thought to play an etiological and maintaining role in depression (Ehlers, Frank, & Kupfer, 1988).

BA directly targets avoidance behavior and routine disruptions. First, therapists focus on establishing a therapeutic relationship and presenting the model of depression. Emphasis is placed on establishing a goal of changing behavior rather than altering mood; clients' tendency to believe they cannot engage in an action until they feel better is gently challenged by requesting that clients try to engage in planned behaviors regardless of how they feel. Time is spent developing collaborative treatment goals, with a distinction made between short-term goals, many of which will be addressed during therapy, and long-term goals, only a few of which will be directly addressed during the course of treatment.

A critical element of this treatment is a focus on functional analysis. Therapist and client explore the triggers for depressive episodes, the nature of depressive symptoms, how the client responds to depressive symptoms, and avoidant behaviors and routine disruptions. Clients are taught to conduct their own functional analyses and encouraged to do so particularly after therapy ends in order to prevent relapse. Based on this functional analysis, the client and therapist develop targets for focused activation. Rather than encouraging activity generally, as many behavioral approaches do, BA focuses on idiographic identification of activities that the client believes will be beneficial. Monitoring forms are used to track actions engaged in, triggers, and consequences, and assignments are modified accordingly.

Avoidance behaviors are modified by helping clients identify the function of these behaviors (both the immediate relief and the longer-term problems) and choose alternative coping responses. The acronym TRAP is used to help identify triggers, responses, and avoidance patterns, whereas the acronym TRAC is used to help generate alternative coping responses to the same triggers and responses. Often alternative coping responses involve approach rather than avoidance behaviors. Attention is also paid to regulating routines and to integrating activation strategies into regular routines, in order to be able to fully evaluate their impact. To maximize the impact of activation strategies, clients are encouraged to attend to their experience, particularly their immediate environment, as they engage in activities. (Jacobson et al. [2001] note that this is somewhat similar to mindfulness training in its emphasis on present-moment experience.) This is thought to increase the impact of present-moment contingencies and also to help circumvent ruminative thinking, which is thought to interfere with engagement in life.

Bipolar Disorder

Although psychopharmacological interventions are clearly the treatment of choice for bipolar disorder, research suggests that adjunctive psychosocial interventions can improve outcome and reduce relapse (see Miklowitz, 2001, for a review). In particular, two randomized controlled trials have demonstrated that family-focused therapy (FFT; Miklowitz, 2001; Miklowitz & Goldstein, 1997) is associated with reduced relapse when compared to either crisis management or an individual case-management and problem-solving intervention. Below we provide a brief summary of FFT.

Adjunctive behavioral interventions for bipolar disorder are based in a vulnerability–stress model of bipolar episodes. Research suggests that stressful life events, disruptions in routines (similar to those described earlier for depression), and family stress all have an impact on bipolar disorder (in addition to the biological/genetic vulnerabilities that have clearly been established). For instance, high levels of expressed emotion (EE; i.e., critical comments, hostility, and emotional overinvolvement) among family members predict a negative course of bipolar disorder (see Miklowitz, 2001, for a review). Research has also shown that these displays are due, in part, to perceiving that clients have control over behaviors associated with their disorder, suggesting that psychoeducation may be an effective intervention in reducing high-EE (Miklowitz, 2001).

FFT is a three-stage intervention that is weekly for the first 3 months, biweekly for 3 months, and monthly for the final 3 months. It is intended for use with clients who are receiving concurrent pharmacotherapy; clients who do not consent to medication are not accepted for treatment. As with all behavior therapies, extensive assessment is conducted initially and continually throughout treatment. In particular, a mood chart is used to track the client's daily mood and its association with events that may be influential (e.g., interpersonal conflict, exercise habits, and sleep–wake cycle). Family assessments are also conducted, assessing EE directly and also more generally assessing familial interaction styles.

The therapist begins treatment by establishing a relationship with the client and family and providing the treatment rationale. In particular, the rationale for family intervention is important, as it begins to involve family members in the treatment. The stated goals for therapy are encouraging the client to work with his or her psychiatrist to stabilize on medication and working with the family to minimize stress through psychoeducation, communication training, and problem-solving training.

The psychoeducational module lasts for approximately seven sessions. Topics covered include symptoms and course of the disorder, the etiology of bipolar disorder, and ways to intervene within the vulnerability–stress model. The client and family are taught how to identify various risk and protective factors for relapse so that all can work together to reduce the risk of relapse. The second module focuses on communication enhancement training and lasts approximately seven sessions. A skills training approach is used to reduce the likelihood that family members will engage in aversive family communication following a bipolar episode. Skills focused on are chosen to match the idiographic needs of the family, based on the family assessment and continued observation of the family throughout treatment. The final module of treatment focuses on problem-solving training and lasts four or five sessions. In this module, the therapist helps family members to communicate about difficult topics and to generate a framework for developing solutions to problems. This also provides a context for sharing their emotional reactions to challenging topics. Termination of treatment includes preparation for relapse (e.g., completing the "relapse drill" in which triggers are identified and each family member has a role to play in reducing the risk of relapse), and review of the important elements of treatment for clients and families to keep attending to in their daily lives (e.g., medication compliance, communication and problem-solving skills).

THE THERAPEUTIC RELATIONSHIP AND THE STANCE OF THE THERAPIST

In 1970, Lang, Melamed, and Hart published a paper on an automated procedure for administering behavioral treatments for fear in 29 female undergraduates. In the abstract, they concluded that "an apparatus designed to administer systematic desensitization automatically was as effective as a live therapist in reducing phobic behavior, suggesting that desensitization is not dependent on a concurrent interpersonal interaction" (p. 220). Since that time, there has been a large number of studies demonstrating the effectiveness of self-administered treatments and treatments with minimal therapist contact. For example, in the case of panic disorder and agoraphobia, a single session of behavioral treatment leads to significant improvements in people who had just presented to an emergency room during a panic attack (Swinson, Soulios, Cox, & Kuch, 1992). Panic disorder can also be treated effectively over the telephone (Swinson, Fergus, Cox, & Wickwire, 1995). Even treatment with a self-help book can be as effective as treatment with a therapist for relieving the symptoms of panic disorder (Gould & Clum, 1995; Hecker, Losee, Fritzler, & Fink, 1996).

Do these findings mean that the therapeutic relationship is unimportant in behavior therapy? Probably not. In most of the studies on self-help treatments, there is a confound—clients are required to have regular contact with a clinician for the study assessments. In fact, recent findings from Febbraro, Clum, Roodman, and Wright (1999) suggest that self-help treatments for panic disorder may be less effective when they are used on their own, without occasional professional contact to monitor the client's progress and treatment compliance. In other words, the therapeutic relationship may be important even for self-help treatments.

An additional limitation of the findings regarding self-administered treatments is that participants in studies of these treatments may be less impaired, on average, than those who present for treatment in routine clinical practice. For example, studies on self-help treatments for anxiety disorders often exclude individuals with severe comorbid depression and suicidal ideation, substance use disorders, bipolar disorder, psychotic disorders, organic impairments, and certain personality disorders. The more impaired a particular person is by his or her problems, the more important the therapeutic relationship likely becomes.

There is no reason to think that developing a good client–therapist relationship necessarily takes a long time. Follette, Naugle, and Callaghan (1996) argue that even a limited amount of therapist–client contact can lead to considerable behavioral change, in part because of the reinforcing nature of the therapeutic relationship. The techniques of behavior therapy can certainly be powerful even outside the context of therapy. However, relevant therapist behaviors may increase the likelihood that a client will complete the necessary practices and take advantage of the treatment to the fullest extent possible.

There is now emerging evidence that therapist behaviors do affect outcome in behavioral treatments (for a review, see Keijsers, Schaap, & Hoogduin, 2000). For example, Keijsers, Schaap, Hoogduin, and Lammers (1995) concluded that therapist empathy, warmth, positive regard, and genuineness assessed early in treatment were predictive of a positive outcome following behavioral treatment for panic disorder and agoraphobia, as was the tendency for clients to rate their therapists as more understanding and respectful. Williams and Chambless (1990) found that individuals with agoraphobia who described their therapists as more confident, caring, and involved, improved more than those who did not describe their therapists in these ways. In addition, there is evidence that therapist style can affect a client's motivation during treatment for problem drinking, and that therapist styles that enhance motivation are particularly useful for alcoholics who are particularly angry and hostile (Miller, Benefield, & Tonigan, 1993).

A study comparing the quality of the therapeutic alliance in single sessions from 18 cognitive-behavioral therapists and 13 psychodynamic-interpersonal therapists found higher scores on the Working Alliance Inventory for the cognitive-behavioral therapists (Raue, Castonguay, & Goldfried, 1993). This finding is interesting in light of the reputation that behavior therapists have for downplaying the importance of the therapeutic relationship, relative to insight-oriented therapists. The relationship between a strong therapeutic alliance and a successful outcome following behavioral treatment is unclear, however. For example, Woody and Adessky (2002) did not find a significant relationship between therapeutic alliance (as measured by the Working Alliance Inventory) and outcome following cognitive-behavioral group treatment for social phobia.

For a long time, the therapeutic relationship has been underemphasized in behavioral writings and in the training of behavior therapists, compared to some other forms of psychotherapy. Instead, researchers have tended to focus more on examining the efficacy of particular behavioral techniques, with little discussion of the context in which behavior therapy occurs. However, in recent years, therapists working within a behavioral framework have become increasingly interested in the role of the therapeutic relationship and in the effects of therapist behavior on the outcome of treatment (e.g., Kohlenberg & Tsai, 1991). The therapist is potentially a powerful source of social reinforcement; thus it makes sense from a behavioral perspective that the therapeutic relationship and therapist behavior would play a role in the process and outcome of treatment.

CURATIVE FACTORS OR MECHANISMS OF CHANGE

Changes in Environmental Contingencies

A central factor thought to underlie change in behavior therapy involves the relationship between behavior and the environment. Given that behavior is thought to be functional, in other words, maintained by contingencies in the environment, behavior change is thought to be due to alterations in environmental contingencies. This may take several different forms. Most obviously, the individual's context may be altered to reduce reinforcement for problematic behavior and increase reinforcement for desired behavior. This may be the case in parent training interventions in which the child's environment is directly altered, or in couple or family therapy where the responses individuals have to one another are a target of intervention. Similarly, in self-management approaches, the client him- or herself may alter the contingencies in his or her environment.

Often the environment is not directly altered, but the client learns to engage in new behaviors, which in turn are reinforced by the existing environmental contingencies. For instance, in social skills training, it is expected that the individual will receive meaningful, natural social reinforcement for new skills, which will increase the frequency of these newly learned behaviors. Similarly, *in vivo* exposure is likely to result in the client's exhibiting new, nonavoidant behaviors (such as attending parties) that will then be maintained by natural reinforcement from the environment. To maximize adaptive responding to new environments, behavior therapy focuses on helping clients to develop flexible behavioral repertoires (Goldiamond, 1974) rather than rigid behavioral patterns based on past learning. These flexible repertoires, along with a decreased emphasis on arbitrary verbal rules (Hayes, Kohlenberg, & Melancon, 1989), are expected to promote continued adaptation after therapy has ended.

Emotional Processing

Exposure-based interventions were initially developed to *extinguish* fearful responses to classically conditioned stimuli. However, research has demonstrated that fearful associations are never unlearned (for instance, individuals can spontaneously recover "extinguished" fearful responses when they are reexposed to the unconditioned stimulus). Based on these findings, newer models suggest that exposure results in learning new, nonfearful associations to previously feared stimuli. According to Foa and Kozak's (1986) now classic emotional processing model, fearful responses are altered when an individual fully accesses the associative fear network (including stimulus, response, and meaning elements of the fear) and incorporates new, nonthreatening information. Foa and Kozak review research that supports the proposed importance of initial activation of the fear structure (indicated by physiological responding to the feared stimulus) as well as habituation within and across sessions for efficacious exposure therapy. However, others have pointed out that not all exposure research supports the emotional processing model (e.g., Craske, 1999; Mineka & Thomas, 1999), leading to some to propose cognitive mechanisms of change for this behavioral intervention.

Cognitive Models

Many researchers have noted that exposure-based treatments may in fact lead to cognitive change for individuals, and this may be the mechanism of change. For instance, Mineka and Thomas (1999) suggest that exposure disconfirms clients' beliefs that they do not have control over anxiety-provoking situations. Similarly, both Zinbarg (1993) and Rachman (1996) note that exposure techniques may alter emotionally relevant cognitive representations. In other words, clients' experiences when engaging in previously avoided activities may challenge their beliefs that such behaviors are dangerous or impossible for them to engage in, leading them to be more likely to continue to engage in such behaviors. Certainly behavioral experiments have long been an integral part of cognitive therapy techniques, suggesting that a client's own experiences may provide particularly salient disconfirming data for clinically relevant cognitions. To date, no research has adequately addressed whether behavioral techniques are efficacious due to their facilitation of cognitive change. Although some data suggest that cognitive techniques do not significantly add to the efficacy of behavioral techniques for depression (Jacobson et al., 1996), this does not mean that the behavioral techniques do not have their effect due to cognitive change.

Biological Changes

Although it is commonly assumed that psychosocial interventions are efficacious through psychological mechanisms, recent research has indicated that psychosocial interventions can lead to biological changes. Most striking have been treatment findings in the OCD literature in which successful behavior therapy has been associated with changes in glucose metabolic rates in the caudate nucleus, comparable to changes found following pharmacotherapy (see Cottraux & Gérard, 1998, for a review). Although this may mean that such biological changes are the mechanisms of change for behavior therapy, they may instead be correlates, rather than causes of, change.

TREATMENT APPLICABILITY AND ETHICAL CONSIDERATIONS

Applicability of Behavioral Treatments

Behavioral interventions have been applied to a wide range of presenting problems including anxiety disorders, mood disorders, substance use disorders, serious mental illness (as an adjunctive treatment), eating disorders, personality disorders, childhood disorders (e.g., anxiety, conduct problems, and autism), and health problems. Behavioral interventions tend to be more effective when clients present with focal target problems (and these types of presentations have been the most commonly studied); however, functional analysis and behavioral principles can be adapted to address a wide range of more diffuse clinical presentations as well. Recent research has also begun to investigate the impact of behavioral interventions targeting a single disorder on comorbid disorders that are not necessarily the focus of treatment. In a number of cases (e.g., Brown et al., 1995), comorbid disorders tend to improve when a target problem is treated, suggesting that the learning that takes place in these interventions may generalize to other, related problems.

Although the idiographic principles underlying behavior therapy make it particularly responsive to variability in client characteristics (e.g., gender, ethnicity, age, class, sexual orientation, and other individual difference variables that may play an important role in understanding the function of specific behaviors and in expectations for therapy), the tendency to investigate efficacy of interventions using standardized protocols, with predominantly white samples, has provided only limited empirical knowledge of the cross-cultural applicability of these intervention techniques (as is true of all modes of therapy). Studies have demonstrated the efficacy of these interventions across gender and a range of age groups (from children to older adults), however.

In the last decade or so, important progress has been made in providing models for how to apply behavioral treatments in culturally diverse groups (see Iwamasa, 1996, for a review of work in this area). A review of cultural considerations suggested for specific groups is beyond the scope of this chapter; readers are encouraged to read the special series cited earlier for more detail. It has been noted that characteristics of (cognitive) behavioral interventions may make them a particularly good match for certain groups (for instance, the problem-focused nature of treatment may fit with certain cultural expectations and with the needs of low socioeconomic status clients), but that treatments also need to be adapted so that they are culturally sensitive (e.g., Organista & Munoz, 1996; Renfrey, 1992). Again, this is consistent with the functional model underlying behavior therapy, which emphasizes the importance of idiographic, contextually sensitive conceptualization and treatment. In fact, Tanaka-Matsumi, Seiden, and Lam (1996) provide an excellent model for incorporating culturally relevant information into a functional assessment of a client. Several case studies suggest that behavior therapy can be effective with clients from culturally diverse backgrounds when this diversity is taken into account (e.g., Fink, Turner, & Beidel, 1996; Toyokawa & Nedate, 1996). Randomized controlled trials are now needed in order to further explore the efficacy of these interventions.

Ethical Issues

In addition to the ethical considerations that are associated with any form of psychotherapy, behavioral approaches raise some specific concerns that should be kept in mind. Given the focus on behavioral change, and the use of strategies that have an intentional impact on the likelihood of certain behaviors, people often express concern that behavior therapy can be coercive and impose change chosen by the therapist rather than client. In fact, this is a consideration in all forms of therapy; contingencies are always present that are likely to affect clients' behavior. In behavior therapy, the goal of behavioral change is made explicit and therapists collaborate with clients to ensure consensus on treatment goals. Progress and goals are continually assessed to provide repeated opportunities for clients to influence the course and direction of their therapy.

Behavior therapy often involves activities that take place outside the clinic, such as riding the subway or elevators with clients. This change in context challenges traditional conceptualizations of the boundaries that surround therapy. For instance, a therapist might eat at a restaurant with a client or visit his or her home, activities that would typically be forbidden in the context of a therapeutic relationship. It is important to be aware of the potential for these activities to be misconstrued by clients as evidence of a different sort of relationship. The clear rationale for the therapeutic utility of these activities assists in clarifying how they fall within the therapeutic, rather than social, domain. Therapists must also be sensitive to any potential danger for clients during exposures, being sure at all times to maintain the safety of clients.

CASE ILLUSTRATION

Background Information and Pretreatment Assessment

Deborah was a 43-year-old woman who worked as an elementary school teacher. She was married and had two children. She reported having difficulties with social anxiety for as long as she could recall. The problem had been particularly bad since college, when she had to drop several courses due to anxiety over giving presentations. Although she could not recall how the problem began, she remembered a number of life events that seemed to lead to exacerbations in her anxiety. For example, during one particularly difficult year in high school, she remembered being teased on a regular basis and pretending to be ill on several occasions so she could stay home from school to avoid being around her classmates. She described her home life while growing up as relatively happy, although she also reported that her parents were critical at times and that she often felt pressure from her parents to meet high standards in school and in other areas of her life.

As part of her initial assessment, Deborah received the SCID-IV (First et al., 1996). DSM-IV criteria were met for a principal diagnosis of social anxiety disorder (generalized). Criteria were also met for a past diagnosis of major depressive disorder, triggered by the loss of a job 10 years earlier. She reported significant fear and avoidance of a wide range of social situations, including parties, public speaking (except when teaching her students), writing in public, speaking to people in authority, meeting new people, being assertive, and having conversations with others. She reported that her social anxiety has prevented her from making friends and from returning to school to complete her master's degree. She finally decided to seek treatment after reluctantly agreeing to be the maid of honor at her sister's wedding, which was approaching in only 3 months.

Deborah reported several characteristic thoughts that seemed to contribute to her social anxiety. Her primary concern in social situations was that she would appear stupid or incompetent in front of others, despite the fact that she almost always receives positive feedback about her performance. Her anxious thoughts were particularly problematic at work and around people who she did not know well. She would become upset if she

perceived even the slightest bit of rejection in these situations. However, she was quite comfortable around her family and her closest friends and was rarely upset if they criticized her behavior. Deborah also reported a fear that she would seem boring to others and that other people would not want to spend time with her if they had the opportunity to get to know her. When asked what types of variables affected her fear, Deborah mentioned that she was more anxious around others who she perceives as better in some way (e.g., more competent, successful, or educated), who she does not know well, or who appeared self-assured. She also reported being particularly anxious in brightly lit places (because others might notice her blushing or shaky hands) and in more formal situations.

As part of her pretreatment assessment, Deborah completed a series of self-report questionnaires, including the Social Interaction Anxiety Scale (SIAS; Mattick & Clarke, 1998) and Social Phobia Scale (SPS; Mattick & Clarke, 1998) to measure her social anxiety, the Depression Anxiety Stress Scales (DASS; Lovibond & Lovibond, 1995) to measure depression and generalized anxiety, and the Illness Attitudes Rating Scale (IIRS; Devins, 1994) as a measure of functional impairment. She also rated her levels of fear and avoidance for each of 12 items from her exposure hierarchy, using scales ranging from 0 (no fear; no avoidance) to 100 (maximum fear; complete avoidance). Her scores on these measures are reported later, in the section on outcome. Finally, Deborah completed a behavioral approach test involving trying to return a sweater to a department store. Deborah was able to wait in line at the store, but when she reached the front of the line, she was too anxious to approach the cashier to ask about returning the sweater.

Behavioral Conceptualization

Deborah's social anxiety seemed, in part, to have been initially exacerbated by some negative experiences she had in social situations. More recently, the anxiety appeared to be maintained by her avoidance of social situations and her exaggerated beliefs about the potential dangers of being around other people. A number of situations appeared to trigger Deborah's anxiety.

Treatment

Deborah received cognitive-behavioral group treatment, similar to that described by Heimberg and Becker (2002). Her group included six other clients, all with a principal diagnosis of social phobia. The group met for 12 weekly sessions, each lasting 2 hours. The first two sessions included psychoeducation regarding the nature of social anxiety and its treatment. These sessions began with a discussion of the notion that anxiety and fear are normal emotions and that attempts to avoid experiencing them can actually increase their frequency and intensity. In addition, the survival value of social anxiety and its associated symptoms was reviewed. Clients in the group were encouraged to recognize that not all social anxiety is problematic. At times, social anxiety can protect us from making mistakes that might otherwise be associated with severe negative social consequences. Clients were also encouraged to conceptualize their social anxiety in terms of three components, including a *physical component* (e.g., blushing, shaking, and sweating), a *cognitive component* (e.g., unrealistic assumptions regarding social situations), and a *behavioral component* (e.g., avoidance and overprotective behaviors). The treatment strategies were reviewed, with an emphasis on how each technique can be used to target particular components of the problem. Homework during these initial sessions involved monitoring anxiety symptoms on diaries and completing assigned readings, including introductory chapters from the *Shyness and Social Anxiety Workbook* (Antony & Swinson, 2000b). Relevant readings from this book were assigned throughout the remaining sessions of treatment as well.

Subsequent sessions included primarily instruction in cognitive restructuring and exposure to feared situations (both during in-session simulated exposures and between-session *in vivo* exposures practiced for homework). Cognitive restructuring involved teaching the group to identify anxiety-provoking beliefs (e.g., "it is important for everyone to like me" and "if my hands shake during a presentation, people will think I am incompetent") and to replace them with more balanced or realistic interpretations regarding social situations, after considering the evidence for the thoughts (for an overview of cognitive therapy techniques, see Reinecke & Freeman, Chapter 7, this volume). For her exposure practices, Deborah was encouraged to confront situations in which she might, in fact, draw attention to herself or look incompetent in front of others. For example, she practiced purposely losing her train of thought during presentations, shopping and then returning items to stores, spilling water on herself in a restaurant, asking for directions, dropping her keys in public, and wearing her dress inside-out at the mall. Each client in the group, including Deborah, developed an individualized hierarchy, which was used to guide his or her exposure practices, as described earlier in this chapter. In addition to cognitive and exposure-based strategies, one session of the group was spent discussing strategies for improving communication skills (see McKay, Davis, & Fanning, 1995).

Outcome

Relative to the other members of the group, Deborah's progress was more gradual. However, she was particularly motivated and completed almost all of her homework assignments. By the end of treatment, she was much less concerned about being judged by others and she reported a reduction in the sensations of blushing and shaking. She had begun a night course in pottery and reported having socialized on a number of occasions with her classmates.

TABLE 6.2. Deborah's Pre- and Posttreatment Assessment Scores

Measure	Pre	Post
SIAS	57	40
SPS	39	24
Mean Hierarchy (fear)	67.5	45.7
Mean Hierarchy (avoid)	67.5	39.3
DASS—Depression	6	6
DASS—Anxiety	6	6
DASS—Stress	12	2
IIRS	40	35

Note. SIAS, Social Interaction Anxiety Scale; SPS, Social Phobia Scale; Mean Hierarchy (fear), mean fear rating on Deborah's 12 hierarchy items; Mean Hierarchy (avoid), mean avoidance rating on Deborah's 12 hierarchy items; DASS, Depression Anxiety Stress Scales; IIRS, Illness Intrusiveness Rating Scale.

Deborah was able to attend her sister's wedding and experienced only moderate levels of anxiety while carrying out her responsibilities as maid of honor. Deborah's pre- and posttreatment scores on various measures are reported in Table 6.2. In addition, at the end of treatment she repeated the behavioral approach test. This time, she was able to return the sweater at the department store, with only minimal anxiety.

CURRENT AND FUTURE TRENDS

Because behavior therapy is grounded in a commitment to scientific inquiry, its practice is constantly evolving and changing. We highlight here a few areas in which it seems the field is most likely to evolve over the next several years. First, it is important to note that an integration of behavioral and cognitive techniques is more common than a separation of these two elements. Thus, integration of cognitive and behavioral interventions is certainly a current (as well as a past) trend. In addition, attention is being paid to the potential utility of integrating other intervention strategies (both psychological and pharmacological) in order to maximize efficacy of interventions. Initial data suggest, somewhat surprisingly, that combined cognitive behavioral and pharmacological interventions may *not* be more efficacious than cognitive-behavioral interventions alone for treating anxiety disorders (Barlow et al., 2000), particularly over the long term, after treatment has ended. Work investigating the efficacy of integrating mindfulness and acceptance-based techniques into behavioral treatments for a range of disorders was described earlier. In addition, a trial is currently under way investigating whether the addition of interpersonal and experiential elements to a cognitive-behavioral protocol increases its efficacy in treating generalized anxiety disorder (Newman, Castonguay, Borkovec, & Molnar, in press). We expect to learn more about the utility of psychotherapy integration in the coming years.

A substantial current and future trend concerns an emphasis on investigating the effectiveness of behavioral interventions in clinical practice, as opposed to research settings. Behaviorists have committed themselves to the importance of "effectiveness" research in order to respond to the criticism that randomized controlled "efficacy" trials are often conducted on a narrow, nonrepresentative sample of clients with a given disorder. Trials now typically use many fewer exclusion criteria and make an effort to include more representative samples. In addition, behaviorists are conducting research in clinical settings in order to investigate the utility of treatments within the context they will be applied. So far, effectiveness research has been promising, suggesting that behavioral techniques are beneficial in treatment-seeking clinical samples (Stuart, Treat, & Wade, 2000; Warren & Thomas, 2001).

Behaviorists are also currently focusing on how to disseminate empirically supported behavioral interventions so they will be more widely used in the community. The effectiveness research described earlier is one method of pursuing this aim. A new journal, *Cognitive and Behavioral Practice,* was developed in an effort to bridge the gap between practitioners and researchers and to provide a forum for clinicians to describe their behavioral applications.

Finally, behaviorists are focusing on developing interventions that target disorders not previously treated effectively, more diverse client samples, and comorbid clinical presentations. As described previously, researchers and clinicians are exploring how behavioral interventions can be used in a culturally sensitive manner and whether these adapted interventions are efficacious. In addition, several protocols have been developed that specifically target comorbid and more complex clinical cases. For instance, Cloitre, Koenen, Cohen, and Han (2002) have developed a treatment that combines emotion regulation and interpersonal skills training with imaginal exposure to treat women with PTSD and emotional dysregulation due to histories of child sexual abuse, and Najavits (2001) has developed an approach that treats substance abuse and PTSD concurrently. These efforts, combined with the focus on effectiveness, will help us continue to develop interventions that can optimally treat the clients presenting for services.

ACKNOWLEDGMENTS

We would like to thank Cynthia E. Crawford and Allison Wagg for their assistance in the preparation of this chapter.

SUGGESTIONS FOR FURTHER READING

Barlow, D. H. (Ed.). (2001). *Clinical handbook of psychological disorders* (3rd ed.). New York: Guilford Press.—This popular edited volume provides detailed, session-by-session, evidence-based protocols for treating a wide range of psychological problems, including anxiety disorders, mood disorders, substance use disorders, eating disorders, and several other conditions.

Caballo, V. E. (Ed.). (1998). *International handbook of cognitive and behavioural treatments for psychological disorders.* Oxford, UK: Pergamon.—Like Barlow's 2001 text, this book offers clinical guidelines for treating a wide range of disorders from a behavioral or cognitive-behavioral perspective. It includes chapters on 22 different disorders, including many that are not typically discussed in handbooks of this type (e.g., hypochondriasis, bidy dysmorphic disorder, problem gambling).

Goldfried, M. R., & Davison, G. C. (1994). *Clinical behavior therapy* (expanded ed.). New York: Wiley.—A classic textbook that provides detailed instructions for and examples of both cognitive and behavioral intervention strategies.

Haynes, S. N., & O'Brien, W. O. (2000). *Principles and practice of behavioral assessment.* New York: Kluwer Academic/Plenum Press.—This book reviews all aspects of behavioral assessment, including historical perspective, theoretical underpinnings, psychometric issues, and detailed practical descriptions of the techniques that are typically used.

Kanfer, F. H., & Goldstein, A. P. (Eds.). (1991). *Helping people change: A textbook of methods* (4th ed.). Needham Heights, MA: Allyn & Bacon.—An edited, practitioner-oriented volume that reviews effective methods of psychological intervention, including many behavioral interventions such as modeling, operant methods, and exposure methods.

Margraf, J. (1998). Behavioral approaches. In A. S. Bellack & M. Hersen (Series Eds.) & P. Salkovskis (Vol. Ed.), *Comprehensive clinical psychology. Vol. 6: Adults: Clinical formulation and treatment* (pp. 25–49). Oxford, UK: Elsevier Science.—This chapter provides a thorough overview of the historical, conceptual, and practical underpinnings of behavior therapy.

O'Donohue, W., & Krasner, L. (Eds.). (1995). *Theories of behavior therapy: Exploring behavior change.* Washington, DC: American Psychological Association.—This large edited volume (more than 750 pages) provides the most comprehensive review available on various theoretical perspectives in behavior therapy

Plaud, J. J., & Eifert, G. H. (Eds.). (1998). *From behavior theory to behavior therapy.* Boston: Allyn & Bacon.—Most of the chapters in this book are organized around particular clinical disorders and issues, and in each case, the emphasis is on understanding the links between behavioral theory and behavioral treatment for that particular problem.

REFERENCES

Abramowitz, J. S. (1996). Variants of exposure and response prevention in the treatment of obsessive–compulsive disorder: A meta-analysis. *Behavior Therapy, 27,* 583–600.

Addis, M. (1997). Evaluating the treatment manual as a means of disseminating empirically validated psychotherapies. *Clinical Psychology: Science and Practice, 4,* 1–11.

Addis, M. E., Wade, W. A., & Hatgis, C. (1999). Barriers to dissemination of evidence-based practices: Addressing practitioners' concerns about manual-based psychotherapies. *Clinical Psychology: Science and Practice, 6,* 430–441.

American Psychiatric Association. (2000). *Diagnostic and statistical manual of mental disorders* (4th ed., text revision; DSM-IV-TR). Washington, DC: Author.

Antony, M. M., & Barlow, D. H. (2002). Specific phobia. In D. H. Barlow (Ed.), *Anxiety and its disorders: The nature and treatment of anxiety and panic* (2nd ed., pp. 380–417). New York: Guilford Press.

Antony, M. M., Craske, M. G., & Barlow, D. H. (1995). *Mastery of your specific phobia (client workbook).* Boulder, CO: Graywind.

Antony, M. M., Downie, F., & Swinson, R. P. (1998). Diagnostic issues and epidemiology in obsessive compulsive disorder. In R. P. Swinson, M. M. Antony, S. Rachman, & M. A. Richter (Eds.), *Obsessive–compulsive disorder: Theory, research, and treatment* (pp. 3–32). New York: Guilford Press.

Antony, M. M., & McCabe, R. E. (in press). Social and specific phobias. In A. Tasman, J. Kay, & J. A. Lieberman (Eds.), *Psychiatry* (2nd ed.), Chichester, UK: Wiley.

Antony, M. M., McCabe, R. E., Leeuw, I., Sano, N., & Swinson, R. P. (2001). Effect of exposure and coping style on *in vivo* exposure for specific phobia of spiders. *Behaviour Research and Therapy, 39,* 1137–1150.

Antony, M. M., Orsillo, S. M., & Roemer, L. (Eds.). (2001). *Practitioner's guide to empirically-based measures of anxiety.* New York: Kluwer Academic/Plenum Press.

Antony, M. M., & Swinson, R. P. (2000a). *Phobic disorders and panic in adults: A guide to assessment and treatment.* Washington, DC: American Psychological Association.

Antony, M. M., & Swinson, R. P. (2000b). *The shyness and social anxiety workbook: Proven, step-by-step techniques for overcoming your fear.* Oakland, CA: New Harbinger.

Bandura, A. (1969). *Principles of behavior modification.* New York: Holt, Rinehart & Winston.

Barlow, D. H. (Ed.). (2001). *Clinical handbook of psychological disorders* (3rd ed.). New York: Guilford Press.

Barlow, D. H. (2002). *Anxiety and its disorders: The nature and treatment of anxiety and panic* (2nd ed.). New York: Guilford Press.

Barlow, D. H., & Craske, M. G. (2000). *Mastery of your anxiety and Panic (MAP-3).* Boulder, CO: Graywind.

Barlow, D. H., Craske, M. G., Cerny, J. A., & Klosko, J. S. (1989). Behavioral treatment of panic disorder. *Behavior Therapy, 20,* 261–282.

Barlow, D. H., Gorman, J. M., Shear, M. K., & Woods, S. W. (2000). Cognitive-behavioral therapy, imipramine, or their combination for panic disorder. *Journal of the American Medical Association, 283,* 2529–2536.

Beck, A. T., Steer, R. A., & Brown, G. (1996). *Manual for Beck Depression Inventory—II.* San Antonio, TX: Psychological Corporation.

Becker, R. E., Heimberg, R. G., & Bellack, A. S. (1987). *Social skills training treatment for depression.* Elmsford, NY: Pergamon Press.

Bellack, A. S., & Hersen, M. (Eds.). (1985). *Dictionary of behavior therapy techniques.* New York: Pergamon Press.

Bellack, A. S., Mueser, K. T., Gingerich, S., & Agresta, J. (1997). *Social skills training for schizophrenia.* New York: Guilford Press.

Bernstein, D. A., Borkovec, T. D., & Hazlett-Stevens, H. (2000). *New directions in progressive relaxation training: A guidebook for helping professionals.* Westport, CT: Praeger.

Borkovec, T. D., Alcaine, O., & Behar, E. (in press). Avoidance theory of worry and gen-

eralized anxiety disorder. In R. G. Heimberg, C. L. Turk, & D. S. Mennin (Eds.),
*Generalized anxiety disorder: Advances in re-
search and practice.* New York: Guilford Press.

Borkovec, T. D., & Newman, M. G. (1998). Worry and generalized anxiety disorder. In A. S.
Bellack & M. Hersen (Series Eds.) & P.
Salkovskis (Vol. Ed.), *Comprehensive clinical
psychology. Vol. 6: Adults: Clinical formulation
and treatment* (pp. 439–459). Oxford, UK:
Elsevier Science.

Bourque, P., & Ladouceur, R. (1980). An investigation of various performance-based treatments with acrophobics. *Behaviour Research
and Therapy, 18,* 161–170.

Brown, T. A., Antony, M. M., & Barlow, D. H.
(1995). Diagnostic comorbidity in panic
disorder: Effect on treatment outcome and
course of comorbid diagnoses following
treatment. *Journal of Consulting and Clinical
Psychology, 63,* 408–418.

Bulik, C. M., Sullivan, P. F., Carter, F. A., McIntosh, V. V., & Joyce, P. R. (1998). The role of
exposure with response prevention in the
cognitive-behavioural therapy for bulimia
nervosa. *Psychological Medicine, 28,* 611–623.

Clark, D. M. (1986). A cognitive approach to
panic. *Behaviour Research and Therapy, 24,*
461–470.

Clark, D. M., Salkovskis, P. M., Hackmann, A.,
Middleton, H., Anastasiades, P., & Gelder,
M. (1994). A comparison of cognitive therapy, applied relaxation and imipramine in
the treatment of panic disorder. *British Journal of Psychiatry, 164,* 759–769.

Clark, D. M., Salkovskis, P. M., Hackmann, A.,
Wells, A., Ludgate, J., & Gelder, M. (1999).
Brief cognitive therapy for panic disorder:
A randomized controlled trial. *Journal of
Consulting and Clinical Psychology, 67,*
583–589.

Cloitre, M., Koenen, K. C., Cohen, L. R., &
Han, H. (2002). Skills training in affective
and interpersonal regulation followed by
exposure: A phase-based treatment for
PTSD related to childhood abuse. *Journal of
Consulting and Clinical Psychology, 70,*
1067–1074.

Cottraux, J., & Gérard, B. (1998). Neuroimaging
and neuroanatomical issues in obsessive
compulsive disorder: Toward an integrative
model—perceived impulsivity. In R. P.
Swinson, M. M. Antony, S. Rachman, & M.

A. Richter (Eds.), *Obsessive–compulsive disorder: Theory, research, and treatment* (pp
154–180). New York: Guilford Press.

Craske, M. G. (1999). *Anxiety disorders: Psychological approaches to theory and treatment.* Boulder, CO: Westview Press.

Craske, M. G., & Barlow, D. H. (2001). Panic disorder and agoraphobia. In D. H. Barlow
(Ed.), *Clinical handbook of psychological disorders* (3rd ed., pp. 1–59). New York: Guilford
Press.

Craske, M. G., Brown, T. A., & Barlow, D. H.
(1991). Behavioral treatment of panic disorder: A two-year follow-up. *Behavior Therapy, 22,* 289–304.

Craske, M. G., Street, L., & Barlow, D. H. (1989).
Instructions to focus upon or distract from
internal cues during exposure treatment of
agoraphobic avoidance. *Behaviour Research
and Therapy, 27,* 663–672.

Devins, G. M. (1994). Illness intrusiveness and
the psychosocial impact of lifestyle disruptions in chronic life-threatening disease.
Advances in Renal Replacement Therapy, 1,
251–263.

Durand, V. M. (1991). *Severe behavior problems: A
functional communication training approach.*
New York: Guilford Press.

D'Zurilla, T. J., & Goldfried, M. R. (1971). Problem-solving and behavior modification.
Journal of Abnormal Psychology, 78, 107–126.

Edelman, R. E., & Chambless, D. L. (1993).
Compliance during sessions and homework in exposure-based treatment of agoraphobia. *Behaviour Research and Therapy,
31,* 767–773.

Ehlers, C. L., Frank, E., & Kupfer, D. J. (1988).
Social zeitgebers and biological rhythms: A
unified approach to understanding the etiology of depression. *Archives of General Psychiatry, 45,* 948–952.

Elias, M. J., & Clabby, J. F. (1992). *Building social
problem-solving skills: Guidelines from a school-
based program.* San Francisco, CA: Josey-
Bass/Pfeiffer.

Emmelkamp, P. M. G., Bruynzeel, M., Drost, L.,
& van der Mast, C. A. P. G. (2001). Virtual
reality treatment in acrophobia: A comparison with exposure *in vivo. Cyberpsychology
and Behavior, 4,* 335–339.

Emmelkamp, P. M. G., Krijn, M., Hulsbosch, A.
M., de Vries, S., Schuemie, M. J., & van der
Mast, C. A. P. G. (2002). Virtual reality treat-

ment versus exposure *in vivo*: A comparative evaluation in acrophobia. *Behaviour Research and Therapy, 40,* 509–516.

Emmelkamp, P. M. G., & Wessels, H. (1975). Flooding in imagination vs. flooding *in vivo*: A comparison with agoraphobics. *Behaviour Research and Therapy, 13,* 7–15.

Eysenck, H. J. (1952). The effects of psychotherapy: An evaluation. *Journal of Consulting Psychology, 16,* 319–324.

Eysenck, H. J. (1959). Learning theory and behavior therapy. *Journal of Mental Science, 195,* 61–75.

Eysenck, H. J. (1960). *Behavior therapy and the neuroses.* Oxford, UK: Pergamon Press.

Febrarro, G. A. R., Clum, G. A., Roodman, A. A., & Wright, J. H. (1999). The limits of bibliotherapy: A study of the differential effectiveness of self-administered interventions in individuals with panic attacks. *Behavior Therapy, 30,* 209–222.

Ferster, C. B. (1973). A functional analysis of depression. *American Psychologist, 28,* 857–870.

Fink, C. M., Turner, S. M., & Beidel, D. C. (1996). Culturally relevant factors in the behavior treatment of social phobia: A case study. *Journal of Anxiety Disorders, 10,* 201–209.

First, M. B., Spitzer, R. L., Gibbon, M., & Williams, J. B. W. (1996). *Structured Clinical Interview for Axis I DSM-IV Disorders Research Version—Patient Edition* (SCID-I/P, ver. 2. 0). New York: New York State Psychiatric Institute, Biometrics Research Department.

Foa, E. B., Blau, J. S., Prout, M., & Latimer, P. (1977). Is horror a necessary component of flooding (implosion)? *Behaviour Research and Therapy, 15,* 397–402.

Foa, E. B., Franklin, M. E., & Kozak, M. J. (1998). Psychosocial treatments for obsessive–compulsive disorder: Literature review. In R. P. Swinson, M. M. Antony, S. Rachman, & M. A. Richter (Eds.), *Obsessive–compulsive disorder: Theory, research, and treatment* (pp. 258–276). New York: Guilford Press.

Foa, E. B., Jameson, J. S., Turner, R. M., & Payne, L. L. (1980). Massed versus spaced exposure sessions in the treatment of agoraphobia. *Behaviour Research and Therapy, 18,* 333–338.

Foa, E. B., & Kozak, M. J. (1986). Emotional processing of fear: Exposure to corrective information. *Psychological Bulletin, 99,* 20–35.

Foa, E. B., & Rothbaum, B. O. (1998). *Treating the trauma of rape: Cognitive behavioral therapy for PTSD.* New York: Guilford Press.

Follette, W. C., Naugle, A. E., & Callaghan, G. M. (1996). A radical behavioral understanding of the therapeutic relationship in effecting change. *Behavior Therapy, 27,* 623–641.

Franklin, M. E., & Foa, E. B. (2002). Cognitive behavioral treatments for obsessive compulsive disorder. In P. E. Nathan & J. M. Gorman (Eds.), *A guide to treatments that work* (2nd ed., pp. 367–386). New York: Oxford University Press.

Franklin, M. E., Jaycox, L. H., & Foa, E. B. (1999). Social skills training. In M. Hersen & A. S. Bellack (Eds.), *Handbook of comparative interventions for adult disorders* (2nd ed.). New York: Wiley.

Goldiamond, I. (1974). Toward a constructional approach to social problems. *Behaviorism, 2,* 1–84.

Gould, R. A., & Clum, G. A. (1995). Self-help plus minimal therapist contact in the treatment of panic disorder: A replication and extension. *Behavior Therapy, 26,* 533–546.

Green, L. (1978). Temporal and stimulus factors in self-monitoring by obese persons. *Behavior Therapy, 9,* 328–341.

Gunther, L. M., Denniston, J. C., & Miller, R. R. (1998). Conducting exposure treatment in multiple contexts can prevent relapse. *Behaviour Research and Therapy, 36,* 75–91.

Haw, J., & Dickerson, M. (1998). The effects of distraction on desensitization and reprocessing. *Behaviour Research and Therapy, 36,* 765–769.

Hawton, K., & Kirk, J. (1989). Problem solving. In K. S. Hawton, P. M. Salkovskis, J. Kirk, & D. M. Clark (Eds.), *Cognitive behaviour therapy for psychiatric problems: A practical guide* (pp. 406–426). Oxford, UK: Oxford University Press.

Hayes, S. C., Follette, V. M., & Linehan, M. (in press). *Mindfulness, acceptance, and relationship: Expanding the cognitive-behavioral tradition.* New York: Guilford Press.

Hayes, S. C., Jacobson, N. S., Follette, V. M., & Dougher, M. J. (1994). *Acceptance and change: Content and context in psychotherapy.* Reno, NV: Context Press.

Hayes, S. C., Kohlenberg, B. S., & Melancon, S. M. (1989). Avoiding and altering rule-control as a strategy of clinical treatment. In S. C. Hayes (Ed.), *Rule-governed behavior: Cognition, contingencies and instructional control* (pp. 359–385). New York: Plenum Press.

Hayes, S. C., Strosahl, K. D., & Wilson, K. G. (1999). *Acceptance and commitment therapy: An experiential approach to behavior change.* New York: Guilford Press.

Hecker, J. E., Losee, M. C., Fritzler, B. K., & Fink, C. M. (1996). Self-directed versus therapist-directed cognitive behavioral treatment for panic disorder. *Journal of Anxiety Disorders, 10,* 253–265.

Heimberg, R. G., & Becker, R. E. (2002). *Cognitive-behavioral group therapy for social phobia: Basic mechanisms and clinical strategies.* New York: Guilford Press.

Hersen, M., & Barlow, D. H. (1984). *Single case experimental designs.* Boston: Allyn & Bacon.

Iwamasa, G. Y. (Ed.). (1996). Special series: Ethnic and cultural diversity in cognitive and behavioral practice. *Cognitive and Behavioral Practice, 3*(2).

Jacobson, E. (1938). *Progressive relaxation.* Chicago: University of Chicago Press.

Jacobson, N. S., & Christensen, A. (1998). *Acceptance and change in couple therapy: A therapist's guide to transforming relationships.* New York: Norton.

Jacobson, N. S., Dobson, K. S., Truax, P. A., Addis, M. E., Koerner, K., Gollan, J. K., Gortner, E., & Prince, S. E. (1996). A component analysis of cognitive-behavioral treatment for depression. *Journal of Consulting and Clinical Psychology, 64,* 295–304.

Jacobson, N. S., Martell, C. R., & Dimidjian, S. (2001). Behavioral activation treatment for depression: Returning to contextual roots. *Clinical Psychology: Science and Practice, 8,* 255–270.

Jones, M. C. (1924a). Elimination of children's fears. *Journal of Experimental Psychology, 7,* 382–390.

Jones, M. C. (1924b). A laboratory study of fear: The case of Peter. *Journal of General Psychology, 31,* 308–315.

Kanfer, F. H., & Gaelick-Buys, L. (1991). Self-management methods. In F. H. Kanfer & A. P. Goldstein (Eds.), *Helping people change: A*

textbook of methods (4th ed., pp. 305–360). Needham Heights, MA: Allyn & Bacon.

Kazdin, A. E. (2002). Psychosocial treatments for conduct disorder in children and adolescents. In P. E. Nathan & J. M. Gorman (Eds.), *A guide to treatments that work* (2nd ed., pp. 57–86). New York: Oxford University Press.

Keijsers, G. P. J., Schaap, C. P. D. R., & Hoogduin, C. A. L. (2000). The impact of interpersonal patient and therapist behavior on outcome in cognitive-behavior therapy: A review of empirical studies. *Behavior Modification, 24,* 264–297.

Keijsers, G. P. J., Schaap, C. P. D. R., Hoogduin, C. A. L., & Lammers, M. W. (1995). Patient–therapist interaction in the behavioral treatment of panic disorder with agoraphobia. *Behavior Modification, 19,* 491–517.

Klosko, J. S., Barlow, D. H., Tassinari, R., & Cerny, J. A. (1990). A comparison of alprazolam and behavior therapy in treatment of panic disorder. *Journal of Consulting and Clinical Psychology, 58,* 77–84.

Kohlenberg, R. J., & Tsai, M. (1991). *Functional analytic psychotherapy: Creating intense and curative therapeutic relationships.* New York: Plenum Press.

Krasner, L., & Ullmann, L. P. (Eds.). (1965). *Research in behavior modification: New developments and implications.* New York: Holt, Rinehart & Winston.

Lang, P. J., Melamed, B. G., & Hart, J. (1970). A psychophysiological analysis of fear modification using an automated desensitization procedure. *Journal of Abnormal Psychology, 76,* 220–234.

Lawrence, E., Eldridge, K., Christensen, A., & Jacobson, N. S. (1999). Integrative couple therapy: The dyadic relationship of acceptance and change. In J. M. Donovan (Ed.), *Short-term couple therapy* (pp. 226–261). New York: Guilford Press.

Lazarus, A. A. (1958). New methods in psychotherapy: A case study. *South African Medical Journal, 33,* 660–664.

Leitenberg, H., Rosen, J. C., Gross, J., Nudelman, S., & Vara, L. S. (1988). Exposure plus response–prevention treatment of bulimia nervosa. *Journal of Consulting and Clinical Psychology, 56,* 535–541.

Leung, A. W., & Heimberg, R. G. (1996). Homework compliance, perceptions of control, and outcome of cognitive behavioral treatment of social phobia. *Behaviour Research and Therapy, 34,* 423–432.

Liberman, R. P., Wallace, C. J., Blackwell, G., Kopelowicz, A., Vaccaro, J. V., & Mintz, J. (1998). Skills training versus psychosocial occupational therapy for persons with persistent schizophrenia. *American Journal of Psychiatry, 155,* 1087–1091.

Lindsley, O. R., Skinner, B. F., & Solomon, H. C. (1953). *Studies in behavior therapy* (Status report 1). Waltham, MA: Metropolitan State Hospital.

Linehan, M. M. (1993). *Cognitive-behavioral treatment of borderline personality disorder.* New York: Guilford Press.

Linehan, M. M., Cochran, B. N., & Kehrer, C. A. (2001). Dialectical behavior therapy for borderline personality disorder. In D. H. Barlow (Ed.), *Clinical handbook of psychological disorders* (3rd. ed., pp. 470–522). New York: Guilford Press.

Lovibond, S. H., & Lovibond, P. F. (1995). *Manual for the Depression Anxiety Stress Scales* (2nd ed.). Sydney: Psychology Foundation of Australia.

Margraf, J. (1998). Behavioral approaches. In A. S. Bellack & M. Hersen (Eds.), *Comprehensive clinical psychology* (Vol. 6, pp. 25–49) (P. M. Salkovskis, Ed.). New York: Elsevier.

Marks, I. M., Swinson, R. P., Basoglu, M., Kuch, K., Noshirvani, H., O'Sullivan, G., Lelliott, P. T., Kirby, M., McNamee, G., Sengun, S., & Wickwire, K. (1993). Alprazolam and exposure alone and combined in panic disorder with agoraphobia: A controlled study in London and Toronto. *British Journal of Psychiatry, 162,* 776–787.

Marlatt, G. A., & Gordon, J. R. (1985). *Relapse prevention: Maintenance strategies in the treatment of addictive behaviors.* New York: Guilford Press.

Martell, C. R., Addis, M. E., & Jacobson, N. S. (2001). *Depression in context: Strategies for guided action.* New York: Norton.

Mattick, R. P., & Clarke, J. C. (1998). Development and validation of measures of social phobia scrutiny fear and social interaction anxiety. *Behaviour Research and Therapy, 36,* 455–470.

McFall, R. M. (1970). Effects of self-monitoring on normal smoking behavior. *Journal of Consulting and Clinical Psychology, 35,* 135–142.

McKay, D., Todaro, J., Neziroglu, F., & Campisi, T. (1997). Body dysmorphic disorder: A preliminary evaluation of treatment and maintenance using exposure and response prevention. *Behaviour Research and Therapy, 35,* 67–70.

McKay, M., Davis, M., & Fanning, P. (1995). *Messages: The communications skills book* (2nd ed.). Oakland, CA: New Harbinger.

Menzies, R. G., & Clarke, J. C. (1993). A comparison of *in vivo* and vicarious exposure in the treatment of childhood water phobia. *Behaviour Research and Therapy, 31,* 9–15.

Miklowitz, D. J. (2001). Bipolar disorder. In D. H. Barlow (Ed.), *Clinical handbook of psychological disorders* (3rd ed., pp. 523–561). New York: Guilford Press.

Miklowitz, D. J., & Goldstein, M. J. (1997). *Bipolar disorder: A family-focused treatment approach.* New York: Guilford Press.

Miller, W. R., Benefield, R. G., & Tonigan, J. S. (1993). Enhancing motivation for change in problem drinking: A controlled comparison of two therapist styles. *Journal of Consulting and Clinical Psychology, 61,* 455–461.

Miltenberger, R. (1997). *Behavior modification: Principles and procedures.* Boston: Brooks/Cole.

Mineka, S., & Thomas, C. (1999). Mechanisms of change in exposure therapy for anxiety disorders. In T. Dalgleish & M. J. Power (Eds.), *Cognition and emotion* (pp. 747–764). New York: Wiley.

Mischel, W. (1968). *Personality and assessment.* New York: Wiley.

Mischel, W. (1984). Convergences and challenges in the search for consistency. *American Psychologist, 39,* 351–364.

Morgan, H., & Raffle, C. (1999). Does reducing safety behaviours improve treatment response in patients with social phobia? *Australia and New Zealand Journal of Psychiatry, 33,* 503–510.

Mowrer, O. H. (1939). Stimulus response theory of anxiety. *Psychological Review, 46,* 553–565.

Mueser, K. T. (1998). Social skills training and problem solving. In A. S. Bellack & M. Hersen (Eds.), *Comprehensive clinical psychology* (Vol. 6, pp. 183–201) (P. M. Salkovskis, Ed.). New York: Elsevier.

Najavits, L. M. (2001). *Seeking safety: A treatment manual for PTSD and substance abuse.* New York: Guilford Press.

Nathan, P. E., & Gorman, J. M. (Eds.). (2002). *A guide to treatments that work* (2nd ed.). New York: Oxford University Press.

Nelson, R. O., & Hayes, S. C. (1986). The nature of behavioral assessment. In R. O. Nelson & S. C. Hayes (Eds.), *Conceptual foundations of behavioral assessment* (pp. 3–41). New York: Guilford Press.

Nemeroff, C. J., & Karoly, P. (1991). Operant methods. In F. H. Kanfer & A. P. Goldstein (Eds), *Helping people change: A textbook of methods* (4th ed., pp. 121–160). Needham Heights, MA: Allyn & Bacon.

Newman, M. G., Castonguay, L. G., Borkovec, T. D., & Molnar, C. (in press). Integrative therapy for generalized anxiety disorder. In R. G. Heimberg, C. L. Turk, & D. S. Mennin (Eds.), *Generalized anxiety disorder: Advances in research and practice.* New York: Guilford Press.

Nezu, A. M. (1986). Efficacy of a social problem solving therapy approach for unipolar depression. *Journal of Consulting and Clinical Psychology, 54,* 196–202.

Norcross, J. C. (2002). *Psychotherapy relationships that work: Therapist contributions and responsiveness to patients.* New York: Oxford University Press.

O'Donohue, W., & Krasner, L. (1995). Theories in behavior therapy: Philosophical and historical contexts. In W. O'Donohue & L. Krasner (Eds.), *Theories of behavior therapy: Exploring behavior change* (pp. 1–22). Washington, DC: American Psychological Association.

Organista, K. C., & Munoz, R. F. (1996). Cognitive behavioral therapy with Latinos. *Cognitive and Behavioral Practice, 3,* 255–270.

Öst, L.-G. (1997). Rapid treatment of specific phobias. In Davey, G. C. L. (Ed.), *Phobias: A handbook of theory research and treatment* (pp. 227–246). New York: Wiley.

Öst, L. -G., Ferebee, I., & Furmark, T. (1997). One-session group therapy of spider phobia: Direct versus indirect treatments. *Behaviour Research and Therapy, 35,* 721–732.

Öst, L.-G., Lindahl, I.-L., Sterner, U., & Jerremalm, A. (1984). Exposure *in vivo* vs. applied relaxation in the treatment of blood phobia. *Behaviour Research and Therapy, 22,* 205–216.

Perpina, C., Botella, C., Banos, R., Marco, H., Alcaniz, M., & Quero, S. (1999). Body image and virtual reality in eating disorders: Is exposure to virtual reality more effective than the classical body image treatment? *Cyberpsychology and Behavior, 2,* 149–155.

Rachman, S. J. (1996). Mechanisms of action of cognitive-behavior treatment of anxiety disorders. In M. R. Mavissakalian & R. F. Prien (Eds.), *Long term treatments of anxiety disorders.* Washington DC: American Psychiatric Press

Rankin, H., Hodgson, R., & Stockwell, T. (1983). Cue exposure and response prevention with alcoholics: A controlled trial. *Behaviour Research and Therapy, 21,* 435–446.

Raue, P. J., Castonguay, L. G., & Goldfried, M. R. (1993). The working alliance: A comparison of two therapies. *Psychotherapy Research, 3,* 197–207.

Renfrey, G. S. (1992). Cognitive behavior therapy and the Native American client. *Behavior Therapy, 23,* 321–340.

Roemer, L., & Orsillo, S. M. (2002). Expanding our conceptualization of and treatment for generalized anxiety disorder: Integrating mindfulness/acceptance-based approaches with existing cognitive-behavioral models. *Clinical Psychology: Science and Practice, 9,* 54–68.

Rothbaum, B. O., Hodges, L. F., Ready, D., Graap, K., & Alarcon, R. D. (2001). Virtual reality exposure therapy for Vietnam veterans with posttraumatic stress disorder. *Journal of Clinical Psychiatry, 62,* 617–622.

Rowe, M. K., & Craske, M. G. (1998). Effects of varied-stimulus exposure training on fear reduction and return of fear. *Behaviour Research and Therapy, 36,* 719–734.

Salkovskis, P. M. (1998). Psychological approaches to the understanding of obsessional problems. In R. P. Swinson, M. M. Antony, S. Rachman, & M. A. Richter (Eds.), *Obsessive–compulsive disorder: Theory, research, and treatment* (pp. 33–50). New York: Guilford Press.

Savard, J., & Morin, C. M. (2002). Insomnia. In M. M. Antony & D. H. Barlow (Eds.), *Handbook of assessment, treatment planning, and outcome evaluation: Empirically supported strategies for psychological disorders* (pp. 523–555). New York: Guilford Press.

Schmidt, N. B., Woolaway-Bickel, K., Trakowski, J., Santiago, H., Storey, J., Koselka, M., & Cook, J. (2000). Dismantling cognitive-behavioral treatment for panic disorder: Questioning the utility of breathing retraining. *Journal of Consulting and Clinical Psychology, 68,* 417–424.

Schwartz, M. S. (Ed.). (1995). *Biofeedback: A practitioner's guide* (2nd ed.). New York: Guilford Press.

Segal, Z. V., Williams, J. M. G., & Teasdale, J. D. (2002). *Mindfulness-based cognitive therapy for depression: A new approach to preventing relapse.* New York: Guilford Press.

Skinner, B. F. (1974). *About behaviorism.* New York: Knopf.

Stern, R., & Marks, I. (1973). Brief and prolonged flooding: A comparison in agoraphobic patients. *Archives of General Psychiatry, 28,* 270–276.

Stern, R., & Marks, I. (1973). Brief and prolonged flooding: A comparison in agoraphobic patients. *Archives of General Psychiatry, 28,* 270–276.

Strosahl, K. D., Hayes, S. C., Bergan, J., & Romano, P. (1998). Assessing the field effectiveness of Acceptance and Commitment Therapy: An example of the manipulated training research method. *Behavior Therapy, 29,* 35–64.

Stuart, G. L., Treat, T. A., & Wade, W. A. (2000). Effectiveness of an empirically based treatment for panic disorder delivered in a service clinic setting: 1-year follow-up. *Journal of Consulting and Clinical Psychology, 68,* 506–512.

Summerfeldt, L. J., & Antony, M. M. (2002). Structured and semi-structured diagnostic interviews. In M. M. Antony & D. H. Barlow (Eds.), *Handbook of assessment, treatment planning, and outcome evaluation: Empirically supported strategies for psychological disorders* (pp. 3–37). New York: Guilford Press.

Swinson, R. P., Fergus, K. D., Cox, B. J., & Wickwire, K. (1995). Efficacy of telephone-administered behavioral therapy for panic disorder with agoraphobia. *Behaviour Research and Therapy, 33,* 465–469.

Swinson, R. P., Soulios, C., Cox, B. J., & Kuch, K. (1992). Brief treatment of emergency room patients with panic attacks. *American Journal of Psychiatry, 149,* 944–946.

Tanaka-Matsumi, J., Seiden, D. Y., & Lam, K. N. (1996). The Culturally Informed Functional Assessment (CIFA) Interview: A strategy for cross-cultural behavioral practice. *Cognitive and Behavioral Practice, 3,* 215–234.

Tarrier, N., Pilgrim, H., Sommerfield, C., Faragher, B., Reynolds, M., Graham, E., & Barrowclough, C. (1999). A randomized trial of cognitive therapy and imaginal exposure in the treatment of chronic posttraumatic stress disorder. *Journal of Consulting and Clinical Psychology, 67,* 13–18.

Telch, M. J., Lucas, J. A., Schmidt, N. B., Hanna, H. H., Jaimez, T. L., & Lucas, R. A. (1993). Group cognitive-behavioral treatment of panic disorder. *Behaviour Research and Therapy, 31,* 279–287.

Terhune, W. S. (1948). The phobic syndrome: A study of eighty-six patients with phobic reactions. *Archives of Neurology and Psychiatry, 62,* 162–172.

Toyokawa, T., & Nedate, K. (1996). Applications of cognitive behavior therapy to interpersonal problems: A case study of a Japanese female client. *Cognitive and Behavioral Practice, 3,* 289–302.

Ullmann, L. P., & Krasner, L. (1965). *Case studies in behavior modification.* New York: Holt, Rinehart & Winston.

Visser, S., & Bouman, T. K. (2001). The treatment of hypochondriasis: Exposure plus response prevention vs. cognitive therapy. *Behaviour Research and Therapy, 39,* 423–442.

Warren, R., & Thomas, J. C. (2001). Cognitive behavior therapy of obsessive compulsive disorder in private practice: An effectiveness study. *Journal of Anxiety Disorders, 15,* 277–285.

Weissman, M. M., Markowitz, J. C., & Klerman, G. L. (2000). *Comprehensive guide to interpersonal psychotherapy.* New York: Basic Books.

Wheeler, J. G., Christensen, A., & Jacobson, N. S. (2001). Couples distress. In D. H. Barlow (Ed.), *Clinical handbook of psychological disorders* (3rd ed., pp. 609—630). New York: Guilford Press.

Williams, K. E., & Chambless, D. L. (1990). The relationship between therapist characteristics and outcome of *in vivo* exposure treatment for agoraphobia. *Behavior Therapy, 21,* 111–116.

Wilson, G. T. (1996). Manual-based treatments: The clinical application of research findings. *Behaviour Research and Therapy, 34,* 295–314.

Wilson, G. T. (1998). Review. Manual-based

treatment and clinical practice. *Clinical Psychology: Science and Practice, 5,* 363–375.

Wolpe, J. (1958). *Psychotherapy by reciprocal inhibition.* Stanford, CA: Stanford University Press.

Woody, S. R., & Adessky, R. S. (2002). Therapeutic alliance, group cohesion, and homework compliance during cognitive-behavioral group treatment of social phobia. *Behavior Therapy, 33,* 5–27.

Woody, S. R., & Sanderson, W. C. (1998). Manuals for empirically supported treatments: 1998 update. *The Clinical Psychologist, 51,* 17–21.

Yartz, A. R., & Hawk, L. W. (2001). Psychophysiological assessment of anxiety: Tales from the heart. In M. M. Antony, S. M. Orsillo, & L. Roemer (Eds.), *Practitioner's guide to empirically-based measures of anxiety* (pp. 25–30). New York: Kluwer Academic/Plenum Press.

Zinbarg, R. E. (1993). Information processing and classical conditioning: Implications for exposure therapy and the integration of cognitive therapy and behavior therapy. *Journal of Behavior Therapy and Experimental Psychiatry, 24,* 129–139.

7

Cognitive Therapy

Mark A. Reinecke
Arthur Freeman

Cognitive therapy has attracted substantial interest from mental health professionals during the 30 years since it was first introduced. The "cognitive revolution" (Mahoney, 1977, 1991), ushered in by a 1956 symposium on information processing at MIT and the publication of seminal works by Bruner, Goodnow, and Austin (1956), Chomsky (1956, 1957), Kelly (1955), Newell and Simon (1956), and Whorf (1956), has matured so that cognitively based therapies have moved to the forefront of professional interest. Cognitive therapy has become a meeting ground for therapists from diverse theoretical and philosophical positions ranging from the psychoanalytic to the behavioral. Psychodynamic therapists find in cognitive therapy a dynamic core that involves working to alter tacit beliefs and interpersonal schemata. Behavioral therapists find in the model a brief, active, directive, collaborative, psychoeducational model of psychotherapy that is empirically based and has as its goal direct behavioral change. The merging of cognitive therapy and behavior therapy has become more the rule than the exception. Behavior therapy associations around the world have added the term "cognitive" to their name and the

prestigious journal *Behavior Therapy* now carries the subtitle, "An International Journal Devoted to the Application of Behavioral and Cognitive Sciences to Clinical Problems." Empirical support, in the form of randomized controlled outcome studies, has led cognitive-behavioral therapy to be identified as a treatment of choice for a range of conditions including depression, eating disorders, panic disorder, generalized anxiety disorder, obsessive–compulsive disorder, and self-mutilation by a number of organizations including the British Health Service (Department of Health, 2000, 2001) and the Agency for Health Care Policy and Research (AHCPR, 1993).

The literature on cognitive therapy has grown in an almost exponential fashion during the past decade. Rooted in the early work of Aaron Beck on the treatment of depression (A. Beck, 1972, 1976; Beck, Rush, Shaw, & Emery, 1979), contemporary cognitive therapy has become a broad-spectrum model of therapy and psychopathology and has been applied to a wide range of problems, patient groups, and therapeutic contexts. There are now centers for cognitive therapy in such widely separated locations as Buenos Aires, Stockholm, and

Shanghai. The basic model has been adapted to a variety of cultures rather easily. Therapists in both Sweden and China claim that there has been interest in cognitive therapy in their country as the model seemed to suit their national character. Given the differences between these cultures, this is a most interesting statement. Cognitive approaches appear to be applicable cross-culturally because they are process focused and phenomenologically based. Helping individuals to develop the ability to examine their beliefs (whatever those beliefs might be) appears to be far more helpful cross-culturally than focusing on specific points of content. The model is respectful of the fact that specific tacit beliefs may be shared by members of particular cultures, and that there are meaningful cross-cultural differences in these beliefs. Cross-cultural differences in tacit beliefs appear to exist with regard to the development of skills or competence, personal responsibility, adaptability or malleability of behavior, and the expression of anger. Western societies, for example, have been characterized by an emphasis on individual autonomy and achievement, whereas Asian societies appear to place a relative emphasis on social cohesion and an individual's responsibility to family and the larger community.

Cognitive models and procedures have been refined during the years since the first edition of this book. As cognitive models have developed they have become more specific, integrated, and differentiated. This has led to the development of alternative cognitive-behavioral "schools" or approaches, and to attempts to develop standards of clinical training in cognitive-behavioral psychotherapy. The Academy of Cognitive Therapy, for example, was established in 1998 to credential mental health professionals who practice empirically supported forms of cognitive therapy. At the same time, cognitive-behavioral strategies and techniques have "diffused" into wider practice—they have been integrated into therapeutic work by clinicians trained in other

approaches. It is not uncommon to encounter clinicians who state that they "conceptualize patients dynamically, but use cognitive techniques." This is interesting in that it reflects an increasing acceptance of the usefulness of cognitive-behavioral approaches. Clinical warmth, empathy, and positive regard, once viewed as characteristics of Rogerian psychotherapy, are now seen as forming a foundation for all effective psychotherapy. In a similar manner, cognitive-behavioral strategies and techniques—including collaborative rapport, development and sharing of a rationale, maintenance of therapeutic structure, the use of homework, monitoring of mood and thoughts, attention to the moment-to-moment experience of the patient, and disputation of distressing thoughts—are becoming part of a general standard of care. Cognitive therapy may, like Rogerian therapy before it, come to be accepted as a foundation for many forms of effective treatment.

This chapter reviews the theoretical bases and history of cognitive therapy. It then discusses specific conceptual and technical issues leading to the various treatment strategies. Finally the chapter presents applications of the cognitive therapy model for treating a range of clinical disorders.

HISTORICAL BACKGROUND

We begin with a brief review of the philosophical foundations of cognitive psychotherapy. Cognitive theory is founded on intellectual traditions dating to the Stoic philosophers, such as Epictetus (1983), who in the first century commented, "What upsets people is not things themselves but their judgments about the things. . . . So when we are thwarted or upset or distressed, let us never blame someone else but rather ourselves, that is, our own judgments" (p. 13)

Contemporary cognitive psychotherapy is founded upon the concept of "psychological constructivism." Michael Mahoney (1991) has defined this as

> a family of theories about mind and mentation that (1) emphasize the active and proactive nature of all perception, learning, and knowing; (2) acknowledge the structural and functional primacy of abstract (tacit) over concrete (explicit) processes in all sentient and sapient experience; and (3) view learning, knowing and memory as phenomena that reflect the ongoing attempts of body and mind to organize (and endlessly reorganize) their own patterns of action and experience—patterns that are, of course, related to changing and highly mediated engagements with their momentary worlds. (p. 95)

The cognitive–constructivist model of human behavior is different from traditional psychodynamic theories in that behavior is not viewed as determined by early experiences or mediated by the regulation of unconscious drives. It may also be contrasted with operant behavioral formulations in that our emotional and behavioral reactions are not viewed simply as the products of our reinforcement histories and current environmental contingencies. Rather, our behavior is seen as goal-directed, purposive, active, and adaptive. Constructivism asserts that individuals do not simply react to events. Rather, individuals are proactive and develop systems of personal meaning that organize their interactions with the world. Constructivists suggest that knowledge (both personal and scientific) is relative insofar as it is based on personal and cultural epistemologies and may not be based on a knowable "objective" reality (Mahoney, 1991; Neimeyer, 1993). In concrete terms, constructivists suggest that there are a virtually limitless number of interpretations that can be derived from any given event. Constructivist models are consonant with recent work examining limits of human reasoning and logic (Fodor, 2000; Gigerenzer & Selton, 2001).

Contemporary cognitive psychotherapy reflects the confluence of several schools of thought and is an extension of the earlier work of Adler (1927, 1968), Arieti (1980), Bowlby (1985), Frankl (1985), Freud (1892), and Tolman (1949). The influence of psychodynamic theory on the evolution of cognitive psychotherapy is perhaps most apparent in the topographic model of personality and psychopathology that they share. Whereas Freud partitioned the psyche into the conscious, preconscious, and unconscious domains, with an individual's behavior primarily mediated by unconscious motives or drives (the id), cognitive theorists partition cognitive processes into "automatic thoughts," "assumptions" and "schemata."

Like dynamic psychotherapists, cognitive therapists recognize the importance of attending to internal dialogues and motivations. Although they explicitly eschew drive-reduction metaphors and the notion that behavior is motivated by defenses against the expression of anxiety-laden impulses, the cognitive therapist nonetheless works to give voice to the unspoken. Explicit attempts are made to identify and change unrecognized beliefs and attitudes that contribute to patients' distress. The role of cognitive variables—including intentions, expectations, memories, goals, and cognitive distortions—in the etiology of emotional disorders has a long tradition in psychology and psychiatry. It dates to Freud, who first acknowledged, and later challenged, the role of rationality in human adaptation.

The influence of the behavioral school of psychology is reflected in cognitive therapy's focus on behavior change, its recognition of social and environmental determinants of behavior, and its use of empirical research as a means of refining both the theory and clinical technique. An empiricist attitude is encouraged for both the therapist and the patient, and behavioral interventions are employed as an integral part of the treatment. An emphasis is placed on identifying discrete problems whose improvement can be objectively assessed.

Many writers have referred to cognitive therapy as a variant or offspring of behavior modification. This is reflected in the widespread use of the term "cognitive-behavioral therapy." As should be clear, however, this does not do justice to the conceptual richness of the model. Moreover, it does not acknowledge the important contributions of other theoretical orientations to its development. Cognitive therapy (Beck et al., 1979) may be viewed as one variant of a larger family of cognitive-behavioral therapies (Dobson & Dozois, 2001).

Cognitive psychotherapy has historically been identified with a specific set of techniques and has been viewed by some as a model whose scope is limited to the treatment of specific emotional disorders. This view, while understandable, reflects an oversimplification of contemporary cognitive theory. The view that the cognitive model is no broader than that which is immediately relevant to the conduct of therapy stems from several historical currents. The model, as it was initially presented, was in fact largely limited to the treatment of major depression among adults. The model was limited in scope and was not intended as a theory of personality or of developmental psychopathology. Although early treatment outcome studies were positive, it was not until the early 1980s that cognitive models of other disorders were developed and the etiology of maladaptive belief systems became a focus of attention. As such, cognitive therapy reflects an evolving model of psychotherapy, psychopathology, and development whose scope of utility is expanding.

The development of cognitive-behavioral psychotherapy encompasses early work by Bandura (1977a, 1977b), A. Beck (1972, 1976), Ellis (1962), Goldfried (see Goldfried & Merbaum, 1973), Kelly (1955), A. Lazarus (1976, 1981), Mahoney (1974), Meichenbaum (1977), Mischel (1973), Rehm (1977), and Seligman (1975). These authors were among the first to incorporate cognitive mediational constructs with behavioral theory. They focused on the role of social learning processes in the development of emotional problems and on the use of cognitive restructuring, the development of social problem-solving capacities, and the

acquisition of behavioral skills in resolving them. Although cognitive models of psychopathology and psychotherapy have been refined and elaborated since that time, the techniques described in those early works continue to serve as the basis of clinical practice and so deserve mention.

Arguably the first contemporary cognitive-clinical psychologist was George Kelly (1955) who, in proposing his "personal construct theory" of emotional disorders, explicitly recognized the importance of subjective perceptions in human behavior. He proposed that individuals actively perceive or "construe" their behavior and generate abstractions about themselves, their world, and their future. An individual's "constructs," as such, can be quite idiosyncratic or personal and represent the ways in which they categorize their experiences. These constructs, in turn, determine how the individual will respond to events. From this perspective, a goal of therapy is to understand patients' subjective judgments about their experiences and to assist patients to construe them in a more adaptive manner. Kelly's therapeutic techniques, while not widely used today, remain an important forerunner of modern "constructivist" or "structural" schools of cognitive therapy (Guidano, 1991, 1995; Guidano & Liotti, 1983, 1985).

The development of cognitive therapy accelerated during the 1970s as information-processing models of clinical disorders were developed, as therapeutic techniques based on cognitive-mediational models were proposed, and as outcome studies documenting the efficacy of the techniques were published. Meichenbaum (1977), for example, described the role of internalized speech in the development of emotional disorders. Meichenbaum's techniques for "self-instructional training" via the rehearsal of "self-statements," modeling, and self-reinforcement have proven particularly useful in treating depressed or impulsive children.

Bandura (1973, 1977a, 1977b) is perhaps best known for developing social learning models of anxiety and aggression and for identifying the central importance of perceptions of "self-efficacy" or personal competence in guiding human behavior.

In reformulations of traditional behavioral theory, a number of authors argued that human behavior is mediated not only by environmental antecedents and contingencies but also by an individual's beliefs and perceptions. The now familiar "ABC" model of the relationships between "Antecedent Events," "Beliefs," "Behavior," and "Consequences" for the individual proposed by Albert Ellis (1962; Ellis & Harper, 1961) suggested that neurotic or maladaptive behaviors are learned and are directly related to irrational beliefs that people hold about events in their lives. Ellis developed a typology of common cognitive distortions, as well as a number of directive therapeutic techniques for changing them. Ellis's model assumes that by identifying and changing unrealistic or irrational beliefs, it is possible to alter one's behavioral or emotional reactions to events. As irrational beliefs are often tightly held and long-standing in nature, highly focused and, at times, confrontationally expressed interventions are necessary to dispute them. Ellis's therapeutic approach is active and pragmatic. Although the basic tenets of rational-emotive behavior therapy (REBT) have not, as yet, been subjected to extensive empirical scrutiny (Engels, Garnefski, & Diekstra, 1993; Haaga & Davison, 1993), his clinical techniques for challenging irrational beliefs are widely used.

In developing a behavioral model of depression, Seligman (1975) proposed that individuals become depressed when they come to believe that they are unable to control important outcomes in their life (including both positive or reinforcing events and negative events or punishments). This "learned helplessness" model of depression was subsequently refined by Abramson, Seligman, and Teasdale (1978) in an "attributional reformulation" of the theory. The model has generated a great deal of empirical interest (Abramson, Alloy, & Met-

alsky, 1988; Abramson, Metalsky, & Alloy, 1989; Alloy, Abramson, Metalsky, & Hartlage, 1988; Peterson & Seligman, 1984; Sweeney, Anderson, & Bailey, 1986) and suggests that attributions made by depressed patients about the causes of events may be an important target of therapy.

Rehm (1977) proposed a cognitive-behavioral model of depressive disorders focusing on deficits in "self-regulation." Specifically, he suggested that depressed individuals manifest impaired self-monitoring (they selectively attend to negative events, and to the immediate rather than the delayed consequences of their behavior), self-evaluation (they are overly self-critical and tend to make inappropriate attributions about their responsibility for negative events), and self-reinforcement (they do not tend to reward themselves for their successes and can be highly self-punitive when they fail to meet their goals). Rehm's model extended earlier behavioral self-regulation models (Kanfer, 1971) and is clinically useful in that it directs clinicians' attention to specific cognitive and behavioral problems experienced by depressed patients (Fuchs & Rehm, 1977).

During recent years additional models focusing on specific cognitive-behavioral deficits associated with psychopathology have been developed, and "integrative" or "modular" cognitive behavioral approaches have been proposed. These approaches attempt to address the full array of cognitive, behavioral, and environmental factors mediating an individual's distress (Curry & Reinecke, 2003; Reinecke, 2002). Cognitive therapies, then, include a diverse array of techniques based on the assumption that behavioral and emotional difficulties stem from the activation of maladaptive beliefs, attitudes, expectations, attributions or schema, or from the use of maladaptive behavioral coping strategies. Cognitive models assume that maladaptive beliefs are learned and reinforced, and that interventions that change these cognitive and behavioral processes can bring about behavioral and emotional improvement. Cognitively focused models emphasize the central role of cognitive and perceptual processes in adaptation and change, whereas the more behaviorally focused models emphasize the role of behavioral skills and reinforcement history. Most contemporary cognitive-behavioral models acknowledge the role of both environmental and cognitive processes in the development of psychopathology and use both cognitive and behavioral techniques. It is worth noting that many forms of cognitive therapy assume that behavioral interventions exert their effects by providing the individual with experiences that are inconsistent with extant maladaptive beliefs.

ASSUMPTIONS OF COGNITIVE THERAPY

Like behavioral, psychodynamic, and systemic models of psychotherapy, cognitive therapy might best be described as a "school of thought" rather than a single theory. As alternative models vary both conceptually and in practice, it can be difficult to define the scope of cognitive-behavioral therapy. Cognitive models might usefully be characterized along a continuum ranging from behaviorally oriented rationalism to radical constructivism. Although these approaches are conceptually somewhat distinct, they share a number of fundamental assumptions. The basic assumptions of cognitive therapy are as follows:

1. The way individuals construe or interpret events and situations mediates how they subsequently feel and behave. Cognitions are postulated to exist in a transactional relationship with affect and behavior and with their consequent effect on events in the individual's environment. As such, human functioning is the product of an ongoing interaction between specific, related "person variables" (beliefs and cognitive processes, emotions, and behavior) and environmental variables. These variables influ-

ence one another in a reciprocal manner over the course of time. None, as a result, is viewed as "primary" or a "first cause." Rather, each is seen as both an initiator and a product of a transactional process.

2. This interpretation of events is active and ongoing. The construing of events allows individuals to derive or abstract a sense of meaning from their experiences and permits them to understand events with the goal of establishing their "personal environment" and of responding to events. Behavioral and emotional functioning, as a result, are seen as goal directed and adaptive.

3. Individuals develop idiosyncratic belief systems that guide behavior. Beliefs and assumptions influence an individual's perceptions and memories and lead the memories to be activated by specific stimuli or events. The individual is rendered sensitive to specific "stressors," including both external events and internal affective experiences. Beliefs and assumptions contribute to a tendency to selectively attend to and recall information that is consistent with the content of the belief system and to "overlook" information that is inconsistent with those beliefs.

4. These stressors consequently contribute to a functional impairment of an individual's cognitive processing and activate maladaptive, overlearned coping responses. A feed-forward system is established in which the activation of maladaptive coping behaviors contributes to the maintenance of aversive environmental events and the consolidation of the belief system. The person who believes, for example, that "the freeway is horribly dangerous" might drive in such a timid manner (20 miles per hour slower than traffic; stopping on the entrance ramp before merging) that he causes an accident, thus strengthening his belief in the danger of freeways and the importance of driving even more defensively.

5. The "cognitive specificity hypothesis" states that clinical syndromes and emotional states can be distinguished by the specific content of the belief system and the cognitive processes that are activated.

The foundation of cognitive therapy is the belief or meaning system. Our knowledge base provides us with a lens through which we interpret our experiences and a set of expectations that guide us in developing plans and goals. Our beliefs may be available to our conscious awareness (as in the case of "automatic thoughts") or may be implicit and unstated (as with schemata). Our use of the term "meaning system" suggests that our knowledge base and ways of processing information are organized and coherent. From this perspective, human behavior is both goal directed and generative. It is based on rules and tacit beliefs that are elaborated and consolidated over the course of an individual's life. Cognitive processes, emotional responses, and behavioral skills are adaptive. Cognitive processes are seen as playing a central role in organizing our response both to daily events and to long-term challenges. Cognitive processes do not function independently of emotional regulation and behavioral action. Rather, they form an integrated adaptive system (R. Lazarus, 1991; Leventhal, 1984). Cognitive processes, emotions, and behavior cannot be divorced from biological and social functioning. Cognitions are dependent on (and influence) the functions of the brain and are acquired in a social context. To understand cognition, then, one must understand action and the uses to which the knowledge will be put. To understand emotion, one must understand cognition and the structure that is imposed by a meaning system.

When we speak of "cognitions" we are not limiting ourselves to "automatic thoughts"—that is, to the thoughts and beliefs that comprise a person's moment-to-moment stream of consciousness. Rather, cognitions include our perceptions, memories, expectations, standards, images, attributions, plans, goals, and tacit beliefs. Cognitive variables, then, include thoughts in our conscious awareness as well as inferred cognitive structures and cognitive processes (Kihlstrom, 1987, 1988; Meichenbaum & Gilmore, 1984; Safran, Vallis, Segal, & Shaw, 1986).

Cognitive therapy has, in the past, been criticized as being both cold (in that it does not attend fully to emotions) and impersonal (in that it does not address the social contexts in which individuals function or the importance of the therapeutic relationship). Both of these criticisms, however, stem from a misunderstanding of cognitive-behavioral models and treatment practices. The importance of emotion in psychotherapy has been noted by Beck from his earliest writings (A. Beck, 1976) and is more fully elaborated in the concepts of "modes" and "affective schema" (Clark & Beck, 1999). The central importance of social factors for understanding the development of psychopathology and its treatment has been noted by a number of cognitive-behavioral writers (Gotlib & Hammen, 1992; Safran & Segal, 1990).

THE BASIC COGNITIVE THERAPY MODEL

The standard cognitive therapy model posits that three variables play a central role in the formation and maintenance of the common psychological disorders: the cognitive triad, schemata, and cognitive distortions (Beck et al., 1979).

The Cognitive Triad

The construct of the cognitive triad was first proposed by Beck as a means of describing the negativistic thoughts and dreams of depressed inpatients (A. Beck, 1963). He observed that the thoughts of depressed individuals typically include highly negative views of themselves, their world, and the future. The thoughts of anxious patients, in contrast, tend to differ from those of depressed individuals in each of these domains. They tend to view the world or others as potentially threatening and maintain a vigilant and wary orientation toward their future. The concept of the cognitive triad, then, serves as a useful framework for examining the automatic thoughts and tacit assumptions that patients describe. Virtually all patient problems can be related to maladaptive or dysfunctional beliefs in one of these three areas. When beginning therapy, as a result, it is often helpful to inquire as to patients' thoughts in each of these areas. As patients' beliefs and attitudes are quite idiosyncratic, we should anticipate that the specific content of their thoughts regarding the self, their world, and the future will differ. By assessing the degree of contribution of thoughts in each of these areas to their distress, the therapist can begin to develop a conceptualization of their concerns.

Schemata

The concept of schemata plays an important role in cognitive models of emotional and behavioral problems. The concept was originally proposed by Kant and has more recently been employed by Piagetian psychologists and associative network theorists to refer to organized, tacit cognitive structures made up of abstractions or general knowledge about the attributes of a stimulus domain and the relationships among these attributes (Horowitz, 1991). Stored in memory as generalizations from specific experiences and prototypes of specific cases, schemata provide focus and meaning for incoming information. Although not in our conscious awareness, they direct our attention to those elements of our day-to-day experience that are most important for our survival and adaptation. Schemata are seen, then, as influencing cognitive processes of attention, encoding, retrieval, and inference. Individuals tend to assimilate their experiences to preexisting schemata rather than to accommodate schemata to events that are unexpected or discrepant (Fiske & Taylor, 1984; Kovacs & Beck, 1978; Meichenbaum & Gilmore, 1984). That is, we tend to make sense of new experiences in terms of what we already believe, rather than by changing our preexisting views. As Paul Simon observed in his

song "The Boxer," "A man hears what he wants to hear and disregards the rest."

In addition to representations and prototypical exemplars of specific events, schemata also incorporate emotions or "affective valences" related to the events. From this perspective, the distinction that is often drawn between "cold," cognitive approaches to psychotherapy and "warm," emotion-focused models is misguided. Rather, cognition and emotion are viewed as interacting components of an integrated, adaptive system (Leventhal, 1984). Events in one's life activate both ideational content and an associated affect. Cognitive schemata, as a result, might more accurately be described as cognitive-emotional structures (Greenberg & Safran, 1987; R. Lazarus, 1991; Turk & Salovey, 1985). As Flavell (1963) succinctly observed, cognitive and emotional reactions are "interdependent in functioning—essentially two sides of the same coin" (p. 80). This notion is clinically useful in that it guides us to examine a patient's thoughts when a strong emotion is expressed and to elicit a patient's feelings when they describe a strongly held, maladaptive belief.

Schemata are established as individuals abstract similarities between events. They are maintained, elaborated, and consolidated through processes of assimilation and are changed through accommodation to novel experiences (Rosen, 1985, 1989). These adaptive processes underlie the effectiveness of behavioral interventions. Behavioral exposure and training provide individuals with experiences and evidence that are inconsistent with their existing beliefs. Behavioral and emotional change is not seen as stemming from associatively based learning and reinforcement. Rather, it is due to the elaboration or adaptation of existing beliefs and the construction of alternative beliefs. In essence, to change an individual's feelings one must change the individual's thoughts or beliefs. As Kegan (1982) observed, behavioral and emotional change involve "an evolution of meaning" (p. 41).

In addition to beliefs about the world

and our social relationships, we also possess stable, unstated beliefs about ourselves. These "self-schemata" include cognitive generalizations that "serve as a template against which individuals perceive and encode information about themselves" (Turk & Salovey, 1985, p. 4). Like other schemata, self-schemata orient one's perception, encoding, retrieval, and utilization of information in a schema-consistent manner. This, along with the fact that they are often highly elaborated and associated with intense affect, can make them difficult to change (Fiske & Taylor, 1984; Markus, 1977; Turk & Salovey, 1985). The precise content of schemata is not typically open to introspection or rational disputation. Nonetheless, basic categories for classifying events can be inferred from monitoring the types of information that are most frequently remembered and used (Kovacs & Beck, 1978; Meichenbaum & Gilmore, 1984).

Highly depressed persons, for example, often maintain schemata that "I'm defective" (self) and "people are unreliable" (social). Although these beliefs may be tacit, in that they are not in the depressed person's conscious awareness, they will, nonetheless, influence the person's perceptions, memories, and social interactions. Highly angry individuals, in contrast, may or may not believe that they are flawed or defective. They do, however, tend to believe that "the world is dangerous" (social), and that "people are malicious" (social). Although these beliefs may not be part of their daily thoughts, they strongly influence their behavior and emotional reactions toward others.

As noted, schemata are developed and consolidated over the course of an individual's infancy and childhood. Maladaptive schemata typically are seen as serving an adaptive function and may represent internalizations of ongoing or repetitious parental behavior. The parent who is unsupportive, punitive, or unpredictable toward his or her infant, for example, will likely behave in a similar manner during later years. The child's nascent beliefs that "my needs won't be met

by others," "I am flawed or inadequate," and "I must submit to the control of others to avoid punishment" are initially represented nonverbally as subjective encodings of interactive experiences and are elaborated and consolidated by later events. They are reified as procedural memories, tacit beliefs, or representations about the self and the world—they become the "givens" of life. Recent research suggests that maladaptive schema can, under some circumstances, develop as the result of a single traumatic experience (see Hembree & Foa, 2003).

Tacit beliefs or schemata are later activated by events that are similar to early experiences that surrounded their development (Ingram, 1984). As the activation of the memory spreads throughout the associative links of the schema's network, other memories, exemplars, expectations, and emotions related to the event will be activated. If the schemata are elaborate, individuals become preoccupied with the event. As thoughts about personal weakness, hopelessness, and unremitting disappointment gain predominance, individuals become less active and socially engaged and their mood becomes increasingly depressed and hopeless. People's observations of themselves in this state only provide further evidence of their inadequacy and contribute to a worsening of their interpersonal problems.

Both behavior and emotions, from this perspective, are adaptive. Individuals behave in terms of outcomes that they desire and expectations that they maintain. Behavior is influenced by the intentions or goals that precede it, the plans or exemplars that accompany and direct it, and the criteria for successful completion against which it is compared. Our behavior, as a result, is responsive to feedback from our environment in that it is compared with a goal or an intended state on an ongoing basis and is adjusted to compensate for discrepancies. Human behavior, from this perspective, is structured and organized. It is guided by tacit rules or cognitive structures.

Schemata play a central role in the expression of clinical disorders and are postulated to account for consistencies in behavior over time and for continuities in one's sense of self through one's life. These tacit rules, assumptions, and beliefs serve as the wellspring of the various cognitive distortions seen in patients. Schemata are often strongly held and are seen as essential for the person's safety, well-being, or existence. Schemata that are consolidated early in life and are powerfully reinforced by significant others are often highly valent in the personality style of the individual (Beck, Freeman, & Associates, 1990; Layden, Newman, Freeman, & Byers, 1993; Young, 1991). Schemata, like other beliefs, rarely function in isolation. Like the cognitive distortions we discuss next, schemata occur in complex combinations and permutations.

Cognitive Distortions

There is a potentially infinite amount of information impinging upon us in our day-to-day lives. As a result, we must selectively attend to those events or stimuli that are most important to our adaptation and survival. Some events will be examined, recalled, and reflected on; others will be overlooked, ignored, and forgotten as uninteresting or unimportant. As our attentional capacities and ability to process information are limited, some distortion of our experiences necessarily *must* occur. Just as there is no perfect lens or mirror, all human perception is influenced by prior experience and by the individual's current emotional state. It seems intuitively reasonable to assert that emotions (at least strong ones) can influence rationality of choice. An individual's perceptions, memories, and thoughts can become distorted in a variety of adaptive and maladaptive ways. Some individuals may, for example, view life in an unrealistically positive way and perceive that they have control or influence that they may not, in reality, possess. They may take chances that most people would avoid—such as starting a new business or investing in a

risky new stock. If successful, the individual is vindicated and may be envied for his or her *chutzpah,* or nerve. Such distortions can, however, be problematic in that they may lead individuals to take chances that may eventuate in great danger, They might, for example, experience massive chest pains and not consult a physician due to the belief that "nothing will happen to me. . . . I'm too young and healthy for a heart attack."

It is the negative or maladaptive distortions that typically become the focus of therapy. One task in treatment is to make these distortions manifest and to assist patients to recognize the impact of the distortions on their life. Distortions, as such, represent maladaptive ways of processing information and may become emblematic of a particular style of behaving or of certain clinical syndromes. Like many constructs, how we define and understand notions such as "rationality," "distortion," "adaptiveness," "maladaptiveness," and "bias" has important philosophical and practical implications. They should be carefully scrutinized.

The distortions and patient styles are presented here in isolation for the sake of discussion. This is not meant to be a comprehensive list but rather is presented for illustrative purposes. Typical distortions and examples of the common clinical correlates include the following:

1. *Dichotomous thinking.* "Things are black or white"; "You're with me or against me." This tendency toward "all-or-nothing" thinking is encountered in borderline and obsessive compulsive disorders.
2. *Mind reading.* "They probably think that I'm incompetent"; "I just know that they will disapprove." This processing style is common to avoidant and paranoid personality disorders.
3. *Emotional reasoning.* "I feel inadequate so I must be inadequate"; "I'm feeling upset, so there must be something wrong." This distortion is common among individuals suffering from anxiety disorders.
4. *Personalization.* "That comment wasn't

just random, I know it was directed toward me." At the extreme, this is common in avoidant and paranoid personality disorders.

5. *Overgeneralization.* "Everything I do turns out wrong"; "It doesn't matter what my choices are, they always fall flat." At the extreme, this is common among depressed individuals.

6. *Catastrophizing.* "If I go to the party, there will be terrible consequences"; "It would be devastating if I failed this exam"; "My heart's beating faster, it's got to be a heart attack." At the extreme, this distortion is characteristic of anxiety disorders, especially social anxiety, social phobia, and panic.

7. *"Should" statements.* "I should visit my family every time they want me to"; "They should do what I say because it is right." At the extreme, this is common in obsessive–compulsive disorders and among individuals who feel excessive guilt.

8. *Selective abstraction.* "The rest of the information doesn't matter. . . . This is the salient point"; "I've got to focus on the negative details, the positive things that have happened don't count." At the extreme, this is common in depression.

Other common cognitive distortions include "disqualifying the positive," "externalization of self-worth," and "perfectionism." The latter cognitive distortion has been associated with vulnerability for relapse of depression, obsessive–compulsive personality, and anorexia. Fallacies and irrational beliefs often center on the desire for control over events, the value of self-criticism, worrying, and ignoring problems and beliefs about fairness and stability in relationships.

EVIDENCE FOR COGNITIVE MODELS OF DEPRESSION

Cognitive therapy makes a number of statements about the phenomenology of depression, its etiology, mediating mechanisms, and processes of change in psychotherapy (Clark & Beck, 1999; Ingram, Miranda, & Segal, 1998). The "standard model" of cognitive therapy for depression (Beck et al., 1979) makes a number of specific predictions that can be framed as hypotheses. The model assumes that (1) rigidly held negativistic beliefs about self-worth and overvaluation of particular outcomes serve as proximal vulnerability factors for depression; (2) these factors interact with social or environmental variables in precipitating the onset of a depressive episode; (3) the beliefs of depression prone individuals are characterized by themes of unlovability and helplessness; (4) the activation of these beliefs by stressful life events or personal losses effects a range of cognitive processes, including memory, appraisal, perception, and problem solving; and (5) that two personality styles—sociotropy and autonomy—serve as mediating variables in determining the ways in which specific life events influence mood. Sociotropic individuals tend to base feelings of personal worth on relationships with others and are sensitive to loss or rejection, whereas autonomous individuals base feelings of worth on accomplishment or achievement and are sensitive to failure. Tacit dysfunctional beliefs are seen, then, as playing a causal role in the onset of depressive episodes, and they are believed to be latent or inactive during periods when the individual is not depressed.

Findings to date are quite supportive of cognitive hypotheses about the nature of clinical depression (for reviews, see Clark & Beck, 1999; Solomon & Haaga, 2003). As predicted, clinically depressed individuals tend to demonstrate negative beliefs about the self, the world, and the future. They demonstrate higher levels of pessimism, a more negative attributional style, impaired social problem solving, negativistic tacit beliefs or schemata, higher levels of sociotropy and autonomy, heightened levels of self-focused attention, and a greater tendency to ruminate than do controls. Their thoughts tend to be characterized by themes of loss, inadequacy, and failure. Moreover, they tend to show lower levels of positive self-referent thinking. These negative patterns of thinking are found in patients with both unipolar and bipolar depression and are characteristic of both melancholic and nonmelancholic depression. To be sure, many of these cognitive deficits are not specific to depression and many are state dependent. That is, they tend to vary with the individual's level of depression. Moreover, there tends to be an overlap in the distributions of cognitive variables for depressed and nondepressed individuals. There are individual differences in the strength of these beliefs and processes among both depressed and vulnerable groups. Finally, these cognitive processes may not be unique to depression. Research is, nonetheless, largely supportive of descriptive aspects of the cognitive model of depression.

Evidence regarding hypotheses about cognitive mediation of depression is supportive but mixed. Early studies tended to rely on self-report measures of mood and cognition and tended to use cross-sectional designs. It was not possible, as such, to draw strong conclusions about whether cognitive factors mediated mood and adjustment. More recent research using experimental measures of cognition (such as the Stroop Task, incidental memory tasks, dichotic listening paradigm), priming procedures, and longitudinal designs has been more supportive (for reviews, see Clark & Beck, 1999; Ingram et al., 1998; Solomon & Haaga, 2003). Depressed individuals tend, for example, to attend to events or stimuli that include themes of loss or failure, and remitted depressed individuals demonstrate higher levels of dysfunctional attitudes or schemata than do never depressed persons. These beliefs are apparent, however, only after they have been brought to awareness by a priming procedure. It appears, then, that dysfunctional beliefs may persist after a depressive episode has ended and may, as predicted by the standard model, be latent much of the time. One may think of latent

depressogenic beliefs and processing styles as similar, in some ways, to software on a computer. They are stored on the hard drive but are not active or apparent (pulled up on the screen) until they are booted up by specific commands. To be sure, there are methodological difficulties with studies of remitted depressed individuals (Solomon & Haaga, 2003). Nonetheless, recent findings are consistent with predictions of the cognitive model regarding cognitive mediation of depression.

As noted, the standard model predicts that tacit depressogenic beliefs serve as proximal risk factors for depression. They are postulated to have developed based on early experience and to play an etiological role in depression. They should, then, precede the onset of an individual's first depressive episode. Demonstrating this precedence, however, has proven quite challenging. To demonstrate cognitive vulnerability it is necessary to assess levels of dysfunctional attitudes or schemata in a sample of "at risk" or "cognitively vulnerable" individuals who have never experienced a depressive episode and follow them over time. The Temple–Wisconsin Cognitive Vulnerability to Depression Study (Abramson et al., 1998; Alloy et al., 2000) has attempted to make such an assessment. Preliminary findings are consistent with predictions made by cognitive theories of depression—never depressed individuals with high levels of dysfunctional attitudes and negativistic attributions were much more likely to experience an episode of major depression than were low-risk controls (17% vs. 1%) during a 2-year follow-up period. Moreover, recent findings indicate that relationships between insecure attachment style and depression are mediated by the occurrence of dysfunctional attitudes, both for clinical (Reinecke & Rogers, 2001) and nonclinical (Roberts, Gotlib, & Kassel, 1996; Whisman & McGarvey, 1995) groups. Although preliminary, these findings are consistent with predictions made by the cognitive theory regarding the etiology of depression (Ingram et al., 1998).

THE EFFICACY AND EFFECTIVENESS OF COGNITIVE THERAPY FOR DEPRESSION

Does cognitive therapy work? The results of empirical outcome studies have generally been both supportive and promising (Agency for Health Care Policy and Research, 1993; Hollon & Shelton, 2001; Robinson, Berman, & Neimeyer, 1990). A number of randomized controlled trials have been published during recent years supporting the utility of cognitive therapy for treating depression among adults (for reviews, see DeRubeis & Crits-Christoph, 1998; Hollon, Thase, & Markowitz, 2002; Lambert & Davis, 2002; Schulberg, Katon, Simon, & Rush, 1998) and youth (Curry, 2001; Harrington, Whittaker, Shoebridge, & Campbell, 1998; Reinecke, Ryan, & DuBois, 1998; Spence & Reinecke, 2003). An early meta-analysis of 28 outcome studies indicated a greater degree of change for cognitive therapy in comparison to a waiting-list or no-treatment control, pharmacotherapy, behavior therapy, or other types of psychotherapies (Dobson, 1989). Moreover, initial findings indicated that relapse and recurrence rates were lower for patients who received cognitive therapy than for those who had received medications. Cognitive therapy appeared, then, to offer lasting benefits to patients (Hollon, Shelton, & Loosen, 1991). Methodological difficulties, however, limited our confidence in many of these early studies. Although the effect sizes reported typically were large, many of the studies did not include clinical samples or more severely depressed patients and tended to rely on self-report measures of mood, and questions were raised about the adequacy of the medication trials against which cognitive therapy was compared.

These concerns were addressed in subsequent research. As in earlier studies, cognitive-behavioral therapy was found to be effective in alleviating mild to moderate clinical depression (Hollon & Shelton,

2001). Not all studies, however, have been entirely supportive. Although cognitive therapy typically has been found to be as effective as medications for the acute treatment of clinical depression, this was not found to be the case in the National Institute of Mental Health (NIMH) Treatment of Depression Collaborative Research Program (TDCRP; Elkin et al., 1989), a multisite clinical trial comparing cognitive therapy (CT), interpersonal therapy (IPT), the antidepressant medication imipramine (IMI), and a placebo control (pill with adjunctive clinical management; PBO-C). Although 50% of subjects who received cognitive-behavioral therapy (CBT) in this study demonstrated a "clinically significant improvement" (Ogles, Lambert, & Sawyer, 1995), CT was found in this study to be less effective than medications and not appreciably better than placebo for patients with severe depression (Elkin et al., 1995). Moreover, CT did not appear to offer lasting benefits relative to other forms of treatment (Shea et al., 1992). Based on these findings, several individuals suggested that CT may not be a treatment of choice for more severely depressed adults (American Psychiatric Association, 2000). Given the attention these findings received, questions about the efficacy of CT for depression arose.

On closer examination, however, these findings become more complex. The results of the TDCRP are inconsistent with those of other controlled outcome studies, and between site differences in response to CBT within the TDCRP suggested that CT may not have been adequately administered at several of the sites. Patients who received CBT at sites with more experienced cognitive therapists tended to do better. In fact, TDCRP patients with more severe depression who received CBT at sites with experienced therapists tended to do as well as those who had received medications. Moreover, when data from the TDCRP are combined with those of other controlled outcome studies, CT appears to be as effective as medications for treating severe depression

(DeRubeis, Gelfand, Tang, & Simons, 1999). Taken together, these findings suggest that the TDCRP may have underestimated the efficacy of CT and that therapist skill may be related to outcome (at least for more severely depressed individuals). CT appears, then, to be useful as a treatment for clinical depression (Hollon & Shelton, 2001). Its effectiveness, however, may be dependent on the skill with which it is used. As Hollon and colleagues (2002) cogently note, "the therapist's expertise makes a greater difference the more difficult the depression is to treat" (p. 62).

This observation is potentially important insofar as many practicing clinicians adopt an "integrative" or "eclectic" stance—introducing cognitive interventions as adjuncts to psychodynamic or humanistically based trials of therapy. This approach is not consistent with standards for empirically supported forms of therapy. Although clinical flexibility can be quite important, eclectic approaches lack fidelity (i.e., they do not adhere to accepted CBT guidelines or protocols) and have not been demonstrated to be effective in either controlled trials or community settings. It has not been shown that that dabbling in cognitive therapy—incorporating CBT techniques into other forms of therapy—is clinically efficacious. In the absence of empirical evidence for the effectiveness of integrative or eclectic forms of psychotherapy for clinical depression, it would seem prudent, when possible, for clinicians to attempt to follow guidelines for CT as closely as possible. This is particularly true when assisting patients with more severe or intractable depressions.

Taken together, the results of randomized controlled trials suggest that CT may be efficacious for treating major depression. CBT has also found to be useful in treating atypical depression (Jarrett et al., 1999; Mercier, Stewart, & Quitkin, 1992) and (in conjunction with medications) chronic depression (Keller et al., 2000). Controlled trials, however, tend to use highly selected samples and typically are carried out in uni-

versity research clinics. The question arises, is CT effective in community settings? Is it useful in treating the broader and more complex range of clinical problems encountered in general clinical practice? Although research is limited, preliminary findings have been positive (Haaga, DeRubeis, Stewart, & Beck, 1991; Persons, Bostrom, & Bertagnolli, 1999; Persons, Burns, & Perloff, 1988). Although there is some evidence that cognitive-behavioral approaches developed in research clinics are effective in private practice settings, additional work is necessary.

Research findings indicate that CT may have enduring effects. The results of several studies suggest that relapse rates after CT are lower than those with antidepressant medications (Evans, Hollon, DeRubeis, & Piasecki, 1992; Hollon, 1990; Hollon et al., 1991; Murphy, Simons, Wetzel, & Lustman, 1984; Simons, Murphy, Levine, & Wetzel, 1986), and that CT may prevent the recurrence of depression after the completion of treatment (Beck, Hollon, Young, Bedrosian, & Budenz, 1985; Blackburn, Eunson, & Bishop, 1986; Kovacs, Rush, Beck, & Hollon, 1981). Moreover, providing CBT booster sessions or maintenance therapy after initial remission can reduce the risk of relapse (Blackburn & Moore, 1997; Jarrett et al., 1998, 2001). Additional research on the ways in which psychotherapy may serve to prevent relapse and recurrence of depression is sorely needed. Studying the course of depression after treatment can be quite difficult insofar as attrition from therapy and seeking additional "out of protocol" treatments can contribute to misleading results. Intent-to-treat designs offer the most stringent test of a treatment. To understand the effects of a treatment on relapse and recurrence, however, it is necessary to compare subjects who have completed and benefited from adequate trials of alternative treatments. Intent-to-treat designs may not be appropriate for this purpose as differential retention or attrition between treatment groups can affect the results obtained. It is difficult, then, to draw firm conclusions about the effects of CBT on relapse. Findings to date suggest, nonetheless, that CT is as effective as pharmacotherapy for treating the acute symptoms of depression, and that it can reduce the risk of relapse or recurrence, at least when it is administered in an appropriate manner. The mechanisms by which it reduces the risk of relapse, however, are not well understood.

Clinical reports suggest that CT and medications can be used together (Wright, 1987, 1992; Wright & Schrodt, 1989), and that a combination of CBT and medications can be useful in treating chronic depression (Keller et al., 2000). Moreover, the results of several studies indicate that CT may be effective in alleviating "biological" symptoms of depression (e.g., insomnia, loss of appetite, and decreased libido) and that it is useful in treating patients from impoverished backgrounds (Blackburn, Bishop, Glen, Walley, & Christie, 1981; Blackburn et al., 1986).

Taken together, findings indicate that CBT can be efficacious in treating clinical depression, and that it can be useful in treating even severe or chronic depression. In addition, CBT appears to reduce the risk of relapse when booster or maintenance sessions are provided. Moreover, providing patients who have received medications with a brief trial of CBT appears to reduce the risk of relapse after medications have been discontinued.

COGNITIVE THERAPY FOR OTHER DISORDERS

Although initially developed as a treatment for depression, cognitive-behavioral models and interventions have been proposed for a range of clinical disorders and conditions. These models have been put to empirical test, and treatments derived from them have received substantial empirical support. Generalized anxiety disorder (GAD), for example, can be understood as stemming from deficits in the regulation of affect in conjunction with a desire to avoid worry (Mennin, Turk, Heimberg, & Carmin, 2003). Controlled outcome studies suggest that cognitive-behavioral interventions may be helpful in alleviating anxiety among patients with GAD, and that gains are maintained over time (Blowers, Cobb, & Matthews, 1987; Borkovec & Costello, 1993; Butler, Cullington, Hibbert, Klimes, & Gelder, 1987; Butler, Fennell, Robson, & Gelder, 1991; White, Keenan, & Brooks, 1992).

Panic disorder can also be conceptualized in cognitive-behavioral terms. Panic attacks occur when individuals make "catastrophic interpretations" to internal, bodily sensations, such as palpitations or breathlessness (Clark, 1986, 1988). This might occur, for example, if a healthy individual were to interpret momentary dizziness as a signal of a heart attack or an impending stroke. A number of CBT protocols have been developed based on this model (Clark, Salkovskis, & Chalkley, 1985; Clark et al., 1994; Craske, Brown, & Barlow, 1991; Telch et al., 1993). These protocols typically include a psychoeducational component in which the panic attacks are explained to the patient, the presentation of a cognitive rationale, cognitive restructuring, relaxation training, controlled breathing, exposure to anxiety-provoking cues, and panic induction (Hofmann, 2003; Hofmann & Spiegel, 1999). The objective are to provide patients with a way of understanding their symptoms, a sense of control over them, and the perception that their somatic symptoms are neither harmful nor indicative of a more significant illness. Controlled outcome studies indicate that these approaches are superior to wait-list, medication, pill placebo, and relaxation training controls (Beck, Sokol, Clark, Berchick, & Wright, 1992; Sokol, Beck, Greenberg, Berchick, & Wright, 1989). Given the strength of these findings, CBT has been recognized as an efficacious treatment for panic by both the American Psychiatric Association (1998) and the Division of Clinical Psychology of the American Psychological Association (Chambless et al., 1996).

A substantial amount of work has been completed during recent years examining cognitive factors associated with posttraumatic stress disorder (PTSD). Cognitive-behavioral models based on information-processing and emotion-processing paradigms (Foa & Kozak, 1986; Foa, Steketee, & Rothbaum, 1989; Resick & Schnicke, 1992) have proven quite useful in providing an understanding of the ways in which traumatic experiences can disrupt core cognitive processes or schemata and may result in the activation of "pathological fear structures" (Hembree & Foa, 2003). These fear structures or schemata are distinguished from other beliefs by the occurrence of excessive avoidance, hyperarousal, pathological memory structures, and maladaptive interpretations and meanings. These pathological structures lead individuals with PTSD to erroneously perceive innocuous events as dangerous and to view themselves as incompetent or vulnerable. These beliefs are both extreme and inflexible. Evidence bearing on this model has recently been reviewed by Hembree and Foa (2003). Treatment strategies based on this model focus on changing memories of the trauma and personal narratives that have been developed to explain the traumatic event (Foa & Rothbaum, 1998). This is accomplished through discussions of the impact of the events, *in vivo* exposure to trauma-related stimuli, imaginal exposure, identification of trauma-related maladaptive beliefs, cognitive restructuring, and training in anxiety management techniques (such as relaxation, thought stopping, and adaptive self-statements). The results of controlled outcome studies suggest that these approaches can be quite helpful in treating individuals with PTSD (Foa & Rothbaum, 1998; Marks, Lovell, Noshirvani, Livanou, & Thrasher, 1998; Tarrier et al., 1999). Given the strength of these findings, CBT has been recommended as a treatment of choice for PTSD (Foa, Davidson, & Frances, 1999).

Social anxiety—a marked or persistent fear of social situations—can develop during childhood or adolescence and often follows a chronic course. It can be quite disabling and is characterized by physiological symptoms of anxiety, avoidance of social situations, and an increased risk of developing a range of comorbid psychiatric disorders. Research on social anxiety completed during recent years has led to important advances in its conceptualization (Clark & Wells, 1995; Rapee & Heimberg, 1997) and treatment (Rapee, 1998). Cognitive factors associated with social anxiety include negative self-evaluations, magnified perceptions of criticism or negative evaluation by others, attentional and memory biases, heightened sensitivity to others' behavior, and the belief that one should be able to control other's reactions and impressions (for a review, see Wilson & Rapee, 2003). Cognitive-behavioral interventions, including psychoeducation, relaxation training, identification of maladaptive thoughts and expectations, rational disputation, social skills training, and *in vivo* exposure, have been developed during recent years (Bates & Clark, 1998; Butler & Wells, 1995; Chambless & Hope, 1996; Clark, 1997; Heimberg & Juster, 1994; Merluzzi, 1996; Wells, 1997). Outcome studies indicate that these approaches are superior to wait-list and supportive therapy controls, and that gains tend to be maintained over time (Taylor, 1996; Wilson & Rapee, 2003).

Cognitive-behavioral models and treatments have also been developed for such diverse problems as body dysmorphic disorder (Kroenke & Swindle, 2000; Veale, 2001; Veale, Gournay, Dryden, & Boocock, 2001; Veale & Riley, 2001), obsessive–compulsive disorder (Clark & Purdon, 2003; Salkovskis & Wahl, 2003; Steketee, 1996), anger management (Dahlen & Deffenbacher, 2001), psychotic disorders (Chadwick, Birchwood, & Trower, 1996; Fowler, Garety, & Kuipers, 1995; Haddock & Slade, 1996; Kingdon &

Turkington, 1994; Tarrier & Haddock, 2002; Tarrier et al., 1998), marital problems (Epstein & Schlesinger, 2003), and eating disorders (Fairburn, 1985; Fairburn, Jones, Peveler, Hope, & O'Conner, 1993; Fairburn et al., 1991, 1995; Fairburn, Shafran, & Cooper, 1998; LeGrange, 2003).

THE PRACTICE OF THERAPY

An element common to the different cognitive-behavioral models is their emphasis on helping patients examine the manner in which they construe or understand themselves and their world (cognitions) and to experiment with new ways of responding (behavioral). By learning to understand the idiosyncratic ways in which they perceive themselves, the world, and their prospects for the future, patients can be helped to alter negative emotions and to behave more adaptively. In practice, cognitive therapy sessions are (1) structured, active, and problem oriented;(2) time limited and strategic; (3) psychoeducational; (4) based on constructivist models of thought and behavior; and (5) collaborative.

Cognitive therapy employs both coping and mastery models and uses a range of approaches to develop adaptive skills.Cognitive therapy attempts to identify specific, measurable goals and moves quickly and directly into those areas that create the most difficulty for the patient. The approach is similar in this regard to contemporary short-term dynamic and interpersonal psychotherapy (Crits-Christoph & Barber, 1991).Cognitive therapy does not presume to protect individuals from experiencing distress in the future. Anxiety, depression, and guilt can play an essential and adaptive role in people's lives. Cognitive therapy endeavors not to alleviate these emotions but to provide patients with skills for understanding and managing them.

One reason that individuals can experience difficulty coping with internal or external stimuli is a lack of adaptive skills. Cog-

nitive and behavioral skills typically develop over the course of one's development through structured interactions with supportive caregivers. Developmentally important competencies include the ability to regulate affective arousal, interpersonal or social skills, the ability to direct and maintain one's attention, and cognitive skills (including executive functions and formal operational thought). An important component of cognitive therapy is to *enhance patients' skills* and sense of personal competence so that they can more effectively deal with the exigencies of life and thereby have a greater sense of control and self-efficacy. Social skills training, relaxation training, and anger control exercises are examples.

The Therapeutic Relationship in Cognitive Therapy

As Truax and Carkhuff (1964) observed, therapists who are "nonpossessively warm," empathetic, and genuine achieve greater gains than do those who are not. Cognitive therapy recognizes the central importance of these nonspecific relationship variables in facilitating change but views them as "necessary but not sufficient" for therapeutic improvement. That is, the development of a warm, empathic, and genuine relationship is not, in our view, necessarily accompanied by behavioral or emotional change.

The therapeutic relationship should be collaborative. The term "therapetic collaboration" refers to a specific form of patient–therapist relationship. The therapist is viewed as a "coinvestigator"—working with patients to make sense of their experiences and emotions by exploring their thoughts, images, and feelings with them. Socratic questioning is often used as a means of providing patients with an understanding of the ways their beliefs influence their feelings and actions. As Beck and colleagues (1979) stated, "The therapeutic relationship is used not simply as *the* instrument to alleviate suffering but as a vehicle to facilitate a common effort in carrying out specific goals" (p. 54). The cognitive therapist does not view the therapeutic relationship as the primary motor of therapeutic change. Whereas psychodynamic and psychoanalytic clinicians view experiences within the therapeutic relationship as singularly important for developing an understanding of internal dynamics, cognitive therapists view the therapeutic relationship as one of three sources of information (the other two being the childhood antecedents of specific beliefs and automatic thoughts that are activated on a day-to-day basis). These dimensions are colloquially referred to as the "three-legged stool" by cognitive therapists. Clinicians are encouraged to attend to each leg of the stool as a means of facilitating change.

The therapist's directiveness can be adjusted over the course of treatment depending on the needs of the patient. With a highly depressed patient who is immobilized by psychomotor retardation and feelings of hopelessness, for example, the therapist may want to adopt a more assertive, directive stance. Behavioral interventions serving to "activate" the patient may be introduced. In contrast, a less directive stance might be employed in working with a highly passive and dependent patient. The man who states, "You're the doctor, just tell me what to do," may feel unable to cope with day-to-day problems on his own and thus seeks guidance and reassurance from others. In this case one may wish to shift to him a greater proportion of the responsibility for identifying problems, identifying and evaluating automatic thoughts, and developing homework assignments. Attempts might be made to encourage him to take responsibility for the direction of the therapy and discuss with him his passivity toward the therapist and toward others in his life.

The transference relationship also plays an important role in cognitive therapy (Reinecke, 2002; Safran & Segal, 1990). The patient's behavior toward the therapist may reflect the activation of schemata (as might the therapist's behavioral and emo-

tional responses to the patient). The patient's experiences during the therapy hour can, as a consequence, serve as evidence to dispute tacit beliefs. Moreover, schemata activated in the therapeutic relationship can be, in many ways, similar to those activated in the patient's relationships with others. The therapist works, through the use of Socratic questioning, to develop greater awareness in patients of their thoughts, feelings, and perceptions—including those about the therapeutic relationship. Cognitive therapy understands transference and countertransference from a social learning perspective and uses experiences within the therapeutic relationship as a means of clarifying and changing tacit beliefs and maladaptive interpersonal patterns (see Leahy, 2001; Reinecke 2002).

Patients' patterns of interaction with others are often recapitulated in their relationship with their therapist. The disorganization, anger, confusion, anxiety, avoidance, envy, helplessness, fear, resentment, and attraction that they exhibit toward the therapist need not be in reaction to specific behaviors on the part of the therapist. In this sense, the cognitive construct of schema activation is similar to the psychodynamic concept of transference. However, cognitive theory does not presume that the elaboration and interpretation of the transference is the principle mechanism of change in therapy, or that patterns of interaction apparent in the therapeutic relationship represent a recapitulation of earlier mother–infant interactions. Although there may be fundamental similarities between the processes of change in psychotherapy and those in development, cognitive therapy does not assume that therapeutic change is based on a reconstruction of developmental experiences in the context of a supportive therapeutic relationship.

Assessment and Treatment Planning

Before therapeutic change can occur, a trusting therapeutic collaboration must be established. The first goal in cognitive therapy, then, is for rapport to be established through empathic, active listening. Patients need to feel that they have been heard, and that their concerns have been understood and acknowledged by their therapist. As is characteristic of other forms of psychotherapy, the cognitive therapist encourages and facilitates patient speech and promotes the experience of affect in the therapy session. The cognitive therapist also identifies recurrent patterns in the patient's behavior and thoughts, points out the use of maladaptive coping strategies or distortions, and draws attention to feelings and thoughts that the patient may find disturbing. Before specific interventions are made, however, a careful review of their developmental, familial, social, occupational, educational, medical, and psychiatric history is completed. These data are useful in helping to turn a patient's presenting complaints into a working problem list and a treatment conceptualization (Persons, 1989). The establishment of a problem list helps both patient and therapist have an idea of where the therapy is going, a general time frame, and a means of assessing therapeutic progress. Having agreed on a problem list, an agenda is set for each session.

The review of the patient's feelings and experiences since the last session flows seamlessly into the development of an agenda. The identification of an agenda item leads directly into an examination of the patient's emotions and thoughts in a recent situation.

The structuring of sessions through the establishment of an agenda helps to maintain the strategic focus of the therapy. Specific problems or issues can be identified so that the therapist and patient can make the most efficient use of their time. Setting an agenda at the beginning of each session allows both patient and therapist to bring out issues of concern for discussion. Moreover, it allows for a continuity between sessions so that sessions are not individual events but rather part of a cohesive whole. A typical agenda might include the following:

1. Discussion of events during the past week and feelings about the prior therapy session.
2. A review of self-report scales filled out by the patient prior to the session.
3. A review of agenda items remaining from the previous session.
4. A review of the patient's homework. The patient's success or problems in doing the homework are discussed, as are the results of the assignment.
5. Current problems are put on the agenda. This might involve the development of specific skills (e.g., social skills, relaxation training, or assertiveness skills) or the examination of dysfunctional thoughts.

Each session concludes with a review or summary of the session, which gives the patient an opportunity to clarify their goals as well as skills, techniques, or insights that have been discussed. A homework assignment for the next session can then be developed. Finally, the patient is asked for his or her response to the session.

Assessment Techniques

Identifying specific problems and objectively evaluating the effectiveness of interventions made to alleviate them is an essential part of cognitive psychotherapy. Assessment instruments, including self-report questionnaires, behavior rating scales, and clinician rating scales, can be quite useful in this regard.

A large number of well-validated rating scales have been developed during recent years, and it would be beyond the scope of this chapter to review them. There are several, however, that we have found to be particularly useful and that deserve note. When depression is a primary concern, the Beck Depression Inventory (BDI) is among the most useful tools available to the therapist (Beck & Steer, 1987; Beck, Ward, Mendelson, Mock, & Erbaugh, 1961). It is among the most widely used self-report measures for depression in the world and is well accepted as reliable and valid measure of depressed mood. The administration of a self-report depression scale, such as the BDI, prior to each session can provide objective data regarding therapeutic progress and can assist in identifying the specific focus of a patient's depression.

When anxiety is a target symptom, the Beck Anxiety Inventory (BAI), a 21–item self-report symptom checklist designed to measure the severity of anxiety-related symptoms (Beck, Epstein, Brown, & Steer, 1988), the Zung Anxiety Scale, or the State–Trait Anxiety Scale may be used. These measures provide a useful, objective measure of the patient's general level of anxiety and can be used both quantitatively and qualitatively as a diagnostic aid.

The Hopelessness Scale (HS) is a brief and highly useful measure of pessimism (Beck, Weissman, Lester, & Trexler, 1974). As levels of hopelessness are often highly correlated with suicidal potential, the HS can be used in conjunction with a measure of depression as a means of estimating suicide risk (Beck, Brown, & Steer, 1989; Drake & Cotton, 1986; Freeman & Reinecke, 1993). Moreover, pessimistic patients often tend to believe that it is not possible for problems in their lives to be resolved and feel personally unable to influence important events. They feel, in short, that they are "ineffective." Given these perceptions and beliefs, such individuals often find it difficult to summon up motivation to participate actively in their treatment. And why should they? They do not perceive that it will be of help. Their hopelessness, then, interferes with their ability to progress. An initial focus of treatment, as a result, might be on the beliefs underlying their hopelessness. As they learn new ways of coping, experience greater self-efficacy, and perceive that change is possible, their level of hopelessness will decrease.

Assessment of Vulnerability Factors

There are circumstances, situations, or deficits that have the effect of decreasing the patient's ability to effectively cope with life's challenges. These factors lower the patient's tolerance for stress and may serve to increase the patient's suicidal thinking, lower threshold for anxiety stimuli, or increase the patient's vulnerability to depressogenic thoughts and situations (Freeman & Simon, 1989). These include (1) acute or chronic illness, (2) hunger, (3) fatigue, (4) major or minor stressful events, (5) loss of social support or an important relationship, (6) alcohol, substance abuse, (7) chronic pain, and (8) new life circumstances.

As Elster (2000) notes, "visceral factors" (such as these) have the effect of limiting rational decision making or voluntary choice. An assessment of these factors allows for a more comprehensive understanding of experiences that may be exacerbating a patient's distress and assists in developing a treatment plan. Interventions can be directed toward increasing supports, alleviating stressors, and improving coping skills.

Diagnosis and Treatment Planning

An initial step in developing a treatment plan involves the establishment of a formulation of the patient's problems. The conceptualization must meet several criteria. It must be (1) useful, (2) parsimonious, and (3) theoretically coherent. It should explain past behavior, make sense of current difficulties, predict future behavior, and yield pragmatic recommendations. The conceptualization process begins with the compilation of a specific, behaviorally based problem list, which is then prioritized. A particular problem may be the primary focus of therapy because of its debilitating effect on the individual. In another case, one may focus on the simplest problem first, thereby giving the patient a sense of confidence in the therapy itself as well as practice in basic problem solving. In a third case, the initial focus might be on a "keystone" problem—that is, a problem whose solution will cause a ripple effect in solving other problems. Having set out the treatment goals with the patient, the therapist can begin to develop strategies and the interventions that will help put them into effect.

Cognitive therapy is proactive in that it endeavors to anticipate problems that may arise and provides patients with skills to cope with them. As such, the therapist must develop hypotheses about what reinforces and maintains dysfunctional thinking and behavior. As noted, beliefs are seen as adaptive and are held with varying degrees of strength. In developing a conceptualization of a particular problem, it is useful to discuss with patients the strength with which they believe key automatic thoughts or assumptions. Automatic thoughts containing the phrase "I am _____" can be particularly difficult to change in that they are often regarded as part of the self. As one young woman, whose frequent and vociferous complaining had led her to be fired at work and to be dropped from the lead role in a theatrical production, stated, "I know I make people defensive, but it's just who I am, and they have to accept me for that. . . . I'm just identifying problems I see for people who are the authorities, so they have to change them. . . . I *can't* change who I am. . . . Even back in high school they voted me 'most likely to complain'."

Chronic behavioral and emotional patterns are often seen by patients as "part of me." Like the woman described previously, they often remark that "this is who I am and this is the way I have always been." Challenges to these core beliefs are often accompanied by anxiety, anger, or avoidance. Attempts to change strongly held beliefs about the self should be patient, incremental, and based on guided discovery rather than direct confrontation or disputation.

Specific Interventions

A range of cognitive and behavioral techniques can be used to identify and change cognitive distortions, maladaptive beliefs, and the schemata that underlie them. These techniques are modeled for patients and practiced in session. The precise mix of cognitive and behavioral techniques used will depend on the patient's abilities, the level of pathology, and the specific treatment goals. When working with severely depressed patients, for example, initial treatment goals might center on facilitating behavioral activity, improving self-care, and reducing social isolation. Graded task assignments can be used to address these problems. Starting at the bottom of a hierarchy of difficulty and moving through successively more challenging tasks can provide patients with a sense of personal efficacy.

Pharmacotherapy may be an important adjunct in the therapy program. Cognitive therapy and pharmacotherapy are not mutually exclusive but can be integrated into an effective treatment program (Wright, 1987, 1992; Wright & Schrodt, 1989). In addition to its value in modifying dysfunctional thoughts or maladaptive behavior that contribute to patients' feelings of dysphoria, anxiety, or anger, cognitive therapy can also be used to improve medication compliance. Maladaptive thoughts such as "this just proves I'm crazy" and "this means there must be something wrong with my brain" can be quite distressing and can undermine treatment compliance. Were pharmacotherapy used alone, these beliefs might not be addressed. Antidepressant medications typically take several weeks before improvement is seen. Cognitive therapy, however, can be helpful in a short period and thus can provide depressed patients with a sense of relief before the medications can be titrated to an effective dose. Moreover, as Wright (1992) observed, cognitive therapy can "arm the patient with problem-solving techniques that can maximize the chances of good psychosocial functioning . . . and can reduce the risk of non-adherence to a long term pharmacotherapy regimen."

Although the empirical evidence is limited, clinical experience suggests that pharmacotherapy may be useful in alleviating biologically based symptoms of depression, such as insomnia, fatigue, and impaired concentration, and thus may help the severely depressed patient to participate more actively in the therapy process. The mechanisms of therapeutic change, however, are not well understood. In a provocative early study of pharmacotherapy and cognitive therapy, Simons, Garfield, and Murphy (1984) found that therapeutic improvement following the administration of tricyclic antidepressant medications was accompanied by changes in dysfunctional thoughts. Medications are clearly indicated in combination with psychotherapy for patients with bipolar disorder or psychosis and for patients who are so depressed that they are unresponsive to verbal or behavioral interventions.

Cognitive Techniques

In practice, cognitive therapy may be defined as a set of techniques designed to alleviate emotional distress by directly modifying the dysfunctional cognitions that accompany them. As such, any intervention or technique that alters a patient's perceptions or beliefs might be viewed as "cognitive." The number of techniques that are potentially available is virtually infinite.

A number of years ago, for example, David Burns reported the case of a patient who was disabled by recurring panic attacks. She feared that any exertion whatsoever would trigger a fatal heart attack and so became quite sensitive to her physical state and assiduously avoided all physical activities. As part of her therapy, Burns asked her to stand and raise her hands over her head, which she did with no difficulty. He then requested that she lower them and raise them again. No problem. Within minutes the patient was vigorously doing jumping jacks in his office and recognized that the sensation of her heart pounding need not signify an impending heart attack. The frequency of her panic attacks subsequently declined. Although we are not presenting jumping jacks as a model for cognitive ther-

apy, the value of this case example still stands. The effective cognitive therapist is able to provide patients with experiences in a creative, flexible manner that will refute their maladaptive beliefs.

A relatively small number of techniques have been found to be useful with a wide range of problems. As with other models of psychotherapy, it is necessary for cognitive therapists to be aware of available interventions and to be able to move skillfully between various techniques. Therapists will be able to teach these skills to their patients so that they can "become their own therapist." Although these techniques have been described in detail elsewhere (J. Beck, 1995; Freeman, Pretzer, Fleming, & Simon, 1990; Persons, Davidson, & Tompkins, 2001), we briefly present them here.

Idiosyncratic Meaning. In many ways, our constructs determine our perceptions. The limits of our words are the limits of our world. The meanings attached to the patient's words and thoughts can be explored. The patient who believes, for example, that he will be "devastated" by his spouse leaving might be asked, in a supportive manner, what he means by "devastated." He may be asked to reflect on exactly how he would be devastated and then on the ways he might be spared from "devastation." All words carry an idiosyncratic or personal meaning. The exploration of these meanings models the need for active listening skills, increased communication, and the value of examining one's assumptions.

Questioning the Evidence. Individuals can be taught the value of questioning the evidence that they are using to maintain their beliefs. This involves systematically examining evidence in support of a belief, as well as evidence that is inconsistent with it. An examination of the reliability of the sources of the information might be made, and the individual might come to recognize that he or she has overlooked information that is inconsistent with their beliefs.

Reattribution. Patients often take responsibility for events and situations that are only minimally attributable to them. The therapist can help the patient distribute responsibility among all relevant parties.

Rational Responding. One of the most powerful techniques in cognitive therapy involves helping the patient to challenge dysfunctional thinking. The Dysfunctional Thought Record (DTR) is an ideal format for testing maladaptive beliefs. The process begins with patients identifying the thought, emotion, or situation that causes them difficulty. If the patient presents with an emotional issue (i.e., "I'm very sad"), the therapist needs to inquire as to the situations that engender the emotion and the attendant thoughts. If the patient presents with a thought (i.e., "I'm a loser"), the therapist ascertains the feelings and the situation. Finally, if the patient presents a situation (i.e., "My husband left me"), the therapist would endeavor to determine the thoughts and emotions that precede, accompany, and follow the event. Statements such as "I feel like a loser" are reframed as thoughts and the accompanying emotions are elicited. After the automatic thought has been identified, a "rational response" can be developed. Rational responding involves four steps: (1) a systematic examination of evidence supporting and refuting the belief, (2) the development of an alternative, more adaptive explanation or belief, (3) decatastrophizing the belief, and (4) identifying specific behavioral steps that can be taken to cope with the problem.

Examining Options and Alternatives. This involves working with patients to generate additional options. Suicidal patients, for example, often see their alternatives as so limited that death becomes a viable solution. Patients can be assisted to develop, and then to evaluate, alternative solutions.

Decatastrophizing. Patients are taught to examine whether they are overestimating the severity of a situation or the likelihood of a negative outcome. Through Socratic questioning they are encouraged to "keep the problem in perspective."

Fantasized Consequences. Patients are asked to describe a fantasy about a feared situation, their images of it, and the attendant concerns. In verbalizing their fantasies, patients can often see the irrationality of their ideas. If the fantasized consequences are realistic, the therapist can work with the patient to assess the danger and develop coping strategies.

Advantages and Disadvantages. By asking the patient to examine both the advantages and the disadvantages of both sides of an issue, a broader perspective can be achieved. This basic problem-solving technique is useful in gaining a perspective and then plotting a reasonable course of action.

Turning Adversity to Advantage. There are times that a seeming disaster can be used to advantage. Losing one's job can be, in some cases, the entry point to a new job or career. Having a deadline imposed may be seen as oppressive and unfair but may be used as a motivator. Patients are assisted in identifying strengths or competencies they have acquired through overcoming past adversities.

Guided Association/Discovery. In contrast to the psychodynamic technique of free association, guided association or discovery involves the therapist working with the patient to identify relationships between ideas, thoughts, and images by means of Socratic questioning. Also referred to as the "vertical" or "downward arrow" technique, the therapist provides conjunctions to patients' verbalizations and thus encourages them to identify a series of automatic thoughts. The use of statements such as "And then what?" or "And that means, what?" allows the therapist to guide patients toward an understanding of themes within their stream of automatic thoughts and to identify possible underlying schemata.

Use of Exaggeration or Paradox. There seems to be room at the extremes for only one position. By taking an idea to its extreme, the therapist can help to move the patient to a more moderate or adaptive position vis-à-vis a particular belief. Given their sensitivity to criticism, however, some patients may experience paradoxical interventions as making light of their problems. As such, the therapist who chooses to use the paradoxical or exaggeration techniques must have (1) a strong working relationship with the patient, (2) good timing, and (3) the good sense to know when to back away from the technique.

Scaling. For those patients who see things as all or nothing, the technique of scaling along a continuum can be quite useful. Scaling of emotions, for example, can lead patients to gain a sense of distance and perspective. A depressed patient who believes that he is "incompetent," for example, might first be asked to rate the strength of his belief in this statement on a 100-point scale. He can then be asked to establish anchor points for his belief—identifying the "most incompetent person in the world" (0) and the "most highly skilled and competent person in the world" (100). When asked to rate himself on the "competence scale" he has developed, he typically would recognize that he is neither entirely incompetent nor the most competent individual but that, like others, he has strengths and weaknesses and has at least a modicum of competence.

Externalization of Voices. Most individuals, when asked to reflect on their thoughts, can "hear" the voice of their thoughts in their head. When patients are asked to externalize these thoughts, they are in a better position to deal with these "voices" and thoughts. By having the therapist take the part of the dysfunctional voice, the patient can gain ex-

perience in responding adaptively. The therapist might begin, for example, by modeling rational responses to patients' verbalizations of their dysfunctional thoughts. After modeling a more adaptive or functional voice, the therapist can, in a graded manner, become an increasingly more difficult and dysfunctional voice for the patient. With practice, patients come to recognize the dysfunctional nature of their thoughts and can become better able to respond adaptively to them.

Self-Instruction. Meichenbaum (1977) and Rehm (1977) developed an extensive battery of self-instruction techniques that are useful in working with depressed or impulsive patients. Patients can be taught, for example, to offer direct self-instructions for more adaptive behavior as well as counterinstructions to avoid dysfunctional behavior.

Thought Stopping. Given the relationship between thoughts and mood, maladaptive automatic thoughts can have a "snowball effect" in that even mild feelings of dysphoria or anxiety can bias subsequent cognitive processes, leading the individual to feel continually more distraught. What started as a small and insignificant problem can easily gather weight, speed, and momentum. Thought stopping is best used when the negative emotional state is first recognized. Anxious patients, for example, can be taught to picture a stop sign or "hear a bell" at the outset of an anxiety attack. This momentary break in the process can allow them to reflect on the origin of the anxiety and to introduce more powerful cognitive techniques (such as rational responding) before their anxiety escalates.

Distraction. This technique is especially helpful for patients with anxiety problems. Because it is almost impossible to maintain two thoughts simultaneously, anxiogenic thoughts generally preclude more adaptive thinking. Conversely, a focused thought distracts from the anxiogenic thoughts. By having patients focus on complex counting, addition, or subtraction, they are rather easily distracted from other thoughts. Having the patient count to 200 by 13s, for example, can be effective, as can reading a page of text upside down. When outdoors, counting cars, people wearing the color red, or any cognitively engaging task will suffice. Distraction or refocusing of attention may be achieved by focusing on some aspect of the environment, engaging in mental exercise or imagery, or initiating physical activity. Although this technique is short term, it is useful to allow patients the time to establish some degree of control over their thinking. This time can then be used to introduce other cognitive techniques.

Direct Disputation. There are times at which direct disputation is helpful. When there is an imminent risk to the patient, as in the case of suicide, direct disputation might be considered. As these approaches are, in some regard, noncollaborative, the therapist risks becoming embroiled in a power struggle or argument with the patient. Disputation of core beliefs may, in fact, engender avoidance or a passive–aggressive response. Disputation, argument, or debate must be used carefully, judiciously, and with skill.

Labeling of Distortions. Fear of the unknown and "fear of fear" (Foa, Steketee, & Young, 1984) can be important concerns for anxious patients. The more that can be done to identify the nature and content of the dysfunctional thoughts and to help label the types of distortions that patients use, the less frightening the entire process becomes. Patients can be taught to identify and label specific distortions during the therapy session and can be asked to practice the exercise at home. This can be accomplished with the aid of a "thought record" on which patients record their automatic thoughts on an ongoing basis during the day, or with a counter with which they simply record the frequency of the thoughts.

Developing Replacement Imagery. Many anxious patients experience vivid images during times of stress. Inasmuch as their anxiety may be exacerbated by these images, patients can be helped by training in the development of "coping images." For example, rather than imagining failure, defeat, or embarrassment, the therapist assists the patient to develop a new, effective coping image. Once well practiced, patients can substitute these images outside the therapy session.

Bibliotherapy. Several excellent books can be assigned as readings for homework. These books can be used to educate patients about the basic cognitive therapy model, emphasize specific points made in the session, introduce new ideas for discussion, or offer alternative ways of thinking about patients' concerns. Some helpful books include *Love Is Never Enough* (A. Beck, 1989), *Feeling Good* (Burns, 1980), *Woulda, Coulda, Shoulda* (Freeman & DeWolfe, 1989), and *Mind over Mood* (Greenberger & Padesky, 1995).

Behavioral Techniques

Behavioral techniques are regularly used in CBT. Behavioral interventions can be used to test the validity of maladaptive thoughts and assumptions. By having the patient attempt feared or avoided behaviors, old ideas can be directly challenged. A second use of behavioral techniques is to practice new, more adaptive behaviors or coping strategies. Specific behaviors can be introduced in the office and then practiced at home. As with cognitive homework assignments, the therapist will want to review the thoughts and emotions experienced by patients as they attempted the behavioral assignment with them. Commonly employed behavioral interventions include the following:

Activity Scheduling. Activity scheduling is among the most widely used techniques in the therapist's armamentarium. For patients who are feeling overwhelmed, the activity schedule can be used to plan more effective time use. The activity schedule is both a retrospective tool to assess past time utilization and a prospective tool to help plan better time use.

Mastery, Pleasure, and Social Ratings. The activity schedule can also be used to assess and plan activities that offer patients a sense of personal efficacy or mastery, pleasure, and social connection. The greater the mastery, pleasure, and connectedness, the lower the rates of anxiety and depression.

Social Skills or Assertiveness Training. If patients lack specific social skills, the therapist helps them to develop them. This may involve anything from teaching patients how to properly shake hands, maintain appropriate eye contact, hold a conversation, or avoid excessively seeking reassurance.

Graded Task Assignments. Graded task assignments involve a series of small sequential steps that lead to the desired goal. By setting out a task and then arranging the necessary steps in a hierarchy, patients can be helped to make reasonable progress with a minimum of stress. As patients attempt each step, the therapist can be available for support and guidance.

Behavioral Rehearsal/Role Playing. Adaptive behaviors are practiced in session with the therapist serving as teacher and model. The therapist can monitor the patient's performance and offer suggestions for improvement. In addition, anticipated road blocks can be identified. There can be extensive rehearsal before the patient attempts the behavior in vivo.

In Vivo Exposure. There are times that therapy must take place outside the consulting room. Although this can be time-consuming, such *in vivo* therapy can be quite powerful. A therapist might, for example, accompany his or her patient into a feared situation, such as a supermarket or crowded shopping center. As noted earlier, the objective of in vivo exposure is not solely to allow patients to "habituate" to the feared setting but to provide them with incontrovertible behavioral evidence that is inconsistent with their dysfunctional beliefs.

Relaxation Training. Anxious and depressed patients often profit from relaxation training. Relaxation training can be taught in the office and then practiced by the patient at home. Although relaxation tapes are commercially available, we have found that therapists can easily create a tape incorporating images that the patient finds most relaxing and that focus on symptoms that are most distressing to these patients.

Homework

No therapy takes place solely within the confines of the consulting room. Insights and skills gained within the therapeutic milieu will, by their nature, be consolidated and employed in the patient's day-to-day life. This consolidation process, while implicit in many models of psychotherapy, is explicitly exploited in cognitive therapy. It is important for the patient to understand that practicing cognitive-behavioral skills at home allows for a greater therapeutic focus and for more rapid gains. As Burns and Auerbach (1992) observed in their review of factors associated with improvement in therapy, "differences in homework compliance are significantly correlated with recovery from depression."

Homework assignments can be either cognitive or behavioral. They might involve having the patient complete an activity schedule (an excellent homework for the first session) or a DTR or try a new behavior. The homework assignment should, when appropriately assigned, flow directly from the session material. It is simply an extension of the skill developed during the therapy hour into the patient's daily life. It is important to review homework assignments each week and reward progress. If completed homework assignments are not regularly discussed, the patient will come to see them as unimportant and will stop doing them.

Even assignments that are failed can be useful. A patient with social anxiety, for example, might anticipate rejection were he to talk to an unfamiliar person. A reasonable assignment might be to "talk to the salesclerks at the 7–11 where you buy your coffee each morning, and note their reactions." If the clerks respond positively to the patient (as one might expect they would) he will have an experience that is inconsistent with his beliefs and will begin to develop a new social skill. Suppose, however, the patient is not able to talk to the clerk but instead runs from the store, shrieking as the hot coffee spills down his shirt. All is not lost. In his recounting the episode in therapy we will gain access to that most important of information—his "hot cognitions"—the automatic thoughts that occur while he is anxious. These, in turn, are submitted to rational refutation and become further grist for the therapeutic mill.

Common Errors in Conducting Cognitive Therapy

To paraphrase Francis Bacon, it is easier to know a bad cake than it is to bake a good one. So it is with psychotherapy—it is often easier to identify shortcomings or difficulties in a therapy session than it is avoid them. There are, nonetheless, a number of common errors made in conducting cognitive therapy. These include (1) inadequate socialization of the patient to the model; (2) failure to develop a specific problem list or to share a rationale with the patient; (3) not assigning appropriate homework (and not following up on homework assignments that have been completed); (4) premature emphasis on identifying schemata; (5) therapist impatience; becoming overly directive during therapy in an attempt to immediately resolve the patient's symptoms; (6) premature introduction of rational techniques

(before a formulation has been completed); (7) lack of attention to developing a trusting collaborative rapport; inadequate attention to "nonspecific factors" of the therapy relationship; and (8) not attending to the therapist's own emotional reactions, automatic thoughts, and schemata—the countertransference.

Termination

Termination in cognitive therapy begins in the first session. As the goal of cognitive therapy is not cure per se but more effective coping, the cognitive therapist does not plan for therapy ad infinitum. As a skills acquisition model of psychotherapy, the therapist's goal is to assist patients in acquiring the capacity to deal with internal and external stressors that are a part of life. When the objective rating scales, patient report, therapist observations, and feedback from significant others confirm improvement and a higher level of adaptive abilities, the therapy can move toward termination. The final sessions typically include a review of the patient's presenting concerns, cognitive and behavioral skills they have developed over the course of treatment, and a discussion of upcoming events that may precipitate a relapse. Patients are taught to distinguish a lapse from a relapse, and coping strategies for managing difficult life circumstances are reviewed and practiced. Particular attention is paid to cognitive and behavioral factors that have been associated with relapse (such as perfectionism, excessive reassurance seeking, negative attributional style, hopelessness, and low personal efficacy). Goals during the final phase of treatment, then, center on consolidating gains and relapse prevention.

Although numerous outcome studies have found that cognitive therapy can be highly effective in 12–15 sessions, there is no typical duration for the treatment. In assisting patients with more severe or chronic difficulties, for example, we have found that meaningful gains can be achieved within several weeks as patients learn cognitive and behavioral techniques for coping with their feelings of depression, anxiety, and anger. Cognitive therapy can profitably continue for 2–3 years, however, as the assumptions and schemata underlying their difficulties are examined and addressed. Nonetheless, studies have failed to find a relationship between duration of therapy and effectiveness (Berman, Miller, & Massman, 1985; Miller & Berman, 1983; Shapiro & Shapiro, 1982). Rather, findings suggest that the significant gains often occur during the first 3 sessions and that benefits of continuing treatment beyond 12–15 sessions are modest. With this in mind, we have often found it useful to discuss the expected duration of therapy with patients at the outset and to negotiate a termination date or a set number of sessions in advance. This process encourages both the therapist and the patient to maintain a problem focus and maintains a sense of urgency in the treatment.

Termination in cognitive therapy is accomplished gradually to allow time for ongoing modifications and corrections. Sessions are tapered off from once weekly to biweekly. From that point, sessions can be set on a monthly basis, with follow-up sessions at 3 and 6 months until therapy is ended. Patients can, of course, still call for an appointment in the event of an emergency. Sometimes patients call simply to get some information or a reinforcement of a particular behavior or to report a success. With the cognitive therapist in the role of a consultant/collaborator, this continued contact is appropriate and important. As the conclusion of treatment nears, the patient's thoughts and feelings about the termination are carefully explored, as are schemata and assumptions regarding separation. The termination of therapy can have important meanings for the patient and can activate memories and schemata about separations from others in the patient's past (Mann, 1973; Safran & Segal, 1990). Termination can afford the therapist an opportunity to explore with patients their thoughts, feel-

ings, and characteristic ways of coping with separations. This is particularly important when working with patients whose histories suggest that they have responded to separations and losses in maladaptive ways. Such reactions are not uncommon among patients with personality disorders.

As noted earlier, it is essential for therapists to attend to their own emotional reactions and thoughts over the course of therapy (Leahy, 2001). This is nowhere more important than during the termination period. In addition to the therapist's feelings and beliefs about separation, one of the difficulties often encountered in doing cognitive therapy is the pressure to achieve significant improvement rapidly. Cognitive therapy, with its focus on strategic, observable gains can leave therapists with the belief that they are responsible for ensuring that the goals of the treatment are met. As is so often the case in life, our expectations and goals may not be fully realized, and important work may remain for the patient after the conclusion of treatment. Cognitive therapy views the mechanisms of therapeutic change as essentially similar to those underlying development over the lifespan. Cognitive and behavioral skills, insights, and new ways of understanding one's life that are acquired during therapy may sow the seeds of further growth after termination. As Safran and Segal (1990) cogently observed, the thoughts and emotions that emerge as the conclusion of therapy approaches have "significance for the patient's internal working model and for his or her relationship with the therapist"—thus, they should be examined carefully and utilized as an important part of the therapy process.

Noncompliance

Noncompliance, sometimes called resistance, often carries the implication that the patient does not want to change or "get well," for either conscious or unconscious reasons. Leahy (2001) defines resistance as "anything in the patient's behavior, thinking, affective response, and interpersonal style that interferes with the ability of that patient to utilize the treatment and to acquire the ability to handle problems outside of therapy. . ." (p. 11). This is, admittedly, a rather imprecise definition. It does, however, direct us to attend to the broad sweep of cognitive, behavioral, and social processes that hinder therapeutic progress. Resistance may be manifested directly (e.g., tardiness or missing of appointments and failure to complete homework) or more subtly through omissions in the material reported in the sessions. Clinically, we can identify several reasons for noncompliance. They can appear in any combination or permutation, and the relative strength of any noncompliant action may change with the patient's life circumstance, progress in therapy, relationship with the therapist, and so on. Several reasons for noncompliance are as follows:

1. Failure to validate the patient's emotional experience and beliefs.
2. Poorly developed adaptive skills (limited coping capacity).
3. Lack of therapist skill to help the patient change.
4. Environmental or social stressors preclude changing.
5. Patient cognitions regarding the possibility of failure.
6. Patient cognitions regarding possible negative consequences of their changing.
7. Patient and therapist distortions are congruent.
8. Poor socialization to the cognitive therapy model.
9. Secondary gain for a dysfunctional behavior.
10. Lack of collaboration in the therapeutic alliance.
11. Poor timing of interventions.
12. Failure to attend to patient's desire to maintain a stable, consistent view of themselves (schema protection)
13. Failure to address patients' "justifying" or "imperative" beliefs

14. Failure to develop a problem list or share therapeutic rationale.

TREATMENT APPLICABILITY

Cognitive Specificity Hypothesis

Of particular importance for the clinician is the "cognitive specificity hypothesis"—the postulate that emotional states (and clinical disorders) can be distinguished in terms of their specific cognitive contents and processes. Cognitive specificity directs our attention toward cognitive and behavioral processes that mediate specific disorders and that may serve as a focus of treatment. As noted, depression is characterized by a number of cognitive processes including the cognitive triad, perceptual and memory biases, negativistic attributional style, and problem-solving deficits. Depressed individuals tend to view themselves as flawed in important ways and lacking the requisite abilities for attaining important goals. They view their future as bleak and view others as uncaring and rejecting. Their views of themselves and their world are filtered through the dark prism of negativistic attributions and expectations. The schemata of depressed persons encompass associations related to themes of deprivation, loss, and personal inadequacy (Guidano & Liotti, 1983; Kovacs & Beck, 1978). Anxiety disorders, in contrast, stem from a generalized perception of threat in conjunction with a belief that one is unable to cope with the impending danger. Each of the specific anxiety disorders (obsessive–compulsive disorder, panic disorder, simple phobia, generalized anxiety disorder, social anxiety) can be distinguished by the nature of the perceived threat (Freeman et al., 1990). Other emotions (including anger, guilt, relief, dissappointment, despair, hope, resentment, jealousy, joy, pity, and pride) and clinical disorders (including personality disorders) also can be distinguished in terms of their specific cognitive contents and processes

(Beck et al., 1990; Ortony, Clore, & Collins, 1988). The cognitive specificity hypothesis is of central importance in the clinical practice of cognitive therapy in that it allows us to provide patients with a rationale for understanding emotional reactions that might otherwise be seen as inscrutable and allows us to target our interventions toward specific central beliefs and attitudes that mediate their distress. Our interventions will vary, as such, depending on the specific constellation of beliefs, expectations, attributions, and skill deficits that the patient demonstrates.

Treatment of Anxiety

This model suggests how cognitive, social, and behavioral factors interact in the development and treatment of disorders. As anxious individuals confront a situation (e.g., an upcoming exam), their perceptions of that event are influenced by their existing beliefs, memories, schemata, and assumptions. In evaluating the situation, they make two judgments—an assessment of the degree of risk or threat (which incorporates assessments of the severity of the outcome and the probability that it will occur) and an assessment of their ability to cope with that risk. If, for example, they believe that they are capable and well prepared and that the exam will have little bearing on their ultimate grade, they will not view the test as a threat but a challenge. If, however, they believe the exam is highly important and that they are not prepared, they will view the situation as threatening and will become anxious. Anxiety may be seen as an adaptive response to a perceived threat. Should the individual cope successfully with the threat (by studying strenuously and passing the exam), this experience will enhance his or her sense of self-efficacy and will inspire confidence in his or her ability to cope with future tests. If, however, the individual fails the exam or avoids the threat (by dropping the course), his or her perception of personal efficacy will decline and the belief that the situation was a legitimate threat will increase. As a consequence, the individual will become vigilant about similar situations in the future and will become more likely to avoid them. Treatment of anxiety disorders, then, involves reexamining beliefs, assumptions, and schemata; developing appropriate coping skills; enhancing perceptions of personal efficacy; decatastrophizing perceived threats; and discouraging avoidance or withdrawal.

Anxious individuals appear to share a number of beliefs and may demonstrate attentional biases toward threat relevant stimuli. Research suggests that anxious patients tend to believe that if a risk exists, it is adaptive to worry about it (anxious over concern), it is necessary to be competent and in control of situations (personal control/perfection), and it is adaptive to avoid problems or challenges (problem avoidance). Moreover, they tend to demonstrate heightened levels of anxiety sensitivity, self-focused attention, and deficits in emotion regulation. As noted, the common themes shared by each of the anxiety disorders are a perception of a threat and a belief that the threat cannot be managed or avoided. The threats may be real or imagined and are most often directed toward the person or the personal domain. Are all anxiety threats from without? Certainly not. Whereas legitimate external threats can contribute to feelings of anxiety—the possibility of losing one's job or spouse or of failing an exam, the large Doberman down the street, an IRS audit, one's brakes on an icy road—there are internal threats as well. These can include somatic sensations and emotions (as occur in panic disorder) and thoughts (as in obsessive–compulsive disorder), as well as images, impulses, and fantasies. All, however, are similar in that they are perceived as endangering our physical, psychological, emotional, or social well-being.

The cognitive model of anxiety involves several elements. Anxiety, being an adaptive response to one's environment, begins with the perception of threat in a specific situation. As noted, the meaning individuals attach to the situation is determined by their schemata and by their memories of similar situations in their past. The individual then makes an assessment of the seriousness of the threat and an evaluation of his or her ability to cope with it. If the situation is viewed as threatening, a sense of danger will ensue. If a mild threat is perceived, the individual will respond to it as a challenge. The individual will feel excitement and enthusiasm. Cognitive and perceptual processes can be affected by an individual's current mood (Bower, 1981). In this case, when an individual begins feeling anxious, he or she is likely to become even more vigilant to perceived threats and will begin to recall threatening experiences in his or her past. The individual may come, as a consequence, to perceive threat where none existed before.

The course of cognitive therapy for anxiety disorders follows from the foregoing discussion of general principles. In conceptualizing an individual's anxiety, we begin by assessing his or her "anxiety threshold" or ability to tolerate anxiety. Each person has a general anxiety threshold as well as an ability to tolerate anxiety in specific situations. These thresholds may shift in response to stresses in the individual's day-to-day life and supports that are available to the individual. The therapist begins, then, by asking what specific events, situations, or interactions trigger the individual to become anxious.

Next, an assessment is made of automatic thoughts accompanying the feelings of anxiety. Although the thoughts of anxious individuals often incorporate themes of threat and vulnerability, their specific content can be quite personal or idiosyncratic and may be related to a specific syndrome. As the cognitive specificity hypothesis suggests, each of the anxiety disorders can be distinguished on the basis of its accompanying cognitive contents and processes. *Panic disorder,* for example, is characterized by a sensitivity or vigilance to physical sensations and

a tendency to make catastrophic interpretations of these somatic feelings. Momentary feelings of dizziness, for example, might be interpreted as evidence of an aneurysm or brain tumor. *Agoraphobia* typically involves a fear of being unable to rapidly reach a "safety zone," such as one's house—leading the individual to avoid cars, planes, crowded rooms, bridges, and other places where ready escape might be blocked. *Phobias,* in contrast, stem from a fear of specific objects (such as a large dog) or a situation (such as speaking in public). *Obsessive–compulsive disorder* is characterized by a fear of specific thoughts or behaviors, whereas *generalized anxiety disorder* involves a more pervasive sense of vulnerability and a fear of physical or psychological danger.

When people enter a situation they make several evaluations. The first is, "What risk do I perceive for myself in this situation." Second is an assessment of the personal or environmental resources that may be available to the individual. If people perceive their resources as adequate to cope with the risk, they typically do not experience anxiety. Cognitive interventions are directed toward reducing the perception of threat and toward increasing an individual's confidence in his or her ability to cope with the situation. Before intervening, however, it is important to assess whether the threat is "perceived or real," whether the individual actually lacks the skills to cope with the situation, and whether the patient's perception of limited resources is veridical.

Personality traits of autonomy and sociotropy/dependence (Beck, Epstein, & Harrison, 1983) appear to influence the ways in which individuals cope with anxiety-provoking situations. Autonomous individuals typically adopt a goal-oriented stance and prefer to "take action," whereas sociotropic individuals typically seek support, reassurance, or protection from others.

The usual responses to stress are fight, flight, or freeze. Highly autonomous individuals, when stressed, will typically attempt to "solve it themselves." They rarely seek help spontaneously and do not come into therapy willingly. They often describe their anxiety in terms of vague physiological symptoms and may feel trapped and encroached on during therapy sessions. The therapist who attempts to engender a warm, close rapport with the autonomous patient, or who gives direct recommendations or homework assignments, may find the patient becoming more anxious and possibly leaving therapy.

Dependent or sociotropic individuals, in contrast, enter therapy willingly. They often feel immobilized by their anxiety and actively seek guidance and support from others. They may ask how often they can come for therapy and may become concerned that if they do not tell the therapist everything, the therapist's ability to help will be impaired. When stressed, dependent patients become vulnerable to feelings of abandonment. They are typically compliant in following therapeutic recommendations and diligent in completing homework assignments. Nonetheless, their tendency to defer to others and to seek reassurance or guidance from others limits their ability to cope with life's problems independently. Thus, a goal of therapy is to encourage them to accept greater responsibility for identifying problems and generating alternative solutions.

Not all anxiety reactions are the same. Rather, symptom patterns vary from person to person. One individual may experience predominantly physical symptoms—such as tachycardia, difficulty breathing, dizziness, indigestion, wobbliness, or hot flashes—necessitating the development of an individualized treatment program. Another individual's anxiety, however, might be characterized by "fears of the worst" happening and thoughts of losing control. Their treatment program would be somewhat different. When treating anxiety disorders, it is helpful to keep this variability in mind and to address each of the component symptoms individually.

As with other clinically important problems, treatment of anxiety begins with the development of a parsimonious case conceptualization. By adopting a phenomenolgical stance, we attempt to understand the individual's thoughts, feelings, and behavioral responses as they are confronted with anxiety-provoking situations. Questions to be addressed include the following:

- Is the patient in real danger, or is his or her response out of proportion to threat?
- What attributions does the patient make as to the cause of the anxiety?
- Has the patient accurately assessed his or her own abilities, or does the therapist hold erroneous and distorted views of personal efficacy and competence?
- What expectations does the patient hold regarding his or her behavior and the behavior of others? Are the expectations for self (or therapist) reasonable?
- What are the dysfunctional automatic thoughts and cognitive distortions that accompany the anxiety?
- What are the schemata and assumptions that maintain the patient's anxiety?
- What behavioral skills are needed to cope more effectively?
- Does the patient engage in maladaptive behaviors (e.g., avoidance, drug use, self-focused attention, or excessive seeking of reassurance) that may be exacerbating his or her feelings of vulnerability?

Consideration of these questions will guide the therapist toward a more systematic and effective treatment program. Interventions would be directed toward addressing the specific beliefs and coping deficits that are identified.

Personality Disorders

Personality disorders refer to enduring patterns of thought, perception, and interpersonal relatedness that are inflexible and maladaptive. They tend to occur in a range of settings and are often accompanied by significant distress. More often than not, they greatly impair the individual's social or occupational functioning. They are both chronic and pernicious. Personality disorders differ from other clinically important problems (e.g., major depression or anxiety disorders) in that they tend not to fluctuate over time and are not characterized by discrete periods of distress.

Like other problems discussed, each of the personality disorders can be described in terms of a specific constellation of cognitive contents and processes (Freeman, 2002; Layden et al., 1993; Sperry, 1999). The schemata of a dependent individual, for example, tend to be characterized by beliefs of the form, "I am a flawed or incapable person" (self), "The world is a dangerous place" (world), and by the assumption, "If I can maintain a close relationship with a supportive person, then I can feel secure." As a consequence, the individual with a dependent personality disorder continually seeks relationships with others, fears the loss of relationships, and feels despondent and anxious when deprived of the support of others.

A schizoid individual, in contrast, may also hold the belief that "the world is a dangerous place" (world), but also maintains the schema, "Others are dangerous or malevolent" (world), and the assumption, "If I can avoid intimate relationships with others, then I can feel secure." The behavioral and emotional responses of such an individual, as a consequence, are quite different. Such an individual tends to be indifferent to the praise or criticism of others, to maintain few close friendships, and to be emotionally aloof from others. As one patient succinctly stated, "My dream is to get through law school so I can get a lot of money . . . then I'd buy an island . . . I'd never have to deal with anyone, that would be ideal."

Personality disorders reflect the activity of maladaptive schemata and assumptions (Beck et al., 1990; Bricker, Young, & Flannagan, 1993; Freeman, 1993, 2002; Young, 1991). Although these schemata may have been adaptive in the context in which they were developed, they have lost their func-

tional value. As the beliefs underlying personality disorders are tacit, they are not open to direct refutation. As a consequence, patients tend (at least initially) not to view their perceptions, thoughts, or behavior as problematic. Their difficulties are ego-syntonic. Rather, they believe that the problems reside in others. As the "complaining woman" described earlier remarked, "I'm just identifying problems . . . *they* have to change them." She believed that her behavior was both appropriate and rational, and that she was doing a service to others by pointing out their shortcomings.

Because their difficulties are ego-syntonic, individuals with personality disorders typically seek treatment due to other concerns—most often feelings of depression, anxiety, or anger or difficulties maintaining jobs or relationships. It is important to remember that the patient's goals in seeking treatment may not be shared with others (including the therapist). If a patient is not willing to work on "core" issues, therapy may still prove useful by providing the patient with techniques for controlling his or her feelings of depression or anxiety and by assisting the patient to develop trusting relationships. Although more time-consuming, the gradual uncovering of schemata through guided discovery and the demonstration that they are maladaptive through Socratic questioning can be far more fruitful than direct confrontation.

Cognitive therapy of personality disorders differs from short-term cognitive psychotherapy in that it incorporates a more comprehensive exploration of the developmental origins of the schemata (a "developmental analysis") and examines the ways in which the schemata are expressed in the therapeutic relationship. Unlike psychodynamic psychotherapy, however, the cognitive therapist does not focus on the transference relationship as a means of permitting interpretation of underlying drives, defenses, or ego functioning. As in other approaches, the development of an angry or depressive relationship with the therapist may undermine therapeutic collaboration. Such negative perceptions, attributions, or expectations are challenged directly and the therapeutic relationship serves as evidence that the tacit belief is not true.

The therapeutic relationship plays a central role in the treatment of personality disorders. The therapeutic relationship serves as a microcosm of the patient's responses to others. The sensitive nature of the relationship means that the therapist must exercise great care. Being even 2 minutes late for a session with the dependent personality may elicit anxiety about abandonment. The same 2-minute lateness will raise the specter of being taken advantage of by the paranoid personality.

It is often valuable to discuss the time frame for treatment with patients at the outset of therapy. Many patients, for example, may have read of cognitive therapy and expect that they will be "cured" in 12–20 sessions. Given the greater severity and chronicity of their difficulties, however, a longer time frame might be anticipated. Although patients may expect some symptomatic improvement within a relatively short period, a longer time is necessary to identify and change tacit beliefs (12–20 months is a far more reasonable time frame).

Cognitive therapy of personality disorders is a rapidly evolving area for clinical theory and research. Although few controlled outcome studies have yet been completed, our clinical experience suggests that the model provides a parsimonious means of understanding a range of persistent and self-defeating patterns of thought, emotion, and behavior. The potential value of cognitive therapy for treating these most challenging patients, though not yet realized, is great.

CASE ILLUSTRATION

Presenting Problems

Bob, 20 years of age, was living with his parents at the time of his referral for cogni-

tive therapy. He was working part-time as a box boy at a local parts warehouse and had recently taken a leave of absence from a prestigious university. Bob was mildly obese and although appropriately attired, had an unkempt, disheveled look—as if he had not showered in several days. He walked with a heavy, plodding gait, and he mumbled, making his speech difficult to understand. Eye contact was poor, and his speech was driven and rambling. His diagnoses at the time of his referral were bipolar disorder and depressed and avoidant personality disorder.

Bob's presenting concerns included a history of severe depression, suicidality, feelings of worthlessness, social anxiety, manic episodes (characterized by decreased sleep, agitation, constant talking, irrational spending, grandiose delusions, and motoric overactivity), and poor social skills. He had participated in psychoanalysis four times a week for several years and had received trials of a number of medications—all to no avail. Although his episodes of mania were reasonably well controlled by lithium (which he took regularly), his feelings of depression continued to worsen. Bob had been hospitalized twice due to suicidal ideations, and his psychiatrist had recommended he be placed in a residential treatment program due to his deteriorating condition. His parents were interested in a second opinion before placing their son in a long-term treatment facility and felt that cognitive therapy was their "last hope."

Initial Assessment

Complete developmental, social, and medical histories were obtained and a battery of objective rating scales were administered in order to gain a clearer idea of his problems. Bob's scores on the BDI, BAI, and HS were 28, 51, and 19, respectively. These scores are indicative of clinically severe depression, anxiety, and pessimism. His responses on the Minnesota Multiphasic Personality Inventory (MMPI) yielded a 2–8–7 profile, with concomitant elevations of scales 3, 4, and 10. His responses on the MMPI were similar to those of persons who are highly anxious, depressed, agitated, and tense. Bob was dependent and unassertive in his relationships with others and felt unable to meet the challenges of day-to-day life. His responses on a series of automatic thought questionnaires revealed that he was highly concerned that others like him, that he experienced difficulty being alone, and that he "could not avoid thinking about his past mistakes."

Background

Bob was the younger of two children and had grown up in an affluent suburb and attended exclusive schools. Although he had done quite well academically during his elementary and high school years, his interpersonal and emotional functioning were quite poor. He was plagued by feelings of self-doubt and worthlessness and made self-critical comparisons with others on an almost continual basis. He believed that others were of "stellar quality" and that he was "stupid and a fraud." When asked to elaborate, Bob noted that although he had graduated near the top of his high school class, his father had written many of his papers. While away at college, Bob began to withdraw. He rarely attended class, and during one fire drill remained in his room "hoping to be killed in the flames." After several weeks of desperate calls to his parents and increasing suicidal ideations, Bob returned home. His father, concerned by possible repercussions of leaving the university, devised an elaborate story that Bob needed to return home as his mother was having brain surgery. When he returned home, his father was disappointed and could not tell anyone in the family or community about it. To protect his secret, whenever they left the house Bob was required to lie on the floor of the car, covered by a blanket.

Although Bob had done well academically and had attempted to be a "perfect child," he struggled internally with feelings of anger, depression, and inadequacy. He reported experiencing sadistic fantasies of attacking children in the neighborhood and recalled having made obscene phone calls to an 8-year-old boy while he was in high school.

Cognitive Formulation

Bob's depression and anxiety were superimposed on a self-critical and perfectionistic personality style. He maintained high, even grandiose, standards for his own performance (e.g., believing that he needed to earn the Nobel Prize in literature) and anticipated rejection from anyone who would come to know him. Bob's beliefs and actions were characteristic of many depressed individuals and fit well with cognitive models of depression. Negative views of the self, world, and future, for example, were readily apparent in thoughts. His social skills were poor, and he tended to behave in ways that led others to withdraw from him. Bob's social problem-solving capacities were poorly developed, and he engaged in few activities that would provide a sense of accomplishment or pleasure. When he did do well on a task, he would minimize the significance of his accomplishment and would begin recounting past failures. He tended to respond to feelings of depression and anxiety though rumination and withdrawal rather than through adaptive coping. Given the information available to this point, one might conceptualize Bob's difficulties as follows:

Behavioral coping strategies
Avoidance or withdrawal
Seeking reassurance from others

Cognitive distortions
Dichotomizing (e.g.,"if I'm not right, I must be wrong . . . I can't even think right").
Selective abstraction (e.g., "I wasn't comfortable in class that first day, it didn't feel right knew it, that just tells you I'll never make it in college").

Personalization (e.g., "Everybody was sitting at other tables in the cafeteria . . . it shows nobody likes me").

"Should" statements (e.g., "I should be smarter and do more . . . I have to").

Magnification/minification (e.g., "I know he sent me a letter about how much he liked my class, but it doesn't mean anything . . . it doesn't count").

Catastrophizing (e.g., "I'm incompetent at life . . . I have no abilities").

Self-critical comparison (e.g., "Everyone is better than me, I can't even blow a bubble").

Automatic thoughts

"I'm so stupid . . . I'm an unintelligent jerk."

"People will discover I'm a fake."

"I'll never be a success."

"My life is meaningless . . . I have no one to share it with."

"I'm really disturbed . . . I have a hollow head."

Assumptions

"If I can avoid others, then I can feel secure."

"If I'm successful, then I can feel good about myself."

Schemata

"I'm fundamentally defective" (self).

"The world is a dangerous place" (world).

"People are unreliable and unsupportive" (social relations).

Course of Therapy

The first goals in treatment were to establish trust and rapport, develop a problem list, and educate Bob about the process of cognitive therapy. During the initial sessions, Bob invariably appeared sad and anxious. He maintained a pessimistic outlook and continually sought reassurance from the therapist that he was "OK." Bob expressed a great deal of anger about his limited progress in psychoanalysis and was skeptical about cognitive therapy. We began, then, with a discussion of his feelings about therapy, what he had learned in his analysis, and what his goals were for the future. He conceded that he had developed a number of important insights during his analysis, and that he "really didn't know much" about cognitive therapy. Bob remarked that he just wanted "to be an average person in college"—a reasonable and appropriate goal—and agreed to read a short book on cognitive therapy before our next session. His first formal homework assignment was to "write down his thoughts when he was feeling upset during the week"—an initial step toward completing a DTR (Beck et al., 1979).

Bob's feelings of dysphoria and anxiety became more severe as he became adept at identifying his automatic thoughts. This is not uncommon and appears to reflect patients' increasing sensitivity to thoughts they had been attempting to avoid. Rational responding, a countering technique (McMullin, 1986), was introduced to alleviate these feelings. Bob was asked to write down his thoughts when he was feeling particularly depressed or anxious. He then systematically examined evidence for and against each of the distressing thoughts (rational disputation), listed alternative ways of thinking about the evidence (reattribution), and developed more adaptive ways of coping with the concerns (decatastrophizing and search for alternative solutions). As noted, for example, Bob felt he was "an unintelligent jerk." A brief review of Bob's recent past revealed that although he had left several schools, he had graduated near the top of his high school class, had received a score of 1580 (out of 1600) on his college entrance exam, and had been admitted to the honors program at an Ivy League university. Taken together, the evidence suggested that Bob was not unintelligent. In fact, he was quite bright. A more parsimonious (and reasonable) interpretation of his experiences was that he lacked confidence in his abilities given events during junior and senior high school, and he was unprepared to cope with the anxiety of moving away from his home and parents. A goal of therapy would be to develop skills to accomplish this goal.

Given his low motivation and social isolation, Bob next was encouraged to begin completing daily "activities schedules" (Beck et al. , 1979). He wrote down his activities on an hour-by-hour basis, then rated them as to their degree of "mastery/sense of accomplishment" and "pleasure/fun." As might be expected, Bob engaged in few activities that provided him with a sense of worth, accomplishment, or enjoyment. Depressed patients such as Bob often avoid challenging tasks and experience difficulty completing tasks they had accomplished with ease before the onset of their depression. Thoughts that "I can't do it" and "What's the point?" inhibit them from engaging in activities that might provide them with a sense of competence or pleasure. Moreover, their avoidance of tasks and impaired performance serves as further evidence that "there's something wrong with me . . . I can't do it." Activity scheduling serves to directly counteract these processes. Bob and his therapist developed a list of simple activities he would attempt each day. He was encouraged, for example, to get out of bed at 10:00 A.M. and take a shower (rather than lounging in bed until midafternoon), to call a friend on the phone, to accept an invitation from a friend to play cards, and to go to the local gym for a swim. As Bob began to employ these techniques, his feelings of anxiety and dysphoria began to decline. These gains were reflected in Bob's improving scores on several objective rating scales. His scores on the BDI, for example, declined from a 28 (severe) at week 2 of treatment to a 9 (mild) at week 23. His scores on the BAI declined from a 51 (severe) to a 3 (negligible anxiety) during this same period.

To paraphrase Freud, the important goals of life are to love and to work. With this in mind, we were not content to note reductions in Bob's feelings of dysphoria and anxiety but wished to address larger issues in his life—his inability to develop close relationships with others and to live independently from his parents. Behavioral interventions (such as modeling appropriate eye contact and role playing basic conversational skills) were introduced to develop Bob's social skills, and a hierarchy of social activities (beginning with playing cards with his friends and concluding with going on a "date" with a woman) was established. Bob was able to progress through the hierarchy over several months but encountered a great deal of anxiety with each new step. Relaxation training, rational responding, guided imagery, and role playing of the activities were useful in helping Bob to develop these skills.

At the same time, Bob was encouraged to consider ways of returning to college. As he was highly anxious about leaving home (his last two attempts to live on his own had ended in psychiatric hospitalizations), Bob began by taking night classes at a local university. Not surprisingly, he did quite well. His tendency to minimize these accomplishments was addressed directly in therapy, as was the effect of these accomplishments on his mood and self-esteem. After approximately 6 months, Bob began discussing the possibility of applying to college once again. His fears of another "breakdown," as well as his uncertainty about possible majors and careers, became the focus of therapy. Once again, he began seeking reassurance from the therapist that he would "be OK." This provided an opportunity for examining experiences that had contributed to the consolidation of his schemata and the ways they were reflected in the therapy relationship. It was noted, for example, that Bob frequently sought reassurance and assistance from his mother during his childhood, and that his father's attempts to assist him with his homework during high school had maintained his belief that he was "incompetent" and "stupid." Bob acknowledged that reassurance (whether from his therapist or his parents) did little to alleviate these feelings, and that his search for support precluded him from solving problems on his own. Experiences during his childhood that were inconsistent with these beliefs were examined, and Bob was encouraged to "test out" the current validity of the beliefs by completing tasks without seeking support or reassurance.

Bob was subsequently accepted at a major university several hundred miles from home. Before leaving for college, however, we felt it would be beneficial for him to have an experience that would give him confidence that he could live alone. Rather than continuing with his job as a box boy, Bob applied for a position as a relief worker in a small South American village. During his 6 weeks away from home, Bob was confronted with numerous challenges that previously he would have felt he could not handle. He returned home with a new (longer) hairstyle, an earring, and a developing sense of identity as an individual who might be able to help others. Bob left for college several weeks later. After a difficult first year, he became a residence hall counselor and his grades began to stabilize. Booster sessions were held approximately once a month. Therapy was concluded after approximately 3 years. Bob graduated from college, began teaching inner-city children in another state, and has been accepted to graduate school. Although he remains somewhat anxious and self-critical, he has become able to function autonomously. The gains made over the course of treatment are reflected not only in his improved scores on objective rating scales but also in the quality of his life. The goals of therapy were not limited to the alleviation of depression and anxiety but included a focus on latent beliefs and the establishment of an adult identity. Individuation from his parents, a return to school, the development of career goals, and the acquisition of social skills were all important objectives.

This case illustrates how strategic interventions can be employed in treating severe and long-standing psychological difficulties.

The treatment of this individual was multifaceted and incorporated traditional cognitive and behavioral approaches, as well as interpersonal interventions focusing on the ways in which unstated beliefs or schemata were expressed in the therapeutic relationship (Safran & McMain, 1992; Safran & Segal, 1990). Social problem solving, rational responding, attributional retraining, behavioral skill training, and developmental analysis of underlying schemata and assumptions all played a role. With the exception of three family sessions, Bob's parents were not included in his treatment. This was explicitly discussed with Bob—a goal of therapy was to encourage him to accept responsibility for the course of his treatment and to function more autonomously.

CONCLUSION

The usefulness of cognitive therapy for treating a range of behavioral and emotional difficulties has been well established. Refined models of depression and the anxiety disorders have been proposed and have generated a great deal of empirical interest. Controlled studies of cognitive therapy's effectiveness in the treatment of other clinically important problems, however, remain to be completed. Moreover, the processes underlying change over the course of therapy are not well understood. What specific cognitive and behavioral techniques, for example, are most closely associated with clinical improvement? Do rationalistic and constructivist variants of cognitive therapy differ with regard to their effectiveness in treating specific disorders? What changes in patients over the course of their treatment? Cognitive models of psychopathology will continue to evolve in response to the needs of our patients and the results of empirical research. Although important practical and conceptual problems remain, cognitive therapy stands as a useful paradigm for understanding human adaptation and for improving the quality of our patients' lives.

SUGGESTIONS FOR FURTHER READING

Beck, A. T., Rush, A. J., Shaw, B. F., & Emery, G. (1979). *Cognitive therapy of depression.* New York: Guilford Press.—The original manual for cognitive therapy of depression and suicide.

Beck, J. (1995). *Cognitive therapy: Basics and beyond.* New York: Guilford Press.—This clinical text reviews strategies and techniques of cognitive therapy and provides practical recommendations for addressing more complex clinical issues.

Dobson, K. S. (Ed.). (2001). *Handbook of cognitive-behavioral therapies* (2nd ed.) New York: Guilford Press.—More than a compendium of techniques, the authors offer critical reviews of recent research and suggest areas of inquiry.

Freeman, A., & Reinecke, M. (1993). *Cognitive therapy of suicidal behavior.* New York: Springer.—These authors propose an expanded cognitive model of suicidality that incorporates developmental, biological, and social factors, and includes numerous case examples and clinical vignettes.

Freeman, A., Simon, K., Beutler, L., & Arkowitz, H. (Eds.). (1989). *Comprehensive handbook of cognitive therapy.* New York: Plenum Press.—An expansive text that lives up to its title. It is comprehensive, scholarly, and, as a handbook, clinically useful.

Guidano, V. F., & Liotti, G. (1983). *Cognitive processes and emotional disorders.* New York: Guilford Press.—A thoughtful, although sometimes dense, introduction to the constructivist school of cognitive therapy. The discussions of depression and obsessive–compulsive disorder are particularly good.

Mahoney, M. (1991). *Human change processes.* New York: Basic Books.—An exceptionally strong discussion of cognitive processes mediating behavior and emotional change. Cognitive therapy is placed in a historical context and its relationship to the fields of philosophy, evolutionary biology, and developmental psychology are reviewed.

Persons, J., Davidson, J., & Tokins, M. (2001). *Essential components of cognitive-behavior therapy for depression.* Washington, DC: American Psychological Association.—This book and its accompanying video provide an overview of empirically supported psychotherapy for depression.

Safran, J., & Segal, Z. (1990). *Interpersonal process in cognitive therapy.* New York: Basic Books.—This book addresses a common criticism of cognitive therapy—that it does not attend to interpersonal factors in psychotherapy. They propose a cognitive-constructivist model for understanding the transference relationship, and provide recommendations for employing the therapeutic relationship to facilitate change.

REFERENCES

Abramson, L., Alloy, L., Hogan, M., Whitehouse, W., Cornette, M., Akhavan, S., & Chiara, A. (1998). Suicidality and cognitive vulnerability to depression among college students: A prospective study. *Journal of Adolescence, 21,* 157–171.

Abramson, L., Alloy, L., & Metalsky, G. (1988). The cognitive diathesis–stress theories of depression: Toward an adequate evaluation of the theories' validities. In L. B. Alloy (Ed.), *Cognitive processes in depression* (pp. 3–30). New York: Guilford Press.

Abramson, L., Metalsky, G., & Alloy, L. (1989). Hopelessness depression: A theory-based subtype of depression. *Psychological Review, 96*(2), 358–372.

Abramson, L., Seligman, M., & Teasdale, J. (1978). Learned helplessness in humans: Critique and reformulation. *Journal of Abnormal Psychology, 87,* 49–74.

Adler, A. (1927). *Understanding human nature.* New York: Fawcett.

Adler, A. (1968). *The practice and theory of individual psychology.* New York: Humanities Press.

Agency for Health Care Policy and Research. (1993). *Depression in primary care: Treatment of major depression.* (AHCPR Publication No. 93-0551). Rockville, MD: U.S. Government Printing Office.

Alloy, L., Abramson, L., Metalsky, G., & Hartlage, S. (1988). The hopelessness theory of depression: Attributional aspects. *British Journal of Clinical Psychology, 27,* 5–21.

Alloy, L., Abramson, L., Hogan, M., Whitehouse, W., Rose, D., Robinson, M., Kim, R., & Lapkin, J. (2000). The Temple–Wisconsin cognitive vulnerability to depression project: Lifetime history of Axis I psychopathology in individuals at high and low cognitive risk for depression. *Journal of Abnormal Psychology, 109*(3), 403–418.

American Psychiatric Association. (1998). Practice guideline for the treatment of patients with panic disorder. *American Journal of Psychiatry, 155,* 1–34.

American Psychiatric Association. (2000). Practice guideline for the treatment of patients with major depressive disorder (rev.). *American Journal of Psychiatry, 157*(Suppl. 4).

Arieti, S. (1980). Cognition in psychoanalysis. *Journal of the American Academy of Psychoanalysis, 8,* 3–23.

Bandura, A. (1973). *Aggression: A social learning analysis.* Englewood Cliffs, NJ: Prentice-Hall.

Bandura, A. (1977a). Self-efficacy: Towards a unifying theory of behavior change. *Psychological Review, 84,* 191–215.

Bandura, A. (1977b). *Social learning theory.* Englewood Cliffs, NJ: Prentice-Hall.

Bates, A., & Clark, D. M. (1998). A new cognitive treatment for social phobia: A single-case study. *Journal of Cognitive Psychotherapy: An International Quarterly, 12,* 289–302.

Beck, A. T. (1963). Thinking and depression: I. Idiosyncratic content and cognitive distortions. *Archives of General Psychiatry, 9,* 324–333.

Beck, A. T. (1972). *Depression: Causes and treatment.* Philadelphia: University of Pennsylvania Press.

Beck, A. T. (1976). *Cognitive therapy and the emotional disorders.* New York: International Universities Press.

Beck, A. (1989). *Love is never enough.* New York: HarperCollins.

Beck, A. T., Brown, G., & Steer, R. (1989). Prediction of eventual suicide in psychiatric inpatients by clinical ratings of hopelessness. *Journal of Consulting and Clinical Psychology, 57*(2), 309–310.

Beck, A. T., Epstein, N., Brown, G., & Steer, R. (1988). An inventory for measuring clinical anxiety. *Journal of Consulting and Clinical Psychology, 56,* 893–897.

Beck, A. T., Epstein, N., & Harrison, R. (1983). Cognitions, attitudes and personality dimensions in depression. *British Journal of Cognitive Psychotherapy, 1*(1), 1–16.

Beck, A. T., Freeman, A., & Associates. (1990).

Cognitive therapy of personality disorders. New York: Guilford Press.

Beck, A. T., Hollon, S., Young, J., Bedrosian, R., & Budenz, D. (1985). Combined cognitive-pharmacotherapy versus cognitive therapy in the treatment of depressed outpatients. *Archives of General Psychiatry, 42,* 142–148.

Beck, A. T., Rush, A. J., Shaw, B. F., & Emery, G. (1979). *Cognitive therapy of depression.* New York: Guilford Press.

Beck, A. T., Sokol, L., Clark, D., Berchick, R., & Wright, F. (1992). A crossover study of focused cognitive therapy for panic disorder. *American Journal of Psychiatry, 149*(6), 778–783.

Beck, A. T., & Steer, R. (1987). *Manual for the revised Beck Depression Inventory.* San Antonio, TX: Psychological Corporation.

Beck, A. T., Ward, C., Mendelson, M., Mock, J., & Erbaugh, J. (1961). An inventory for measuring depression, *Archives of General Psychiatry, 4,* 561–571.

Beck, A. T., Weissman, S., Lester, D., & Trexler, L. (1974). The measurement of pessimism: The hopelessness scale. *Journal of Consulting and Clinical Psychology, 42,* 861–865.

Beck, J. (1995). *Cognitive therapy: Basics and beyond.* New York: Guilford Press.

Berman, J., Miller, R., & Massman, P. (1985). Cognitive therapy versus systematic desensitization: Is one treatment superior? *Psychological Bulletin, 97,* 451–461.

Blackburn, I., Bishop, S. Glen, A, I., Walley, L., & Christie, J. (1981). The efficacy of cognitive therapy in depression: A treatment using cognitive therapy and pharmacotherapy, each alone and in combination. *British Journal of Psychiatry, 139,* 181–189.

Blackburn, I., Eunson, K., & Bishop, S. (1986). A two year naturalistic follow-up of depressed patients treated with cognitive therapy, pharmacotherapy, and a combination of both. *Journal of Affective Disorders, 10,* 67–75.

Blackburn, I., & Moore, R. (1997). Controlled acute and follow-up trial of cognitive therapy and pharmacotherapy in outpatients with recurrent depression. *British Journal of Psychiatry, 171,* 328–334.

Blowers, C., Cobb, J., & Mathews, A. (1987). Generalized anxiety: A controlled treatment study. *Behavior Research and Therapy, 25,* 493–502.

Borkovec, T., & Costello, E. (1993). Efficacy of applied relaxation and cognitive-behavioral therapy in the treatment of generalized anxiety disorder. *Journal of Consulting and Clinical Psychology, 61,* 611–619.

Bower, G. (1981). Mood and memory. *American Psychologist, 36,* 129–148.

Bowlby, J. (1985). The role of childhood experience in cognitive disturbance. In M. Mahoney & A. Freeman (Eds.), *Cognition and psychotherapy* (pp. 181–200). New York: Plenum Press.

Bricker, D., Young, J., & Flannagan, C. (1993). Schema-focused cognitive therapy: A comprehensive framework for characterological problems. In K. Kuehlwein & H. Rosen (Eds.), *Cognitive therapy in action: Evolving innovative practice* (pp. 88–125). San Francisco: Jossey-Bass.

Bruner, J., Goodnow, J., & Austin, G. (1956). *A study of thinking.* New York: Wiley.

Burns, D. (1980). *Feeling good.* New York: Morrow.

Burns, D., & Auerbach, A. (1992). Does homework compliance enhance recovery from depression. *Psychiatric Annals, 22*(9), 464–469.

Butler, G., Cullington, A., Hibbert, G., Klimes, I., & Gelder, M. (1987). Anxiety management for persistent generalized anxiety. *British Journal of Psychiatry, 151,* 535–542.

Butler, G., Fennell, M., Robson, P., & Gelder, M. (1991). Comparison of behavior therapy and cognitive behavior therapy in the treatment of generalized anxiety disorder. *Journal of Consulting and Clinical Psychology, 59*(1), 167–175.

Butler, G., & Wells, A. (1995). Cognitive-behavioral treatments: Clinical applications. In R. G. Heimberg, M. R. Liebowitz, D. A. Hope, & F. R. Schneier (Eds.), *Social phobia: Diagnosis, assessment, and treatment* (pp. 310–333). New York: Guilford Press.

Chadwick, P., Birchwood, M., & Trower, P. (1996). *Cognitive therapy for delusions, voices, and paranoia.* Chichester, UK: Wiley.

Chambless, D. L., & Hope, D. A. (1996). Cognitive approaches to the psychopathology and treatment of social phobia. In P. M. Salkovskis (Ed.), *Frontiers of cognitive therapy* (pp. 345–382). New York: Guilford Press.

Chambless, D. L., Sanderson, W. C., Shoham, V. Johnson, S. B., Pope, K., S., Crits-

Christoph, P., Baker, M., Johnson, B., Woody, S. R., Sue, S., Beutler, L., Williams, D. A., & McCurry, S. (1996). An update on empirically validated therapies. *The Clinical Psychologist, 49*(2), 5–18.

Chomsky, N. (1956). Three models for the description of language. *IRE Transactions on Information Theory, 2*(3), 113–124.

Chomsky, N. (1957). *Syntactic structures.* The Hague, Netherlands: Mouton.

Clark, D. A., & Purdon, C. (2003). Cognitive theory and therapy of obsessions and compulsions: A critical re-examination. In M. Reinecke & D. Clark (Eds.), *Cognitive therapy across the lifespan* (pp. 90–116). Cambridge: Cambridge University Press.

Clark, D. M. (1986). A cognitive approach to panic. *Behavior Research and Therapy, 24,* 461–470.

Clark, D. M. (1988). A cognitive model of panic attacks. In S. Rachman & J. D. Maser (Eds.), *Panic: Psychological perspectives* (pp. 71–89). Hillside, NJ: Erlbaum.

Clark, D. M. (1997). Panic disorder and social phobia. In D. M. Clark & C. G. Fairburn (Eds.), *Science and the practice of cognitive-behavior therapy* (pp. 119–153). Oxford, UK: Oxford University Press.

Clark, D. C., & Beck, A. T. (1999). *Scientific foundations of cognitive theory and therapy of depression.* New York: Wiley.

Clark, D. M., Salkovskis, P. M., & Chalkley, A. J. (1985). Respiratory control as a treatment for panic attacks. *Journal of Behavior Therapy and Experimental Psychiatry, 16,* 23–30.

Clark, D. M., Salkovskis, P. M., Hackman, A., Middleton, H., Anastasiades, P., & Gelder, M. (1994). A comparison of cognitive therapy, applied relaxation, and imipramine in the treatment of panic disorder. *British Journal of Psychiatry, 164,* 759–769.

Clark, D. M., & Wells, A. (1995). A cognitive model of social phobia. In R. G. Heimberg, M. R. Liebowitz, D. A. Hope, & F. R. Schneier (Eds.), *Social phobia: Diagnosis, assessment, and treatment* (pp. 69–93). New York: Guilford Press.

Craske, M. G., Brown, T. A., & Barlow, D. H. (1991). Behavioral treatment of panic disorder: A two-year follow-up. *Behavior Therapy, 22,* 289–304.

Crits-Christoph, P., & Barber, J. (Eds.). (1991). *Handbook of short-term dynamic psychotherapy.* New York: Basic Books.

Curry, J. (2001). Specific psychotherapies for childhood and adolescent depression. *Biological Psychiatry, 49,* 521–533.

Curry, J., & Reinecke, M. (2003). Modular therapy for adolescents with major depression. In M. A. Reinecke, F. M. Dattilio, & A. Freeman (Eds.), *Cognitive therapy with children and adolescents: A casebook for clinical practice* (2nd ed., pp. 95–127). New York: Guilford Press.

Dahlen, E., & Deffenbacher, J. (2001). Anger management. In W. Lyddon & J. Jones (Eds.), *Empirically supported cognitive therapies: Current and future applications* (pp. 163–181). New York: Springer.

Department of Health. (2000). *National service framework for mental health.* London: HMSO.

Department of Health. (2001). *Treatment choice in psychological therapies and counseling.* London: HMSO.

DeRubeis, R., & Crits-Christoph, P. (1998). Empirically supported individual and group psychological treatments for adult mental disorders. *Journal of Consulting and Clinical Psychology, 66,* 37–52.

DeRubeis, R., Gelfand, L., Tang, T., & Simons, A. (1999). Medication versus cognitive behavior therapy for severely depressed outpatients: Mega-analysis of four randomized comparisons. *American Journal of Psychiatry, 156,* 1007–1013.

Dobson, K. S. (1989). A meta-analysis of the efficacy of cognitive therapy for depression. *Journal of Consulting and Clinical Psychology, 57*(3), 414–419.

Dobson, K. S., & Dozois, D. (2001). Historical and philosophical bases of the cognitive-behavioral therapies. In K. Dobson (Ed.), *Handbook of cognitive-behavioral therapies* (2nd ed., pp. 3–39). New York: Guilford Press.

Drake, R., & Cotton, P. (1986). Depression, hopelessness, and suicide in chronic schizophrenia. *British Journal of Psychiatry, 148,* 554–559.

Elkin, I., Gibbons, R., Shea, M., Sotsky, S., Watkins, J., Pilkonis, D., & Hedeker, D. (1995). Initial severity and differential treatment outcome in the National Institute of Mental Health Treatment of Depression Collaborative Research Program. *Journal of Consulting and Clinical Psychology, 63,* 841–847.

Elkin, I., Shea, M., Watkins, J., Imber, S., Sotsky, S., Collins, J., Glass, D., Pilkonis, D., Leber, W., Docherty, J., Fiester, S., & Parloff, M. (1989). National Institute of Mental Health Treatment of Depression Collaborative Research Program: General effectiveness of treatments. *Archives of General Psychiatry, 46,* 971–982.

Ellis, A. (1962). *Reason and emotion in psychotherapy.* New York: Lyle Stuart.

Ellis, A., & Harper, R. (1961). *New guide to rational living.* New York: Crown.

Elster, J. (2000). *Strong feelings: Emotion, addiction, and human behavior.* Cambridge, MA: MIT Press.

Engels, G., Garnefski, N., & Diekstra, R. (1993). Efficacy of rational-emotive therapy: A quantitative analysis. *Journal of Consulting and Clinical Psychology, 61,* 1083–1090.

Epictetus. (1983). *The handbook of Epictetus* (N. White, Trans.). Indianapolis, IN: Hackett.

Epstein, N., & Schlesinger, S. (2003). Treatment of family problems. In M. A. Reinecke, F. M. Dattilio, & A. Freeman (Eds.), *Cognitive therapy with children and adolescents: A casebook for clinical practice* (2nd ed., pp. 304–337). New York: Guilford Press.

Evans, M., Hollon, S., DeRubeis, R., & Piasecki, J. (1992). Differential relapse following cognitive therapy and pharmacotherapy for depression. *Archives of General Psychiatry, 49*(10), 802–808.

Fairburn, C. G. (1985). Cognitive-behavioral treatment for bulimia. In D. M. Garner & P. E. Garfinkel (Eds.), *Handbook of psychotherapy for anorexia nervosa and bulimia* (pp. 160–192). New York: Guilford Press.

Fairburn, C. G., Jones, R., Peveler, R. C., Carr, S. J., Solomon, R. A., O'Connor, M. E., Burton, J., & Hope, R. A. (1991). Three psychological treatments for bulimia nervosa. *Archives of General Psychiatry, 48,* 463–469.

Fairburn, C. G., Jones, R., Peveler, R. C., Hope, R. A., & O'Connor, M. (1993). Psychotherapy and bulimia nervosa: The longer term effects of interpersonal psychotherapy, behavior therapy and cognitive-behavior therapy. *Archives of General Psychiatry, 50,* 419–428.

Fairburn, C. G., Norman, P. A., Welch, S. L., O'Connor, M. E., Doll, H. A., & Peveler, R. C. (1995). A prospective study of outcome in bulimia nervosa and the long-term effects of three psychological treatments. *Archives of General Psychiatry, 52,* 304–312.

Fairburn, C. G., Shafran, R., & Cooper, Z. (1998). A cognitive behavioral theory of anorexia nervosa. *Behavior Research and Therapy, 37,* 1–13.

Fiske, S., & Taylor, S. (1984). *Social cognition.* Reading, MA: Addison-Wesley.

Flavell, J. (1963). *The developmental psychology of Jean Piaget.* New York: Van Nostrand.

Foa, E., Davidson, J., & Frances, A. (1999). The Expert Consensus Guidelines Series: Treatment of posttraumatic stress disorder. *Journal of Clinical Psychiatry, 60*(16), 4–76.

Foa, E. B., & Kozak, M. J. (1986). Emotional processing of fear: Exposure to corrective information. *Psychological Bulletin, 99,* 20–35.

Foa, E. B., & Rothbaum, B. O. (1998). *Treating the trauma of rape: Cognitive behavioral therapy for PTSD.* New York: Guilford Press.

Foa, E. B., Steketee, G., & Rothbaum, B. (1989). Behavioral/cognitive conceptualizations of post-traumatic stress disorder. *Behavior Therapy, 20,* 155–176.

Foa, E., Steketee, G., & Young, M. (1984). Agoraphobia: Phenomenological aspects, associated characteristics, and theoretical considerations. *Clinical Psychology Review, 4,* 431–457.

Fodor, J. (2000). *The mind doesn't work that way: The scope and limits of computational psychology.* Cambridge, MA: MIT Press.

Fowler, D., Garety, P. & Kuipers, E. (1995). *Cognitive-behavior therapy for psychosis: Theory and practice.* Chichester, UK: Wiley.

Frankl, V. (1985). Cognition and logotherapy. In M. Mahoney & A. Freeman (Eds.), *Cognition and psychotherapy* (pp. 259–276). New York: Plenum Press.

Freeman, A. (1993). A psychosocial approach for conceptualizing schematic development for cognitive therapy. In K. Kuehlwein & H. Rosen (Eds.), *Cognitive therapies in action: Evolving innovative practice* (pp. 54–87). San Francisco: Jossey-Bass.

Freeman, A. (2002). Cognitive-behavioral therapy for severe personality disorders. In S. G. Hofmann & M. C. Tompson (Eds.), *Treating chronic and severe mental disorders: A handbook of empirically supported interventions* (pp. 382–402). New York: Guilford Press.

Freeman, A., & DeWolfe, R. (1989). *Woulda, coulda, shoulda.* New York: HarperCollins.

Freeman, A., Pretzer, J., Fleming, B., & Simon, K. (1990). *Clinical applications of cognitive therapy.* New York: Plenum Press.

Freeman, A., & Reinecke, M. A. (1993). *Cognitive therapy of suicidal behavior: Manual for treatment.* New York: Springer.

Freeman, A., & Simon, K. (1989). Cognitive therapy of anxiety. In A. Freeman, K. Simon, L. Beutler, & H. Arkowitz (Eds.), *Comprehensive handbook of cognitive therapy* (pp. 347–366). New York: Plenum Press.

Fuchs, C., & Rehm, L. (1977). A self-control behavior program for depression. *Journal of Consulting and Clinical Psychology, 45,* 206–215.

Gigerenzer, G., & Selton, R. (Eds.). (2001). *Bounded rationality: The adaptive toolbox.* Cambridge, MA: MIT Press.

Goldfried, M., & Merbaum, M. (Eds.). (1973). *Behavior change through self-control.* New York: Holt, Rinehart & Winston.

Gotlib, I. & Hammen, C. (1992). *Psychological aspects of depression: Toward a cognitive-interpersonal integration.* New York: Wiley.

Greenberg, L. S., & Safran, J. D. (1987). *Emotion in psychotherapy.* New York: Guilford Press.

Greenberger, D., & Padesky, C. A. (1995). *Mind over mood: A cognitive therapy treatment manual for clients.* New York: Guilford Press.

Guidano, V. F. (1991). *The self in process: Toward a post-rationalist cognitive therapy.* New York: Guilford Press.

Guidano, V. F. (1995). A constructivist outline of human knowing processes. In M. Mahoney (Ed.), *Cognitive and constructive psychotherapies: Theory, research and practice* (pp. 89–102). New York: Springer.

Guidano, V. F., & Liotti, G. (1983). *Cognitive processes and emotional disorders: A structural approach to psychotherapy.* New York: Guilford Press.

Guidano, V. F., & Liotti, G. (1985). A constructivist foundation for cognitive therapy. In M. Mahoney & A. Freeman (Eds.), *Cognition and psychotherapy* (pp. 101–142). New York: Plenum Press.

Haaga, D., & Davison, G. (1993). An appraisal of rational-emotive therapy. *Journal of Consulting and Clinical Psychology, 61*(2), 215–220.

Haaga, D., DeRubeis, R., Stewart, B., & Beck, A. (1991) Relationship of intelligence with cognitive therapy outcome. *Behavior Research and Therapy, 29,* 277–281.

Haddock, G., & Slade, P. (Eds.). (1996). *Cognitive-behavioural interventions with psychotic disorders.* London: Routledge.

Harrington, R., Whittaker, J., Shoebridge, P., & Campbell, F. (1998). Systematic review of efficacy of cognitive behaviour therapies in childhood and adolescent depressive disorder. *British Medical Journal, 316,* 1559–1563.

Heimberg, R. G., & Juster, H. R. (1994). Treatment of social phobia in cognitive-behavioral groups. *Journal of Clinical Psychiatry, 55*(6, Suppl.), 38–46.

Hembree, E., & Foa, E. (2003). Promoting cognitive change in posttraumatic stress disorder. In M. Reinecke & D. Clark (Eds.), *Cognitive therapy across the lifespan* (pp. 231–257). Cambridge: Cambridge University Press.

Hofmann, S. (2003). The cognitive model of panic. In M. Reinecke & D. Clark (Eds.) *Cognitive therapy across the lifespan* (pp. 117–137). Cambridge, UK: Cambridge University Press.

Hofmann, S. G., & Spiegel, D. A. (1999). Panic control treatment and its applications. *Journal of Psychotherapy Practice and Research, 8,* 3–11.

Hollon, S. (1990). Cognitive therapy and pharmacotherapy for depression. *Psychiatric Annals, 20*(5), 249–258.

Hollon, S., & Shelton, R. (2001). Treatment guidelines for major depressive disorder. *Behavior Therapy, 32,* 235–258.

Hollon, S., Shelton, R., & Loosen, P. (1991). Cognitive therapy and pharmacotherapy for depression. *Journal of Consulting and Clinical Psychology, 59*(1), 88–99.

Hollon, S., Thase, M., & Markowitz, J. (2002). Treatment and prevention of depression. *Psychological Science in the Public Interest, 3*(2), 39–77.

Horowitz, M. (Ed.). (1991). *Person schemas and maladaptive interpersonal patterns.* Chicago: University of Chicago Press.

Ingram, R. (1984). Toward an information processing analysis of depression. *Cognitive Therapy and Research, 8,* 443–478.

Ingram, R. E., Miranda, J., & Segal, Z. V. (1998). *Cognitive vulnerability to depression.* New York: Guilford Press.

Jarrett, R., Basco, M., Riser, R., Ramanan, J., Marwill, M., & Rush, A. (1998). Is there a role for continuation phase cognitive therapy for depressed outpatients? *Journal of Consulting and Clinical Psychology, 66,* 1036–1040.

Jarrett, R., Kraft, D., Doyle, J., Foster, B., Eaves, G., & Silver, P. (2001). Preventing recurrent depression using cognitive therapy with and without a continuation phase: A randomized clinical trial. *Archives of General Psychiatry, 58,* 381–388.

Jarrett, R., Schaffer, M., McIntire, D., Witt-Browder, A., Kraft, D., & Risser, R. (1999). Treatment of atypical depression with cognitive therapy or phenelzine: A double-blind, placebo-controlled trial. *Archives of General Psychiatry, 56*(5), 431–437.

Kegan, R. (1982). *The evolving self.* Cambridge, MA: Harvard University Press.

Keller, M., McCullough, J., Klein, D., Arnow, B., Dunner, D., Gelenberg, A., Markowitz, J., Nemeroff, C., Russell, J., Thase, M., Trivedi, M., Zajecka, J., Blalock, J., Borian, F., DeBattista, C., Fawcett, J., Hirschfeld, R., Jody, D., Keitner, G., Kocsis, J., Koran, L., Kornstein, S., Manber, R., Miller, I., Ninan, P., Rothbaum, B., Rush, A., Schatzberg, A., & Vivan, D. (2000). A comparison of nefazodone, the cognitive behavioral-analysis system of psychotherapy, and their combination for the treatment of chronic depression. *New England Journal of Medicine, 342*(20), 1462–1470.

Kelly, G. (1955). *The psychology of personal constructs.* New York: Norton.

Kihlstrom, J. (1987). The cognitive unconscious. *Science, 237,* 1445–1452.

Kihlstrom, J. (1988). Cognition, unconscious processes. In G. Adelman (Ed.), *Neuroscience year: The yearbook of the encyclopedia of neuroscience* (pp. 34–36). Boston: Birkhauser.

Kingdon, D. G., & Turkington, D. (1994). *Cognitive-behavioral therapy of schizophrenia.* New York: Guilford Press.

Kovacs, M., & Beck, A. (1978). Maladaptive cognitive structures in depression. *American Journal of Psychiatry, 135*(5), 525–533.

Kovacs, M., Rush, A., Beck, A., & Hollon, S. (1981). Depressed outpatients treated with cognitive therapy or pharmacotherapy: A one year follow-up. *Archives of General Psychiatry, 38,* 33–39.

Kroenke, K., & Swindle, R. (2000). Cognitive-behavioral therapy for somatization and symptom syndromes: A critical review of controlled clinical trials. *Psychotherapy and Psychosomatics, 69*(4), 205–215.

Lambert, M., & Davis, M. (2002). Treatment for depression: What the research says. In M. Reinecke & M. Davison (Eds.), *Comparative treatments of depression* (pp. 21–46). New York: Springer.

Layden, M., Newman, C. Freeman, A., & Byers, S. (1993). *Cognitive therapy of the borderline patient.* Boston: Allyn & Bacon.

Lazarus, A. (Ed.). (1976). *Multimodal behavior therapy.* New York: Springer.

Lazarus, A. (1981). *The practice of multimodal therapy.* New York: McGraw-Hill.

Lazarus, R. (1991). *Emotion and adaptation.* New York: Oxford University Press.

Leahy, R. L. (2001). *Overcoming resistance in cognitive therapy.* New York: Guilford Press.

LeGrange, D. (2003). The cognitive model of bulimia nervosa. In M. A. Reinecke & D. Clark (Eds.), *Cognitive therapy across the lifespan* (pp. 293–314). Cambridge, UK: Cambridge University Press.

Leventhal, H. (1984). A perceptual motor theory of emotions. In K. Scherer & P. Ekman (Eds.), *Approaches to emotion* (pp. 271–291). Hillsdale, NJ: Erlbaum.

Mahoney, M. (1974). *Cognition and behavior modification.* Cambridge, MA: Ballinger.

Mahoney, M. (1977). Reflections on the cognitive-learning trend in psychotherapy. *American Psychologist, 32,* 5–13.

Mahoney, M. (1991). *Human change processes.* New York: Basic Books.

Mann, J. (1973). *Time-limited psychotherapy.* Cambridge, MA: Harvard University Press.

Marks, I., Lovell, K., Noshirvani, H., Livanou, M., & Thrasher, S. (1998). Treatment of posttraumatic stress disorder by exposure and/or cognitive restructuring. *Archives of General Psychiatry, 55,* 317–325.

Markus, H. (1977). Self-schemata and processing information about the self. *Journal of Personality and Social Psychology, 35,* 63–78.

McMullin, R. E. (1986). *Handbook of cognitive therapy techniques.* New York: Norton.

Meichenbaum, D. (1977). *Cognitive behavior modification.* New York: Plenum Press.

Meichenbaum, D., & Gilmore, J. (1984). The nature of unconscious processes: A cognitive-behavioral perspective. In K. Bowers & D. Meichenbaum (Eds.), *The unconscious reconsidered* (pp. 273–298). New York: Wiley.

Mennin, D., Turk, C., Heimberg, R., & Carmin, C. (2003). Focusing on the regulation of emotion: A new direction for conceptualizing and treating Generalized Anxiety Disorder. In M. A. Reinecke & D. Clark (Eds.), *Cognitive therapy across the lifespan* (pp. 60–89). Cambridge, UK: Cambridge University Press.

Mercier, M., Stewart, J., & Quitkin, F. (1992). A pilot sequential study of cognitive therapy and pharmacotherapy of atypical depression. *Journal of Clinical Psychiatry, 53,* 166–170.

Merluzzi, T. (1996). Cognitive assessment and treatment of social phobia. In P. W. Corrigan & S. C. Yudofsky (Eds.), *Cognitive rehabilitation for neuropsychiatric disorders* (pp. 167–190). Washington, DC: American Psychiatric Press.

Miller, R., & Berman, J. (1983). The efficacy of cognitive behavior therapies: A quantitative review of the research evidence. *Psychological Bulletin, 94,* 39–53.

Mischel, W. (1973). Toward a cognitive social learning reconceptualization of personality. *Psychological Review, 80,* 252–283.

Murphy, G. E., Simons, A. D., Wetzel, R. D., & Lustman, P. J. (1984). Cognitive therapy versus tricyclic antidepressants in major depression. *Archives of General Psychiatry, 41,* 33–41.

Neimeyer, R. (1993). An appraisal of constructivist psychotherapies. *Journal of Consulting and Clinical Psychology, 61*(2), 221–234.

Newell, A., & Simon, H. (1956). The logic theory machine: A complex information processing system. *IRE Transactions on Information Theory, 2*(3), 61–79.

Ogles, B., Lambert, M., & Sawyer, J. (1995). Clinical significance of the National Institute of Mental Health Treatment of Depression Collaborative Research Program data. *Journal of Consulting and Clinical Psychology, 63,* 321–326.

Ortony, A., Clore, G., & Collins, A. (1988). *The cognitive structure of emotions.* Cambridge: Cambridge University Press.

Persons, J. (1989). *Cognitive therapy in practice: A case conceptualization approach.* New York: Norton.

Persons, J., Bostrom, A., & Bertagnolli, A. (1999). Results of randomized controlled trials of cognitive therapy for depression generalize to private practice. *Cognitive Therapy and Research, 23,* 535–548.

Persons, J., Burns, D., & Perloff, J. (1988). Predictors of dropout and outcome in private practice patients treated with cognitive therapy for depression. *Cognitive Therapy and Research, 12,* 557–575.

Persons, J., Davidson, J., & Tompkins, M. (2001). *Essential components of cognitive-behavior therapy for depression.* Washington, DC: American Psychological Association.

Peterson, C., & Seligman, M. (1984). Causal explanations as a risk factor for depression: Theory and evidence. *Psychological Review, 91,* 347–374.

Rapee, R. M. (1998). *Overcoming shyness and social phobia: A step-by-step guide.* Killara, Australia: Lifestyle Press.

Rapee, R., & Heimberg, R. (1997). A cognitive-behavioral model of anxiety in social phobia. *Behaviour Research and Therapy, 35,* 741–756.

Rehm, L. (1977). A self-control model of depression. *Behavior Therapy, 8,* 787–804.

Rehm, L. (1995). Psychotherapies for depression. In K. Craig & K. Dobson (Eds.), *Anxiety and depression in adults and children* (pp. 183–208). Thousand Oaks, CA: Sage.

Reinecke, M. (2002). Cognitive therapies of depression: A modularized treatment approach. In M. Reinecke & M. Davison (Eds.), *Comparative treatments of depression* (pp. 249–290). New York: Springer.

Reinecke, M., & Rogers, G. (2001). Dysfunctional attitudes and attachment style among clinically depressed adults. *Behavioural and Cognitive Psychotherapy, 29,* 129–141.

Reinecke, M., Ryan, N., & DuBois, D. (1998). Cognitive-behavioral therapy of depression and depressive symptoms during adolescence: A review and meta-analysis. *Journal of the American Academy of Child and Adolescent Psychiatry, 37*(1), 26–34.

Resick, P. A., & Schnicke, M. K. (1992). Cognitive processing therapy for sexual assault victims. *Journal of Consulting and Clinical Psychology, 60,* 748–756.

Roberts, J., Gotlib, I., & Kassel, J. (1996). Adult attachment security and symptoms of depression: The mediating roles of dysfunctional attitudes and low self-esteem. *Journal of Personality and Social Psychology, 70,* 310–320.

Robinson, L., Berman, J., & Neimeyer, R. (1990). Psychotherapy for the treatment of depression: A comprehensive review of controlled outcome research. *Psychological Bulletin, 108,* 30–49.

Rosen, H. (1985). *Piagetian concepts of clinical relevance.* New York: Columbia University Press.

Rosen, H. (1989). Piagetian theory and cognitive therapy. In A. Freeman, K. Simon, L. Beutler, & H. Arkowitz (Eds.), *Comprehensive handbook of cognitive therapy* (pp. 189–212). New York: Plenum Press.

Safran, J., & McMain, S. (1992). A cognitive-interpersonal approach to the treatment of personality disorders. *Journal of Cognitive Psychotherapy: An International Quarterly, 6*(1), 59–67.

Safran, J., & Segal, Z. (1990). *Interpersonal process in cognitive therapy.* New York: Basic Books.

Safran, J., Vallis, T., Segal, Z., & Shaw, B. (1986). Assessment of core cognitive processes in cognitive therapy. *Cognitive Therapy and Research, 10*(5), 509–526.

Salkovskis, P., & Wahl, K. (2003). Treating obsessional problems using cognitive-behavioral therapy. In M. A. Reinecke & D. Clark (Eds.), *Cognitive therapy across the lifespan* (pp. 138–171). Cambridge, UK: Cambridge University Press.

Schulberg, H., Katon, W., Simon, G., & Rush, A. (1998). Treating major depression in primary care practice: An update of the Agency for Healthcare Policy and Research Guidelines. *Archives of General Psychiatry, 55,* 1121–1127.

Segal, Z. (1988). Appraisal of the self-schema construct in cognitive models of depression. *Psychological Bulletin, 103,* 147–162.

Seligman, M. (1975). *Helplessness: On depression, development, and death.* San Francisco: Freeman.

Shapiro, D., & Shapiro, D. (1982). Meta-analysis of comparative therapy outcome studies: A replication and refinement. *Psychological Bulletin, 92,* 581–604.

Shea, M., Elkin, I., Imber, S., Sotsky, S., Watkins, J., Collins, J., Pilkonis, D., Beckham, E., Glass, D., Dolan, R., & Parloff, M. (1992). Course of depressive symptoms over follow-up: Findings from the National Institute of Mental Health Treatment of Depression Collaborative Research Program. *Archives of General Psychiatry, 49,* 782–787.

Simons, A., Garfield, S., & Murphy, G. (1984). The process of change in cognitive therapy and pharmacotherapy of depression: Changes in mood and cognition. *Archives of General Psychiatry, 41,* 45–51.

Simons, A., Murphy, G., Levine, J., & Wetzel, R. (1986). Cognitive therapy and pharmacotherapy for depression: Sustained improvement over one year. *Archives of General Psychiatry, 43,* 43–48.

Sokol, L., Beck, A., Greenberg, R., Berchick, R., & Wright, F. (1989). Cognitive therapy of panic disorder: A non-pharmacological alternative. *Journal of Nervous and Mental Disease, 177*(12), 711–716.

Solomon, A., & Haaga, D. (2003). Cognitive theory and therapy of depression. In M. A. Reinecke & D. Clark (Eds.), *Cognitive therapy across the lifespan* (pp. 12–39). Cambridge, UK: Cambridge University Press.

Spence, S., & Reinecke, M. (2003). Cognitive-behavioral approaches to understanding and treating child and adolescent depression. In M. A. Reinecke & D. Clark (Eds.), *Cognitive therapy across the lifespan* (pp. 358–395). Cambridge, UK: Cambridge University Press.

Sperry, L. (1999). *Cognitive behavior therapy of DSM-IV personality disorders.* Philadelphia: Brunner/Mazel.

Steketee, G. S. (1996). *Treatment of obsessive compulsive disorder.* New York: Guilford Press.

Sweeney, P., Anderson, K., & Bailey, S. (1986). Attributional style in depression: A meta-analytic review. *Journal of Personality and Social Psychology, 50,* 974–991.

Tarrier, N., & Haddock, G. (2002). Cognitive-behavioral therapy for schizophrenia: A case formulation approach. In S. G. Hofmann & M. C. Tompson (Eds.), *Treating chronic and severe mental disorders: A handbook of empirically-supported interventions* (pp. 69–95). New York: Guilford Press.

Tarrier, N., Pilgrim, H., Sommerfield, C., Fragher, B., Reynolds, M., Graham, E., & Barrowclough, C. (1999). A randomized trial of cognitive therapy and imaginal exposure in the treatment of chronic post-traumatic stress disorder. *Journal of Consulting and Clinical Psychology, 67,* 8–13.

Tarrier, N., Yusupoff, L., Kinney, C., McCarthy, E., Gledhill, A., Haddock, G., & Morris, J. (1998). Randomised controlled trial of intensive cognitive behaviour therapy for patients with chronic schizophrenia. *British Medical Journal, 317,* 303–307.

Taylor, S. (1996). Meta-analysis of cognitive-behavioral treatments for social phobia. *Journal of Behavior Therapy and Experimental Psychiatry, 27,* 1–9.

Telch, M. J., Lucas, J. A., Schmidt, N. B., Hanna, H. H., Jaimez, T. L., & Lucas, R. (1993). Group cognitive-behavioral treatment of panic disorder. *Behaviour Research and Therapy, 31,* 279–287.

Tolman, E. (1949). *Purposive behavior in animals and men.* Berkeley: University of California Press.

Truax, C., & Carkhuff, R. (1964). Significant developments in psychotherapy research. In L. Abt & B. Reiss (Eds.), *Progress in clinical psychology* (Vol. 6, pp. 124–155). New York: Grune & Stratton.

Turk, D., & Salovey, P. (1985). Cognitive structures, cognitive processes, and cognitive-behavior modification: I. Client issues. *Cognitive Therapy and Research, 9,* 1–17.

Veale, D. (2001). Cognitive-behaviour therapy for body dysmorphic disorder. *Advances in Psychiatric Treatment, 7,* 125–132.

Veale, D., Gournay, K., Dryden, W., & Boocock, A. (1996). Body dysmorphic disorder: A cognitive-behavioural models and a pilot randomized controlled trial. *Behaviour Research and Therapy, 34,* 717–729.

Veale, D., & Riley, S. (2001). Mirror, mirror on the wall, who is the ugleiest of them all? The psychopathology of mirror gazing in body dysmorphic disorder. *Behavior Research and Therapy, 39,* 1381–1393.

Wells, A. (1997). *Cognitive therapy of anxiety disorders.* Chichester, UK: Wiley.

Whisman, M., & McGarvey, A. (1995). Attachment, depressotypic cognitions, and dysphoria. *Cognitive Therapy and Research, 19,* 633–650.

White, J., Keenan, M., & Brooks, N. (1992). Stress control: A controlled comparative investigation of large group therapy for generalized anxiety disorder. *Behavioural Psychotherapy, 20,* 97–113.

Whorf, B. (1956). *Language, thought, and reality.* Cambridge, MA: MIT Press.

Wilson, J., & Rapee, R. (2003). Social phobia. In M. A. Reinecke & D. Clark (Eds.), *Cognitive therapy across the lifespan* (pp. 258–292). Cambridge, UK: Cambridge University Press.

Wright, J. (1987). Cognitive therapy and medication as combined treatment. In A. Freeman & V. Greenwood (Eds.), *Cognitive therapy: Applications in psychiatric and medical settings* (pp. 36–50). New York: Human Sciences Press.

Wright, J. (1992). Combined cognitive therapy and pharmacotherapy of depression. In A. Freeman & F. Dattilio (Eds.), *Comprehensive casebook of cognitive therapy* (pp. 285–292). New York: Plenum Press.

Wright, J., & Schrodt, G. (1989). Combined cognitive therapy and pharmacotherapy. In A. Freeman, K. Simon, L. Beutler, & H. Arkowitz (Eds.), *Comprehensive handbook of cognitive therapy* (pp. 267–282). New York: Plenum Press.

Young, J. (1991). *Cognitive therapy for personality disorders: A schema-focused approach.* Sarasota, FL: Professional Resource Exchange.

8

Postmodern Approaches to Psychotherapy

ROBERT A. NEIMEYER
SARA K. BRIDGES

Postmodern, constructivist therapies draw on several therapeutic traditions—particularly the humanistic, systemic, and feminist—while also reinterpreting and extending these traditions in light of characteristically postmodern themes, having to do especially with the primacy of personal meaning, the construction of identity in a social field, and the revision of life narratives that are incoherent or restrictive. Indeed, as we use the term, "postmodern therapy" is itself a pastiche of perspectives, subsuming a variety of specific constructivist, social constructionist, and narrative approaches that share several basic philosophic similarities, as we discuss later. For this reason, we use the term "postmodern" when we explicitly wish to emphasize the broad range of this orientation, and the terms "constructivist," "narrative," and "social constructionist" when we are speaking principally about one of its variants, which themselves subsume many specific therapies. However, we are less interested in getting bogged down in terminological nuances than in conveying the sorts of ideas and practices associated with this perspective, and we refer the interested reader to scholarly descriptions of the defining features and

emphases that differentiate these approaches for details (Botella, 1995; Chiari & Nuzzo, 1996; Lyddon, 1995; Neimeyer, 1995a).

Although this immense variety of postmodern approaches frustrates any attempt to offer a single definition of their features, in general they tend to be more collaborative than authoritarian, more developmental than symptom oriented, more process oriented than content focused, and more reflective than psychoeducational. Our goal in this chapter is to demystify many of the concepts and practices associated with this loose confederation of contemporary approaches, providing a foothold in the sometimes daunting postmodern terrain for those students and professionals intrepid enough to explore them. We begin by considering the intellectual and historical backdrop that informs these perspectives, and that helps shape their distinctive orientation to the conceptualization and treatment of psychosocial problems.

HISTORICAL BACKGROUND

No intellectual development arrives on the scene as a result of the "immaculate conception" of its founder. Instead, each inevitably arises from the commingling of concepts from previous generations, representing the fertile marriage of ideas having different intellectual pedigrees. Extending and adapting this "marriage" metaphor, we might even say that every nascent theory represents "something old, something new, something borrowed, and something 'true'"—at least to its adherents! In other words, every emerging perspective repackages the wisdom of earlier thinkers, adds its own insights and innovations, draws on other streams of thought (with or without crediting the source), and then propounds this complex mixture as in some sense a valid reflection of "reality"—at least within the constraints imposed by present knowledge.

If postmodern theories of psychotherapy represent a partial exception to these general rules, it is only in the self-awareness with which postmodernists recognize that their theories exemplify these inevitable features of all social constructions. Thus, in this opening section we offer an admittedly selective reading of a few of the historical people and processes that have contributed to the growing group of constructivist, narrative, and social constructionist approaches to therapy that together have come to be called postmodern—with full awareness that rather different historical introductions to the field might well be written (Fransella, 1996; Mahoney, 1991; Neimeyer, 2000a).

The Intellectual Backdrop

Newcomers to postmodern therapies are typically of two types: those who are closet philosophers and share a fascination with theory, and students of a more practical bent who are frustrated with this same tendency toward abstraction. Our goal in this chapter is to provide just enough orientation to the philosophic frameworks that support postmodern practice to highlight its distinctiveness, taking care to ground some of the loftier concepts in concrete clinical illustra-

tions and methods. Thus, if we sometimes simplify the daunting complexity of postmodern discourse, we hope we can be forgiven. Fortunately, high-level discussions of the theoretical underpinnings of the therapies discussed here are in good supply, and we point toward several of these throughout the chapter for those readers who want to delve more deeply into the concepts behind the clinical practice.

If there is a unifying theme that links postmodern forms of psychotherapy, it is at the level of their *epistemology,* or theory of knowledge. Although most therapists who work within this perspective acknowledge that a "real world" exists outside human consciousness or language, they are much more interested in the nuances in people's construction of the world than they are in evaluating the extent to which such constructions are "true" in representing a presumably external reality. This emphasis on the active, form-giving nature of the mind dates back at least to the Italian historian Giambattista Vico (1668–1744), who traced the development of thought to the attempt to understand the world by projecting on it human motives, myths, fables, and linguistic abstractions. The German philosopher Immanuel Kant (1724–1804) likewise emphasized the transformative character of the mind, which necessarily imposes spatial, temporal, and causal order on the phenomena of experience. From these philosophers, constructivists borrowed a model of knowledge as an active structuring of experience, rather than a passive assimilation of "things in themselves," uncontaminated by human knowing.

At the threshold to the 20th century, these themes were elaborated by the German analytic philosopher Hans Vaihinger (1852–1933), whose *Philosophy of "As If"* asserted that people develop "workable fictions" (e.g., of mathematical infinity or God) to order and transcend the hard data of experience, and establish uniquely human goals. A similar emphasis on the distinction between our linguistic "map" of experience and the "territory" of the world was made by the Polish intellectual Alfred Korzybski (1879–1950), whose system of general semantics focused on the role of the speaker in assigning meanings to events. From these thinkers, constructivists drew the implication that human beings operate on the basis of symbolic linguistic constructs that help them navigate in the world without contacting it in any simple, direct way. Stated differently, proponents of postmodernism argue that people live in an interpreted world, one organized as much by their individual and collective categories of meaning as by the structure of an "objective" world of external stimuli. In practice, this carries the implication that therapy is more a matter of *intervening in meaning* than it is a procedure for ameliorating unwanted symptoms or training people in more adequate coping skills.

Toward a Constructivist Psychology

By the 1930s, these and parallel philosophical influences began to find expression in psychology, inspiring a focus on the ways in which people actively *construct* experience, rather than simply "register" environmental stimuli in a *tabula rasa* fashion. Among the psychologists to take this avowedly "constructivist" turn were the Swiss developmental psychologist, Jean Piaget, who traced the qualitative transformations through which children schematized the physical and social world, and the British experimental psychologist Fredric Bartlett, who demonstrated that memories did not simply entail recalling stored events but instead were constructed in light of present motives through the guidance of mental *schemas*. Both influences continue to be felt in contemporary research on autobiographical memory, which examines the construction and periodic consolidation of a shifting sense of identity throughout adult life (Neisser & Fivush, 1994).

The first person to develop a thoroughgoing theory of psychotherapy that drew on these philosophic ideas was the American clinical psychologist George Kelly. Working in the relative isolation of rural Kansas in the 1930s and 1940s, Kelly confronted the overwhelming psychological needs of farming communities that had been devastated by the twin crises of the Dust Bowl and the Great Depression (Neimeyer, 2000b). This experience prompted Kelly to design efficient psychotherapeutic procedures in which clients were coached to enact carefully constructed fictional identities in their daily lives for a fixed period (usually only 2 or 3 weeks), as a way of helping people free themselves from the press of circumstances and experiment with quite different ways of living. Kelly's *fixed role therapy*—which we explore in more detail in a later section—was therefore the first form of brief therapy and foreshadowed the use of dramatic and narrative strategies of change incorporated in many contemporary constructivist therapies. Eventually, Kelly (1955/1991) drafted a comprehensive *psychology of personal constructs* that placed these procedures in a rigorous theoretical context and suggested diagnostic, therapeutic, and research methods targeting the unique personal construct systems that individuals devised to structure and anticipate the themes of their lives.

The Postmodern Trend

Although interest in personal construct theory grew slowly in the decades that followed the publication of his work, Kelly was in a sense ahead of his time. Certainly, an emphasis on the role of personal systems of meaning and the fictional construction of identities seemed an odd fit in a field dominated by a concern with unconscious motives on the one hand and the modification of observable behavior on the other. Consequently, it was not until a postmodern *Zeitgeist* began to work its way into the human sciences and the helping professions some 30–40 years later that significant numbers of psychotherapy theorists began to rediscover Kelly's insights and to extend them in radically new directions.

But what is *postmodernism,* and what is its relevance for clinical practice? As the term suggests, "posties" can best be defined in relation to the traditional intellectual framework that they strive to succeed, undermine, or critique, namely, *modernism.* Modernism is a broad concept, almost too broad to define with any precision, because it encompasses so many domains of social life. However, as applied to the human sciences, modernism embodies the Enlightenment faith in technological and human progress through accumulation of legitimate knowledge. Throughout its century-long history, psychology has for the most part followed this paradigm through the development of logical, experimental, and statistical methods presumed to yield objective data, providing a secure foundation for theories that were assumed to reflect, with as little distortion as possible, the universal and timeless "realities" of human behavior. "Truth," in this view, is discovered, a bit at a time, whether the "truth" concerned general laws of human behavior, or concrete historical determinants of that behavior in the lives of individuals in psychotherapy. At the core of this program is the belief in a knowable world, and with it a knowable self.

Dissenting from this traditional view, postmodernism calls into question the concept of timeless certainty, asserting that all human "realities" are necessarily personal, cultural, and linguistic constructs—although they are no less substantial or important for this reason (Appignanesi & Garratt, 1995). "Truth," in this view, is actually constituted by individuals and social groups and reflects the dominant social ideologies of the day, however fallible these turn out to be in the hindsight of later generations. For example, cultural assumptions about the appropriate roles of women or ethnic minorities, laws that prohibit and punish certain behavior, and even psychiatric diagnoses can all be considered historically situated (and changing) social constructions, but this does not mitigate their impact on those subjected to them. Scholars working from a postmodern perspective therefore seek to reveal the often hidden ways in which reality and power is constructed in the course of social life (Derrida, 1978; Foucault, 1970). Therapists and activists animated by this spirit attempt to analyze and *deconstruct* these same patterns when they function to limit or constrain the possibilities for a given person or community. This spirit of "resistance" against the taken-for-granted assumptions of cultural "texts" in the service of personal or social transformation is especially evident in some postmodern approaches, like the narrative and radical–critical therapies to be discussed later.

Rather than elaborate further at this point on the implications of constructivist epistemology for postmodern practice, we revisit these themes in the sections that follow, considering some of their concrete expressions in the conceptualization of personality, psychopathology, psychological assessment, and therapeutic practice.

THE CONCEPT OF PERSONALITY

The concept of "personality" is a two-edged sword. At one level, it serves a useful integrative function, helping explain how the myriad forms and facets of human functioning are organized into a larger and potentially more holistic pattern. Personality, in this sense, is what makes you *you,* a self both distinguishable from others and recognizable, with meaningful variations and developments, across time. As such, the personality or "self" has played a central role in the history of psychotherapy, serving as an orienting concept for clinical diagnosis, as well as a target for clinical interventions. From Freud's classic structural formulation of ego functioning (Freud, 1940/1964) to its elaboration by object relations (Kernberg, 1976) and self-theorists (Kohut, 1971), and from early conceptions of the "proprium" (Allport, 1961) to humanistic theories of self-development (Rogers,

1961), various models of personality have provided a foundation for theories of psychotherapy. Even scientifically parsimonious cognitive-behavioral therapies (e.g., Beck, 1993) implicitly presume a foundational role for the self in their focus on training clients in self-monitoring, recording of self-talk, and similar procedures. Viewed in a critical sociohistorical perspective, such models can be seen as expressing a modernist discourse in which the self is viewed as individualistic, singular, essential, stable, and knowable, at least in principle (Neimeyer, 1998). It follows that psychotherapy, as a series of authoritative technical procedures to bring about self-change, would focus chiefly on disorders of individuals that impair adaptation and then treat them in such a way as to enhance the client's self-actualization, self-control, self-efficacy, and the like.

In a sense, postmodern approaches to psychotherapy both extend and problematize this conception of selfhood. On the one hand, the self retains its role as an organizing concept in many constructivist theories, which focus on the "core ordering processes" (Mahoney, 1991) by which individuals construct a sense of personal identity in an intersubjective field (Guidano, 1991). Moreover, in keeping with humanistic personality theories, constructivists typically emphasize the role of personal meanings in shaping people's responses to life events and regard human beings as capable of at least a bounded agency in determining the course of their lives (Kelly, 1955/1991). In this view, we *are* our constructs: Personality can be seen as the composite of our myriad ways of interpreting, anticipating, and responding to the social world. For example, early abusive experiences in intimate relationships might have made it compellingly important for me to discriminate between *people who are safe to be close to* and *those who are dangerous.* Once this "personal construct" is integrated into my system, however, it says as much about me as it does about my world, as I vigilantly (if often un-

consciously) screen possible relational partners in terms of the safety or danger that they represent and behave toward them accordingly. Ultimately, Kelly argued that some constructs become "superordinate" or central to our systems of living, creating hierarchical matrices of meaning that he termed "personal construct systems." Viewed from this perspective, the "self" is not constituted by any set of inherent, essential inner qualities or fixed traits but instead simply represents the distillation of our shifting efforts to engage the social world. This conception of personality in terms of a developing system of idiosyncratic constructs has given rise to several distinctive methods of clinical assessment, which are reviewed later in this chapter.

On the other hand, some postmodern theorists regard even this conception of personality as suspiciously romantic, expressing the cognitivism and individualism of Western culture, with its emphasis on "well integrated" and sovereign selves as the hallmark of personal identity. In this more radical and critical vision, identity is far less stable and coherent, at best comprising a "dialogical self" whose distinguishable parts vie for voice in our inner world (Hermans, 2003), and in its more extreme forms herald the "death of the self" altogether (Lather, 1992). Considering personality as simply a linguistic construction, a view of the "saturated self" as populated by the contradictory discourses in which one is immersed threatens the very conception of the individual as a coherent entity with identifiable boundaries and properties (Gergen, 1991). Thus, in this version of *social constructionism,* it is little wonder that we as individuals are fraught with uncertainty, conflict, and contradiction, insofar as our individual lives are merely the sites of incompatible discourses of identity (e.g., about the requirements for being a good partner, parent or professional, all anchored in diverse conversations and media images), each of which "positions" us as a certain kind of person but in ways that typically make competing demands of us (Efran & Cook, 2000). Such a perspective further tempers the traditional, modernist assumption of the ultimate knowability of the self, and with it the relevance of rationalistic self-analysis and self-control procedures (R. Neimeyer, 1993a, 1995a). Instead, it follows from this more socialized view of selfhood that psychotherapeutic procedures for fostering change would need to tack between the self and social system, helping clients articulate, elaborate, and negotiate those (inter)personal meanings by which they organize their experience and action, as well as the sometimes oppressive or conflictual role of cultural discourses that "colonize" their lives (R. Neimeyer, 1995b). This attention to the processes by which identity is constructed and maintained in a social field is evident in several of the family and systemic expressions of postmodern therapies that are covered later.

Placed in a larger perspective, these relative emphases on the personal versus social construction of identity can be seen as expressions of a broader "epigenetic systems" model that views human meaning and action as the emergent outcome of a series of hierarchically embedded systems and subsystems (Mascolo, Craig-Bray, & Neimeyer, 1997). In biology, epigenesis stands in contrast to theories that view an organism's structures, behaviors, or capacities as either essential and inborn, or as the simple and predictable result of maturational unfolding. Instead, new structures are seen as emerging through the interaction of a multileveled organism–environment system, in which the functioning of each constituent feature (e.g., chromosomes) is shaped through transactions of more basic levels (e.g., genes) and higher-order ones (e.g., cell matrices). As applied to human functioning, epigenesis implies that meaning and action emerge from a similarly multilayered system of systems, which include biogenetic, personal–agentic, dyadic–relational, and social–cultural levels. *Biogenetic* systems refer to all systems below the level of the organ-

ism-as-agent (genetic, cellular, and organ systems). The *personal–agentic* level refers to functioning of the organism as a personality, having a bounded degree of choice in determining its own development. *Dyadic–relational* systems emerge out of co-actions between two or more individuals (e.g., family systems), which are further nested within larger *social–linguistic* systems of cultural patterns, institutions, discourses, and beliefs. In this integrative model, all psychologically significant structures and symptoms emerge from the complex interaction of all levels of this comprehensive system, rather than from a given level considered in isolation. For example, a young man's experience of depression can best be understood not simply as an expression of a biogenetic predisposition to mood disorder but also as an experience that compels exploration of its significance for his developing personality (or sense of inner division), his relationships (particularly with his family, peers, and employer), and cultural scripts or narratives (especially those concerned with what it means to be a "man" and dominant and perhaps oppressive discourses of what it means to be "mentally ill").

Although many different processes and structures might be studied within this broad epigenetic approach, several constructivist and postmodern psychologies converge in taking as their unit of analysis the *situated interpretive activity* of individuals and groups (Mascolo et al., 1997). This carries four specific implications that have relevance for psychotherapy. First, the concept of *interpretation* suggests that all psychological and social activity involves assessments of the meaning that events have for people, in keeping with the emphases of most contemporary constructivist theorists (Neimeyer & Mahoney, 1995). Second, the focus on interpretive *activity* suggests that interpretation is an active rather than a passive process; both "doing" and "construing" are ways of accomplishing something in the world. Third, the emphasis on *situated* interpretive activity implies that human activity always emerges in a context that typically involves other people or has been structured by previous social or linguistic activity. Human functioning always requires coordinating with the demands of this larger social context, as this evolves across the lifespan and across history. And finally, the emphasis on the situated character of activity suggests that individuals are not naturally unified beings but instead adapt to different contexts by developing specialized modules of meanings and competencies that might or might not be integrated into more comprehensive systems.

PSYCHOLOGICAL HEALTH AND PATHOLOGY

In general, postmodern psychotherapists shy away from traditional diagnosis, although they recognize its necessity to satisfy the demands of insurance companies and managed health care organizations. This cautiousness about formal diagnosis is in reaction to an objectivistic, modernist way of defining people by their disorder rather than by their unique ways of approaching life difficulties. Although linguistically it may be convenient to refer to a client with profound difficulties with interpersonal relationships, fear of real or imagined abandonment, and self-harm tendencies as a "borderline," doing so does little to expand the choices available to this client or to the therapist who works with the client (Harter, 1995). Stated differently, postmodern psychotherapists reject the view that diagnosis should be viewed as an objective procedure to benefit the therapist, and instead view it as useful only to the extent that it suggests helpful possibilities for the client and therapist to address the problem in more hopeful terms.

This ambivalence about traditional diagnosis notwithstanding, postmodern psychotherapists make use of a number of distinctive problem formulations at different levels of the epigenetic hierarchy from the biogenetic to the cultural. However, they do so with the awareness that these diagnoses themselves are human constructions (Raskin & Lewandowski, 2000) that are helpful to some clients and not others, and to some therapists and not others. It is the interplay between the client and the therapist that guides the utility of formal diagnoses for a particular client, and an interplay between the different levels of the hierarchy that informs the diagnostic process. The tendency of postmodern psychotherapy to consider how these levels interact distinguishes it from psychiatric and psychotherapeutic approaches that focus on only the lower end of the continuum—the biogenetic and the personal–agentic levels. Understanding that a combination of factors may be contributing to personal difficulties allows the psychotherapist multiple avenues for problem exploration, as illustrated in the discussion of assessment that follows. Thus, in this section we describe a general approach to understanding "disorder" at all four levels, deferring discussions of specific problem conceptualizations associated with various constructivist, social constructionist, and narrative perspectives until later in the chapter, when they can be anchored in detailed case examples.

At the biogenetic level, postmodern psychotherapists recognize that some personal difficulties can have physiological origins. As is true with all "best practices" of psychotherapy, it is important for postmodern practitioners to identify physiological causes of distress (thyroid difficulties in mood disorder, blood flow problems in erectile dysfunction, etc.). For this reason, referrals for medical evaluation may be quite appropriate, although pharmacological treatment is rarely regarded as sufficient in itself. This was illustrated by work with a client whose mood swings were usefully regulated by pharmacotherapy for her bipolar disorder. However, both the psychosocial precipitants for her mood fluctuations (e.g., the stillbirth of her child and her husband's drinking) and the effects of her emotional lability (e.g., poor relationships in the workplace) still required a good deal of therapeutic attention at individual and systemic levels.

On the personal–agentic level, diagnostic attention is paid to personal ways of making meaning that have not been revised to meet the changing needs of lived experiences. Indeed, the founding figure of clinical constructivism, George Kelly (1955/1991), described disorder as any construction that continues to be used despite repeatedly having proven itself a failure. Often personal constructions of "how things work" in the world were created during the individual's early years of meaning making, and although they may have been useful guides at that time, they may have lost their utility in current life situations. For example, a child may learn early on that having someone get angry with her means a loss of love or attention, so she works to be "good" and not misbehave. Yet, as an adult avoiding all anger from anyone may result in nonassertive behavior, feelings of low self-worth, and relational difficulties. Thus, a revision of the initial construction of "anger means loss" may lead to a more adaptive way of making life meaning. Note that the revision of life meanings is a co-constructed process between the client and the therapist, although the choice of revision (and the direction it takes) is the propriety of the client.

One critical guide to therapeutic work at the personal–agentic level is provided by the client's emotional experience in and between sessions. In a constructivist view, problematic emotions such as panic are seen as signals of significant shifts in or challenges to the client's meaning-making process (Kelly, 1955/1991), rather than problems to be eliminated or controlled. For example, high levels of *anxiety* reflect the experience of "being caught with our constructs down," unable to anticipate and interpret a compellingly important experience, whereas *guilt* describes the awareness of behaving in a way that conflicts with our core sense of self. The wife of a minister, for instance, experienced recurrent panic

symptoms upon leaving her tightly knit extended family and community to follow her husband's "calling" to another state, a move that thrust her into a new and unfamiliar social world, deprived of familiar supports. This jarring transition was further complicated by keen feelings of guilt and disloyalty when she was tempted to pursue her own dreams of advanced education, which were apparently at odds with core constructs concerning her roles in her family and the African American church community to which she belonged. Finding ways of restoring a sense of connection to her distant family of origin and negotiating a wider range of options for her position as the "first lady" of her congregation lessened both her anxiety attacks and feelings of guilt about how she enacted her role in her church and family.

Like the personal–agentic level, the dyadic–relational level is concerned with meaning-making processes. However, at this level diagnostic attention is paid to the interaction between clients and those most relevant to them in their current life or in the past. In particular, the ability (or inability) of the client to enter into genuine role relationships (Leitner, Faidley, & Celantana, 2000) entailing the cultivation of deep and meaningful intimacies with another person is explored. In addition, the ways in which each partner either validates or invalidates the meaning-making processes of the other can disclose destructive patterns in a couple's relationship, as depicted in the section "The Process of Clinical Assessment." Importantly, relational difficulties do not have to be with people currently in the client's life, as a problematic relationship can still exist with someone who is no longer living. For the minister's wife mentioned earlier, for example, her "abandonment" of the city that was filled with concrete reminders of the life of her recently deceased beloved father complicated her adjustment to her new community, exacerbating both her panic over loss of a symbolic bond with him and her guilt over "leaving him behind." Fostering an emotionally vivid "dialogue" with him by placing him symbolically in an empty chair in the therapy room allowed her to restore a sense of connection to and support from him, freeing her to have a more "real" life with those around her.

At the cultural–linguistic level, postmodern therapists pay particular attention to the cultural embeddedness of difficulties in a client's life. Like all embracing meaning systems, the vast and implicit system of signs, symbols, rules, and roles that constitutes culture is a two-edged sword, on the one hand providing a supportive framework within which people can construct a viable sense of identity, but on the other hand limiting the repertoire of possibilities that they can endorse, or even perceive. In the case of the African American minister's wife, the guilt she experienced for having desires (for advanced education) that did not fit with the "dominant narrative" of her community (White & Epston, 1990) became a focus of concern as she sought ways of drawing on her faith tradition while also finding her unique "voice." As discussed further in the section "Treatment Applicability and Ethical Considerations," this implies that postmodern therapists often function as agents of social change, helping clients reinterpret or resist those features of their cultural frameworks that are oppressive for themselves and others. At the same time, postmodern therapists seek not to impose their own preferred culture on the persons with whom they work, instead focusing on and "deconstructing" the inherent contradictions and possibilities that reside within any given cultural framework.

Finally, we should emphasize the optimism about human potential that underpins many expressions of postmodern therapy. Although the complexity of life—not to mention the complexity of the self—persistently challenges our adaptation, people are ultimately regarded as resourceful in engaging life's inevitable challenges. Postmodern therapists therefore view clients as "incipient scientists" devising ever more compre-

hensive and adequate theories of life (Kelly, 1955/1991), as authoritative "authors" of their own life stories (White & Epston, 1990), or as deliberate "discourse users" (Harré & Gillett, 1994) who selectively draw on the storehouse of available cultural forms to craft satisfying ways of "moving forward" at individual and social levels. This respectful stance toward clients finds expression in all aspects of therapy, from spontaneous forms of assessment in sessions to carefully planned experiments with alternative identities in daily life, as illustrated next.

THE PROCESS OF CLINICAL ASSESSMENT

In keeping with the epigenetic model, constructivist assessment ranges across the entire spectrum of the person–environment system, with a concentration on those mid-level systems (i.e. the personal–agentic and dyadic–relational) that are of most practical relevance to psychotherapy. However, the focus of clinical work is also informed by assessments conducted at concretely biological and abstractly cultural levels, as it is sometimes critical to understand specific organic etiology (e.g., in cases of neurological impairment, physical illness, or disposition to mood disorder) and broad social factors (e.g., economic disadvantage or racial or gender-based oppression) in order to work effectively with individuals and groups struggling with intransigent problems. But even in these cases, constructivist and social constructionist approaches are characterized by attention to the personal and social meanings that characterize and constrain clients presenting for help, as illustrated by Sacks's (1998) evocative exploration of the phenomenological worlds of patients with brain injury, or Brown's (2000a) insightful critique of broad social and linguistic factors that limit the identity options available to women.

In the clinical context, this inclination toward multisystemic assessment means that postmodern therapists sometimes use conventional diagnostic categories (e.g., bipolar disorder and schizophrenia), particularly when these help sensitize the clinician to biogenetic features of the problem that might require attention. But this is typically done only cautiously and conditionally, with the recognition that psychiatric diagnoses are themselves fallible human constructions that provide only a crude orientation to the client's difficulties (Raskin & Lewandowski, 2000). As a result, much more fine-grained assessment of the client's world of meaning is required to reveal his or her individuality, distinctive difficulties, and relevant resources. Our goal in this section is to introduce several such procedures, pointing the reader toward additional sources (G. Neimeyer, 1993) for a fuller presentation of related methods.

As is true for proponents of many other process-oriented approaches to psychotherapy, postmodern therapists prefer to blur the distinction between evaluation and intervention, arguing that the most useful forms of assessment enhance the awareness of both client and therapist regarding relevant themes, issues, difficulties, and resources (Neimeyer, 1993c). As such, they rarely take the form of "stand-alone" procedures completed prior to therapy but instead tend to be introduced in the course of therapy at points at which they have the potential to be not only clarifying but also change generating. Here we present and illustrate a few of the methods used by constructivist, narrative, and social constructionist therapists, some of which also play a role in the detailed case study presented later in the chapter.

Laddering

First introduced by Hinkle (1965), laddering represents an assessment strategy at the personal–agentic level that directly elicits hierarchical features of the individual's personal construct system, linking concrete perceptions, behaviors, or role descriptions with the higher-order issues they imply. As

such, it is frequently helpful in the course of therapy for deepening a client's inquiry into a particular complaint, revealing subtle ways in which a person's sense of self becomes tied up with a symptom. Conversely, as is true for most constructivist methods, it can also help identify important client values and strengths that can provide anchoring points for elaborating a "preferred self" (Eron & Lund, 1996). This is in keeping with the basic precept that every meaning system embodies both problems and prospects, and the most effective therapy entails drawing on the latter to address the former.

Laddering can begin with nearly any personal construct (Kelly, 1955/1991), or significant personal contrast, that is of interest in the course of therapy. For example, in discussing an ongoing conflict between her parents, a client might describe her father as the *rational* one. Sensitized to the implicit contrast, the therapist might then prompt, "whereas your mother is more . . . ," to which the client might reply, "Well, she's more *controlled by her emotions.*" This construct, *rational versus controlled by emotions,* might then become the first "rung" in a ladder that could be "climbed" further through the pattern of questioning described and illustrated later. Alternatively, a client could describe paralyzing indecision about whether to *stay in a familiar job* (or relationship) or *pursue something different.* Again, this contrast could be explored through the laddering procedure, tracing the implications of each alternative. Finally, laddering can be useful in exploring conflicting aspects of oneself, such as antagonistic feelings, actions, or features of one's personality.

Essentially, laddering consists of a series of straightforward, recursive questions in which the therapist first identifies an initial bipolar construct and then asks with which of the poles the client prefers to associate him- or herself. The therapist writes down the construct, notes the client's preference, and then asks either "Why?" or "What is the advantage of that?" (or a linguistic variation) to elicit the higher-order implication of this choice. Connecting the preferred pole to its implied higher-order construct with an arrow, the therapist then requests the opposite or contrast and aligns it with the previous nonpreferred pole. The therapist continues in this way, inquiring about a preference, a reason, or an advantage and its contrast in a cyclical pattern of questioning until the client begins repeating responses or finds it difficult to formulate a further construct. The depiction of the final ladder then can be shared with the client to further mutual inquiry into this hierarchy of meanings and what they imply for his or her behavior. Figure 8.1 depicts the ladder resulting from the interview segment that follows:

Michael was a married, 45-year-old salesman who sought therapy for a nagging depression, which he related to the "emptiness" of his life. Although remarkably buoyant and jocular with office staff, he soon responded to the sympathetic seriousness of the therapist (R.A.N.) by hesitantly acknowledging his loneliness and avoidance of close relationships. When asked for his "personal theory" about the persistence of this problem in his life, Michael responded by saying that he thought it was related to his tendency to "play a role" with everyone he knew, even in supposedly intimate relationships, such as his marriage. Seeking clarification of this important construct through contrast, the therapist asked, "And what would be the opposite of that stance, playing a role?" Michael quickly glanced away, and after a few seconds of silence, again met the therapist's eyes and said, "Just letting people see who I am." Tears immedi-

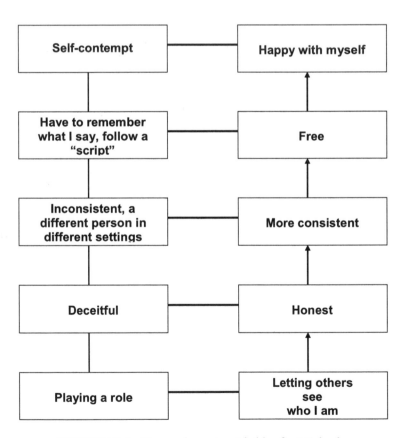

FIGURE 8.1. Personal construct ladder for Michael.

ately followed. Struck by the emotional poignancy of this experiential contrast, the therapist decided to tease out the deeper implications of this construct for Michael through the use of the laddering interview.

THERAPIST: Michael, if you were able to choose between *playing a role* and *letting people see who you are,* which would you prefer?

CLIENT: I guess I'd really want to be someone who *let people see me for who I am,* as hard as that is.

THERAPIST: Can you say why? What would be the advantage of that?

CLIENT: It would be more *honest,* more *real.*

THERAPIST: And that would contrast with . . . ?

CLIENT: Just being *deceitful.*

THERAPIST: And faced with a choice between being *honest* and *deceitful,* you'd prefer. . . .

CLIENT: To be honest.

THERAPIST: Why is that?

CLIENT: Because it would let me be more *consistent.* I feel like I'm *inconsistent, a different person in every setting*—at work, at home, and in social relationships. It's like I don't carry the same person from place to place.

THERAPIST: Hmm. And so faced with the alternatives of being *consistent* or *inconsistent* in that sense, you'd rather . . . ?

CLIENT: Be consistent.

THERAPIST: Because. . . .

CLIENT: (*thoughtful pause*) Because then I would feel *free,* instead of feeling like I have to remember what I said in each relationship, like I have to remember my *script.*

THERAPIST: And choosing between that *scripted* kind of interaction, and that sort of *freedom* . . .

CLIENT: I'd want to be *free.*

THERAPIST: Can you say why?

CLIENT: Hmm . . . (*long pause*). Because then I could be . . . *happy with myself.*

THERAPIST: And the contrast to that is. . . .

CLIENT: Just . . . *self-contempt.* The truth is, I have contempt for people who are like I am. Someday I'd like to be able just to laugh genuinely and not have to work at it, force it for, um, social effect.

Concluding the ladder, Michael then confessed, tears rolling down his cheeks, "You're the first person in 45 years I've ever told, ever acknowledged that my life is a lie."

Once completed, the ladder can flow smoothly into discussion of its deeper themes (in Michael's case, touching on his self-contempt about his ultimate deceitfulness, and his yearning for a sense of freedom from the artificiality of his contrived self-presentations to others). Alternatively, the therapist can sharpen the focus on the client's sense of self-congruence or self-contradiction by going back and asking the client where he or she *actually* would place him- or herself on each of the constructs, revealing points of compatibility or conflict between actual and preferred self-views. Finally, the therapist could draw selectively on any of a number of "facilitative questions" for prompting further processing of the ladder with the client, either in session or in the form of written "homework" between appointments (Neimeyer, Anderson, & Stockton, 2001). These include:

- What central values are implied by the ideas you align yourself with at the upper end of your ladder? How would these expressed in specific behaviors, traits, or roles at the lower end of the ladder? Who in your life best exemplifies your "preferred self" view?
- Were there points at which you hesitated before assigning a pole preference? What might have been going on for you at that point?
- Who in your life most supports/most resists the preferences you describe?
- Which of these preferences are visible/invisible to others? To whom? What

might this say about your important relationships?

- Have there ever been times in your life when you would have placed yourself or your values at the opposite poles of these constructs? What was your life like at that time?
- What could be some positive connotations for your non-preferred poles? Are there any cases in which you could see a value in integrating these opposites in some fashion? What might such a life look like?

Significantly, some of these questions nudge this personal–agentic assessment technique in the direction of a dyadic–relational exploration.

Bow-Tie Interviews

First developed by Procter (1987), the bow-tie interview is situated at the juncture of the personal–agentic and dyadic–relational levels of the epigenetic model, linking personal processes of meaning making to the delicate social ecology of intimate interpersonal relationships that sustain them. It is particularly useful as a means of clarifying complex interactive sequences in conflicted couples and families and in suggesting a road map for intervention. As such, it might be viewed as a variety of *circular questioning*—therapeutic questions that reveal relationships between members of a family—as pioneered by family therapists sharing a concern with the social construction of meaning (Hoffman, 1992). Like the strategies of these postmodern family therapists, bow-tie work entails elaborating the *position* of each member of the problematic system or subsystem, defined as the integrated stance that each person takes at the levels of construction and action. That is, at any given moment of interaction, family members both construe the self and other in certain ways and behave in a way that is coherent with that construction. At the same time, the behaviors or actions of each serve to validate or invalidate the other's construction of their relationship, in a seamless cycle of meaning and action that has no clear beginning or end.

An illustration of this method of assessment is provided with Ken and Donna, a low- to moderate-income white couple in their 20s who sought treatment from a university counseling center for explosive arguments that were threatening their 2-year-old marriage.

Rather than a standard series of questions like those that constitute the laddering interview, bow-tie interviews are structured more fluidly, beginning with any of the four foci that together comprise the bow-tie of the problem (i.e., the constructions or actions that characterize either of the partners). In this case, the obvious starting point was provided by the complaint with which Donna opened their first therapy session, a session she had pushed her accountant husband to attend despite his initial reluctance. Clearly frustrated with Ken's sullen silence, Donna detailed her concerns, which focused on his "shutting her out" and "pushing her away." As a psychology major, she said, she knew that healthy relationships needed to include the sharing of feelings, but she felt increasingly that she had to "dig to reach him on an emotional level." As the therapist explored what Donna was seeking in the relationship, she emphasized her need for "real companionship," something that she more consistently found with friends in the university drama club than with her husband. In response to the therapist's inquiry about how she found herself acting on the basis of these perceptions of the relationship, Donna acknowledged that she would often "press Ken to discuss their problems," and, as he stonewalled her efforts, she would spend more time with university friends to meet her social needs.

Turning to Ken, the therapist then inquired how he made sense of his wife's behavior. Ken's frustration was palpable as he replied, "All she does is complain about our marriage. It's clear that she cares more about her friends than she does about me." Gently prompted to put into words his concerns about the relationship, Ken further disclosed his fear that his wife was "probably having an affair and planning to desert him." In response to the therapist's query about how he found himself acting on the basis of this interpretation of the relationship, Ken conceded that he would withdraw angrily and then periodically explode when Donna would spend evenings away from home. Both partners acknowledged that this cycle had amplified in recent months, though each characteristically blamed the other for its occurrence.

Figure 8.2 diagrams the bow tie of Donna and Ken's positions. Although the natural structure of the session led the therapist to start with Donna's level of the construction of the relationship, in fact the cycle had no clear point of origin that would lead to the attribution of blame to either partner. Instead, each had done his or her part in maintaining the predictable "dance" of their interaction, as the actions of each validated the constructions of the other, which led coherently to that individual's further actions, which further validated the partner's anticipations and interpretations, and so on, without interruption. Looking at the diagram offered by the therapist, both partners felt understood and sensed that an apparently chaotic marriage actually had a clear, if painful predictability. Each also began to grasp, at least in a preliminary way, the meanings of the partner's actions in his or her own terms, and each was more ready to consider thinking about ways to "break the cycle." Indeed, the bow-tie diagram provided a kind of template for further intervention, insofar as altering any aspect of the cycle—whether at the level of behavior change in either partner, reframing the meaning of their interaction, empathically entering the partner's interpretation of their respective actions, or developing more complex "hybrid" interventions across levels or partners—would interrupt the pernicious

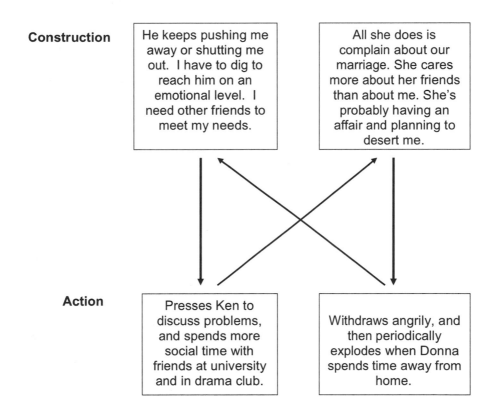

FIGURE 8.2. "Bow tie" linking levels of construction and action for a distressed couple.

pattern and offer "news of a difference" in the relationship (Bateson, 1972). Detailed case studies involving multiple family members are provided by Feixas (1995) and R. Neimeyer (1993c).

Other Assessment Techniques

In keeping with a constructivist emphasis on the structures and processes of meaning making, a broad and growing range of procedures focuses on the content and organization of personal construct systems, the thematic significance people attribute to life experiences, and the style and form of their self-narratives. Here space considerations only permit us to touch on a few of these additional strategies by way of illustration.

First proposed by Kelly (1955/1991) and elaborated by subsequent generations of personal construct theorists, *repertory grid technique* represents a flexible method for eliciting those personal dimensions of meaning that a client uses to structure some important domain of experience. By requesting that the respondent compare and contrast a relevant set of "elements" (e.g., family members, alternative careers, or parts of the body), grid technique prompts the person to articulate personal constructs that he or she uses to organize that aspect of life. Although the resulting constructs can be revealing at a clinical or impressionistic level (e.g., finding that a preponderance of one's constructs are concerned with themes of estrangement or insufficiency versus their contrasts), reliable formal systems of content coding have been devised to analyze construct content into categories (e.g., moral, emotional, relational, and concrete) for both clinical and research purposes (Feixas, Geldschlager, & Neimeyer, 2002). Furthermore, by rating each element on the respondent's own construct dimensions and analyzing the resulting ratings using any of a number of automated programs (Sewell, Adams-Webber, Mitterer, & Cromwell, 1992), the clinician can obtain a quick and comprehensive visual mapping of meaning that the client uses to structure his or her experience of a relevant domain, such as the interpersonal world (Fransella & Bannister, 1977). Thus, rather than having the client respond to standardized questions, grid technique in essence invites clients to construct their own questionnaire through first determining the constructs and then using them to rate or rank the relevant elements. This capacity to yield a highly personal but systematic glimpse of the client's construction of the world, in combination with the ease of administration of computerized grid analysis programs available at no cost through the Internet,[1] helps account for the technique's widespread usage in both clinical and nonclinical applications, ranging from cognitive psychology (Adams-Webber, 2001) to vocational development (G. Neimeyer, 1992). For our purposes, it is also worth noting that grid techniques have been used to assess aspects of all four levels of the epigenetic model, spanning bodily experiences such as the body constructs of cancer patients (Weber, Bronner, Their, Kingreen, & Klapp, 2000), self-roles of depressed clients (Neimeyer, Klein, Gurman, & Greist, 1983), family relationships (Feixas, 1992), and broad cultural attitudes (Neimeyer & Fukuyama, 1984). Variations on the method, such as *implications grids* and *resistance-to-change grids* (Dempsey & Neimeyer, 1995; Hinkle, 1965), provide additional means of identifying core constructs that define the client's key value commitments, which, paradoxically, often constrain their change in psychotherapy.

A somewhat related technique is the *self-confrontation method* (SCM) (Hermans, 2002), a method of personality investigation in which clients are asked to formulate "valuations" or positive/negative assessments of important events and circumstances in their lives and then rate them on a set of provided scales that measure a range of emotional responses to these events, as well as the degree of personal agency or communion with others implied by them. This assessment begins with certain prompting questions to elicit a set of six or eight valuations, such as "Was there something in your past that has been of major importance for your life and that still plays an important part today?" or "Is there a goal or objective that you expect to play an important role in your future life?" In response to the first question, for example, a client might say, "I've always tried to maintain a sense of choice and freedom, and resist attempts on the part of others to determine my actions." Ratings on the provided scales might then suggest that this valuation is associated with strong positive emotions and high levels of personal agency or self-enhancement. In contrast, the same client might assign quite different meanings to the competing valuation, "I am having to compromise my career goals as an artist for the sake of my marriage and step-parenting of my husband's children," rating it as involving strong negative affect (e.g., despondency, disappointment, and unhappiness) and low self-enhancement (e.g., low pride, strength, and self-esteem). Completion of the self-confrontation method at various points across the course of counseling can therefore help crystallize issues demanding therapeutic attention, while also inviting the client to function as a co-investigator in the therapeutic relationship, as illustrated by Hermans and Hermans-Jansen (1995). In this way the SCM functions as a clinical assessment technique situated principally at the personal–agentic level of the epigenetic model.

As presented by Zumaya, Bridges, and Rubio (1999), *sexual holonic mapping* represents an assessment strategy that spans all four levels of the epigenetic model. A *holon* can be defined as a part of a larger system that has sufficient internal complexity to be considered a system in and by itself. In terms of the holonic sexual model, these include systems of *reproduction,* concerned with the significance of procreation; *eroticism,* pertaining to sexual pleasure; *interpersonal bonding,* the capacity for love and attachment; and *gender,* one's identification

with cultural definitions of femininity; masculinity; lesbian, gay, bisexual, or transgendered identities; and so on. By dividing sexuality into holons and inquiring about their unique significance to the client(s), both the therapist and the client(s) are able to obtain a more complete picture of the many interrelated meanings associated with sexuality and how they mesh or conflict with each other. In keeping with a postmodern emphasis on personal and interpersonal meaning making, framing therapeutic inquiries about not only the individual holons but also their points of conflict can reveal a detailed and clinically useful picture of the sexual lives of both individuals and couples. Bridges and Neimeyer (2003) provide a systematic interview format for eliciting this network of holonic meanings, as well as detailed case studies illustrating their application in the context of gay and lesbian relationships. Examples of holonic inquiries include the following:

- What forms of sexual interaction would fit with your preferred gender role? What forms of interaction would not fit? How have you seen these changing across time? (Gender)
- What meanings or fantasies enhance or intensify your excitement and erotic potential? What meanings inhibit it? (Eroticism)
- What role, if any, does having or raising children play in your identity as a person? Has this changed over time, and if so, how? (Reproduction)
- Is the form of closeness sought by both of you similar or dissimilar? How might you signal your need for greater connection or space in a way that is constructive for you both? (Interpersonal bonding)

Thus, through inquiry, creation of sexually related ladders, narrative exploration, and other constructivist techniques, holonic maps are created and sexual meanings are more clearly understood. In the map itself, the holons can be represented as circles of different sizes relative to their importance to the clients, and lines of connection are drawn between the holons to represent their relative impact on the other holons, as illustrated by Zumaya and colleagues (1999) and Bridges and Neimeyer (2003).

Whereas repertory grids, the SCM, and sexual holonic mapping assess the content and structure of a client's meanings, the *Narrative Process Coding System* assesses the topical and stylistic shifts that characterize client accounts of their experience (Angus, Levitt, & Hardke, 1999). First, an investigator using the system segments the dialogue of a transcribed therapy session into topic units that are identified through changes in characters and themes. For instance, a client may begin a session by discussing painful aspects of her divorce and then shift to an examination of disappointing interactions with her parents in childhood. Second, the researcher codes these topic segments into one of three narrative processes. *External* narrative sequences are dominated by event description. An account of how the client put her ex-husband through medical school would be an example of this narrative form. *Internal* narrative sequences focus on emotional and experiential states. A description of the client's anger at his then filing for divorce would illustrate this narrative process. Finally, *reflexive* narrative sequences entail analysis and interpretation of events and internal reactions in order to understand their significance. An exploration of the meaning of "betrayal" in this client's life would be classified as reflexive.

Through the assessment of narrative processes, researchers can trace how client's storytelling about life events evolves across therapy and in response to therapeutic interventions. For example, investigators have found that experiential therapists tend to shift discourse from external event descriptions toward internal and reflexive processes to promote self-exploration and meaning making, while clients tend to shift into a more external process, to integrate their therapeutic insights into their daily life experiences. Likewise, narrative process assessment of various types of treatment could suggest what forms of client processing are associated with more favorable outcomes in different forms of therapy. For instance, research suggests that prompting clients toward an narrating experiences of self and others in an "external" voice (e.g., by communicating childhood events that are then interpreted by the therapist), seems to facilitate progress in psychodynamic therapy, whereas encouraging a more "reflexive," interpretive style appears to promote more rapid gains in a cognitive treatment (Angus et al., 1999). Other constructivist methods for assessing different dimensions of clients' self-narratives include various *content scales* for coding the extent to which people feel like "origins" of life choices or "pawns" of fate, as well as their level of "cognitive anxiety" associated with the diagnosis of serious illness, culture shock, or other unanticipated life transitions (Gottschalk, Lolas, & Viney, 1986). Narrative and content coding of this kind concentrates on the personal–agentic and dyadic–relational levels of the epigenetic model, depending on whether one is coding client monologues (or journals, etc.) or the dialogic interplay of therapeutic discourse.

THE PRACTICE OF THERAPY

As a trend that has influenced many contemporary psychotherapies rather than a single distinct "school" or method, postmodern practices vary widely in their structure, orientation to goal setting, and therapeutic processes. In the following sections we describe the range of approaches to each of these features and underscore the overarching similarities that typify these broadly constructivist forms of therapy.

Basic Structure of Therapy

There is no preferred timetable for therapy that characterizes all postmodern practice.

Several contemporary constructivist therapists have followed Kelly's lead in advocating that therapy be as efficient as possible, as the one to six sessions that characterize depth-oriented brief therapy (DOBT) illustrate (Ecker & Hulley, 1996). On the other hand, some constructivist practitioners adopt the model of therapy as "intermittent long-term consultation," in which the therapist remains available as a guide or "fellow traveler" from time to time, as the client encounters unexpected detours or impasses along life's journey (Mahoney, 1991). Some developmentally oriented constructivist therapists even plan intensive, long-term therapies that can span years of work, seeking to reveal and restructure the client's basic affective stance in intimate relationships (Arciero & Guidano, 2000; Guidano, 1995).

The timing of sessions is similarly variable. Kelly's (1955/1991) fixed role therapy typically involves multiple sessions of practice and processing across a 2- or 3-week period as clients confront the challenge of enacting new roles or identities in their social world, whereas family therapies that adopt a postmodern emphasis often are conducted on a monthly basis, allowing members time to integrate the changes provoked by sessions in the weeks between (Procter, 1987). As these examples imply, *who* attends sessions can be as variable as *when* they do so, with many postmodern practitioners moving smoothly from an individual to a relational focus and back again, with shifting participation within a given therapy in keeping with immediately relevant goals (Efran, Lukens, & Lukens, 1990). Likewise, innovative group therapy formats, such as the Interpersonal Transaction Group (R. Neimeyer, 1988), systematically promote engagement in intimate dyadic conversations within the group, followed by whole-group processing of discoveries made about self and others in the one-on-one conversations. Indeed, some postmodern practices blur the boundaries of conventional therapy altogether, as in the community development work that charac-

terizes social therapy with disadvantaged youth, wartorn communities, and other neglected populations (Newman & Holzman, 1999). Accordingly, the degree of structure within sessions varies widely, although a general precept of seeking minimum sufficient structure to serve therapeutic goals is typically advocated.

Goal Setting

Therapeutic objectives in postmodern therapies are rarely imposed by the therapist and, indeed, are often imprecisely understood even by the client prior to engagement in the therapeutic process. What is typically clear to both is that the client is in some form of distress; something about the client's means of engaging the social world is painful, and perhaps recurrently so. But aside from alleviating this distress, the implications of the initial complaint for their work together will often require further elaboration, during which the problem is likely to undergo change and redefinition (Kelly, 1955/1991). Thus, in sharp contrast to therapeutic perspectives that emphasize the importance of establishing clearly defined target goals from the outset of therapy, postmodern perspectives typically seek to foster a sense of "spaciousness" in the therapeutic hour, a minimally structured encounter in which the initially vague "felt sense" of the problem can be carefully articulated in a way that yields greater clarity and direction (Gendlin, 1996).

But the general distrust of agenda-driven sessions in no way suggests that constructivist therapies are wandering, inefficient, or directionless. On the contrary, the therapist is at every moment of therapeutic contact seeking to focus on precisely that "growing edge" of the client's feelings, concerns, understanding, or preparedness for action that is most ready for attention and extension. For example, this stance might find expression in therapist inquiries at the start of a session, such as "What do you feel ready to accomplish today?" "What would you like this session to do for you?" or "What has become clearer for you since the last time we met?" In addition, it suggests the relevance of looking for specific "markers" of implicit "tasks" that clients are ready to undertake in just this moment of therapy (Greenberg, Elliott, & Rice, 1993), such as the "unfinished business" with her father that suggested the relevance of an imaginal two-chair dialogue in the case of the African American minister's wife cited earlier in this chapter. Thus, a delicate and precise attention to the client's use of *language*—with all the coverbal signals (e.g., shifts in vocal tone, pace, and intonation) and nonverbal nuances (e.g., facial expressions and gestures) that modulate its meaning—characterizes postmodern therapy, such that each moment of interaction suggests what form of conversational intervention is most appropriate to foster the deepening, unfolding, or reconstruction of meaning concerning the problem under discussion (R. Neimeyer, 2001). Such an approach uses the moment-to-moment interaction between client and therapist as the surest and most efficient guide to identifying *process goals* of immediate relevance to the therapy, rather than generically relevant agendas for gross classes of problems (e.g., depression and social anxiety) or clients (e.g., "borderlines" and trauma survivors). Thus, to use Mahoney's (1988) terms, postmodern therapies are less "teleological"— oriented toward some preenvisioned objective—than they are "teleonomic"— displaying meaningful evolution across time, even though the final outcome cannot be forecast in advance (as in child development). This effort to maintain relational responsiveness to the implicit questions or tasks being posed by the client's presentation at each moment of therapy helps ensure that the therapist is attending at the appropriate level of the epigenetic model, with due attention to personal, interpersonal, and cultural factors of relevance to their immediate work.

At an abstract level, however, postmodern therapies can be said to have certain *outcome goals,* which include enhancing client reflexivity, or self-awareness and capacity for self-change (Rennie, 1992), relational responsiveness and openness to others at core levels (Leitner, 1995), empowerment or a sense of clients' "voice" in their lives (Brown, 2000b), and the enactment and social affirmation of a preferred self-narrative (Eron & Lund, 1996). Several of these goals are evident in the illustrations of therapeutic strategies that follow.

Process Aspects of Treatment

As noted by Kelly (1955/1991), constructivist therapies tend to be "technically eclectic but theoretically consistent," promoting the use of diverse change strategies within a coherent but evolving understanding of each case. In this section we sample this diversity of therapeutic methods, suggesting principles that characterize their use, or argue for the addition of collateral forms of treatment, such as psychotropic medication. Later sections on the therapeutic relationship and mechanisms of change then provide a broader context for appreciating their role in therapy, as illustrated in the extended case study later in the chapter.

Depth oriented brief therapy (DOBT; Ecker & Hulley, 1996) is an approach to treatment that also falls under the rubric of postmodern psychotherapy. Its central assumption is that of *symptom coherence,* the idea that at the level of higher-order, unconscious constructions of reality, the client is compelled to have the problem, despite the real pain and trouble it is causing within his or her life. In this view, clients begin therapy consciously identified with an *anti-symptom position,* in which they view the symptom as an unnecessary impediment in their lives. In many therapies the therapist and client would work together against the symptom, in an attempt to eliminate it directly or develop compensatory cognitive, behavioral, or social skills for managing it. In contrast, in DOBT the counselor works experientially with the client to identify the emotional truth of the symptom—the unconscious *pro-symptom position* that makes the symptom vitally necessary to maintain. Only by fully integrating this position into conscious awareness can the client either recognize that it no longer has relevance to his or life or, alternatively, acknowledge its adaptive value in the present and realign goals so that the "symptom" becomes a *choice,* rather than a problem. Thus, DOBT represents a deep implementation of the personal–agentic premises of the epigenetic framework, by bringing to life the hidden agency that perpetuates the symptom.

There are four main aspects of DOBT (Ecker & Hulley, 2000). First, the therapist needs to empathically engage and validate the real suffering of the client in relation to the symptom. Second, the unconscious pro-symptom position that requires the symptom needs to be discovered experientially by the client, prompted by any of several forms of "radical questioning" by the therapist. Third, it is vital to fully integrate the specific themes and purposes of that emotional reality into the consciousness of the client, sometimes underscoring them through an index card task at the end of the session, as in the case vignette that follows. Finally, there is the transformation of previous meaning making to be more congruent with the main themes and purposes underlying the presenting symptomatology. A brief case example helps to clarify this method.

> Carol, a woman in her mid–30s, initially brought her 11-year-old daughter, Dana, to therapy in a community mental health clinic. After several sessions, Carol asked to be seen individually (by SKB), stating that despite their emotional closeness in other respects, she had always felt cold and distant toward her husband sexually. Her only explanation for this situation was that she just didn't like to have sex very much, although she reported that she truly wanted to enjoy the sexual dimension of her marriage, a conscious view that represented the anti-symptom position. As a means of *radical*

questioning—so-called because of its intent to get to the root of the problem—the therapist asked her to complete a sentence stem several times aloud with the first thing that came to her mind: "If I were to like having sex with my husband, I'd feel _____." Carol first stated that she would feel "great" without the symptom, then upon repetition of the stem, "happy," and then after a prolonged silence and with an almost confused look on her face, she voiced the word "embarrassed" hesitantly. Sensing that she was getting close to the pro-symptom position, the therapist asked her to stay in that embarrassed state and to complete the sentence, "I feel embarrassed even thinking about enjoying sex with Franklin. . . ." Doing so, rather than intellectualizing about her experience, Carol suddenly flashed to a series of memories that ushered in the emotional truth of her sexual difficulties, which had their origin in her parents' openly erotic behavior with one another during her adolescence. In a quiet tone, with her legs crossed and her head in her hands, Carol then recalled a time when she was about 15 years old when her mother walked into the bathroom and found her masturbating. Far from being angry, her mother was so pleased that she not only told Carol's father but also called several friends and told them about this "beautiful good news." Carol identified her decision to shut out sexual feelings from that very point. Discussing this series of memories and associated feelings, she also realized that enjoying sex with her husband subjectively meant becoming like her mother, and closer to risking mortifying her own daughter, Dana, in the same way. At the end of the powerful session, the therapist wrote the following pro-symptom position statement on a card to underscore for Carol the compelling purpose that necessitated her sexual neutrality—"I hate to admit it, but experiencing sexual pleasure with my husband makes me more like my mother. So, even though it is hurting my marriage, I will continue to avoid sexual contact, because it is better to sacrifice pleasure and intimacy than to risk doing to Dana what my mother did to me." Prompted by the therapist, Carol read the card aloud and stated that she didn't like what it said but agreed that it was accurate. The therapist then asked Carol to read it twice a day in the week between sessions, with no other attempt to change her sexual behavior with her husband. In the next session, Carol reported that the statement began to seem almost silly to her during the week, and although she knew it would take time and practice, finding a new way to understand her sexuality as her own and not her mother's was a freeing experience for her and also for her relationship with her husband. Once held as a conscious rather than unconscious position, the previously prevailing view soon lost much of its power, permitting the client to relinquish it as her governing emotional reality.

Fixed role therapy (FRT; Kelly, 1955/1991) is a technique used in postmodern psychotherapy (particularly personal construct therapy) to increase the permeability or flexibility of the client's construct system, to enhance awareness of alternative constructions of identity and social relationships, and to aid in the validation of new constructs. As such, it is positioned at the interface of the personal–agentic and dyadic–relational spheres of the epigenetic model. This technique begins with an evaluation of the client's current construct system by asking her to write a self-characterization sketch from the perspective of someone who knows her intimately and sympathetically, perhaps better than anyone actually does know her. After analyzing the sketch to get a sense of the client's core role constructs (R. Neimeyer, 1993c), the therapist then writes a script of an alternative identity or role for the client to enact for a fixed 2- or 3-week period. The role is carefully constructed and needs to be radically different than the current behaviors of the client, without representing their polar opposites (i.e., an introverted client might be coached to take on the role of "Dee Tective," someone who subtly tries to ferret out the motivations of others, rather than someone who

is simply a social extrovert). In addition, it should be in keeping with the basic needs and values of the client.

The client attempts to enact this role within the therapy session first, and then transfers this role to the outside world. The purpose of FRT is to loosen the client's identification with old constructs and open the possibility for new ways of interacting and making life meanings. In fact, it is not uncommon for the client to report that the new ways of interacting feel almost "natural" after the 2-week period, a period filled with practicing the new role with the therapist, and performing it between sessions in the context of an increasingly intimate set of "real life" relationships. A particularly successful FRT outcome was seen with Mayishai, an Asian American college student, whose (abbreviated) self-characterization sketch described her as follows:

> Mayishai is an extremely generous, loving and passive person. Because she wants to make friends quickly, she often lets people take advantage of her and always puts herself last. She is comfortable in this role because it is the role that she plays in her family. However when she uses her generosity to become friends with those outside her culture, they do not understand her and take advantage of her. She does not feel able to tell people that they have hurt her feelings and will simply make excuses not to see these people again. She has become untrustworthy and more withdrawn lately and finds that she has even fewer friends than she did before.

As a provisional alternative, her fixed role enactment sketch read in part as follows:

> Mai Life is a wise and insightful person who, like a fortune-teller, can often know what people are made of within the first few moments of meeting them. She uses the life skills she has gained from helping others to recognize their needs right away and then decides for herself whether she will be the person to meet these needs or not, realizing that at times they will grow more by relying

on others rather than only on her. She is kind while being assertive and direct in her communication with others and although she likes to be around people, she is very choosy about her friends.

In this particular enactment sketch, it was important to pay attention to the role of culture in the client's life and not to move to an extreme that would be in conflict with her family and cultural responsibilities. However, the fixed role allowed Mayishai to use her life skills differently and see herself as a capable and insightful person, one who was desirable as a friend and one who could make choices about her interactions with others. After the role enactment had finished, the client reported that she felt like she was "a better judge of character" and had found more satisfying friendships. She did report that saying "no" to others was still difficult, but now she felt that she had an active choice in when to say "yes" or "no" rather than simply acquiescing to everyone. Importantly, FRT explicitly invites the client to "derole" after the weeks of enactment, carrying forward her or his discoveries on an elective basis. In this sense, the most profound lesson of FRT may be not a particular new role to retain but the deep experiential recognition that one's identity in a social field is an invention, and one that can be reconstructed on an ongoing basis.

Narrative therapy, spanning the cultural–linguistic, dyadic–relational, and personal–agentic levels of the epigenetic model, seeks to reveal the narrow societal prescriptions and assumptions that constrain people's ability to recognize the options open to them (Winslade & Monk, 2001). Because problematic identities are inevitably constructed in social contexts and sustained in repetitive interactions between people, it is these very patterns or *dominant narratives* that become the initial focus of therapeutic attention, as the therapist works with the client to make more visible the influence of the problem-saturated story in his or her

life. Using *curious questions,* the therapist then helps the client "deconstruct" the dominant account of his or her problem and begin to recognize his or her influence on the problem itself. By gradually noticing, historicizing, documenting, and circulating the client's steps toward a preferred story of life and relationships, the therapist helps him or her consolidate an alternative self-narrative, one more rich in possibility (White & Epston, 1990).

Like feminist therapists, narrative therapists are especially vigilant in detecting the roles of cultural discourses that reinforce problematic identities or relational practices, such as the prescriptions for acceptable appearance that engender anorexic behaviors among young women or discourses of personal entitlement that induce couples into conflict-saturated exchanges in divorce mediation contexts. By first *externalizing* these discursive patterns, the therapist helps clients recognize that *they* are not the problem but that the *problem* is the problem, and that they can take an active role in resisting its influence.

The typical steps entailed in this narrative approach can be illustrated by the case of David, a young man in his early 20s, who struggled with depression to such an extent that he dropped out of school, although he was a capable student, was becoming estranged from his family, and was beginning to call in sick consistently to his place of employment. When he began to isolate himself in his room and make indirect allusions to suicide, his parents pressed him to seek therapy (with RAN).

Accompanied to his first therapy session by his father, David immediately conveyed the impression of a young man in torment, whose obvious suffering elicited helpless expressions of concern by his father, expressions that David consistently rebuffed. I therefore focused principally on David, asking his permission to interview him in more detail about the problem while his father remained in the room as a silent witness. David readily agreed. As David recounted the story of his struggle with the problem in outline form, I asked him, "What would you call this problem that seems to have enveloped your life and obscured your future?" David's immediate answer, "a black fog," was more evocative than the clinical term "depression," and it provided a first approximation to naming the problem as something that seemed to have taken on a life of its own over the last several years. Continuing this *externalizing conversation,* I asked David to say more about the history of the problem, prompting him occasionally with questions such as, "When did this black fog first creep into your life?" "What were things like before it arrived?" "When did you first notice it darkening your perception of the world?" David responded that the fog made its first appearance when he was in high school, when the promise of a brilliant athletic career began to dim, despite his father's and coach's faith in his abilities. I gradually shifted toward mapping the "real effects" of the fog in his life through the use of *relative influence questioning*: "What effect would you say the fog has had on your view of yourself and your abilities?" "What plans does the fog have for your educational and occupational future?" "To what extent has the fog seeped into your home life?" "Who in the family seems to be most lost in the fog with you?" David responded to these inquiries with increasing animation, noting how "different" they felt from the internalizing conversations with other professionals that implicitly lodged the problem *inside* him, in terms of cognitive distortions, behavioral deficits, and biochemical imbalances. As a result of this changed perspective, he began to recognize the impact the problem had had on his darkening view of himself, and how it also was making him and his family more and more "invisible" to one another. With these effects in full view, David was ripe for considering questions about *his* influence on the *problem,* using metaphors both implicit in his description of the problem and derived from his athletic background: "What actions have you taken to try to cut through the fog?" "Are there times that you have been able to score points against it, even when you feel like the underdog? Are there others who

seem to be playing on your team at those times? Who in your life is most convinced that you can make a comeback?" Gradually, David began to identify a handful of *unique outcomes* (White & Epston, 1990), "sparkling moments" in which he was able to resist the influence of the dominant narrative of depression, and touchingly reached out to his father in response to the questions regarding valued teammates.

In our next session David brought me a remarkable personal journal he was writing, titled "Lost in the Fog: A Portrait of Depression." As he began to make tangible gains in returning to work and opening to conversations with family members—both in extended family therapy sessions and in his daily life—we began to historicize this *preferred story* of David as resilient and resourceful, someone who was increasingly able to glimpse the outlines of a more satisfying future through the thinning fog of his depression. Selected readings, such as Parker Palmer's (2000) *Let Your Life Speak: Listening to the Voice of Vocation,* offered David alternative and more affirmative understandings of his years of impasse and career indecision, a general narrative frame that he readily appropriated and extended in personal directions. With his family's assent, David expressed confidence in his ability to continue to resist depression's influence after six sessions of therapy, and follow-up contact suggested that he continued to make positive strides several months later.

Detailed procedures for conducting narrative therapy have been drafted for a great diversity of problems, ranging from conflict mediation (Winslade & Monk, 2001) to stuttering (DiLollo, Neimeyer, & Manning, 2002), and for both children (Freeman, Epston, & Lobovits, 1997) and adults (Monk, Winslade, Crocket, & Epston, 1996).

Homework

As suggested by these three representative therapeutic methods, between-session activities are considered a useful adjunct to some, but by no means all, forms of post-modern practice. When they occur, they are more likely to stem from the initiative of the client than from the explicit assignment of the therapist (as in David's case above), although "awareness homework" such as the index card task of DOBT might occasionally be given. By comparison, detailed homework assignments such as the between-session enactment featured in FRT are relatively rare and carefully monitored by the therapist when used. The general skepticism about the heavy use of therapist-assigned homework among postmodern practitioners reflects their conviction that change emerges more as a result of client activity than of therapist design (Bohart & Tallman, 1999), and hence change should not typically be engineered by a high level of therapist prescription.

Resistance to Change

In many postmodern psychotherapy traditions resistance is viewed as an adaptive response to the threat of change to core ways of understanding the world (Kelly, 1955/1991). It is for this reason that specialized assessment techniques have been devised to identify constructs that are likely to be resistant to change (see earlier), and that approaches like FRT seek to mitigate the threat of change by allowing clients to wear the protective mask of "make believe" as they experiment with new roles that do not contradict their previous constructions of self and others. In fact, resistance is usually more apparent when superordinate constructs are being challenged, and as such, it can provide a window into the symptom-maintaining processes of the client. For example, DOBT welcomes the resistance that often arises when therapists ask clients to view themselves in a familiar problem situation (e.g., in Carol's case, having sex with her husband), but without resorting to the usual symptomatic behavior. In such instances, clients often find themselves unable to step into a symptom-free position, even

in their imagination, allowing the therapist to interview them directly about what makes it essential to retain the consciously problematic but unconsciously essential symptomatic way of being. "Befriending" the resistance in this way, rather than merely interpreting it or seeking compliance with therapist requests, can thereby lead to greater therapeutic progress.

Technical Errors

As approaches to therapy that emphasize delicate attunement to the flow of client language during the session, constructivist and narrative therapies require a shifting attention to client metaphors, meanings, and narratives, which suggest precisely which therapeutic task the client is ready to undertake at a given moment (Greenberg et al., 1993). For example, attending to a succession of *quality terms* in the client's speech—phrases or expressions that reveal the client's position with particular power or clarity—helps establish a progressive focus for the therapeutic negotiation of meaning (R. Neimeyer, 2001), as does mutual elaboration of self-descriptive metaphors (Martin, 1994) and provision of "space" for the articulation of implicit meanings not yet symbolized in words (Gendlin, 1996). This close following and amplification of client meaning making suggests that the fundamental technical problems that can arise in such therapies are *tracking errors* in which the therapist moves too far beyond the client's expressed meaning, typically in the direction of the therapist's own agenda. For example, at a transitional moment in a long-standing relationship, a client offered the following metaphor to describe her changing position in the world, a metaphor in which the therapist attempted to join her:

CLIENT: It's strange, but it's like the walls that have defined my boundaries in relation to Karen are beginning to shift, to move right before my eyes. . . .

THERAPIST: Hmm. . . . So it almost seems that your space for living is growing, that the boundaries are opening up in some way.

CLIENT: Umm . . . well, not really opening up, but just shifting, like they are dunes of sand being blown in a desert storm, and I'm not quite clear where they'll end up.

THERAPIST: Ah, so it's not clear at this point in what direction the dunes are moving, whether they're closing in or opening up. . . . Can you say something about the feeling that comes up for you as you visualize yourself in the middle of that stormy movement?

CLIENT: (*closing her eyes; 3-second pause*) Umm, yea . . . it just feels scary, uncertain . . .

In this instance the overeager therapist was in the general "ballpark" of the client's meaning but initially overextended its leading edge in an optimistic direction. Fortunately, clients are adept at providing *process validation* for each move that the therapist makes, moving toward greater intimacy, depth of disclosure, and affirmation of emerging meanings when the intervention is "on target," and hesitating, shifting to more superficial levels, and becoming more symptomatic when their therapists lose attunement (Leitner, 1995). Process invalidation provided by the client in the second conversational turn discussed previously allowed the therapist to once again find the leading edge of the client's meaning making and to make a useful contribution to its elaboration.

Psychotropic Medication

Although the focus of constructivist, social constructionist, and narrative therapies is on the conversational reconstruction of meaning (and its "performance" in action), there are times when adjunctive treatment such as psychotropic medication is both appropriate and desirable. A case in point is the treatment of serious psychosis, in which an identified patient's constructions are so shifting and disorganized that few stable meanings can be identified (Bannister, 1963), or when a delusional system is so entrenched that it precludes the minimal level of trust and openness required for therapeutic conversation (Lorenzini, Sassaroli, & Rocchi, 1989). For instance, the work of Seikkula and his colleagues in Finland with families experiencing the psychotic deterioration of one of their members relies principally on the use of "open dialogue," in which integrated teams of professionals work intensively with families in their homes to foster deep-going discussions of the significance of the distressing symptoms, with full participation of the identified patient (Seikkula, Alakare, & Aaltonen, 2001a). However, in approximately 25% of cases neuroleptic medication was deemed appropriate to make the patient's coherent participation in the dialogue process possible, although pharmacotherapy itself did not appear linked to more favorable outcomes in their research (Seikkula, Alakare, & Aaltonen, 2001b).

Termination

In postmodern perspectives such as narrative therapy, termination is a mutually decided on process that is viewed as a graduation or a rite of passage (Epston & White, 1995) to a preferred identity, a transition that is in itself therapeutic. Consolidating gains made over the course of therapy can be accomplished through the use of a variety of questions, such as the following:

- If you were to write a manual for how to overcome the problem you've just conquered, what sort of ideas would it include? What personal and relationship qualities allowed you to identify this know-how and put it to use? How could you keep this knowledge alive in your own life in the future?

- If someone else consulted me for a problem like the one that once dominated your life, what advice might you offer about how to overcome its influence? Could you as a veteran of this battle write a letter of encouragement that I might share with such a person?

- What might we have seen in your previous life that would have tipped us off to your ability to break free of the problem now?

- What has this experience taught you about the kind of person you are and the kind of life story you want to live in the future?

- How would the knowledge you now have about yourself influence your next step forward? What would the person you will be a few years from now have to say to the person who is sitting here today about what is possible in his life?

- Now that you have reached this point of graduation into a different kind of life, who else should know about it? What difference do you think it would make in their attitude toward you if they had this news?

Such questions can also be augmented by any of a number of creative documents offered by the therapist to acknowledge this passage (e.g., Declarations of Independence from the problem, Certificates of Special Knowledge recognizing major insights, or diplomas signaling graduation from therapy). Final sessions can also be planned as ritual or celebratory occasions in which key support figures in the individual's life might be invited to a social occasion that honors the client's achievements (White & Epston, 1990). Thus, far from traditional conceptions of termination as loss of a special relationship with the therapist or a hazardous transition in the generalization of therapist-taught skills, the completion of therapy can itself help empower the client in pursuing a more satisfying life narrative in the future.

THE THERAPEUTIC RELATIONSHIP AND THE STANCE OF THE THERAPIST

The dialogical conception of identity endorsed by most postmodern approaches carries implications for our understanding of a responsive psychotherapy—simply stated, the therapeutic relationship represents the medium in which the client encounters and performs a new sense of self (R. Neimeyer, 2002). As Shotter (2000) notes, "we continuously shape, build, or construct our performance in our daily affairs as we 'act into' opportunities offered us" (p. 102). In the "joint action" of psychotherapy, the therapist and client engage in "continuous process communication" (Fogel, 1993), in which partners are simultaneously active in responding in gestural, coverbal, and verbal modes to the overlapping expressive behavior of the other(s). A puzzled or distracted look on the visage of the client, for example, sends a "back channel" communication to the speaking therapist to modify or interrupt his or her speech act to take into account the activity of the client. Likewise, transcripts of psychotherapy consistently document the "piggybacking" of client and therapist verbalizations, each elaborating the preceding thought of the other. In this dynamic dialogical interplay, "it becomes meaningless to ask who is the initiator or receiver of the message; both self and other are continuously affected by the exchange of information. . . . The 'message' is socially constructed and negotiated in the very process of communication" (Mascolo et al., 1997, p. 16). Like cooperative soccer players who pass a ball back and forth down field until one scores a goal, developmentally significant insights in psychotherapy are irreducible to the achievement of therapist or client considered alone.

Because much of the change that happens in the meaning-making processes of the client is thoroughly dialogical, the nuanced interbraiding of client and therapist meanings is not easily "decomposed" into a constituent set of relational techniques. However, something can be said about the basic stance of the therapist, and some of the general strategies by which therapists help "sculpt" the malleable medium of therapeutic discourse while respecting the substance of the client's meaning system (see Table 8.1 for details).

In keeping with the collaborative, reflective, and process-directive approach that is central to postmodern psychotherapy, the stance of the therapist is one of respectful, empathic engagement in the client's evolving narrative of self and world. The therapist does not decide what new meanings will be created but instead assists clients in recognizing incompatible old meanings or constructs and works with them as they endeavor to find alternatives. Kelly (1955/1991) believed meanings are created and re-created through interactions between the client and the social surround (Leitner & Faidley, 2002) and that the therapist serves as a representative of the social world in therapy. For this reason, clients often enact *transference* patterns with therapists. For Kelly, transference was understood not as an inherently pathological intrusion into therapy but rather as an inevitable outcome of hu-

TABLE 8.1. Selected Process Interventions in Constructivist Psychotherapy

Intervention	Description
Orienting	Establishing the client's readiness for a specific therapeutic task
Centering	Attending quietly to that which seems most important at a particular therapeutic moment
Focusing	Articulating the "felt sense" of a problem or issue, first contacted as a bodily awareness
Empathizing	Working within the client's meaning system and communicating an understanding of it
Analogizing	Developing figuratively rich language to capture an experience
Nuancing	Highlighting an aspect of the client's communication to invite further elaboration
Dilating	Widening the field of discussion to include broader implications
Constricting	Narrowing discussion to a single focal issue
Tacking	Shifting back and forth dialectically between two poles of the client's experience (e.g., past to present, or from self to social surround) to assess continuity of client's experience across time or contexts
Contrasting	Exploring a sensed conflict in the client's experience
Structuring	Articulating or organizing diffuse material in a way that clarifies its implications for action
Ambiguating	Fostering a looser or more approximate meaning
Weaving	Overlaying or connecting strands of related material
Enacting	Performing one or more "I-positions" in therapeutic monologue or dialogue in the session
Externalizing	Discursively reconstructing a problem as something separate from the client, whose influence can be explored
Witnessing	Serving as an audience for the client's experimentation with a new self-narrative

man meaning making. Upon encountering the therapist for the first time, the client (like anyone else attempting to engage in a new relationship) will import into it those constructions of broadly similar relationships—as he or she sees them—in order to anticipate and "act into" the opportunities the therapist affords. For example, a client might initially anticipate that the therapist will respond like a nurturing mother, a judgmental father, a forgiving priest, a skilled physician, or a sometimes understanding, sometimes fickle lover. However, when constructions transferred from old relationships to new ones are too impermeable or inflexible to meet the uniqueness of the new relationship and to be modified accordingly, difficulties can arise. In particular, for clients with deeply disturbed personal histories, the core of psychotherapy may consist in offering them a reparative relationship in which they are able to risk letting therapists have access into their core understanding of self (Leitner & Faidley, 1996). The creation of this *role relationship* (in which one person attempts to construe the deepest meaning-making process of another) is vital, as both client and therapist seek to establish a reverential *I–Thou* relationship that acknowledges the uniqueness of the other (Buber, 1958). This reciprocal connection does not ordinarily imply that the therapist discloses personal *content* in the therapeutic relationship, although the disclosure of the therapist's *process responses* to the client's behavior (e.g., feeling moved by the client's courageous confrontation of a difficult issue, or feeling distanced by a client's shift toward apparently superficial content) can play a useful role in fostering client awareness and enhancing the intensity of the therapeutic connection.

Like all evolving relationships, that between a given client and therapist will be unique, and will follow its own trajectory. But in general, there will be a shift from early high levels of therapist engagement in process interventions that help co-construct the therapeutic discourse (see Table 8.1) to

the later role of being an active audience to the client's performance of new possibilities. As therapeutic gains are anchored in the responses of relevant others beyond the therapeutic dialogue, the therapist typically recedes into a supporting role for the enactment of the client's new narrative, remaining available for future consultation as necessary as a given episode of therapy reaches its natural conclusion.

CURATIVE FACTORS OR MECHANISMS OF CHANGE

In a sense, neither the concept of "curative factors" nor the concept of "mechanisms of change" fits comfortably within a postmodern framework, deriving as they do from medical and mechanistic metaphors that poorly describe the practice of constructivist, social constructionist, and narrative therapies. However, a concern with human change processes pervades this chapter, as discussed and illustrated in sections on assessment, the therapeutic relationship, the practice of therapy, and in several of the case vignettes offered to exemplify these principles in practice. For this reason, we comment here only briefly on those factors that are presumed to facilitate change in a range of postmodern approaches.

In general, postmodern psychotherapy, like many humanistic approaches, construes change as arising largely from the client's meaning-making capabilities (Bohart & Tallman, 1999). Although new possibilities are brought forth in the dialogic relationship between the client and the therapist, it is client activity and insight that ultimately produce lasting life adaptations. Thus, therapist designs and interventions have only an instigating role as curative factors, serving mainly to highlight client resources, (mal)adaptive core meaning-making processes, and modes of relating that have lost their utility. As such, specific techniques are primarily useful in that they help to elaborate personal meaning-making activities of the client rather than producing change in and of themselves.

The client reflexivity regarding problematic constructions or life narratives that is valued by most postmodern therapists is sometimes, but by no means routinely, supported by historical interpretations of how those patterns came into existence in formative experiences in the client's life. However, the "interpretation" that is crucial here is rarely that of the therapist—instead, it is the meaning attributed to such patterns by the client that triggers insight and possible behavior change. Therapists working within such an understanding therefore typically avoid highly interpretive interactions with clients. Instead, they concentrate on experiential interventions (as illustrated in case examples of DOBT elsewhere in this chapter) that assist the client in encountering those circumstances that contributed to the adoption of a self-limiting pattern that has been perpetuated in current situations. Ultimately, in keeping with constructivist metatheory, the interpretations placed on the client's life experiences need not be *literally* true (such as determining whether a parent was or was not in fact abusive), as long as they correspond to the *emotional* truth of the client (Ecker & Hulley, 1996) and carry helpful implications for approaching the future in a new way (Kelly, 1969). A similar orientation to the "narrative truth" rather than the "historical truth" of the client's experience is evident in constructivist variations of contemporary psychodynamic therapy (Spence, 1982).

If there are "skills" that are relevant to the promotion of self-change in postmodern therapies, they would focus primarily on the client's abilities to explore the subtle interbraiding of personal and social meaning making and the capacity to symbolize, articulate, and renegotiate those constructions of self and world that promote or impede adaptation to shifting life experiences (R. Neimeyer, 1995b). In this sense, an ultimate goal of constructivist psychotherapies is helping clients become *connoisseurs of their*

experience, leaving them better positioned to grasp the entailments of their current self-narratives and to craft and perform new ones.

In the collaborative context of psychotherapy, the person of the therapist plays a vital part in postmodern practice, as has been discussed previously. In general, practitioners who are self-reflective, comfortable with exploring ambiguity, skilled in the use of language and metaphor, and inclined toward deeply intimate therapeutic encounters will be drawn to constructivist and narrative practices. A postmodern penchant for cultural critique will further support working with the broader social contexts within which clients function. Because having an egalitarian, respectful, and supportive relationship is such a vital aspect of functioning from within a postmodern theoretical framework, a constructive working alliance is an expected outcome of psychotherapy regardless of unique therapist personality traits. Thus, both common factors having to do with the construction of the therapeutic relationship as well as more distinctive strategies for promoting the client's reconstruction of meaning play an important role in instigating therapeutic change.

TREATMENT APPLICABILITY AND ETHICAL CONSIDERATIONS

Because of the broad set of approaches and methods that fall under the postmodern umbrella, it is difficult to identify a population to which such approaches have *not* been applied. Indeed, one of the great strengths of this orientation is its internationality, with active research and practice groups animated by postmodern ideas literally spanning the globe, from the United States, Canada, and United Kingdom to Australia and New Zealand. Nor is the theory group confined principally to English-speaking countries, as innovative developments are burgeoning in such countries as

Germany, Italy, Portugal, Serbia, Norway, and Sweden. The Hispanic world is particularly "constructivized," with major training centers being found in Spain, Argentina, Brazil, Chile, and Mexico. The result is a rich blending of traditions, many of which draw inspiration from indigenous cultures such as the Maori of New Zealand, whose communal practices of respectful negotiation and conflict resolution can be read between the lines of many narrative approaches to therapy and mediation (White & Epston, 1990; Winslade & Monk, 2001). A similar diversity of inspiration and application is evident even within North America, where therapists of a constructivist and social constructionist bent have supported members of disadvantaged communities such as inner-city youth in their efforts to develop a sense of identity, voice, and initiative (Holzman & Morss, 2000; Saleebey, 1998).

Postmodern therapists are less enthusiastic, however, about defining diagnostic "categories" of clients to whom their approaches are particularly relevant. In part, this reluctance is an expression of their commitment to individuality, and the recognition that generic categories of clients provide little useful guidance in how to intervene with a given client confronting specific difficulties in meshing with the social world. It is for this reason that constructivist assessment techniques and therapeutic interactions consistently seek to identify that unique set of resources and restrictions embodied in the client's situated interpretive activity, so that the therapist and client can draw on relevant strengths to address limitations. Sometimes, clients' construction of their selves and situations might suggest the relevance of therapeutic techniques that are less favored by postmodern therapists, such as psychoeducational interactions, which cast therapists in an authoritative teaching role, or behavior therapy, which might encourage the monitoring and modification of molecular behaviors. Although constructivist therapists can be both flexible and

forceful in their intervention style (Efran & Fauber, 1995), studies have shown that most prefer a more reflective, participatory style of therapy (Mahoney, 1993; Vasco, 1994). Accordingly, research on treatment acceptability suggests that potential clients who have an internal locus of control tend to prefer constructivist therapies, whereas those with a more external orientation are attracted more toward traditional cognitive or behavioral therapies (Vincent & LeBow, 1995). Likewise, those clients who are inner-directed, open to experience, and define their problems in interpersonal terms tend both to be drawn to and to respond favorably to reflective interventions such as those emphasized in this chapter, whereas those persons who are outer-directed, closed to experience, and conservative—and who correspondingly view their problems as discrete symptoms to be eliminated—have been found to display an affinity for behavior therapy approaches (Winter, 1990).

It therefore seems entirely appropriate for a constructivist therapist to appraise the client's dominant modes of experiencing both the self and symptom, and in those instances in which these personal factors suggest a mismatch with the therapist's style of work, to recommend referral to another mode of therapy. At times, of course, no therapy of any kind might be called for, as when a client experiencing normal grief over a loss might seek consultation about whether such a reaction is in some sense pathological. In such instances, data suggest that careful assessment of personal and social functioning, combined with reaffirming indigenous support systems, might be all that is called for, and that commencing therapy of any kind in such cases might be associated with poorer, rather than better, outcome (R. Neimeyer, 2000d).

In two respects at least, postmodern therapies raise ethical questions that are subtly but significantly different than those raised by traditional perspectives. First, the high respect for the client's world of meaning, combined with the lack of any fixed external reference point for what constitutes psychopathology, can confront the postmodern practitioner with ethical dilemmas in treating clients who do not seek therapy voluntarily, and who experience their behavior and feelings as unproblematic. For example, working with eating disorders such as anorexia can be complicated in this way, as clients who organize their world around the relentless pursuit of thinness may view their "disorder" as entirely congruent with their preferred self-image (Fransella, 1993). However, some social constructionist counselors have devised creative and demonstrably effective ways of dealing with such problems, by helping clients recognize the destructive role of "dominant narratives" or oppressive cultural discourses about weight in their lives, which can be externalized and resisted (White & Epston, 1990).

The second ethical issue that characterizes postmodern work, especially that of a narrative, feminist, or culturally informed type, is the necessity to place personal problems in broader social contexts, in keeping with the overarching emphasis on cultural–linguistic features of problem construction featured in the epigenetic systems model (Mascolo et al., 1997). From this perspective it becomes ethically essential to critique and "deconstruct" oppressive discourses in the broader culture, including the "culture" of our own profession (Holzman & Morss, 2000). A radical example of this is the organization of "anti-anorexia" leagues, in which clients struggling with eating disorders join together to deface billboards glorifying anorexic models (Madigan & Goldman, 1998).

RESEARCH SUPPORT

Research has not been kind to advocates of particular therapeutic approaches who claim superiority for their preferred school over others. Although such claims continue to be propounded, a great deal of evidence now suggests that most of the variance in outcome in psychotherapy is attributable to client variables, such as psychological mindedness, and factors common to most or all therapies, such as the quality of the working alliance (Messer & Wampold, 2002). Indeed, quantitative reviews of controlled outcome studies report that once investigator allegiance is taken into account, apparent differences favoring the efficacy of one approach over another vanish (Robinson, Berman, & Neimeyer, 1990), and it has been found that the lion's share of the difference in efficacy observed in primary studies is accounted for by the advocacy of the researcher for one treatment over another (Luborsky et al., 2002). Underscoring this conclusion, carefully randomized comparative trials in which investigators did not favor one treatment (e.g., cognitive-behavioral therapy) over the other (e.g., mutual support groups) report no differences in the outcome of the treatment conditions (Bright, Baker, & Neimeyer, 1999).

In keeping with this growing evidence base, constructivist psychotherapy researchers have generally been less interested in "horserace" comparisons of their preferred approaches and competitors and more oriented toward conducting basic research on those psychological structures and change processes that are relevant to the refinement of all therapy, regardless of its pedigree. For example, researchers have focused on adducing evidence for the reliability and validity of such constructivist assessment techniques as laddering (Neimeyer et al., 2001), repertory and implications grids (Dempsey & Neimeyer, 1995; Feixas, Moliner, Montes, Mari, & Neimeyer, 1992; Fransella & Bannister, 1977), and various forms of content and narrative coding (Angus, 1992; Viney, 1988). In addition to reassuring clinicians about the psychometric adequacy of these assessment methods, such studies also lend credibility to constructivist models of meaning systems, whose structure and change across the course of therapy have been traced in literally hundreds of studies (Winter, 1992). Significantly, constructivist researchers have been as active in investigating change processes in other therapeutic modalities (e.g., psychodynamic, group, and behavioral) as in their own (Greenberg, Elliott, & Lietaer, 1994; Levitt & Angus, 1999). For example, although both constructivist and process-oriented approaches to group therapy with incest survivors are demonstrably effective (Alexander, Neimeyer, & Follette, 1991; Alexander, Neimeyer, Follette, Moore, & Harter, 1989), further study of the group dynamics in each condition indicates that over a quarter of the variance in outcome reflects processes of identification first with group members and then with group therapists over time (Neimeyer, Harter, & Alexander, 1991). Such a strategy of investigating basic change processes is arguably more relevant to improving our understanding of the mechanisms of action in psychotherapy than a single-minded attempt to demonstrate the superiority of a preferred treatment.

The growing contributions of constructivism to the empirical study of psychotherapy notwithstanding, some postmodern theorists and practitioners are skeptical of the relevance of much psychotherapy research, viewing it as more concerned with advancing the power and prestige of professionals than with serving the interests of clients (Parker, 2000). Even from the standpoint of loyal scientist practitioners working from a constructivist base, there is reason to acknowledge the uncomfortable "essential tension" between the necessary simplification and formalism of outcome research and the slippery subtlety of that relational renegotiation of meaning called psychotherapy (R. Neimeyer, 2000c). Perhaps the most realistic expectation is that research can tell us something of a general sort about the "active ingredients" of therapeutic change, although the delicate dance of connection between a given client and therapist will always require an intuitive

"read" of what is possible and necessary at each moment of therapeutic encounter (R. Neimeyer, 2002).

CASE ILLUSTRATION

Bill was a 43-year-old midlevel manager who was referred to therapy by his company's employee assistance program (EAP) when his symptoms of anxiety proved unresponsive to the brief, cognitive-behavioral therapy he had been offered. On his first consultation with me (RAN), Bill described his life as a "roller coaster" over the last 5 years, culminating in his leaving his wife, Sally, after some 17 years of marriage. Importantly, the fault lines of the divorce also opened a structural chasm within the family, as the couple's 15-year-old son, Randy, remained with his father while their 12-year-old daughter, Cassie, moved with her mother to a distant state. Bill was candid in his first session about the immediate precipitant for the divorce: his clandestine relationship with Delanie, a 39-year-old divorced employee in the same firm who "knew how to treat him," in contrast to the "forceful, argumentative, confrontational" interactions he had long had with Sally. Although the distance from his ex-wife mitigated the friction between them, a number of other problems had seemed to crowd in to take its place, including increasingly "testy" interactions with Randy, whose grades were slipping at school, a recent mediocre annual evaluation that served as a "wake-up call" about his own performance on the job, and above all, the escalating anxiety that had broken through in the form of a handful of anxiety attacks. Having no previous experience in therapy beyond the brief EAP contact, Bill was nonetheless eager to "figure out what was happening to him" with the assistance of an "objective observer," given his conviction that "talking helped." Thus began a complex therapeutic journey that spanned some 18 months of approximately biweekly sessions, which focused principally on the dyadic–relational and personal–agentic spheres of his life.

In subsequent sessions, Bill soon elaborated on his presenting problems, noting how he was "running behind schedule" with Delanie, who was eager for a more open and public relationship, and one that might eventually lead to greater commitment. Despite the "solid ground" on which Bill felt their relationship was built, he confessed to a strong reluctance to move more visibly in this direction, a reluctance that was only partly explainable in terms of the anti-nepotism rules at work that led them to keep their intimacy a secret. At the same time, Bill could feel his daughter Cassie growing "cooler and more distant" with each passing month, particularly as his anxiety had peaked in preparation for his driving to visit her, leading him to cancel the trip. Observing Bill's seeming impasse at this dyadic–relational level, I suggested that he invite Delanie to join us for the fourth session as a "consultant" to his therapy, an invitation she accepted on the condition that therapy remain focused on "his problems."

The session that followed was enlightening, as Delanie eagerly shared her impression of Bill as a "procrastinator" who was "dragging his feet" in committing to her. For her own part, Delanie described herself as a "risk taker" who was eager to "move ahead" in their relationship and saw a greater involvement between Bill's children and herself to be the next crucial step in that direction. My efforts to allow each to articulate his or her view of both the problem and their visions of their future prompted mutual statements of caring and respect and a sense of "closeness" that Bill underscored in his opening remarks in our subsequent individual session. At the same time, however, Bill had experienced still greater distance with Cassie, precipitated by guilt over being unable to fly to visit her on her birthday because of a crippling flight phobia. Further inquiry confirmed what I had suspected: for Bill the problems of his relationship to Delanie and Cassie were in-

tricately interwoven, as he could not imagine forcing his reluctant daughter to meet the woman she blamed for ending her parents' marriage. As he began to voice this sentiment explicitly, Bill remarked that "a part of [him] would feel relieved to break up with Delanie," apparently as a way of resolving his standoff with his daughter. Although he quickly drew back from this conclusion, it was clear that the prospect of marriage was freighted with important emotional meanings that made remaining single the preferred, if denied option. I therefore sought to tease out the higher-order implications of this choice using laddering technique, the results of which are summarized in Figure 8.3.

As the laddering revealed, the unspoken implications of remaining single for Bill included being free, having fewer hassles, feeling productive, and experiencing life as good, the way things ought to be. In contrast, marriage for him entailed the subjective meanings of being constrained, experiencing conflicts, feeling destructive, and regarding life as stressful and uncomfortable. Immediately after completing this hierarchy of constructs, Bill jolted upright and stated, "It just occurred to me that I'm describing my first marriage!" There then followed a probing discussion on how the sense of constriction and conflict in Bill's relationship with Sally was "bleeding over" into his relationship with Delanie, paralyzing him from "moving forward" as, at a more conscious level, he apparently wanted. As the session neared its close, Bill noted enthusiastically, "Now I really feel like I'm in therapy!"

Despite this important step, Bill made little progress in the coming few sessions toward committing more clearly to Delanie or promoting her greater involvement with his children. The tension—both intrapersonal and interpersonal—over this deadlock mounted with a second impending trip to visit Cassie some 500 miles away. As Bill identified his "mysterious jitteriness" over the trip, I took this as an implicit request for help in understanding its meaning and

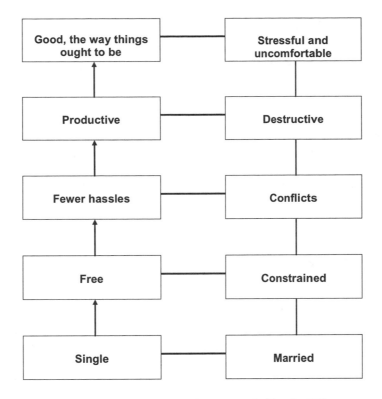

FIGURE 8.3. Personal construct ladder for Bill.

asked him to close his eyes and direct his attention to the bodily "felt sense" associated with the emotion. Drawing on Gendlin's (1996) focusing technique, I asked him to "stay with" the feeling and attempt to give it voice. Bill sat quiet for a moment, then noted that he felt "alone," then "lonesome," despite Delanie's having volunteered to drive the distance with him and stay supportively in the hotel room as Bill went to spend the day with his daughter. Wrinkling his brow, Bill then became aware of the inner complexity of the feeling that was emerging: the "jitteriness" also carried emotional connotations of "undermining Delanie's trust in [him]" as he flashed to an image of becoming too anxious to be able to drive. Further processing of this self-awareness led Bill to identify and articulate his sense of not only losing self-control but also letting down those he loved, including "disappointing God."

The subsequent joint session with Delanie corroborated this relational tension, as Bill tearfully acknowledged "feeling stuck in the middle" in relation to Delanie and Cassie, risking losing one if he moved closer to the other. The tragic dynamic was underscored by Delanie, who emphasized that "only a part of this is about Cassie—the rest is about Bill," adding through her own tears that she "deserved better than to spend the rest of [her] life alone." Under Delanie's ultimatum that they make the trip together, and that Bill arrange at least fleeting contact between her and Cassie, Bill capitulated. However, this plan, though technically successful, precipitated deep fears of marginalization on Delanie's part, expressed in the form of such uncontrolled sobbing on the drive home that she experienced trouble breathing. Thus, it was little surprise that she began distancing self-protectively in the ensuing week.

At this unfortunate juncture, I found myself verging on departure for a planned monthlong professional trip to Australia, with only a single session with Bill left before my leave taking. I therefore sensed that we were at a choice point—should we delve deeply into the source of Bill's torment at the risk of leaving him vulnerable and unsupported during my absence or focus on reinforcing Bill's means of coping with his distressing situation until I could return? Prompted by Bill's apparent readiness (and need) to "understand what was happening to him," I opted for the former. Perhaps influenced by my pending visit to narrative therapy colleagues, I began a sustained externalizing conversation with Bill about the "guilt" that he blamed for "making it impossible for him to look at Randy and Cassie and tell them [he] was going to marry Delanie." The result was a powerful review, prompted by my "curious questioning" about the influence of guilt in Bill's life, but given direction by his detailed and evocative replies. Following the session, I drafted and mailed Bill a letter that captured the essence of our interview, drawing heavily on his own expressions of his situation and integrating the insights that had emerged for him in the course of our conversation. The letter, in its entirety, read:

Dear Bill,

After our session today I found myself thinking more about your bold recognition that guilt is at the core of your difficulties, and needed to be dealt with directly if you are going to get your life back on track. As you said, "I can't continue with my life the way I have been going with my life. Until I take care of myself, I can't deal with anyone else." You went on to note quite a few ways that guilt was having a negative impact on your life:

1. It requires you to be uncomfortable in all of your close relationships.
2. It prevents you from enjoying yourself with abandon with Delanie.

3. It forces you to "distance" yourself from Delanie, and remain uncommitted about the future of your relationship.
4. It keeps you from "taking a position" with your kids.
5. It forces you to conceal the history of your relationship with Delanie, and to keep secrets from those you love.
6. It condemns you to doing unending penance for the "sin" you have committed.

I was very moved by your declaration that "I'm reaching a point that I can't take it anymore; I'm tired of everybody beating on me, and I've got to do something about it." I'm sure you are right about this and that you are indeed correct in directly confronting the destructive influence of guilt on your life. Discussing with your minister the nature of your "sin," as you suggested, and the actions necessary for forgiveness seems to be a bold and creative step in this direction. I was also struck by your idea of talking quite forthrightly with the kids about your history with Delanie, although it might be wise not to move too quickly in eliminating guilt in this way, given the important role that it has played in your life up until this time.

As I leave to spend some time in Australia, I will take with me a good deal of curiosity about these intriguing developments in your life, and I look forward to an update when we get back together. Good luck.

Yours,

Bob Neimeyer

The following session, held just over 1 month later upon my return, was something of a turning point. Bill opened with the remark that the letter I had sent him was "great," because "it recapped our last meeting better than [he] ever could." He then recounted an impressive series of "unique outcomes," instances in which he was "winning [his] life back from guilt" through undertaking small carpentry projects, going camping, and doing other things he had long neglected because they seemed "selfish." At the same time, he announced that he felt "some of the fire coming back" to see Delanie, who continued to interpose some distance between them. Interestingly, he also had spontaneously showed the letter to Delanie, who responded by taking it to discuss with her own EAP counselor, because she suspected it had actually been written as an indirect therapeutic communication to describe her! As a result, she had asked Bill's permission to join him for the next session, so that she could uncover the role of guilt in her own life and her relationship to Bill and his children.

The next session was relationally clarifying but initially stalemated: Bill increasingly resented Delanie's demands to be more involved with his children, which echoed for him some of the worst aspects of his previous marriage. Likewise, Delanie increasingly questioned Bill's commitment to her because of his unwillingness to "bring together [his] two separate lives." As a result, each intensified his or her behavior in a way that was coherent with his or her construction of the situation but that also validated the partner's interpretation. This pernicious validational cycle is depicted in the bow-tie diagram in Figure 8.4. Mapping this "dance of despair" for them, I was gratified by Bill's response that it was "a recipe for a holding pattern if ever there was one. The stability makes sense, because the pattern gets reinforced over time." Delanie concurred, and added that it felt good to know that "it's not just that one of us is flawed or crazy."

The next several sessions continued this

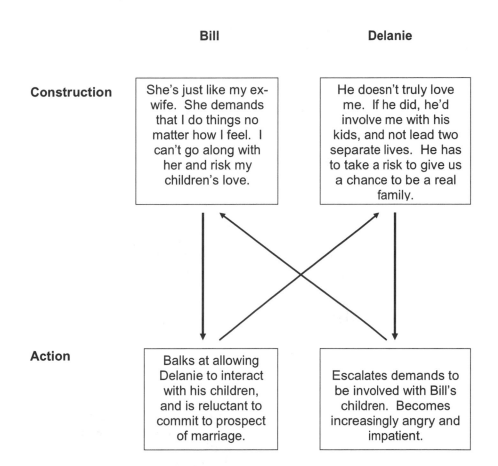

FIGURE 8.4. "Bow tie" linking levels of construction and action for Bill and Delanie.

progress, though with occasional setbacks. For example, Bill reported "feeling more and more like [his] old self, more relaxed and focused," to the point of taking Delanie on a public date, the first in their 2-year relationship. Furthermore, he even courageously had a heart-to-heart talk with his preacher about his affair and divorce, characterizing the minister as "tacitly forgiving." The one domain in which little headway was made was in involving Delanie with Cassie, as he planned a solo visit to see his daughter. As a father–daughter visit, the trip was remarkable for Bill's degree of risk taking; he even read Cassie a carefully prepared letter in his hotel room reaffirming his love for her and asking her to forgive him for the divorce "when she was ready." A subsequent, nonaccusatory letter followed to his ex-wife, Sally, explaining the reasons for their estrangement in terms of their "basically different views of life." Gradually, Delanie softened, moving slowly from feeling "totally excluded, almost invisible" in the realignment of Bill's family, to a more empathic stance. Couple sessions were often marked by poignant emotion but also deepened connection. As Bill formulated it through a haze of tears in one session, "Delanie's willingness to compromise and understand is exactly what made me fall in love with her." As Delanie moved close to him and wiped her own eyes, he added, "She gives me power through her love."

The remaining months of this episode of therapy were characterized by growing closeness between Bill and Delanie—both agreed that the relationship was "stronger than ever"—although the rare visits to or from Cassie remained fraught with anxiety. This was compounded by an intensification of Bill's long-standing flight phobia, which he described as a "fear of being closed in, unable to get out." Not only was his inability to travel by air complicating his executive work life, but it was also, and even more seriously, slowing his reconnection with his daughter. Bill therefore eagerly accepted my referral to a behavioral colleague who offered an *in vivo*

desensitization program for flight phobia in the hope of freeing himself of the constraints it imposed in both the personal and professional spheres. Our planned contact ended on this relatively optimistic note, with Bill noting in his closing session, "It is silly to lose my relationship with Delanie over my reluctance to commit."

I heard nothing more from Bill over the ensuing 4 years, until he called to request another session. In many respects, Bill had consolidated his therapeutic gains over this interval: He and Delanie had been happily married for nearly 3 years, he credited his stronger parenting with Randy with helping his son straighten out his school problems and get through a difficult breakup with his girlfriend, and he and Delanie had worked out their respective careers in a way that supported their continued professional development. But two problems stubbornly persisted: the flight phobia, as Bill did not feel sufficient "trust" in the behavior therapist to continue beyond four sessions, and the "tug of war" between Cassie and Delanie, which had contributed to his having no contact with his daughter except through correspondence for 3 years. Indeed, despite the civility of their earlier contacts, Cassie's letters had been unequivocal in stating that she "could never accept Delanie, and did not want to see her." Thus, Bill was left in a deep quandary and was seeking my help "to stand up, be a man, and do what's right."

Of course, Bill was not the only one of us to experience personal and professional growth during the hiatus in our relationship. I, too, had developed as a postmodern therapist, incorporating new concepts and methods—such as DOBT—that were coherent with my earlier ways of working while moving them in a more consistently experiential direction. In the terms of the narrative process model, our earlier sessions had tacked back and forth between Bill's initially *external* narratives and my frequently *reflexive* interventions, helping him shift from the brute "facts" of his problem to their meaning. Now, however, I was more inclined to promote a sustained *internal* exploration of a problematic position in order to help clients encounter and articulate the powerful but unstated premises that sustained their symptomatic behavior. Viewing Bill's chronic complaint from a DOBT perspective, I now more clearly construed his motivation to transcend the pattern of anxious avoidance of Cassie as an *anti-symptom position* that motivated his return to therapy. The pain this "standoff" caused him was very real, and my first tasks in the session were to help him articulate it and to respond to it with genuine empathy. But my ultimate task was to help him encounter the problem's higher-order, hidden purpose, that system of meanings and intentions that constituted his unconscious *pro-symptom position.* Much of the session therefore consisted of *radical inquiry* whose goal was to quickly lead Bill to "bump into" these deeply embedded constructs in an experientially vivid way, without in any way attempting to interpret, invalidate, or challenge them. Once both the anti-symptom and pro-symptom stances were in clear view, I hoped his painfully repetitive story of his relationship with his daughter would make a new kind of sense, setting the stage for the conscious affirmation of one position or the other, or the possible integration of both into a more comprehensive self narrative.

Using the technique of *symptom deprivation,* I began by asking Bill to close his eyes and "get a clear visual picture of Delanie and Cassie together, engaged in some ordinary, day-to-day activity," to prompt his awareness of how he would experience "reality" deprived of the customary distance he maintained between them. After a moment of silence, Bill visibly winced, and said, "I wanted to say it would be wonderful, but my first reaction was to break out into a cold sweat. I immediately flashed to a big confrontation between two stubborn people." Intrigued, I instructed him to simply sit with this scene for a few more moments, and to "let me know if anything else came

up." This triggered the *serial accessing* of felt meanings in which Bill first noted with a trembling jaw that the emotion that washed over him "felt exactly like the internal panic over getting on board a plane." He then swallowed hard, opened his eyes, and said, "It may not even be Delanie and Cassie together—it may be *me* and Cassie together that's the problem." He fell silent for a moment more, then added, "I've got something I can't break through here."

Rather than shifting to an abstract discussion of this impasse, I used the technique of *sentence completion* to keep Bill in contact with the further implications of this pro-symptom position. This involved my inviting him, without prereflection, to complete the stem, "If Cassie were to come here, then. . . ." His first response was predictable and safe: "we'd be happy to see her." His second went deeper: "I'd be nervous about losing one or both of them." As his eyes moistened, I prompted him with a third, more personal stem, to which he replied, "If Cassie were to come here, then *I* . . . might see her walk out of my life." Wiping away tears, Bill then flashed to an image of Cassie at age 9, as he sat snuggled up with her, telling her she'd soon be a teenager and "all grown up." Putting her arms around his neck, she had lovingly reassured him, "I'll always be your little girl." Tears welled in Bill's eyes, and he removed his glasses to wipe them away, sobbing silently.

With all of the elements of his pro-symptom position now in view, Bill's deeper purpose in maintaining the distance with Cassie became clear, despite its great costs in their relationship as well as his marriage. Bringing the session to a close, I formulated this stance in sharply etched words on an index card, which I handed to Bill and asked him to read slowly aloud: "As painful as this present standoff is, I would rather suffer this terrible distance from Cassie than to have her walk away, and never feel her arms around my neck, never hear her say, 'I'm still your little girl.'" Choking on the word "arms," Bill stammered out the sentence and, drying his tears, quietly noted that inhabiting this position consciously "made me understand the things I've been doing in a whole different light." My request that he simply read the card a few times a day, with no attempt to change his behavior, cultivated a deeper appreciation of his intentions, whose fruits became evident in our final follow-up session scheduled for 1 month later.

Bill returned for our final session looking somehow younger and stronger, with the deep lines of worry I had grown accustomed to seeing now less visibly etched on his brow. Behavioral progress was, if anything, even more visible: he had sent direct but compassionate letters to Sally, urging her to "bury the hatchet" for the sake of the children; to Randy, expressing his need for the young man to "respect" Delanie, for the sake of their "special father–son relationship"; and to Delanie, offering comfort and perspective on various concerns and feelings she had had since the death of her beloved father some 2 years before. Most remarkably, he had also drafted a letter to Cassie, raising the topic of another visit, promising to continue the weekly phone calls he had initiated since our last session, and noting that future letters would be sent from him and Delanie together. Significantly, Bill noted that he was "doing this because he could no longer live with the standoff, not because of pressure from Delanie." These clear shifts suggested that the pro-symptom position brought to light in the previous session had now begun to be dissolved in the light of Bill's awareness, opening as real behavioral options actions that were previously "off limits" at an unconscious level.

A follow-up phone call from Bill 3 months later confirmed this progress and provided evidence of a further surprising development: Bill had actually taken an airplane—his first in over a decade—for his work, and had scheduled a flight to visit Cassie as well. Somehow, he said, he no longer felt the fear of "enclosure" as intensely, though he could not say why. Bill's

therapy therefore illustrates both the explicit and unspecifiable processes of therapeutic change, as well as the use of a number of postmodern procedures to map a client's meaning system, clarify his relational patterns, instigate deepened reflexivity, and consolidate the emerging contours of a preferred life narrative. It also underscores the extent to which therapists no less than clients grow as persons and professionals, a growth that is supported and prompted by the continuously evolving practice of postmodern psychotherapy.

CURRENT AND FUTURE TRENDS

As philosophically sophisticated, practically useful, and empirically responsive orientations to clinical practice, postmodern therapies seem likely to continue to prosper in the 21st century. However, factors both internal to these approaches and external to them are likely to affect the speed and direction of such growth, fostering the extension of these perspectives in some areas while inhibiting them in others.

Facilitative factors that are likely to promote the further extension of constructivist, social constructionist, and narrative approaches include their remarkable flexibility in conceptualizing constraints on people's lives that originate at many levels, ranging from the individual through the cultural, and their creative generation of a broad and expanding array of techniques for assessing and enlarging systems of meaning. These same factors make these approaches congenial to both humanistic psychologists who cherish client uniqueness and radical–critical therapists who strive to deconstruct the role of oppressive cultural discourses that subjugate individuals and groups. This dual focus also helps account for the immense appeal of postmodern therapies far beyond the borders of the United States, as literally dozens of major conferences and training centers have developed throughout Europe, Australasia, and Central and South America to explore their implications in quite different cultural contexts.

External factors, such as the increasing ethnic, cultural, and lifestyle diversity of most Western nations also encourage the development of perspectives that make fewer assumptions about what constitutes "normal" or "abnormal" behavior but that instead offer a subtle range of concepts and methods for respectfully engaging the diversity of human experience. The push for briefer therapies, a topic considered in detail by Hoyt (Chapter 10, in this volume) further bodes well for postmodern approaches to working with individuals, families, and groups that share an optimistic emphasis on human change processes and their facilitation through efficient experiential procedures. Finally, the current trend toward integration of diverse psychotherapies is congenial to a multifaceted postmodern perspective, which has influenced contemporary developments in traditions ranging from the psychodynamic to the humanistic, and in contexts embracing individuals, families, and groups. However, the strong epistemological orientation of constructivist and social constructionist theorists also leads them to caution against an indiscriminate gallimaufry of principles and procedures and instead to advocate only selective integration of perspectives that share key metatheoretical commitments (Messer, 1987; R. Neimeyer, 1993b).

On the other hand, the same richness and subtlety that makes postmodern ideas attractive to seasoned clinicians of several schools probably also impedes their acceptance by developing student clinicians, who often prefer the apparent simplicity of more rule-governed, prescriptive approaches. Likewise, the commitment to the delicate interplay of client and therapist meanings in the process of therapy that characterizes constructivist and social constructionist work poses challenges to psychotherapy researchers who prefer to test the average benefit of standardized interventions to a defined diagnostic category of clients. Although those con-

structivist approaches whose efficacy has been assessed have fared favorably (Greenberg et al., 1994), the tendency of constructivist researchers to group patients by issues (e.g., "unfinished business") rather than psychiatric diagnosis (e.g., generalized anxiety disorder) militates against their inclusion in approved lists of "empirically supported treatments" for particular disorders, no matter how many such controlled studies are conducted. More seriously, perhaps, the revolutionary spirit of "resistance" against aspects of mainstream approaches that postmodernists consider oppressive and pathologizing can prove threatening to powerful interests in the traditional mental health disciplines, which tend to gravitate toward more conservative, replicable forms of therapy that seem to offer the twin advantages of mass dissemination and differentiation from the "products" offered by other competing therapeutic professions.

In summary, postmodern approaches to clinical practice, like all models of psychotherapy, offer a unique and evolving distillation of intellectual and cultural trends, which are turned toward the practical goal of improving the human condition. We hope that the concepts, procedures, and case illustrations discussed in this chapter offer something of value to readers as they engage the problems and prospects in the lives of the individuals, families, and communities with which they work.

NOTE

1. See, for example, the popular WebGrid program available at *http://gigi.cpsc.ucalgary.ca/*.

SUGGESTIONS FOR FURTHER READING

Ecker, B., & Hulley, L. (1996). *Depth-oriented brief therapy.* San Francisco: Jossey-Bass.—A comprehensive and readable orientation to this constructivist hybrid of dynamically-informed and brief therapies, complete with extensive case studies.

Hermans, H. J. M., & Kempen, H. J. G. (1993). *The dialogical self.* New York: Academic Press.—Summarizes the theory of the self as constituted in dialogue, and presents a detailed self-confrontation method for studying "valuations" formulated by clients facing a variety of life problems.

Monk, G., Winslade, J., Crocket, K., & Epston, D. (1996). *Narrative therapy in practice.* San Francisco: Jossey Bass.—A readable introduction to the principles of narrative therapy, as well as detailed discussions of its applications in supervision and psychotherapy for a broad range of problems.

Neimeyer, R. A., & Mahoney, M. J. (Eds.). (1995). *Constructivism in psychotherapy.* Washington, DC: American Psychological Association.—A comprehensive survey of constructivist, social constructionist, and narrative approaches to psychotherapy written by leading representatives of each perspective.

Neimeyer, R. A., & Raskin, J. (Eds.). (2000). *Constructions of disorder: Meaning-making frameworks for psychotherapy.* Washington, DC: American Psychological Association.—Acquaints the reader with the alternative approaches to clinical diagnosis or case conceptualization featured in each of the major orientations to postmodern therapy, organized around discussions of actual cases.

Winter, D. A. (1992). *Personal construct psychology in clinical practice.* London: Routledge.—A detailed survey of research conducted within a personal construct theory framework, much of which uses adaptations of repertory grid technique to study the relationship of construct system structure to various diagnostic groups, and its change over the course of treatment using a variety of therapeutic models.

REFERENCES

Adams-Webber, J. R. (2001). Prototypicality of self and evaluating others in terms of "fuzzy" constructs. *Journal of Constructivist Psychology, 14,* 315–324.

Alexander, P. C., Neimeyer, R. A., & Follette, V. M. (1991). Group therapy for women sexually abused as children: A controlled study and investigation of individual differences. *Journal of Interpersonal Violence, 6,* 219–231.

Alexander, P. C., Neimeyer, R. A., Follette, V. M., Moore, M. K., & Harter, S. L. (1989). A comparison of group treatments of women sexually abused as children. *Journal of Consulting and Clinical Psychology, 57,* 479–483.

Allport, G. W. (1961). *Pattern and growth in personality.* New York: Holt.

Angus, L. E. (1992). Metaphor and the communication interaction in psychotherapy. In S. G. Toukmanian & D. L. Rennie (Eds.), *Psychotherapy process research* (pp. 187–210). Newbury Park, CA: Sage.

Angus, L., Levitt, H., & Hardke, L. (1999). Narrative processes and psychotherapeutic change: An integrative approach to psychotherapy research and practice. *Journal of Clinical Psychology, 55,* 1255–1270.

Appignanesi, R., & Garratt, C. (1995). *Postmodernism for beginners.* Cambridge, UK: Icon/Penguin.

Arciero, G., & Guidano, V. (2000). Experience, explanation, and the quest for coherence. In R. A. Neimeyer & J. C. Raskin (Eds.), *Constructions of disorder* (pp. 91–117). Washington, DC: American Psychological Association.

Bannister, D. (1963). the genesis of schizophrenic thought disorder: A serial invalidation hypothesis. *British Journal of Psychiatry, 109,* 680–686.

Bateson, G. (1972). *Steps to an ecology of mind.* New York: Dutton.

Beck, A. T. (1993). Cognitive therapy: Past, present, and future. *Journal of Consulting and Clinical Psychology, 61,* 194–198.

Bohart, A. C., & Tallman, K. (1999). *How clients make therapy work.* Washington, DC: American Psychological Association.

Botella, L. (1995). Personal construct theory, constructivism, and postmodern thought. In R. A. Neimeyer & G. J. Neimeyer (Eds.), *Advances in personal construct psychology* (Vol. 3, pp. 3–35). Greenwich, CT: JAI Press.

Bridges, S. K., & Neimeyer, R. A. (2003). Exploring and negotiating sexual meanings. In J. S. Whitman & C. J. Boyd (Eds.), *The therapist's notebook for lesbian, gay and bisexual clients: homework, handouts, and activities for* use in psychotherapy. New York: Hawthorne Press.

Bright, J. I., Baker, K. D., & Neimeyer, R. A. (1999). Professional and paraprofessional group treatments for depression: A comparison of cognitive-behavioral and mutual support interventions. *Journal of Consulting and Clinical Psychology, 67,* 491–501.

Brown, L. (2000a). Discomforts of the powerless. In R. A. Neimeyer & J. Raskin (Eds.), *Constructions of disorder* (pp. 287–308). Washington, DC: American Psychological Association.

Brown, L. S. (2000b). Feminist therapy. In C. R. Snyder & R. E. Ingram (Eds.), *Handbook of psychological change* (pp. 358–380). New York: Wiley.

Buber, M. (1958). *I and thou* (2nd ed.). New York: Charles Scribner's Sons.

Chiari, G., & Nuzzo, M. L. (1996). Psychological constructivisms: A mettheoretical differentiation. *Journal of Constructivist Psychology, 9,* 163–184.

Dempsey, D. J., & Neimeyer, R. A. (1995). Organization of personal knowledge: Convergent validity of implications grids and repertory grids as measures of system structure. *Journal of Constructivist Psychology, 8,* 251–261.

DiLollo, A., Neimeyer, R. A., & Manning, W. H. (2002). A personal construct psychology view of relapse: Indications for a narrative therapy component to stuttering treatment. *Journal of Fluency Disorders, 27,* 19–42.

Ecker, B., & Hulley, L. (1996). *Depth-oriented brief therapy.* San Francisco: Jossey-Bass.

Ecker, B., & Hulley, L. (2000). The order in clinical "disorder": Symptom coherence in depth-oriented brief therapy. In R. A. Neimeyer & J. Raskin (Eds.), *Constructions of disorder* (pp. 63–90). Washington, DC: American Psychological Association.

Efran, J. S., & Cook, P. F. (2000). Linguistic ambiguity as a diagnostic tool. In R. A. Neimeyer & J. D. Raskin (Eds.), *Constructions of disorder* (pp. 121–143). Washington, DC: American Psychological Association.

Efran, J. S., & Fauber, R. L. (1995). Radical constructivism: Questions and answers. In R. A. Neimeyer & M. J. Mahoney (Eds.), *Constructivism in psychotherapy* (pp. 275–302). Washington DC: American Psychological Association.

Efran, J. S., Lukens, M. D., & Lukens, R. J. (1990). *Language, structure, and change.* New York: Norton.

Epston, D., & White, M. (1995). Termination as a rite of passage: Questioning strategies for a therapy of inclusion. In R. A. Neimeyer & M. J. Mahoney (Eds.), *Constructivism in psychotherapy* (pp. 339–356). Washington, DC: American Psychological Association.

Eron, J. B., & Lund, T. W. (1996). *Narrative solutions in brief therapy.* New York: Guilford Press.

Feixas, G. (1992). Personal construct approaches to family therapy. In R. A. Neimeyer & G. J. Neimeyer (Eds.), *Advances in personal construct psychology* (Vol. 2, pp. 217–255). Greenwich, CT: JAI Press.

Feixas, G. (1995). Personal constructs in systemic practice. In R. A. Neimeyer & M. J. Mahoney (Eds.), *Constructivism in psychotherapy* (pp. 305–337). Washington, DC: American Psychological Association.

Feixas, G., Geldschlager, H., & Neimeyer, R. A. (2002). Content analysis of personal constructs. *Journal of Construcivist Psychology, 15,* 1–20.

Feixas, G., Moliner, J. L., Montes, J. N., Mari, M. T., & Neimeyer, R. A. (1992). The stability of structural measures derived from repertory grids. *International Journal of Personal Construct Psychology, 5,* 25–40.

Fogel, A. (1993). *Development through relationships.* Chicago: University of Chicago Press.

Foucault, M. (1970). *The order of things.* New York: Pantheon.

Fransella, F. (1993). The construct of resistance in psychotherapy. In L. M. Leitner & N. G. M. Dunnett (Eds.), *Critical issues in personal construct psychotherapy* (Vol. 15, pp. 117–134). Malabar, FL: Krieger.

Fransella, F. (1996). *George Kelly.* London: Sage.

Fransella, F., & Bannister, D. (1977). *A manual for repertory grid technique.* New York: Academic Press.

Freeman, J., Epston, D., & Lobovits, D. (1997). *Playful approaches to serious problems.* New York: Norton.

Freud, S. (1940). An outline of psycho-analysis. *Standard Edition, 23,* 144–207. London: Hogarth Press, 1964.

Gendlin, E. T. (1996). *Focusing-oriented psychotherapy.* New York: Guilford Press.

Gergen, K. J. (1991). *The saturated self.* New York: Basic Books.

Gottschalk, L. A., Lolas, F., & Viney, L. L. (1986). *Content analysis of verbal behavior in clinical medicine.* Heidelberg: Springer Verlag.

Greenberg, L., Elliott, R., & Lietaer, G. (1994). Research on experiential therapies. In A. E. Bergin & S. L. Garfield (Eds.), *Handbook of psychotherapy and behavior change* (4th ed., pp. 509–539). New York: Wiley.

Greenberg, L., Elliott, R., & Rice, L. (1993). *Facilitating emotional change.* New York: Guilford Press.

Guidano, V. F. (1995). Constructivist psychotherapy: A theoretical framework. In R. A. Neimeyer & M. J. Mahoney (Eds.), *Constructivism in psychotherapy* (pp. 93–108). Washington, DC: American Psychological Association.

Harré, R., & Gillett, R. (1994). *The discursive mind.* Thousand Oaks, CA: Sage.

Harter, S. L. (1995). Construing on the edge. In R. A. Neimeyer & M. J. Mahoney (Eds.), *Constructivism in psychotherapy* (pp. 371–383). Washington, DC: American Psychological Association.

Hermans, H. J. M. (2002). The person as a motivated storyteller. In R. A. Neimeyer & G. J. Neimeyer (Eds.), *Advances in personal construct psychology* (Vol. 5, pp. 3–38). Westport, CT: Praeger.

Hermans, H. J. M. (2003). The construction and reconstruction of the dialogical self. *Journal of Constructivist Psychology, 16,* 89–130.

Hermans, H. J. M. & Hermans-Jansen, E. (1995). *Self-narratives: The construction of meaning in psychotherapy.* New York: Guilford Press.

Hinkle, D. (1965). *The change of personal constructs from the viewpoint of a theory of implications.* Unpublished dissertation, Ohio State University, Columbus.

Hoffman, L. (1992). A reflexive stance for family therapy. In S. McNamee & K. J. Gergen (Eds.), *Therapy as social construction* (pp. 7–24). Newbury Park, CA: Sage.

Holzman, L., & Morss, J. (Eds.). (2000). *Postmodern psychologies, societal practice, and political life.* New York: Routledge.

Kelly, G. A. (1991). *The psychology of personal constructs.* New York: Routledge. (Original work published 1955)

Kelly, G. A. (1969). The language of hypothesis. In B. Mahrer (Ed.), *Clinical psychology and personality* (pp. 147–162). New York: Wiley.

Kernberg, O. F. (1976). *Object relations theory and psychoanalysis.* Northvale, NJ: Jason Aronson.

Kohut, H. (1971). *The analysis of the self.* New York: International Universities Press.

Lather, P. (1992). Postmodernism and the human sciences. In S. Kvale (Ed.), *Psychology and postmodernism* (pp. 88–109). Newbury Park, CA: Sage.

Leitner, L. M. (1995). Optimal therapeutic distance. In R. A. Neimeyer & M. J. Mahoney (Eds.), *Constructivism in psychotherapy* (pp. 357–370). Washington, DC: American Psychological Association.

Leitner, L. M., & Faidley, A. J. (1996). The awful, aweful nature of ROLE relationships. In R. A. Neimeyer & G. J. Neimeyer (Eds.), *Advances in personal construct psychology* (Vol. 3). Greenwich, CT: JAI Press.

Leitner, L. M., & Faidley, A. J. (2002). Disorder, diagnosis, and the struggles of humanness. In J. D. Raskin & S. K. Bridges (Eds.), *Studies in meaning* (pp. 99–121). New York: Pace University Press.

Leitner, L. M., Faidley, A., & Celentana, M. (2000). Diagnosing human meaning making. In R. A. Neimeyer & J. C. Raskin (Eds.), *Constructions of disorder* (pp. 175–203). Washington, DC: American Psychological Association.

Levitt, H., & Angus, L. (1999). Psychotherapy process measure research and the evaluation of psychotherapy orientation. *Journal of Psychotherapy Integration, 9,* 279–300.

Lorenzini, R., Sassaroli, S., & Rocchi, M. T. (1989). Schizohrenia and paranoia as solutions to predictive failure. *International Journal of Personal Construct Psychology, 2,* 417–431.

Luborsky, L., Rosenthal, R., Diguer, L., Andrusyna, T. P., Berman, J. S., Levitt, J. T., Seligman, D. A., & Krause, E. D. (2002). The dodo bird verdict is alive and well—mostly. *Clinical Psychology: Science and Practice, 9,* 2–16.

Lyddon, W. J. (1995). Forms and facets of constructivist psychology. In R. A. Neimeyer & M. J. Mahoney (Eds.), *Constructivism in psychotherapy* (pp. 69–92). Washington, DC: American Psychological Association.

Madigan, S. P., & Goldman, E. M. (1998). A narrative approach to anorexia. In M. F. Hoyt (Ed.), *Handbook of constructive therapies* (pp. 380–700). San Fransisco: Jossey Bass.

Mahoney, M. J. (1988). Constructive metatheory

I: Basic features and historical foundations. *International Journal of Personal Construct Psychology, 1*, 299–315.

Mahoney, M. J. (1991). *Human change processes.* New York: Basic Books.

Mahoney, M. J. (1993). Theoretical developments in the cognitive psychotherapies. *Journal of Consulting and Clinical Psychology, 61*, 187–193.

Martin, J. (1994). *The construction and understanding of psychotherapeutic change.* New York: Teachers College Press.

Mascolo, M. F., Craig-Bray, L., & Neimeyer, R. A. (1997). The construction of meaning and action in development and psychotherapy: An epigenetic systems approach. In G. J. Neimeyer & R. A. Neimeyer (Eds.), *Advances in personal construct psychology* (Vol. 4, pp. 3–38). Greenwich, CT: JAI Press.

Messer, S. B. (1987). Can the Tower of Babel be completed? A critique of the common language proposal. *Journal of Integrative and Eclectic Psychotherapy, 6*, 195–199.

Messer, S. B., & Wampold, B. E. (2002). Let's face facts: Common factors are more important than specific therapy ingredients. *Clinical Psychology: Science and Practice, 9*, 21–25.

Monk, G., Winslade, J., Crocket, K., & Epston, D. (1996). *Narrative therapy in practice.* San Francisco: Jossey-Bass.

Neimeyer, G. J. (1992). Personal constructs and vocational structure: A critique of poor reason. In R. A. Neimeyer & G. J. Neimeyer (Eds.), *Advances in personal construct psychology* (Vol. 2, pp. 91–120). Greenwich, CT: JAI Press.

Neimeyer, G. J. (Ed.). (1993). *Constructivist assessment: A casebook.* Newbury Park, CA: Sage.

Neimeyer, G. J., & Fukuyama, M. (1984). Exploring the content and structure of cross-cultural attitudes. *Counselor Education and Supervision, 23*, 214–224.

Neimeyer, R. A. (1988). Clinical guidelines for conducting Interpersonal Transaction groups. *International Journal of Personal Construct Psychology, 1*, 181–190.

Neimeyer, R. A. (1993a). Constructivism and the cognitive therapies: Some conceptual and strategic contrasts. *Journal of cognitive psychology, 7*, 159–171.

Neimeyer, R. A. (1993b). Constructivism and the problem of psychotherapy integration. *Journal of Psychotherapy Integration, 3*, 133–157.

Neimeyer, R. A. (1993c). Constructivist approaches to the measurement of meaning. In G. J. Neimeyer (Ed.), *Constructivist assessment: A casebook* (pp. 58–103). Newbury Park, CA: Sage.

Neimeyer, R. A. (1995a). Constructivist psychotherapies: Features, foundations, and future directions. In R. A. Neimeyer & M. J. Mahoney (Eds.), *Constructivism in psychotherapy* (pp. 11–38). Washington, DC: American Psychological Association.

Neimeyer, R. A. (1995b). An invitation to constructivist psychotherapies. In R. A. Neimeyer & M. J. Mahoney (Eds.), *Constructivism in psychotherapy* (pp. 1–8). Washington, DC: American Psychological Association.

Neimeyer, R. A. (1998). Social constructionism in the counselling context. *Counselling Psychology Quarterly, 11*, 135–149.

Neimeyer, R. A. (2000a). Constructivist psychotherapies. In *Encyclopedia of psychology* (Vol. 2, pp. 287–290). Washington, DC: American Psychological Association.

Neimeyer, R. A. (2000b). George Kelly. In *Encyclopedia of psychology* (Vol. 2, pp. 805–807). Washington, DC: American Psychological Association.

Neimeyer, R. A. (2000c). Research and practice as essential tensions: A constructivist confession. In L. M. Vaillant & S. Soldz (Eds.), *Empirical knowledge and clinical experience* (pp. 123–150). Washington, DC: American Psychological Association.

Neimeyer, R. A. (2000d). Searching for the meaning of meaning: Grief therapy and the process of reconstruction. *Death Studies, 24*, 541–558.

Neimeyer, R. A. (2001). The language of loss: Grief therapy as a process of meaning reconstruction. In R. A. Neimeyer (Ed.), *Meaning reconstruction and the experience of loss* (pp. 261–292). Washington, DC: American Psychological Association.

Neimeyer, R. A. (2002). The relational co-construction of selves: A postmodern perspective. *Journal of Contemporary Psychotherapy, 32*, 51–59.

Neimeyer, R. A., Anderson, A., & Stockton, L. (2001). Snakes versus ladders: A validation of laddering technique as a measure of hierarchical structure. *Journal of Constructivist Psychology, 14*, 85–105.

Neimeyer, R. A., Harter, S., & Alexander, P. C. (1991). Group perceptions as predictors of outcome in the treatment of incest survivors. *Psychotherapy Research, 1,* 149–158.

Neimeyer, R. A., Klein, M. H., Gurman, A. S., & Greist, J. H. (1983). Cognitive structure and depressive symptomatology. *British Journal of Cognitive Psychotherapy, 1,* 65–73.

Neimeyer, R. A., & Mahoney, M. J. (Eds.). (1995). *Constructivism in psychotherapy.* Washington, DC: American Psychological Association.

Neisser, U., & Fivush, R. (Eds.). (1994). *The remembering self.* Cambridge, UK: Cambridge University Press.

Newman, F., & Holzman, L. (1999). Beyond narrative to performed conversation. *Journal of Constructivist Psychology, 12,* 23–40.

Palmer, P. J. (2000). *Let your life speak.* San Francisco: Jossey-Bass.

Parker, I. (2000). Four story-theories about and against postmodernism in psychology. In L. Holzman & J. Morss (Eds.), *Postmodern psychologies* (pp. 29–47). New York: Routledge.

Procter, H. G. (1987). Change in the family construct system. In R. A. Neimeyer & G. J. Neimeyer (Eds.), *Personal construct therapy casebook* (pp. 153–171). New York: Springer.

Raskin, J. D., & Lewandowski, A. M. (2000). The construction of disorder as human enterprise. In R. A. Neimeyer & J. D. Raskin (Eds.), *Constructions of disorder* (pp. 15–39). Washington, DC: American Psychological Association.

Rennie, D. L. (1992). Qualitative analysis of the client's experience of psychotherapy. In S. G. Toukmanian & D. L. Rennie (Eds.), *Psychotherapy process research* (pp. 211–233). Newbury Park, CA: Sage.

Robinson, L. A., Berman, J. S., & Neimeyer, R. A. (1990). Psychotherapy for the treatment of depression: A comprehensive review of controlled outcome research. *Psychological Bulletin, 108,* 30–49.

Rogers, C. R. (1961). *On becoming a person.* Boston: Houghton Mifflin.

Sacks, O. (1998). *The man who mistook his wife for a hat.* New York: Touchstone.

Saleebey, D. (1998). Constructing the community: Emergent uses of social constructionism in economically distressed communities. In C. Franklin & P. S. Nurius (Eds.), *Constructivism in practice* (pp. 291–310). Milwaukee, WI: Families International.

Seikkula, J., Alakare, B., & Aaltonen, J. (2001a). Open dialogue in psychosis I: An introduction and case illustration. *Journal of Constructivist Psychology, 14,* 247–266.

Seikkula, J., Alakare, B., & Aaltonen, J. (2001b). Open dialogue in psychosis II: A comparison of good and poor outcome cases. *Journal of Constructivist Psychology, 14,* 267–283.

Sewell, K. W., Adams-Webber, J., Mitterer, J., & Cromwell, R. L. (1992). Computerized repertory grids: Review of the literature. *International Journal of Personal Construct Psychology, 5,* 1–24.

Shotter, J. (2000). From within our lives together. In L. Holzman & J. Morss (Eds.), *Postmodern psychologies and societal practice.* New York: Routledge.

Spence, D. (1982). *Narrative and historical truth.* New York: Norton.

Vasco, A. B. (1994). Correlates of constructivism among Protuguese therapists. *Journal of Constructivist Psychology, 7,* 1–16.

Vincent, N., & LeBow, M. (1995). Treatment preference and acceptability: Epistemology and locus of control. *Journal of Constructivist Psychotherapy, 8,* 81–96.

Viney, L. L. (1988). Which data-collection methods are appropriate for a contructivist psychology? *International Journal of Personal Construct Psychology, 1,* 191–203.

Weber, C., Bronner, E., Their, P., Kingreen, D., & Klapp, B. (2000). Body construct systems of patients with hematological malignancies. In J. W. Scheer (Ed.), *The person in society: Challenges to a constructivist theory* (pp. 328–339). Giessen, Germany: Psychosozial Verlag.

White, M., & Epston, D. (1990). *Narrative means to therapeutic ends.* New York: Norton.

Winslade, J., & Monk, G. (2001). *Narrative mediation.* San Francisco: Jossey-Bass.

Winter, D. A. (1990). Therapeutic alternatives for psychological disorder. In G. J. Neimeyer & R. A. Neimeyer (Eds.), *Advances in personal construct psychology* (Vol. 1, pp. 89–116). Greenwich, CT: JAI Press.

Winter, D. A. (1992). *Personal construct psychology in clinical practice.* London: Routledge.

Zumaya, M., Bridges, S. K., & Rubio, E. (1999). A constructivist approach to sex therapy with couples. *Journal of Constructivist Psychology, 12,* 185–201.

9

Integrative Approaches to Psychotherapy

GEORGE STRICKER
JERRY GOLD

HISTORICAL BACKGROUND

An Introduction to Integrative Approaches to Psychotherapy

Integrative psychotherapies result from an explicit attempt to synthesize theoretical constructs and clinical interventions that are drawn from two or more traditional schools of psychotherapy (such as Gestalt therapy, cognitive-behavioral therapy, and psychoanalysis) into one therapeutic approach. It is hoped these efforts will lead to the development of therapeutic systems that will be more effective and applicable to a wider range of clinical populations and problems than were the individual models of psychotherapy that were integrated. Therefore, it is impossible to discuss any one version of integrative psychotherapy as the definitive version, as these approaches are highly varied and, optimally, are in a continuous state of evolution. In this chapter we discuss those contemporary integrative approaches that generally are considered most influential, and we attempt to describe the com-

monalities and consistencies among these models when possible.

Integrative Psychotherapy and Psychotherapy Integration: A Distinction

The term "psychotherapy integration" refers to a philosophical, conceptual, and clinical orientation to the study of psychotherapy. This perspective is defined by openness to understanding the convergences and commonalities among the vast array of sectarian psychotherapies, and by an interest in promoting dialogue among therapists of all orientations. Psychotherapy integration is defined also by a willingness to learn from all therapies and therapists, rather than to declare exclusive loyalty to one school or model of psychotherapy. Our preference is for a process of integration that guides psychotherapy rather than any single product or integrative psychotherapy that might become yet another sectarian approach with all the limitations attendant upon that status (Stricker, 1994).

Historical Antecedents to Contemporary Psychotherapy Integration

The first precursor to contemporary integrative approaches to psychotherapy might well be an article in which French (1933) alerted psychoanalysts to the need for psychoanalytic theory and practice to account for the findings of Pavlov in the area of classical conditioning. This would have anticipated developments in behavior therapy and produced an early version of theoretical integration. A second seminal contribution was Rosenzweig's (1936) introduction of the hypothesis that the many varieties of psychotherapy shared a limited number of essential effective ingredients, or common factors. This article is the foundation of contemporary versions of common factors integration.

During the 1940s and 1950s, several efforts at integrating then current versions of psychoanalytic theory and learning theory were proposed. Sears (1944) was among the first authors to write in this area, but the most extensive, influential, and long-lasting contribution was made by Dollard and Miller (1950), who integrated central psychoanalytic ideas about unconscious motivation and conflict with concepts drawn from the learning theories of Hull, Spence, Tolman, and Mowrer. Though orthodox psychoanalysts often were scornful and dismissive of this model, other psychoanalytic thinkers who were open to contributions from other theories and from empirical research found inspiration in Dollard and Miller's unique synthesis.

Another highly important work, one that was not specifically integrative but that was an influence on many integrative clinicians, was the book *Psychoanalytic Therapy*, by Alexander and French (1946). This volume introduced the concept of the corrective emotional experience, referring to an event that takes place between therapist and patient. During the course of the therapeutic interaction, certain attitudes, emotions, and

behaviors of the therapist were found to modify, powerfully and immediately, unconscious assumptions and perceptions derived from the patient's early development and interpersonal history. The formulation of the corrective emotional experience, and its prescriptive perspective on interventions, expanded the psychoanalysts' role from the provision of insight via interpretation to the inclusion of behavioral interaction and the provision of new experience as valid therapeutic endeavors.

In the 1960s the first explicit attempts at integrating two or more psychotherapeutic systems were published. Most of these focused on combining concepts and methods drawn from behavioral and psychoanalytic models. An early and neglected classic of this type was the marriage of Freud and Skinner proposed by Beier (1966), who described the role that reinforcement and operant conditioning processes played in the shaping, maintenance, and extinction of unconscious conflict and motivation.

The most successful example of psychotherapy integration was accomplished by Beck (Beck, Rush, Shaw, & Emery, 1979), who introduced the relatively new field of cognitively oriented psychotherapy to the practice of behavior therapy. The integrative result, cognitive–behavioral therapy, has obtained the status of an independent school of psychotherapy and has gained clear ascendancy over behavior therapy in contemporary practice.

In the next decade several efforts appeared that crossed the boundaries of the traditional psychotherapies and created integrative, or eclectic (as they were more often known at that time), psychotherapies. Examples of these explorations were the papers published by Marmor (1971) and by Feather and Rhodes (1973), who found that unconscious issues could be treated through the use of behavioral methods such as desensitization to the core conflict.

This trend culminated in the publication of *Psychoanalysis and Behavior Therapy: Towards an Integration,* by Paul Wachtel (1977), which was, and remains today, perhaps the single most important and influential work on the theoretical integration of various psychotherapies. This book, and the positive response it generated, opened the floodgates in the field of psychotherapy integration. During the 1980s many prominent psychotherapy scholars and clinicians explored the technical, theoretical, and philosophical possibilities of integrating therapies in a newly invigorated and enthusiastic way (Arkowitz & Messer, 1984). The Society for the Exploration of Psychotherapy Integration (SEPI)[1] was founded in the early 1980s, and, after a brief affiliation with the *Journal of Eclectic and Integrative Psychotherapy,* began to publish the *Journal of Psychotherapy Integration* in 1991. Two thorough handbooks on psychotherapy integration, which included many of the most important integrative therapies then available, were published in the early 1990s as well (Norcross & Goldfried, 1992; Stricker & Gold, 1993). They demonstrated that integrative thinking had progressed beyond an exclusive focus on the synthesis of psychoanalytic and behavioral models. Current integrative therapies combine cognitive, humanistic, experiential, and family systems models and techniques in ever more complex permutations. It was during the last decade of the 20th century that psychotherapy integration truly came of age (Arkowitz, 1992).

Why is it that psychotherapy integration as a perspective, and integrative psychotherapies as therapeutic models, became so widely accepted in the last 15 to 20 years? Most students of the history of psychotherapy suggest (Gold, 1993; Goldfried & Newman, 1992; Norcross & Newman, 1992) that the failure of any traditional model of psychotherapy to "win all the prizes" and to establish itself as clearly superior to the others had much to do with this change. Another important group of factors were external to psychotherapeutic practice but affected psychotherapists most profoundly. These included the rise of biological models of psychopathology, the introduction of

new generations of increasingly effective psychiatric drugs, and new requirements by the public, the government, and insurance companies for therapists to demonstrate the effectiveness of their methods. Suddenly, the "enemy" was no longer the psychoanalyst, the cognitive-behaviorist, or the Gestalt therapist across the road or in the next state. As people have always done when under siege, therapists put aside their differences and began to work together and to learn from each other.

Other, more positive events may be responsible for the rapid rise of interest in integrative therapies. Most of the founding schools of psychotherapy had their origins 50 to 100 years ago. The founders and founding generations are gone, and the succeeding generations may be more confident in crossing boundaries and assimilating new, "foreign," ideas than were those early therapists who were struggling to establish a new therapeutic position. As the world has become smaller and more integrated, dissemination of ideas and communication among contributors occurs more rapidly. The decades of the 1960s, 1970s, and 1980s saw a questioning of traditional authority in academics and in politics, integration in the social realm, as well as the cross-fertilization of many aspects of Western culture, including music, visual arts, literature, sports, and science.

The Modes of Psychotherapy Integration

Traditionally, there have been three commonly accepted modes or forms of psychotherapy integration (Gold, 1996), although now it is more accurate to speak of four. These modes define general ways in which theory and technique have been integrated and are known as technical eclecticism, the common-factors approach, theoretical integration, and assimilative integration. The ongoing process of psychotherapy integration relies on these modes, and each established approach to integrative psychotherapy can be considered an example of one of these modes.

Technical Eclecticism

Technical eclecticism is the most clinical and technically oriented form of psychotherapy integration but involves the least amount of conceptual or theoretical integration. Clinical strategies and techniques from two or more therapies are applied sequentially or in combination, usually following a broad and comprehensive assessment of the patient. This assessment describes the interconnections between the problems to be addressed and the cognitive, behavioral, emotional, and interpersonal characteristics of the patient. Techniques are chosen on the basis of the best clinical match to the needs of the patient, as guided by clinical knowledge and research findings, regardless of their theoretical origin. The most important examples of this type of integrative psychotherapy are multimodal therapy (Lazarus, 1992, 2002) and prescriptive psychotherapy (Beutler, Alomohamed, Moleiro, & Romanelli, 2002). The former grew out of Lazarus's dissatisfaction with traditional behavior therapy and relies on supplementing behavioral interventions with cognitive, imagery-based, and experiential techniques. Prescriptive psychotherapy does not limit the schools of therapy from which it draws its techniques, aiming at the best match of techniques to problems. For example, the more resistive the patient is, the less directive the therapist will be.

Common-Factors Approaches to Integration

Common-factors integration starts from the identification of effective ingredients that are held in common by any group of therapies. This way of thinking has its origins in Rosenzweig's (1936) seminal discovery that all therapies shared certain change processes, despite their idiosyncratic theories and techniques. Also central to common-factors thinking was J. Frank's (1961) observation

that all systems of psychological healing share certain common, effective ingredients, such as socially sanctioned rituals, the provision of hope, and the shaping of an outlook on life that offers encouragement to the patient. Messer and Wampold (2002), on the basis of several research studies and meta-analyses, concluded that there is a far more convincing argument for common factors as being critical to therapeutic change than for any specific treatment effects.

Integrative therapists who use a common-factors approach try to identify which of the several known common factors will be most important in the treatment of a particular individual. Once the most salient common factors are selected, the therapist reviews the array of interventions and psychotherapeutic interactions to find those that have been found to promote and contain those ingredients. The integrative therapies that result from this process are structured around the goal of maximizing the patient's exposure to the unique combination of therapeutic factors that will best ameliorate his or her problems. Garfield's (2000) common-factors integrative therapy, which relies on the combination of insight, exposure, and the provision of new experience and hope through the therapeutic relationship, is one well-known form of common-factors integration.

Theoretical Integration

Theoretical integration is the most complex, sophisticated, and difficult mode of psychotherapy integration. Psychotherapies that are theoretically integrated rely on a process of synthesizing aspects of varied personality theories, combining models of psychopathology, and integrating various mechanisms of psychological change from two or more traditional systems. These novel integrative theories may indicate the mutual influence of environmental, motivational, cognitive, and affective variables.

Theoretically integrated systems of psychotherapy use interventions from each of the component theories, as well as proposing original techniques that may be added to the technical selection of the traditional therapeutic schools that are the basis of this new approach. Superficially, the clinical choices derived from a theoretically integrated system may resemble the choice of techniques that are suggested by a technically eclectic model. However, important distinctions may be found in the conceptualizations and belief systems that guide the choice of clinical strategies and techniques on the part of the respective therapists. Theoretical integration extends beyond technical eclecticism in clinical practice by increasing the number and type of intrapsychic and behavioral variables that can be targeted therapeutically. Subtle interactions among various levels and spheres of behavior; interpersonal interactions; and motivational, cognitive, and affective and internal states and processes can be evaluated and treated from several complementary therapeutic perspectives. This expanded conceptual framework allows problems at one level or in one sphere of psychological life to be addressed in ways previously considered incompatible. That is, the therapist might intervene in a problem in affect tolerance not only to help the patient be more comfortable emotionally but to promote change in motivation, or to rid the patient of a way of thinking about emotion that maintained powerful unconscious feelings. For example, an intervention that increases the patient's control over impulsive behavior may also open the door to considering the ways in which impulsivity functions in the patient's interpersonal relationships.

Wachtel's cyclical psychodynamic theory and its integrative therapy was the first fully developed form of theoretical integration. He developed a psychodynamically based model of personality, psychopathology, and change that acknowledged and used reinforcement and social learning principles along with traditional psychoanalytic exploration (Wachtel, 1997). The usual model of exploration leading to understanding and then change was supplemented by an understanding that behavioral change, produced by behavioral interventions, might lead to increased understanding. As in the previous example, changing impulsive behavior may not require prior understanding, but understanding might follow from behavioral change.

Assimilative Integration

Assimilative integration has been the focus of much recent interest (Messer, 2001b; Stricker & Gold, 2002) and can be seen as a derivative of both theoretical integration and technical eclecticism. Messer (1992) introduced this concept into the field of psychotherapy integration when he noted that all actions are defined and contained by the interpersonal, historical, and physical context in which those acts occur. As any therapeutic intervention is an interpersonal action (and a highly complex one at that), those interventions are defined, and perhaps even re-created, by the larger context of the therapy. Certain theoretically integrative approaches may be understood to be assimilative as they incorporate new techniques into the existing conceptual model of therapy. When techniques are applied clinically within a theoretical context that differs from the context in which they were developed, the meaning, impact, and use of those interventions may be modified in powerful ways. When interventions such as the use of systematic desensitization within the context of client-centered therapy are assimilated into this different model, their nature is altered by this new context and by the alternative purposes of the therapist. Thus, a behavioral method such as systematic desensitization will mean something entirely different to a patient whose ongoing therapeutic experience has been defined by experientially oriented exploration than that same intervention would mean to a patient in traditional behavior therapy. The psychodynamically based integrative therapy proposed by Stricker and Gold (1996; Gold &

Stricker, 2001) is an example of this form of integrative therapy. In this approach, therapy proceeds according to standard psychodynamic guidelines, but methods from other therapies are used when called for, and they may advance certain psychodynamic goals indirectly at the same time as being effective in treating the target problem. McCullough and Andrews (2001) treat affect phobias using an approach (short-term dynamic psychotherapy) that assimilates techniques from several orientations to the psychodynamic focus of understanding. For further examples of assimilative integration, see the special issue of the *Journal of Psychotherapy Integration* (Messer, 2001b).

THE CONCEPT OF PERSONALITY

Personality as an explanatory or organizing construct (i.e., as an implicit or inferred set of psychological constructs and behaviors) is very much a part of certain integrative psychotherapies. Other systems of psychotherapy integration barely acknowledge the notion of personality or exclude it completely. *Attention to personality is omitted from most integrative models that are based on common factors integration or on technical eclecticism.* The prescriptive focus of these psychotherapies, in which symptoms and targeted problems are matched with therapeutic ingredients (common factors) or with assumed effective techniques (technical eclecticism), means that the therapist uses a narrower lens to understand the patient and his or her behavior and experience. An inferred conceptual system or model of personality presumably would add little to the effectiveness of the prescriptive power of these psychotherapies and might, in fact, serve as an intellectual distraction for the therapist.

One exception to this point is multimodal therapy, the most frequently used form of technical eclecticism (Lazarus, 2002). Assessment in this psychotherapy proceeds from a broad framework that guides the therapist in identifying strengths, weaknesses, and idiosyncrasies in seven areas: Behavior, Affect, Sensation, Imagery, Cognition, Interpersonal Relationships, and Drugs and Biology (the BASIC ID). Lazarus (1992) has noted that these areas of functioning are comprehensive enough to account for the individual's entire personality, especially when his or her concept of the "firing order" is taken into account. This refers to the understanding that these seven areas are dynamically interrelated, and that most complex behaviors and psychological difficulties need to be understood as resulting from the interaction of two or more of the areas in the BASIC ID.

Personality is a much more important concept in those integrative psychotherapies that are based on theoretical or assimilative integration. Assimilative integration has a single personality theory and theory of therapy as its organizing feature. Theoretical integration involves the synthesis of two or more independent personality theories into a novel model of personality. A critical assumption behind this theoretical amalgamation is that this new, integrative personality theory is an improvement over the component theories in its ability to inform the therapist's understanding of psychological development, psychopathology, and, most important, the best and most efficacious choice of interventions.

Integrative theories of personality are employed in two ways, the first of which is similar to the manner that traditional theories of personality are used in pure forms of psychotherapy: as a guide in the identification of psychological structures (e.g., schemata and defense mechanisms) and other features (e.g., anxiety, unconscious motivation, and affect) that need to be influenced and changed by therapy. Second, and uniquely, these theories posit and explain the relationship between psychological phenomena that are ignored or considered irrelevant by traditional theories. Such explanations illustrate an extremely important and singular characteristic of integrative models of personality: *integrative theories substitute circular conceptualizations of causation for the linear views of causation that are typical of traditional personality theories.* Circular views of causation suggest that there are no levels or areas of psychological life that are unimportant or that should be understood merely as superficial, as may result from the more narrow views inherent in older models of personality.

Westen (1988) and Gold (1996) have pointed out that the personality theories that support contemporary integrative approaches share a number of common assumptions and emphases, regardless of deviations in the specific terminology used in each contribution. Integrative personality theories share a deep concern for the way the individual comes to understand his or her experience and for those core meaning structures that compose the person's sense of self and representation of significant relationships. For a more complete discussion of integrative contributions to this area, see Gold (1996).

There are several highly influential integrative theories of personality. As mentioned earlier, the most comprehensive and influential is Wachtel's (1977, 1997) theory of cyclical psychodynamics. The publication of this theory was a watershed event in the history of psychotherapy integration in that Wachtel (1977) demonstrated that a clinically viable and conceptually elegant synthesis of psychoanalytic and learning theories could be achieved. Cyclical psychodynamic theory presented a model of personality that emphasized the mutually and reciprocally determining nature of behavior, interpersonal relationships, and unconscious motivation and conflict. The theory assisted therapists in understanding how changes in psychodynamics could both lead to and follow from changes in behavior and in interactions with others. The latest iteration of cyclical psychodynamics has expanded the theory to include concepts drawn from family systems theory, relational

psychoanalysis, experiential theories, and cognitive theory (Wachtel, 1997).

The procedural sequence object relations model (Ryle & Low, 1993) is another integrative approach to personality. This model informs cognitive-analytic therapy (CAT) and is a synthesis of concepts drawn from cognitive psychology, cognitive therapy, and psychoanalytic object relations theory. The theory describes the complex interrelationships between the way that the individual consciously processes information about the self and others and the unconscious developmental antecedents of the person's cognitive structures, beliefs, assumptions, and role definitions.

A final example of this type of integrative personality is the one proposed by Greenberg, Rice, and Elliott (1993), which integrates ideas from client-centered therapy, cognitive therapy, and experiential therapies. These authors see personality as the meaning-retention and meaning-generation structures through which persons come to understand, remember, and respond to the world. This theory serves as a foundation for therapeutic interventions drawn from the three aforementioned source therapies, all of which can address the modification of pathological meanings.

PSYCHOLOGICAL HEALTH AND PATHOLOGY

Few integrative approaches specifically offer a comprehensive psychological model of health. This omission is not limited to integrative psychotherapies, as many writers within and outside the psychotherapeutic literature have discussed the "disease orientation" of the vast majorities of psychotherapies (Bohart & Tallman, 1999). Moreover, most integrative therapies contain within them the definitions and conceptualizations of health and pathology that derive from the specific component therapies (psychodynamic, cognitive-behavioral, experiential, etc.) that are amalgamated. However, a careful reading of the psychotherapy integration literature suggests strongly that many integrationists share certain critical assumptions about the nature and appearance of psychological health.

Psychological health seems to consist of freedom from psychological constraints on the perception and construction of meaning and experience (Bohart, 1992; Greenberg et al., 1993); repetitive, dysfunctional patterns of thought and of the organization of cognitive data (Guidano & Liotti, 1983); redundant and maladaptive ways of engaging and relating to others (K. Frank, 1999); and the unwitting repetition and maintenance of developmental traumata, conflict, and attachments (Stricker & Gold, 2002). For example, Andrews (1993) described the ultimate goal of his integrative psychotherapy as the consolidation of the "active self," which captures the essence of the kind of psychological freedom that embodies health. He described the "active self" as resulting from people's ability to maintain a stable self-image while being open to, and searching out, novel experiences and flexibly expanding their cognitive, behavioral, emotional, and interpersonal repertoires. In other words, integrationists seem to characterize psychological health as the ability to define one's goals; successfully jettison, modify, or retain goals depending on their (individual and social) adaptive benefit; develop plans to obtain and actively seek out these goals; learn from self-generated and other-generated feedback; and attain them without intrapersonal or interpersonal interference.

It stands to reason, then, that an integrative perspective on the development and maintenance of psychopathology would focus on those psychological and environmental factors that inhibit the individual's freedom of experience and responsiveness and eventuate in psychological and behavioral redundancy. Most integrative theorists work from a developmental framework in that they emphasize the role of childhood and adolescent events in laying down the foundations of perception, thinking, and

motivation that lead to psychopathology (Wachtel, 1977). Essentially, these theorists posit that negative, painful, anxious, and defeated familial and social interactions are internalized and become part of the patient's cognitive and emotional representational systems. This negatively toned representational system, which consciously and unconsciously leads to ongoing predictions and construal of danger (shame, guilt, humiliation, abandonment, etc.) in many, if not most, important interpersonal situations, cannot help but lead the patient into avoidant, defensive, and ultimately self-defeating and self-replicating patterns of construing reality and of social relatedness (Allen, 1993; Wachtel, 1977). These "vicious circles" (Wachtel, 1977) or self-fulfilling and self-defeating prophecies (Andrews, 1993) are central and critical variables in most integrative accounts of psychopathology. Such linked sequences of motivation, conflict, emotion, cognition, and social behavior thus maintain the underlying pathogenic meaning structures (schemata, object representations, procedural sequences, narratives, etc., depending on the theory) that gave rise to them in the first place. These circular, self-confirming sequences limit the patient's ability to see alternatives and lead to the patient unwittingly working his or her way deeper and deeper into a corner, psychologically speaking. As a result, he or she becomes more negative, fearful, anxious, enraged, rigid, or disorganized, and these cognitive and emotional states eventuate in the appearance of symptoms such as panic, anxiety, depression, substance abuse, or the interpersonal disturbances associated with personality disorders.

Thus, most integrative theories of psychopathology operate within what Messer (1992) has identified as the "ironic vision"; that is, things come out badly and redundantly despite the person's best efforts to achieve a new result or experience (Wachtel, 1977). Few persons are aware of the restricting power of their representational systems, or of the ways in which we

unwittingly reproduce past hurts and disappointments in the present. We are aware, however, of the cognitive, emotional, and interpersonal sequelae of those hurts, and it is this distress that often eventuates in the decision to enter therapy.

The various models of integrative psychotherapy rely on several diagnostic systems, some of which are generic (i.e, fourth edition of *Diagnostic and Statistical Manual of Mental Disorders* [DSM-IV; American Psychiatric Association, 1994]) and others of which are uniquely associated with the particular psychotherapy in which it is used. We have already described the diagnostic model (BASIC ID) that is at the heart of multimodal therapy (Lazarus, 1992, 2002). Ryle's (1997) CAT is built around a detailed and formal assessment of the patient's cognitive functioning or procedural sequences, with particular attention paid to "traps" (dysfunctional assumptions and beliefs), "dilemmas" (polarized alternative conceptualizations of experience), and "snags" (aims that are abandoned due to the anticipation of negative consequences). Added to this level of diagnosis is an evaluation of the object representations that were the developmental forerunners of the patient's cognitive difficulties, and that, in turn, are maintained by these cognitive patterns and their behavioral consequences.

Another example of an integrative model of psychotherapy that is built around its own specialized diagnostic system is transtheoretical therapy (Prochaska & DiClemente, 2002). In this approach, the patient is evaluated on a three dimensional matrix. This evaluation matrix includes the *stage of change* at which the patient currently stands (essentially, how ready the person is to change and to take an active part in changing), the *level of change* that is most advantageous or necessary (psychodynamic, experiential, cognitive, behavioral, familial, or environmental), and the *change processes* (e.g., reinforcement, abreaction, or unconditional positive regard) that are most likely to be effective.

THE PROCESS OF CLINICAL ASSESSMENT

Assessment in most integrative approaches is based on the methods that are typical of the component therapies that make up each integrative method. This is most often the case for those integrative therapies that are exemplars of either theoretical or assimilative integration, as these therapies tend to be more long term and more concerned with "deeper" or more complex changes (e.g., in personality structure and representational systems). Thus, an integrative therapy that leans heavily on a psychodynamic foundation, such as cyclical psychodynamics (Wachtel, 1977) or assimilative psychodynamic psychotherapy (Gold & Stricker, 2001), for example, will assess patients initially and primarily with regard to psychodynamic issues such as conflict, character, resistance, and object representations. These therapies also will include ongoing, process-oriented assessments, as do traditional psychodynamic treatments: the patient is evaluated, and the therapist's understanding is revised and reformulated on an ongoing basis throughout therapy, based on the patient's responses and form of participation.

The integrative assessment is expanded to include evaluation of the person's functioning at the cognitive, experiential, and behavioral levels and the mutual influence of those levels on each other and with psychodynamic issues and structures. Similarly, a theoretically integrated therapy that primarily is behaviorally based, such as Fensterheim's (1993) behavioral psychotherapy, would assess the usual behavioral variables in a context that included an ongoing evaluation of the variables that are considered critical from the additional and integrated therapeutic orientation. Where integrative assessment differs from a traditional assessment is in the therapist's awareness of, and attention to, the possibility and advantage of using an intervention from another therapeutic system (in this example, from cognitive-behavioral therapy, or experiential therapy, among others). The parameters of assessment are expanded to include an ongoing evaluation of the benefits and limitations of the "home" or foundation therapy, and of the patient's individualized needs, goals, strengths, and weaknesses, all of which may best be met by an integrative shift. Certain integrationists (Bohart, 2000; Duncan & Miller, 2000; Gold, 2000; Rennie, 2000) also advocate the ongoing assessment of the patient's conscious assessment of the therapy and his or her ideas about which techniques and strategies would be most helpful.

Because most integrative therapies are oriented to the individual, the "unit" of assessment is the individual person, with awareness that this person cannot be understood separately from the interpersonal context in which he or she is located. There are, however, exceptions to this individual focus, as certain writers have made important contributions to the integration of individual therapy with couples, family, and group psychotherapies (Allen, 1993; Gerson, 1996; Gurman, 2002; Pinsof, 1995). In these therapies, assessment is directed toward individual and systemic functioning, and particularly toward the interaction and mutual influence of the two levels upon each other.

As described previously, and as would be expected, *the focus of integrative assessment usually is broader and deeper than assessment in any single pure-form therapy,* including interest in intrapsychic, cognitive, behavioral, experiential, and interpersonal variables. Again, the emphasis on each class of variables is determined by the weighting of the component therapies. As an example of the breadth and depth of integrative assessment, we might consider Andrews's (1993) description of assessment within the active self model. He indicates that the following nine variables are included: Self-concept, Motivations (conscious and unconscious), Expectancies and Plans, Behavior, Awareness of Impressions of Others, Awareness of Responses of Others, Selective Perceptions of

Interpersonal Experiences, Selective Interpretations of Interpersonal Experiences, and Reactive Emotions.

Interest in assessing the individual within a contextual framework is an intrinsic part of many integrative approaches. Assessment of context includes an evaluation of past and current interpersonal relationships and the ways in which others in the patient's life become "neurotic accomplices" (Wachtel, 1977). This term refers to the way in which significant persons contribute to the maintenance and exacerbation of patients' problems by confirming their fears and their problematic representational processes. Assessment of context has been extended by some to include much broader issues as well. Wachtel (1989) has illustrated the need to account for the effect of racial discrimination, poverty, and social disenfranchisement on individual psychology and psychopathology. Gold (1992) extended Wachtel's cyclical psychodynamic thinking to include evaluation of the effects of gender discrimination and political disempowerment on psychological suffering and psychotherapy.

Most integrative therapists explicitly describe an assessment of patients' strengths as an integral part of their work. These strengths often become the basis of interventions, as patients are helped to take on challenges and areas of weakness by using and extending skills in which they are already proficient. As noted earlier, certain theorists (e.g., Bohart, 2000; Duncan & Miller, 2000) have suggested that patients often know best what they need, and may even have the skills to change but are unaware of the ways in which those skills could be best applied or in which situations these efforts would be most productive.

Certain integrative approaches that are examples of technical eclecticism or of common-factors integration are based on an immediate, comprehensive assessment of the patient that leads directly into the selection of therapeutic interventions. These therapies are almost entirely driven by this assessment. We have already discussed two examples of this type of integrative therapy: multimodal therapy (Lazarus, 2002) and transtheoretical therapy (Prochaska & DiClemente, 2002). Another important version of an assessment driven integrative therapy is systematic treatment selection (Beutler et al., 2002), in which the explicit goal is the matching of empirically tested techniques to the needs of each patient. Several basic variables are assessed prior to the selection of therapeutic strategies and techniques. These variables include predisposing client characteristics, such as level of impairment and coping style; the treatment context, meaning the intensity, setting, modality, and format of treatment; and the qualities of the therapeutic relationship, such as the attitude, knowledge, tools, and techniques proffered by the therapist. Once these variables are evaluated, the assessment moves on to consider the other, more discrete issues. These include the identification of specific goals of treatment or focal objectives, the level of intervention, any subsidiary or mediating goals that might interfere with or synergize the attainment of focal objectives, and ongoing assessment of the patient's ability to comply and cooperate with the treatment plan. This assessment must be completed before techniques are selected and employed, and of course the evaluation is revised on an ongoing basis. Transtheoretical therapy, multimodal therapy, and systematic treatment selection (STS) freely and frequently use standardized psychological tests to conduct assessments. For example, Beutler and colleagues (2002) mention such specific instruments as the STS Clinician Rating Form, the Patient Compliance Scale, and the STS Therapy Process Rating Scale as essential and regular sources of data that inform the process through which prescriptive treatment plans evolve. Variables such as the stages of change and processes of change are assessed in transtheoretical therapy through the use of self-report measures (the URICA, or University of Rhode Island Change Assess-

ment, and the POC, or Processes of Change measure; Prochaska & DiClemente, 2002). Few integrative systems that are based on theoretical integration include such heavy reliance on standardized tests, though individual therapists may use some or many at their discretion.

Few integrative therapies rely heavily on formalized psychiatric typologies such as DSM-IV. Those that do typically use psychiatric diagnosis as a starting point for a more intensive and psychologically oriented assessment. An example of this approach is cognitive-behavioral analytic systems psychotherapy (CBASP), which is an integrative therapy developed for the treatment of dysthymic disorder (depression) by McCullough (2001). In this model, the psychiatric diagnosis is the entry point, which indicates that this therapy is appropriate for this patient. However, the assessment that is crucial to the progress of the treatment goes beyond diagnosis and into the spheres of cognition, behavior, and interpersonal skills.

THE PRACTICE OF THERAPY

Basic Structure of Therapy

There is considerable variation in the basic structure of therapy across the many varieties of integrative psychotherapies. As has been stressed in this chapter, the characteristics of each approach are determined largely by its component therapies. Thus, it is a general rule, though one with more than enough exceptions, that those integrative therapies that are more heavily psychodynamic are longer in term (2 or more years) and tend to meet at least on a weekly basis, with two or even three sessions per week being far from unknown. Integrative approaches that give more emphasis to cognitive-behavioral and experiential schools tend to be shorter in length and to meet once a week or even less frequently. Typically sessions last from 45 minutes to 1 hour.

In the last few years several integrative therapies have been described that are specifically identified as *short term*. These include time-limited dynamic psychotherapy (Levenson, 1995), accelerated experiential–dynamic psychotherapy (Fosha, 2000), and short-term restructuring psychotherapy (Magnavita & Carlson, in press). These integrative therapies are designed to be completed in 20 to 30 weekly sessions. Most integrative therapies are individually focused and therefore attendance in sessions is limited to patient and therapist. However, there is a great deal of flexibility in this arrangement. As mentioned earlier, certain integrative therapies merge individual and systems approaches and hold sessions with individuals, couples, families, subsystems within families, and groups, as dictated by clinical necessity. The degree to which any session is structured or governed by a predetermined agenda is a function of the theoretical slant of the specific integrative model. Therapies that lean heavily on humanistic, experiential, or psychoanalytic foundations are less likely to be highly structured than are those that are more cognitive-behavioral in orientation. For example, CBASP (McCullough, 2001) resembles standard cognitive-behavioral approaches much more than other integrative therapies in its extensive use of homework assignments and goal setting for each session and in the therapist's active direction of the content and process of each session.

Goal Setting

The various integrative therapies differ significantly with regard to the nature and specifics of the goals that are determined for each patient. Those approaches that are based on a psychoanalytic or humanistic-experiential foundation posit that most patients can benefit from certain broadly defined changes, regardless of the particular presenting problems. These universal goals include changes in underlying meaning or representational structures, character structure, and the patient's ability to be open to the symbolization and integration of new experiences. Those therapies that are more prescriptive or shorter term tend to avoid such general, shared goals and to focus more specifically on what ails this particular person at this specific time.

Most integrative models stress that goal setting is best accomplished through a process of collaboration in which the therapist may take the lead through the assessment process but is open and respectful of the patient's needs, wishes, and ideas, particularly as these may reflect the patient's efforts to revise or reject the therapist's formulation and treatment plan. Most integrative therapists emphasize overt discussion of some, if not all, therapeutic goals. This is an essential part of establishing trust, respect, and a therapeutic alliance. Goals that are more likely to be discussed are those that are connected to the patient's overt behavior, conscious thoughts and feelings, and relationships. For example, the wish to deal with uncomfortable affect or the problem caused by repetitive difficulty in relationships may be discussed and provide clear goals for the patient and the therapist. Goals that may guide the therapist, but which refer to psychic processes and structures, probably are discussed less frequently with patients. It would be possible to place the many integrative therapies on a continuum of goals that, at one end, would be described as therapist driven, and at the other, patient driven. Those therapies that would be found at the patient-driven end are typically those that are more short term, concerned with the resolution of the presenting problem, and give less emphasis to inferred intrapsychic issues. This patient-specific approach to goals is most evident in the model of client-directed therapy developed by Miller, Duncan, and Hubble (2002), in which patient and therapist collaborate in developing therapeutic strategies and selecting interventions based on the patient's theory of change and his or her plan for achieving those changes.

Advocates of psychotherapy integration argue emphatically that one of the main advantages of this attitude is that *integrative models allow goals to be established at any level,* or in any realm of psychological experience: relational, behavioral, cognitive, affective, motivational, and characterological. Goals do not have to be excluded, overlooked, or characterized as "shallow" or inconsequential due to a preordained theoretical position. Of course, every integrative therapy has its limits, broad as they may be. For example, Lazarus (1992) has made it clear that patients who understand their problems as reflecting unconscious psychosexual conflicts, and who wish to work on such issues, would be best referred to a therapist who could concur with those goals.

Process Aspects of Treatment

As must be evident by now, almost any form of conventionally accepted therapeutic intervention may be used when deemed clinically appropriate. As discussed previously, the choice of intervention may combine theory and the needs of the clinical situation (in theoretical or assimilative integration) or may reflect the clinical assessment of the patient and the process of matching (as in technical eclecticism and common factors integration).

Interpretation of unconscious processes is used in those therapies that integrate psychodynamic principles, when the therapist hypothesizes that insight into unwitting motives, conflicts, resistances, and self- and object representations would be helpful to the patient. For example, a patient who had suddenly developed doubts about an ongoing intimate relationship in which he had been feeling quite comfortable was offered an interpretation of the possible unconscious meanings and functions of these doubts. It was suggested that this process of doubting, as painful as it was, helped him to avoid other deeper uncertainty about important decisions that were looming for him, such as whether to get married. These,

in turn were stimulating vulnerable images of himself in relation to his father, who had committed suicide after a troubled marriage, and were also evoking unresolved feelings of anger and sadness connected to that relationship. As these meanings and emotions became more accessible to awareness, the patient's anxiety and rumination about his current relationship gradually evaporated.

Besides interpretation, integrative therapists use cognitive restructuring, skill-building interventions, and exposure techniques from cognitive-behavioral approaches; experiential techniques such as the empty-chair and two-chair dialogue methods from Gestalt therapy; and empathy, prizing, and reflection of feeling from client-centered therapy, to name just a few of the more prominent types of interventions. At one point in a session the patient may work on tolerating anxiety generated by a feared confrontation with a boss (imaginal desensitization), practice a conversation with someone he or she would like to date (assertiveness training), or work on resolving a long-standing grief reaction by conversing with a deceased parent who has been placed in the empty chair across the room. At other times during a session, or in later sessions, the focus might be on alleviating the patient's overly harsh self-criticism by pointing out the "shoulds" and "musts" that dominate his or her thinking, and by helping the patient to keep track of these thoughts and to substitute more soothing and realistic ideas. Had these interventions been selected in the context of a therapy that was defined as technically eclectic or as a common-factors approach, the selection would have been guided by the central, pressing clinical need and by the identification of the technique that would best meet that need. Selection of that technique in a theoretically or assimilatively integrated theory would be based also on the effect of that technique on the recognition of the meaning of the psychological experience, as well as on the problem.

As an example, consider the case of Mr. C, who sought out therapy for severe social anxiety bordering on agoraphobia and that threatened his job security. Mr. C reported that he had always been an anxious person, but that his anxiety in social situations had increased enormously in the last few months. He was most distressed by his discomfort at his job, where he had previously felt more comfortable than in most other social situations. The data of these initial sessions had suggested to the therapist that Mr. C had become very angry at his coworkers for what he had perceived to be their indifference during a recent crisis in Mr. C's family, and that the upsurge of this anger had stimulated conflicts over the overt expression of anger and hostility that were present in Mr. C's early relationships with his parents. After a few sessions, an interpretation was offered to Mr. C. The patient reported that this interpretation felt "right" to him, and he felt somewhat relieved as this issue continued to be explored. These psychodynamic components of the therapy alternated with periods of more active intervention during which Mr. C practiced confronting some of his colleagues with his hurt and anger, examined and attempted to modify his thinking about anger by keeping a diary of his thoughts (or, a "thought log"), and eventually worked on some of the relational sources of these conflicts by engaging in a (Gestalt-oriented) dialogue with the forbidding images of his parents.

Homework is a central feature of most integrative therapies, even those that have a psychodynamic foundation (Stricker, in press). Sometimes the homework assignments, which usually are developed collaboratively, are traditional applications of cognitive, behavioral, or experiential exercises in the context of another theoretical orientation: Patients whose in-session work leads to psychodynamic insights about their avoidant behavior challenge themselves to face new social situations or to modify the thoughts that drive the anxiety. Other instances of homework are more assimilative and integrative in nature: Homework exercises are used to provoke changes in areas of psychological life other than those with which they usually are associated. For example, patients may be taught relaxation techniques not only because these methods lead to the expected reduction in anxiety but also because successfully lessening those symptoms will lead to changes in their self-image and perception of the therapist (Gold & Stricker, 2001). Patients might be asked to evaluate the effects of the relaxation when entering situations about which they are ordinarily fearful (going through a tunnel in a train, for instance) and to see if their lessened anxiety might lead to increased awareness about feelings, thoughts, memories, and conflicts that are associated with that event. For example, a patient who suffered severe bouts of claustrophobia when flying home from visits to his family, but not on other airplane flights, was taught to modulate his anxiety through a series of cognitive and imagery-based exercises. He then was asked to practice at home, evoking the claustrophobia by imagining himself taking leave of his family and boarding the plane. To his surprise, and eventual great benefit, he discovered that when his symptoms were under control, he was filled with a range of feelings and impressions that were generated by being with his family (sadness, guilt, anger, and fear) that seemed to be the warded-off source of the symptoms. This homework-based discovery became the basis of a great deal of in-session emotional exploration and work on accepting and tolerating painful emotion.

Perhaps the most critical strategic and technical questions in any integrative psychotherapy are when to move from one technique to the next and, correspondingly, to shift orientations and strategies from the behavioral to the experiential to the psychodynamic, and so on. The answers are easier and more straightforward in those technically eclectic and common-factors-based integrative models that feature a comprehensive and specific assessment that is geared to prescriptive matching. In these therapies a shift in technique occurs when the clinical focus changes. For example, as the patient gains certain skills through a behavioral approach (perhaps, as in Mr. C's case, is enabled to be more assertive when angry), other issues, of a cognitive or emotional nature, may emerge. After patient and therapist agree on the next issue to be addressed, the process of prescriptive matching is reapplied and may occur many times until the completion of therapy.

Knowing when to make an integrative shift in a theoretically or assimilatively integrated therapy is more difficult and usually is guided by immediate process observations made by the therapist, often as a reflection of his or her subjective experience of the therapeutic relationship and alliance. K. Frank (1999), Gold and Stricker (2001), and Marcotte and Safran (2002) all have suggested some guidelines for such integrative shifts. Essentially, these writers agree that movement from one orientation and set of therapeutic techniques to another (perhaps from the psychodynamic to cognitive-behavioral) is indicated when the initial way of working has become uncongenial to the patient, is overtaxing the patient's ability to cope, or cooperate, with therapy, requires skills that the patient has not yet developed, or unwittingly is damaging to the patient.

Gold and Stricker (2001), among others, have suggested that certain patients, especially those who are more fragile, less trusting, and less psychologically sophisticated, often make more rapid progress in therapy when the first techniques that are used are more concrete and pragmatic (i.e., more cognitive-behavioral). These patients seem to make better use of psychodynamic exploration when it is introduced after the patient's presenting problems have been ameliorated to some degree, and after the therapist has been established in the patient's perception as helpful and trustworthy. A shift away from a psychodynamic to a more immediately pragmatic form of therapy often may help the patient avoid or alleviate feelings of being confused, mystified, and frustrated by the more subtle goals and methods of psychodynamic therapy and can give these individuals a critically important boost in self-esteem when they have used a cognitive, behavioral, or other technique to solve a problem.

Resistance to change in integrative therapies is conceptualized as resulting from a single factor or a combination of psychological and social factors. The psychodynamic component of many models suggests that resistance occurs when the patient feels frightened of some internal state that is about to emerge into awareness, or is pained, guilty, or ashamed about some past experience, or about the prospect of leaving old ways of living and former attachments behind. The cognitive and behavioral contributions to understanding resistance allow the therapist and patient to look at the contribution of each member of the dyad. Has the therapist asked too much of the patient, or has he or she underestimated the impact of a suggestion or intervention? On the patient's side, resistance may arise from a lack of understanding of the tasks that are posed, by an unwillingness to be open to the therapist's suggestions and interventions, or by a lack of investment in actively changing. Resistance shows itself in myriad forms, from the subtle, characterological patterns with which psychodynamic therapists are familiar to the more overt types of reactance or noncompliance described by cognitive-behavioral therapists (Dowd, 1999). Examples of the former are the patient consistently missing a few minutes of the session, engaging the therapist in an overcompliant, hostile, or idealizing manner, or avoiding certain key subjects by substituting others. On the more obvious side is a failure to keep appointments, a disregard for agreed-on homework assignments, and an unwillingness to fully participate in active interventions of whatever type.

Resistance is resolved clinically by exploration of the meaning of the problem at any level that is necessary (interpersonal, psychodynamic, systemic, cognitive, affective, or behavioral), interpretation, shifting the tone and stance of the therapeutic relationship, or rethinking the choice and intensity of the interventions that are suggested. Integrative therapists who understand individual functioning in a contextual, interpersonal context are acutely aware of those "accomplices in neurosis" who unwittingly or knowingly interfere with the patient's progress in therapy (Wachtel, 1977). This term refers to significant persons in the patient's life who are threatened by his or her attempts to change, and who therefore pressure the patient to remain in old patterns of relating. Integrative therapists will work directly with these significant others on occasion, while at other times the therapeutic focus will be on helping the patient to develop the necessary interpersonal skills to overcome the influence of an accomplice, or to end the relationship if all else fails.

The most common errors that are made by therapists and that are unique to integrative models are the failure to make an integrative shift when it is called for and the too rapid use of an integrative shift when ongoing work within one theoretical and technical framework is a better fit. The first type of error seems to occur frequently because of the somewhat vague guidelines for timing shifts, and sometimes occurs when the therapist is still bound up by loyalties and anxieties about his or her allegiance to one therapy school. Overly rapid shifting, or the overuse of integration, may also occur due to (countertransferential) anxiety on part of the therapist. For example, the therapist may feel too uncomfortable to continue working with a particular issue and therefore may suggest a shift in strategy or technique.

Psychotropic medications are often a part of integrative therapy. When the therapist is a psychiatrist, or psychopharmacologist, he or she may integrate biological and psychological components of the therapy, or may refer the patient to a colleague for a medication consult. Otherwise, medication is handled much as it is in any traditional therapy.

Termination of therapy usually results from a mutual decision made by patient and therapist that the treatment has reached its end. Some of the specifically short-term integrative models mentioned earlier specify a number of sessions at the start. Other integrative therapies do not, particularly those that have a significant psychodynamic component. In this latter group of therapies termination often is considered a significant event that is explored for several weeks or months, with particular concern for the developmental issues around separation and loss that are evoked.

THE THERAPEUTIC RELATIONSHIP AND THE STANCE OF THE THERAPIST

The therapeutic relationship is one of the central common factors that produces changes in virtually all forms of psychotherapy (Rosenzweig, 1936; Weinberger, 1993). On this point most therapists of most orientations agree. Where and how the various therapies deviate from each other is in their relative emphasis on the many effective ingredients of the therapeutic relationship that make it so potentially potent, and on how to maximize the impact of the relationship.

The therapeutic relationship is central to most integrative psychotherapies as well. The central theme of this chapter is highly applicable here: Integrative therapies aim to expand the therapeutic relationship as fully as possible to make that relationship as effective as possible. Again, the particular conceptualization of the relationship in each specific integrative therapy is guided by the way the relationship is construed and used in the major component therapies. Thus, an integrative therapy that is heavily interpersonal (Safran & Segal, 1990), psychodynamic (K. Frank, 1999; Wachtel, 1977), or client centered (Greenberg et al., 1993) will emphasize, respectively, identifying and resolving enactments, the interpretation of transference, or prizing, empathy, and warmth. These variables are considered the most im-

trated, both conceptually and visually, the dilemma of the psychotherapy patient in a cartoon that he included with an article that was concerned with the advantages of psychotherapy integration. This cartoon depicts the first meeting of a therapist and a patient. While this duo is shaking hands in greeting, the thoughts of each are revealed in bubbles above the head of each person. The patient privately frets, "I wonder if he can treat what I have?" The therapist, equally troubled, ponders the question, "I hope he has what I treat!"

In large part, interest in psychotherapy integration, and in specifically integrative therapies, evolved in order to solve this problem. Integrative psychotherapies seem, at least in theory, to be uniquely suited to the needs of patients with diverse backgrounds and problems, those whose lives, personalities, and psychopathology deviate from the "ideal types" that are most easily treated by one of the sectarian therapies. Among the most obvious and important characteristics of successful integration are the flexibility of the therapist and of the therapeutic approach and the overarching concern for the uniqueness of the patient. As was discussed previously, several integrative systems, such as the transtheoretical model and STS are geared completely toward developing the most efficacious patient–technique match possible. Common-factors integration, theoretical integration, and assimilative integration, although not based on explicit prescriptive matching, still guide the therapist toward an interventive focus that is broader and more individualized than is possible in any traditional psychotherapeutic system.

The literature on integrative approaches demonstrates the broad spectrum of patient populations, psychological problems, and psychopathological disorders to which these methods have been successfully applied. As the basic premise of integrative psychotherapy is using the best of what works, any therapeutic approach to any problem may, at least in theory, be improved by the addition of active ingredients from other models.

Integrative approaches have been applied to panic and anxiety disorders (Chambless, Goldstein, Gallagher, & Bright, 1986; Wolfe, 1992) and to obsessive–compulsive disorder (McCarter, 1997). These contributions differ in many ways but share a concern with the provision of a combination of behaviorally oriented exposure techniques with psychodynamically and experientially oriented interventions. In this way, these integrative therapies go farther than traditional therapies in ensuring that "all the bases are covered" with regard to the levels of psychological activity that are implicated in this group of disorders.

Depression has been the focus of much effort on the part of integrationists. This interest applied to depression in its acute and chronic (dysthymic) forms. We have already described Klerman's (Klerman, Weissman, Rounsaville, & Chevron, 1984) integrative, interpersonal psychotherapy for depression. Arkowitz (1992) described a common-factors-based integrative approach to depression. Hayes and Newman's (1993) integrative treatment for depression combined techniques from cognitive therapy, behavior therapy, interpersonal therapy, psychodynamic therapy, experiential therapy, and biological psychiatry. As discussed earlier, McCullough's (2001) integrative CBASP model is the most effective therapy for chronic depression that has been introduced to date.

More severe forms of psychopathology that often are refractory to traditional psychotherapies also have been treated with integrative therapies. Linehan's (1987) dialectical behavior therapy for borderline personality disorder is a prominent example. Gold and Stricker (1993) explored the integration of cognitive-behavioral and psychodynamic therapies for the treatment of personality disorders, an effort that strongly resembled Ryle's (1997) application of CAT to borderline and narcissistic disorders. Cummings (1993) offered an integrative psychotherapy for substances abusers, Tobin (1995) used an integrative therapy for bulimia, and Hellcamp (1993) and Zapparoli and Gislon (1999) explored integrative therapies for schizophrenia. The reader also is referred to the "Goal Setting" section for a description of other populations for whom integrative methods have been developed.

This description of the wide applicability of the integrative therapies may make it seem as though it is the treatment of choice for all patients. Although it may be more widely applicable than any other single approach, because it can go beyond that single approach, no treatment can be all things to all people. The type of integration that is practiced and the presenting problem and goal of the patient establish the limits of the integrative therapies. For example, a patient who is interested solely in self-exploration and has no focal symptom would be best treated by a person with a psychodynamic or a humanistic orientation, whether the therapist is working with a pure or an integrated model. On the other hand, a patient who has a focal symptom and has no interest in self-exploration or change beyond the presenting problem would be best treated by a person with a behavioral or cognitive-behavioral orientation, whether that therapist is working with a pure or an integrated model. Of course, the patient who presents with one and only one interest, be it self-exploration or symptom alleviation, is unusual, comorbidity is more likely than unidimensional problems, and the integrative therapies, because of their breadth and flexibility, have much to recommend them.

Several integrative therapists also have developed models of therapy that account specifically for the unique goals, experiences, needs, and perspectives of particular patient populations. Fodor's (1993) integrative model uses concepts and methods from Gestalt therapy and cognitive-behavioral therapy, along with feminist theory and therapy. Integrative models have been developed for persons of color who live in the United States (Franklin, Carter, & Grace, 1993) and for patients who are members of traditional African societies. Madu (1991) and Pelzer (1991) introduced integrative models that combined traditional African modes of healing with Western psychotherapies. Other integrative approaches are aimed at patients for whom spirituality and religion are important (Healey, 1993; Sollod, 1993). Wachtel (1989), Gold (1992), and Butollo (2000) have demonstrated how an understanding of the economic, political, and ethnic situations in which patients live can be incorporated in therapies that also integrate psychodynamic, cognitive-behavioral, and systems components.

Integrative models have been developed for virtually all age groups and for individuals, couples, and families. Coonerty (1993) described an integrative therapy for children that synthesizes behavioral, family systems, and psychodynamic elements. Several integrative approaches are focused on adolescents and their families (e.g., adolescents with anxiety disorders and depression [Fitzpatrick, 1993], high-risk adolescents [Alexander & Sexton, 2002], and adolescent substance abusers [Rowe, Liddle, McClintic, & Quille, 2002]). Papouchis and Passman (1993) described an integrative model of psychotherapy specifically designed to meet the needs of geriatric patients, involving a judicious integration of cognitive-behavioral techniques into a psychodynamically oriented psychotherapy.

Pinsof (1995) and Gerson (1996) have described their integrative work with families, and Heitler (2001) and Gurman (2002) have offered integrative models for work with couples. Finally, several integrative group psychotherapies exist that have been applied to disparate and important problems and populations (MacKenzie, 2002).

RESEARCH SUPPORT

Chambless and colleagues (1986) compared an integrative approach to treating agoraphobia that combined behavioral, systemic, and psychodynamic theories and techniques to drug therapy and behavior therapy. These researchers found that their integrated model led to marked or great improvement for almost 65% of the patients. Specific treatment effects included lessened avoidance, depression, social phobia, and agoraphobic symptoms and enhanced assertiveness for their patients. This integrative therapy had a much lower dropout rate then either of the other therapies, but there was no direct comparison of effectiveness with other treatments.

Linehan (1987) developed an integrative therapy known as dialectical behavior therapy (DBT), which is aimed at alleviating the symptoms of borderline personality disorder. DBT is an amalgam of skills training, cognitive restructuring, and collaborative problem solving from cognitive-behavioral therapy with relationship elements (such as warmth, empathy, and unconditional positive regard) from client-centered therapy, and with Buddhist meditative practices, especially mindfulness. DBT has gained wide acceptance among clinicians in recent years, due in great part to the research support for its effectiveness. Patients who received DBT demonstrated better treatment retention, had fewer suicide attempts and episodes of self-injury, fewer hospitalizations, decreased anger, greater social adjustment, and more improved general adjustment when compared with those who received standard therapies as practiced in the community (Linehan, 1987).

Research on prescriptive therapy (Beutler & Hodgson, 1993) demonstrated the validity of the strategy of matching patient characteristics and specific therapeutic interventions. Cognitive therapy was most effective for those patients who externalized responsibility for their depressions, whereas those patients with an internal locus of control showed the greatest improvement in the insight-oriented, focused expressive psychotherapy. Patients with higher levels of defensiveness and with greater resistance to

authority were helped most by a self-directed therapy—that is, one in which the patient was given a variety of cognitive-behavioral and experiential exercises from which to choose. This therapy was also the focus of a major study ($n = 248$; Beutler et al., 2002) in which six patient variables were identified that are predictive of success in psychotherapy, and which could be used clinically to match the patient to the most effective interventions. Although there were no specific comparisons to other treatments, the internal success of the approach was clear.

Transtheoretical therapy (Prochaska & DiClemente, 2002), which also focuses intensively on prescriptive matching, has been demonstrated repeatedly to be a highly effective form of therapy with a variety of populations. The use of the stage-of-change model is an important addition to a treatment program and is helpful in predicting change.

Empirical evaluations of integrative psychotherapies that combine psychodynamic components with behavioral, cognitive, or experiential interventions have yielded preliminary but positive results. Klerman and colleagues (1984) found that an integrative, interpersonal psychotherapy for depression repeatedly outperformed medication in the long run and other psychological interventions.

Similarly, Ryle (1995) found that CAT was more effective than purely psychodynamic or behaviorally oriented approaches, although random assignment was not part of the research design. Marcotte and Safran (2002) also have reported that a therapy that integrates cognitive therapy with interpersonal therapy is more effective for depression and generalized anxiety disorder than is traditional cognitive therapy. And, finally, these research results are supplemented by the findings of Shapiro and Firth-Cozens (1990), who studied the impact of two sequences of combined psychodynamic and cognitive-behavioral therapy for depression: dynamic work followed by active intervention or vice versa. Patients in the dynamic–behavioral sequence obtained the greatest improvement and reported the most comfortable experiences of treatment. Patients in the behavioral–dynamic sequence more frequently deteriorated in the second part of the therapy and did not maintain their gains over time as often as did patients in the other group.

Another theoretically integrated approach that has been tested empirically is Process–experiential therapy, an integration of principles and methods derived from client-centered, Gestalt, and cognitive therapies (Greenberg et al., 1993). This therapy has been found to be more efficacious than behavior therapy. The effectiveness of this integrative model has been demonstrated with individuals on a short-term basis for problems such as anxiety and depression, as compared to client-centered or cognitive-behavioral therapy alone.

CBASP (an integration of cognitive, behavioral, analytic, and systems psychotherapy; McCullough, 2001) is the first psychotherapy that has been demonstrated empirically to be effective for treating dysthymic disorder. CBASP has been found to be as effective as antidepressant medication and traditional forms of psychotherapy in alleviating the symptoms and interpersonal problems involved in chronic depression. Also, the results from this integrative therapy are more enduring and more resistant to relapse than are other treatments.

CASE ILLUSTRATION

In our assimilative psychodynamic model of integrative psychotherapy (Gold & Stricker, 2001; Stricker & Gold, 1996) we base our assessment and interventions on an expanded, psychoanalytically oriented framework that we call the three-tier model. We consider detailed evaluations of behavior and social interactions (Tier 1) and of cognitive activity and emotional experience (Tier 2), and we share the traditional psychoanalytic

concern with unconscious processes, mental representations, and character traits (Tier 3). We also assess the interactions between issues at these three levels of experience in an attempt to understand the vicious circles (Wachtel, 1977) and relationship patterns that maintain problems at any of the tiers. We conduct psychotherapy according to psychodynamic principles of exploration, clarification, confrontation, and interpretation and are especially concerned with observing the interaction between patient and therapist and with identifying transference phenomena. However, we often intervene directly at the levels of Tier 1 and Tier 2 when it is clinically advantageous to do so. We use interventions from many therapies, including cognitive-behavioral, humanistic, and systems approaches, within an assimilative perspective: We include these interventions for their direct utility in changing behavior, thinking, and emotion and also for their possible effects on unconscious sources of resistance, transference, conflict, and on unconscious representational systems. We also believe that it is critical to help the patient extricate him- or herself from those relationships and situations that exert a reinforcing influence on the patient's psychopathology.

Integrative interventions are assimilated carefully into the therapy. We always suggest an integrative shift in a tentative way, as an experiment for the patient to try out, evaluate, retain, or toss away, as he or she deems best. We also attend to cognitive, emotional, and dynamic reactions to an integrative shift, and to the success or failure of the technique after the fact. As Wachtel (1977) and other integrative therapists have noted, the impact of the technique on the therapeutic relationship and on the transference–countertransference situation must be continuously monitored.

Ms. F was a woman in her 30s who was referred to psychotherapy by her internist because of chronic anxiety that was punctuated by periodic panic attacks, and episodes of depression. Her DSM-IV Axis I diagnoses

portant in producing change. Integrative therapies that are more cognitive-behavioral or systemic in orientation (Fensterheim, 1993; Pinsof, 1995) do not ignore the therapeutic relationship and its effectiveness but see it as one factor among several that can lead to change, and as a platform for the active learning that takes place in the more technical parts of the therapy.

Many integrative forms of therapy converge around the concept of the therapeutic alliance, as most integrative approaches are founded on the view that effective change occurs best when patient and therapist are bonded in a mutually agreed-on set of goals, within the context of a positively toned and perceived interaction. For the ways in which the alliance is achieved, see chapters in this volume on each therapeutic school. However, the process of integration, and the notion of the integrative shift in particular, seems to some integrative writers (K. Frank, 1999; Gold & Stricker, 2001; Marcotte & Safran, 2002) to be particularly effective in establishing an alliance firmly and quickly and is a way to reestablish or repair the alliance when it has been strained or ruptured. K. Frank (1999) noted that the inclusion of cognitive and behavioral techniques in a psychoanalytic therapy is not only a technical shift but constitutes an interpersonal communication to the patient, one that in effect says, "I'm aware of your suffering with these thoughts, actions, and feelings, and I will try actively to help. I won't let you sit there alone." Along these same lines, Gold and Stricker (2001) point out that skill-building techniques such as assertiveness training, and self-soothing cognitive techniques may enhance the patient's self-esteem and can assist the patient in overcoming negatively toned perceptions of his or her experience in therapy, thus enhancing the therapeutic alliance.

Some of the strengths of integrative therapy also carry the seeds of potential shortcomings. For example, the flexibility and creativity that can be exercised by the integrative therapist also open the door to more undisciplined approaches, particularly when there is no theoretical rationale for the intervention. Messer (2001a; Messer & Winokur, 1980) has also presented a significant challenge to integration. He has spelled out what he refers to as visions of reality, taking the terminology from literary criticism. Different visions characterize different therapeutic orientations, and sometimes different versions of the same orientation. For example, an extended psychodynamic treatment can be described as tragic because of its recognition of human limitations, whereas briefer psychodynamic therapy and behavioral approaches are more readily described as comic because of the focus on a happy ending. An integrative therapist often shifts from one approach to another, but with the shift in technique there also is a shift between what may be incompatible visions of the nature of reality.

Integrative therapists sometimes take active control of the sessions. This is the case when the therapist suggests an integrative shift, or a homework assignment. The therapist shifts from an exploratory, facilitative role when he or she introduces an active intervention into psychodynamic or experientially oriented psychotherapy. Certainly, therapists who identify themselves as multimodal or prescriptive, and those who work from a common-factors perspective, often are active and directive in sessions. However, active and directive do not mean dictatorial and authoritarian. The key phrase used a few sentences ago was, "the therapist suggests." Most integrative therapists view their patient or client as a collaborator and partner. (In fact, we think all good therapists share this perspective, regardless of orientation.) Thus, the patient's sense of what will work for him or for her, the patient's own theory of change (Duncan & Miller, 2000), and the patient's right to refuse a suggestion must be respected. It is the therapist's task to provide the conditions in which change is most likely to occur. It is the therapist's responsibility to know of and to offer the patient a variety of ideas, experiences, tasks, and resources that may lead to change. It is the patient's task and opportunity to attempt to make use of these conditions and experiences to see if he or she can and will change. The therapist may work with those issues (anxiety, resistance, neurotic accomplices, or lack of skill) that interfere with the patient's ability to change, but, ultimately, progress comes from the patient's efforts (Bohart, 2000).

The therapist's experience of the patient and his or her own history as a person and professional obviously enter into any therapy to some degree. As well versed as any clinician may be in theory and technique, ultimately, he or she will understand the patient and his or her situation and needs from a personal point of view. Once again, it must be reiterated that how an integrative therapy makes use of such issues as therapeutic self-disclosure, countertransference, and the "person" of the therapist varies from system to system. These issues are most evident in models that are concerned with interpersonal issues such as enactment: an event within the therapeutic relationship where the therapist is "hooked" into replaying with the patient the kinds of interactions that affected the patient negatively in the past, or that currently are dysfunctional (K. Frank, 1999; Safran & Segal, 1990). There is no way to know that an enactment is occurring without examining one's feelings, thoughts, and experiences, and often these must be shared with the patient before the enactment can be resolved.

As an example, consider the following interaction. A therapist had begun to experience therapy sessions with Mrs. X as dry and repetitive. The therapist would hope that he would receive a call canceling the session. The therapist initially was puzzled by this pattern, as previously he had been pleased by the progress of the therapy, liked and respected Mrs. X, and had found the work stimulating. An examination of previous sessions pointed out the potential enactment. The interaction had slipped into a repetitive and unproductive pattern: Mrs. X

would come in, express her discontent and helplessness with some issue in her life, and the therapist would somewhat reluctantly, and with considerable resentment that was denied and suppressed, step in with a solution that Mrs. X would halfheartedly accept. As the therapist considered this formulation, and his role in it, he was able to recapture his enthusiasm for the therapy.

At their next meeting, the therapist asked if he could share an observation about the therapy and the relationship with Mrs. X. When she agreed, he queried, "I wonder if you've noticed that we seem to be a little worn out with each other? " Upon her agreement, he continued with, "Do you think that could be because we're in some kind of rut? It seems like every session is the same. You come in feeling upset and helpless, and I rush in to fix things. Neither of us is doing what we used to do well, which is look at what is going on. What do you think?" After some discussion, the patient was able to voice her agreement, and the exploration continued, as the therapist added, "You know, this kind of thing probably makes us both kind of annoyed with each other, and then we cover it up by doing the same thing over again. I wonder if this has happened in other relationships as well?" As this discussion continued, present-day and historical sources of the enactment were identified. The patient was assisted in understanding the ways in which this pattern reflected and reproduced aspects of her relationship with her mother, in which the patient had felt that the only moments of intimate contact had occurred when mother was placed in the role of rescuer. She also became aware of the frequency with which her friendships and other current relationships were organized around this issue. The alliance thus was repaired, the patient eventually expressed a good deal of affect, and the work resumed at an effective level of cooperation.

As therapy progresses, and especially as termination of therapy nears, most integrative models suggest that the therapist turn responsibility for decision making about the sessions, homework, and integrative shifts over to the patient. This reinforces autonomy and a sense of self-efficacy, minimizes the patient's anxiety about life after therapy, and allows the patient to practice the "self-therapy" that he or she will need in the future.

It is daunting to work as a therapist in any form of therapy. It may be more daunting, and personally demanding, to work as an integrative therapist. The integrationist must be able to intellectually master the concepts and methods of two or more systems. He or she also must be able to stay free of the common human desire to align oneself with one school of thought and to tolerate the ambiguity that lurks in all psychotherapies. The therapist must be able to straddle the roles of authority, participant, collaborator, and follower and must not either idealize or devalue his or her technical, interpersonal, and experiential expertise. Along this line, integrative therapists might consider following a suggestion originally made by Liddle (1982) for family therapists, that they engage in a periodic epistemological declaration by means of which they regularly review such factors as their theoretical position, therapeutic goals, and methods of treatment evaluation.

CURATIVE FACTORS OR MECHANISMS OF CHANGE

Integrative psychotherapies explicitly are designed to include as many relevant change factors as are possible, and therefore to broaden the likelihood that patients will be exposed to those factors that will best meet their needs. Any change mechanism that has been described consistently in the psychotherapy literature may be found to play a prominent role in one version or another of integrative psychotherapy. Most integrative models stress some combination of the following: insight into, or increased awareness of, conscious and unconscious psychological processes, exposure to anxiety-generating stimuli, learning of new behavioral skills and correction of behavioral dysfunctions, cognitive restructuring and modification of deep meaning structures (schemata, object representations, models of attachment, etc.), enhancing one's capacity to symbolize experience and to experience emotion by directing the focus of inquiry in this direction and to bring about change in repetitive and destructive patterns of interpersonal relatedness. This last mechanism includes the provision of new experiences within the therapeutic relationship through the "corrective emotional experience," or through such relational conditions as prizing, warmth, and genuineness on the part of the therapist.

The particular emphasis given to each of the several mechanisms of change is determined by the specific nature of the integrative model, and by the theories and methods that are combined in that model. For example, as we have discussed previously, therapies based on technical eclecticism or on common-factors integration attempt to match the patient's problems with those curative factors that have been demonstrated to be most effective. Theoretical integration and assimilative integration add to this prescriptive focus a certain number of a priori assumptions about which of the many change factors are likely to be most important, stemming from the home theory.

For example, psychodynamically influenced integrative therapies proceed from the assumption that insight is an important change factor but expand the therapy to include other change factors, such as direct exposure, learning new interpersonal skills, and direct intervention in the patient's family system. Wachtel's (1977) cyclical psychodynamic therapy and Gold and Stricker's (2001) assimilative psychodynamic therapy are examples of this way of thinking. In addition, virtually all integrative therapists agree that there are "Many roads to Rome": that several types of interventions can lead to the same change factor becoming operative, and that change factors can be linked. Wachtel has discussed the important observation that insight often follows behavioral change, rather than always preceding it. Similarly, Safran and Segal (1990) base their cognitive-interpersonal therapy on the premise that important cognitive structures can and will change only after the ongoing interpersonal patterns that maintain them have changed. The notion of a cyclical rather than a linear direction of change is an important one.

Because change in interpersonal skills is considered to be crucial to change at every level of psychological life, any legitimate technique may be applied. Certain integrative approaches emphasize change within the therapeutic relationship, asserting that the most problematic interpersonal patterns and skill deficits will appear in the therapeutic interaction. Not surprisingly, these therapies tend toward the interpersonal, humanistic, and psychodynamic. Didactic instruction in interpersonal functioning tends to be more typical of models that slant toward the cognitive-behavioral, though these boundaries frequently are crossed, as is the wont in integrative therapies. It often is the case that changes will be experienced first in the therapeutic relationship but then will be generalized, with the active assistance of the therapist, to relationships outside therapy.

Most integrative therapies include as significant change factors the impact of the therapist's personality and of the therapeutic relationship. The many lists of common factors that are available (Weinberger, 1993) never fail to include these variables prominently. Those integrative therapies that are based heavily on person-centered therapy (e.g., Bohart's, 1992, experiential approach to integration and Greenberg et al., 1993, process-experiential therapy) stress the classical Rogerian conditions of unconditional positive regard, accurate empathy, and warmth as critical change factors, though not to the exclusive degree that Rogers did. In many ways, a unifying goal of psychotherapy integration is the attempt to go beyond the therapeutic relationship, and the impact of the therapist as a person, by iden-

tifying and including technical interventions that have positive influence as well.

In this regard, integrative therapists have stressed client or patient factors as a central element in change more clearly and frequently than has any single school of psychotherapy. Bohart and Tallman (1999) suggested that client involvement and effort is the single most important factor in any form of psychotherapy. They reported that research has indicated that up to 30% of change may be accounted for by the client's active participation. Bohart (2000), Duncan and Miller (2000), Gold (1994, 2000), and Rennie (2000) have discussed this curative factor in the context of several different forms of integrative therapy, ranging from therapies based on strategic models (Duncan & Miller) to experientially and humanistically oriented approaches (Bohart, Rennie) to a model that is psychodynamically informed (Gold).

To summarize, there is little about curative factors in psychotherapy integration that is unique, almost by definition, because the integrative process draws on other approaches to treatment. Some approaches to integration, such as the common-factors approach, are composed entirely of the general rather than the unique. Technical eclecticism is made up entirely of interventions drawn from other approaches. Both theoretical and assimilative integration are based on at least one other major approach, but the uniqueness they might share with this other approach is reduced by the willingness to incorporate constructs or interventions from other approaches. *The uniqueness of psychotherapy integration rests in the breadth of the process rather than in any theoretical or technical aspect of the treatment.*

TREATMENT APPLICABILITY AND ETHICAL CONSIDERATIONS

Goldfried (1999), drawing on an earlier informal communication from Stricker, illus-

cording to the immediate preferences, preferably empirically based, of the psychotherapist. Both theoretical integration and assimilative integration have theory at their center, and the further developments of these approaches also rest on theoretical advances.

Assimilative integration has been identified as a fourth approach to psychotherapy integration, joining the three that previously were cited as independent approaches. There have been some well-developed assimilative systems that have been presented (e.g., Gold & Stricker, 2001; Stricker & Gold 1996), and we can anticipate that more will follow. However, the challenge for each of these systems is not only how to assimilate techniques from other systems but how to make accommodations in the theory to reflect the value of the foreign techniques (Gold & Stricker, 2001; Wolfe, 2001).

Finally, we would like to close by reiterating a distinction between psychotherapy integration and integrative therapies. This chapter has focused on the integrative therapies, but our preference remains for the process of psychotherapy integration rather than the product per se. Safran and Messer (1997) reach a similar conclusion by endorsing pluralism, emphasizing the dialogue among proponents of the various approaches rather than an ultimate goal of achieving a single correct system of psychotherapy. We see the future of psychotherapy integration as lying with an ongoing consideration of the challenges of psychotherapy without regard to disciplinary boundaries, whether those boundaries are established by traditional sectarian approaches or by newer integrative approaches. We applaud all the gains made by stretching these boundaries, as indicated by the innovative integrative therapies. However, we hope that these do not become frozen but remain open to consideration by the therapist, functioning in a thoughtful and creative way as a local clinical scientist, and also by the results of ongoing psychotherapy research.

NOTES

1. For information about SEPI and an application for membership, send a note to stricker@adelphi.edu

SUGGESTIONS FOR FURTHER READING

Glass, C., Arnkoff, D., & Rodriguez, B. (1998). An overview of directions in psychotherapy integration research. *Journal of Psychotherapy Integration, 8,* 187–210.—An extensive review of the empirical support for many of the approaches described in this chapter.

Lazarus, A. A. (1992). Multimodal therapy: Technical eclecticism with minimal integration. In J. C. Norcross & M. R. Goldfried (Eds.), *Handbook of psychotherapy integration* (pp. 231–263). New York: Basic Books.—A comprehensive summary of an important technically eclectic approach with relevant case material.

Lebow, J. (Ed.). (2002), *Comprehensive handbook of psychotherapy: Vol. 4. Integrative–eclectic.* New York: Wiley.—A compendium of up-to-date reports on a number of influential integrative therapies.

Messer, S. B. (2000). Applying the visions of reality to a case of brief therapy. *Journal of Psychotherapy Integration, 10,* 55–70.—An application of the perspectives of a number of therapeutic systems to a case example.

Wachtel, P. L. (1997). *Psychoanalysis, behavior therapy, and the representational world.* Washington, DC: American Psychological Association.—An expanded edition of a classic in psychotherapy integration that remains the most complete and influential version of theoretical integration.

REFERENCES

Alexander, F., & French, T. (1946). *Psychoanalytic therapy.* New York: Ronald Press.

Alexander, J. F., & Sexton, T. L. (2002). Functional family therapy: A model for treating high-risk, acting out youth. In J. Lebow (Ed.), *Comprehensive handbook of psychothera-*

py, Vol. Four: Integrative–eclectic (pp.111–132). New York: Wiley.

Allen, D. M. (1993). Unified psychotherapy. In G. Stricker & J. R. Gold (Eds.), *Comprehensive handbook of psychotherapy integration* (pp. 125–138). New York: Plenum Press.

American Psychiatric Association. (1994). *Diagnostic and statistical manual of mental disorders* (4th ed.). Washington, DC: Author.

Andrews, J. D. W. (1993). The Active Self model: A paradigm for psychotherapy integration. In G. Stricker & J. R. Gold (Eds.), *Comprehensive handbook of psychotherapy integration* (pp. 165–186). New York: Plenum Press.

Arkowitz, H. (1992). A common factors therapy for depression. In J. C. Norcross & M. R. Goldfried (Eds.), *Handbook of psychotherapy integration* (pp. 402–432). New York: Basic Books.

Arkowitz, H., & Messer, S. (Eds.). (1984). *Psychoanalytic therapy and behavioral therapy: Is integration possible?* New York: Plenum Press.

Beck, A.T., Rush, A.J., Shaw, B.F., & Emery, G. (1979). *Cognitive therapy of depression.* New York: Guilford Press.

Beier, E. G. (1966). *The silent language of psychotherapy.* Chicago: Aldine.

Beutler, L. E., Alomohamed, S., Moleiro, C., & Romanelli, R. (2002). Systematic treatment selection and prescriptive therapy. In J. Lebow (Ed.), *Comprehensive handbook of psychotherapy: Vol. 4. Integrative–eclectic* (pp. 255–272). New York: Wiley.

Beutler, L. E., & Hodgson, A. B. (1993). Prescriptive psychotherapy. In G. Stricker & J. R. Gold (Eds.), *Comprehensive handbook of psychotherapy integration* (pp. 151–163). New York: Plenum Press.

Bohart, A. C. (1992). An integrative process model of psychopathology and psychotherapy. *Revista de Psicoterapia, 9,* 49–74.

Bohart, A. C. (2000). The client is the most important common factor: Clients' self-healing capacities and psychotherapy. *Journal of Psychotherapy Integration, 10,* 127–150.

Bohart, A. C., & Tallman, K. (1999). *How clients make therapy work.* Washington, DC: American Psychological Association.

Butollo, W. (2000). Therapeutic implications of a social interaction model of trauma. *Journal of Psychotherapy Integration, 10,* 357–374.

Chambless, D., Goldstein, A., Gallagher, R., & Bright, P. (1986). Integrating behavior therapy and psychotherapy in the treatment of agoraphobia. *Psychotherapy, 23,* 150–159.

Coonerty, S. (1993). Integrative child therapy. In G. Stricker & J. R. Gold (Eds.), *Comprehensive handbook of psychotherapy integration* (pp. 413–426). New York: Plenum Press.

Cummings, N. (1993). Psychotherapy with substance abusers. In G. Stricker & J. R. Gold (Eds.), *Comprehensive handbook of psychotherapy integration* (pp. 337–352). New York: Plenum Press.

Dollard, J., & Miller, N. E. (1950). *Personality and psychotherapy.* New York: McGraw-Hill.

Dowd, E. T. (1999). Why don't people change? What stops them from changing? An integrative commentary on the special issue on resistance. *Journal of Psychotherapy Integration, 9,* 119–131.

Duncan, B. L., & Miller, S. D. (2000). The client's theory of change: Consulting the client in the integrative change process. *Journal of Psychotherapy Integration, 10,* 169–188.

Feather, B. W., & Rhodes, J. W. (1973). Psychodynamic behavior therapy I: Theory and rationale. *Archives of General Psychiatry, 26,* 496–502.

Fensterheim, H. (1993). Behavioral psychotherapy. In G. Stricker & J. R. Gold (Eds.), *Comprehensive handbook of psychotherapy integration* (pp. 73–86). New York: Plenum Press.

Fitzpatrick M. (1993). Adolescents. In G. Stricker & J. R. Gold (Eds.), *Comprehensive handbook of psychotherapy integration* (pp. 427–436). New York: Plenum Press.

Fodor, I. (1993). A feminist framework for integrative psychotherapy. In G. Stricker & J. R. Gold (Eds.), *Comprehensive handbook of psychotherapy integration* (pp. 217–236). New York: Plenum Press.

Fosha, D. (2000). *The transforming power of affect.* New York: Basic Books.

Frank, J. (1961). *Persuasion and healing.* Baltimore: Johns Hopkins University Press.

Frank, K. (1999). *Psychoanalytic participation.* Hillsdale, NJ: Analytic Press.

Franklin, A.J., Carter, R. T., & Grace, C. (1993). An integrative approach to psychotherapy with Black/African Americans. In G. Stricker & J. R. Gold (Eds.), *Comprehensive handbook of psychotherapy integration* (pp. 465–482). New York: Plenum Press.

French, T. M. (1933). Interrelations between

psychoanalysis and the experimental work of Pavlov. *American Journal of Psychiatry, 89,* 1165–1203.

Garfield, S. (2000). Eclecticism and integration: A personal retrospective view. *Journal of Psychotherapy Integration, 10,* 341–356.

Gerson, M.-J. (1996). *The embedded self.* Hillsdale, NJ: Analytic Press.

Glass, C., Arnkoff, D., & Rodriguez, B. (1998). An overview of directions in psychotherapy integration research. *Journal of Psychotherapy Integration, 8,* 187–210.

Gold, J. (1992). An integrative-systemic approach to severe psychopathology in children and adolescents. *Journal of Integrative and Eclectic Psychotherapy, 11,* 67–78.

Gold, J. R. (1993). The sociohistorical context of psychotherapy integration. In G. Stricker & J. R. Gold (Eds.), *Comprehensive handbook of psychotherapy integration* (pp. 3–8). New York: Plenum Press.

Gold, J. (1994). When the patient does the integrating: Lessons for theory and practice. *Journal of Psychotherapy Integration, 4,* 133–154.

Gold, J. (1996). *Key concepts in psychotherapy integration.* New York: Plenum Press.

Gold, J. (2000). The psychodynamics of the patient's activity. *Journal of Psychotherapy Integration, 10,* 207–220.

Gold, J. R., & Stricker, G. (1993). Psychotherapy integration with personality disorders. In G. Stricker & J. R. Gold (Eds.), *Comprehensive handbook of psychotherapy integration* (pp. 323–336). New York: Plenum Press.

Gold, J., & Stricker, G. (2001). Relational psychoanalysis as a foundation for assimilative integration. *Journal of Psychotherapy Integration, 11,* 47–63.

Goldfried, M. (1999). A participant-observer's perspective on psychotherapy integration. *Journal of Psychotherapy Integration, 9,* 235–242.

Goldfried, M., & Newman, C. (1992). A history of psychotherapy integration. In J. C. Norcross & M. R. Goldfried (Eds.), *Handbook of psychotherapy integration* (pp. 46–93). New York: Basic Books.

Greenberg, L. S., Rice, L. N., & Elliott, R. (1993). *Facilitating emotional change.* New York: Guilford Press.

Guidano, V. F., & Liotti, G. (1983). *Cognitive processes and emotional disorders: A structural approach to psychotherapy.* New York: Guilford Press.

Gurman, A. S. (2002). Brief integrative marital therapy: A depth behavioral approach. In A. S. Gurman & N. S. Jacobson (Eds.), *Clinical handbook of couple therapy* (3rd ed., pp. 180–200). New York: Guilford Press.

Hayes, A., & Newman, C. (1993). Depression: An integrative perspective. In G. Stricker & J. R. Gold (Eds.), *Comprehensive handbook of psychotherapy integration* (pp. 303–322). New York: Plenum Press.

Healey, B. J. (1993). Psychotherapy and religious experience: Integrating psychoanalytic psychotherapy with Christian religious experience. In G. Stricker & J. R. Gold (Eds.), *Comprehensive handbook of psychotherapy integration* (pp. 267–276). New York: Plenum Press.

Heitler, S. (2001). Combined individual/marital therapy: A conflict resolution framework and ethical considerations. *Journal of Psychotherapy Integration, 11,* 349–384.

Hellcamp, D. (1993). Severe mental disorders. In G. Stricker & J. R. Gold (Eds.), *Comprehensive handbook of psychotherapy integration* (pp. 385–400). New York: Plenum Press.

Klerman, G., Weissman, M., Rounsaville, B., & Chevron, E. (1984). *Interpersonal psychotherapy of depression.* New York: Basic Books.

Lazarus, A. A. (1992). Multimodal therapy: Technical eclecticism with minimal integration. In J. C. Norcross & M. R. Goldfried (Eds.), *Handbook of psychotherapy integration* (pp. 231–263). New York: Basic Books.

Lazarus, A. A. (2002). The multimodal assessment treatment method. In J. Lebow (Ed.), *Comprehensive handbook of psychotherapy: Vol. 4. Integrative–eclectic* (pp. 241–254). New York: Wiley.

Lebow, J. (Ed.). (2002). *Comprehensive handbook of psychotherapy: Volume 4. Integrative–eclectic.* New York: Wiley.

Levenson, H. (1995). *Time-limited dynamic psychotherapy.* New York: Basic Books.

Liddle, H A. (1982). On the problems of eclecticism: A call for epistemologic clarification and human-scale theories. *Family Process, 21,* 243–250.

Linehan, H. (1987). Dialectical behavior therapy for borderline personality disorder. *Bulletin of the Menninger Clinic, 51,* 261–276.

MacKenzie, K. R. (2002). Effective group psycho therapies. In J. Lebow (Ed.), *Comprehensive handbook of psychotherapy: Vol. 4. Integrative–eclectic* (pp. 521–544). New York: Wiley.

Madu, S. (1991). Problems of "western" psychotherapy practice in Nigeria. *Journal of Integrative and Eclectic Psychotherapy, 10,* 68–75.

Magnavita, J., & Carlson, R. (in press). Short-term restructuring psychotherapy. *Journal of Psychotherapy Integration.*

Marcotte, D., & Safran, J. D. (2002). Cognitive-Interpersonal psychotherapy. In J. Lebow (Ed.), *Comprehensive handbook of psychotherapy: Vol. 4. Integrative–eclectic* (pp. 273–294). New York: Wiley.

Marmor, J. (1971). Dynamic psychotherapy and behavior therapy: Are they reconcilable? *Archives of General Psychiatry, 24,* 22–28.

McCarter, R. (1997). Directive activity and repair of the self in the cognitive behavior treatment of obsessive compulsive disorder. *Journal of Psychotherapy Integration, 7,* 75–88.

McCullough, J. P., Jr. (2000). *Skills training manual for diagnosing and treating chronic depression: Cognitive behavioral analysis.* New York: Guilford Press.

McCullough, L., & Andrews, S. (2001). Assimilative integration: Short-term dynamic psychotherapy for treating affect phobias. *Clinical Psychology: Science and Practice, 8,* 82–97.

Messer, S. B. (1992). A critical examination of belief structures in integrative and eclectic psychotherapy. In J. C. Norcross & M. R. Goldfried (Eds.), *Handbook of psychotherapy integration* (pp. 130–168). New York: Basic Books.

Messer, S. B. (2001a). Applying the visions of reality to a case of brief therapy. *Journal of Psychotherapy Integration, 10,* 55–70.

Messer, S. B. (Ed.). (2001b). Assimilative integration [Special issue]. *Journal of Psychotherapy Integration, 11*(1).

Messer, S. B., & Wampold, B. E. (2002). Let's face facts: Common factors are more potent than specific therapy ingredients. *Clinical Psychology: Science and Practice, 9,* 21–25.

Messer, S. B., & Winokur, M. (1980). Some limits to the integration of psychoanalytic and behavior therapy. *American Psychologist, 35,* 818–827.

Miller, S. D., Duncan, B. L., & Hubble, M. A. (2002). Client-directed, outcome-informed, clinical work. In J. Lebow (Ed.),

Comprehensive handbook of psychotherapy: Vol. 4. Integrative–eclectic (pp. 185–212). New York: Wiley.

Norcross, J. C., & Goldfried, M. R. (Eds.). (1992). *Handbook of psychotherapy integration.* New York: Basic Books.

Norcross, J. C., & Newman, C. (1992). Psychotherapy integration: Setting the context. In J. C. Norcross & M. R. Goldfried (Eds.), *Handbook of psychotherapy integration* (pp. 3–46). New York: Basic Books.

Papouchis, N., & Passman, V. (1993). An integrative approach to the psychotherapy of the elderly. In G. Stricker & J. R. Gold (Eds.), *Comprehensive handbook of psychotherapy integration* (pp. 437–452). New York: Plenum Press.

Pelzer, K. (1991). Cross-cultural psychotherapy in an African context. *Journal of Integrative and Eclectic Psychotherapy, 10,* 75–80.

Pinsof, W. (1995). *Integrative problem-centered therapy.* New York: Basic Books.

Prochaska, J. O., & DiClemente, C. C. (1992). The transtheoretical approach. In J. C. Norcross & M. R. Goldfried (Eds.), *Handbook of psychotherapy integration* (pp 300–334). New York: Basic Books.

Prochaska, J. O., & DiClemente, C. C. (2002). Transtheoretical therapy. In J. Lebow (Ed.), *Comprehensive handbook of psychotherapy: Vol. 4. Integrative–eclectic* (pp. 165–184). New York: Wiley.

Rennie, D. L. (2000). Aspects of the client's conscious control of the psychotherapeutic process. *Journal of Psychotherapy Integration, 10,* 151–168.

Rowe, C., Liddle, H., McClintic, K., & Quille, T. (2002) Integrative treatment development: Multidimensional family therapy and adolescent substance abuse. In J. Lebow (Ed.), *Comprehensive handbook of psychotherapy: Vol. 4. Integrative–eclectic* (pp. 133–164). New York: Wiley.

Rosenzweig, S. (1936). Some implicit common factors in diverse methods of psychotherapy. *American Journal of Orthopsychiatry, 6,* 412–415.

Ryle A. (1995). *Cognitive analytic therapy: Developments in theory and practice.* Chichester, UK: Wiley.

Ryle, A. (1997). *Cognitive analytic therapy and borderline personality disorder.* New York: Wiley.

Ryle, A., & Low, J. (1993). Cognitive analytic

were generalized anxiety disorder (300.02), panic disorder without agoraphobia (300.01), and major depression (296.3). She also described ongoing discomfort in social situations and a pattern of managing that discomfort by maintaining superficial and distant relationships, especially with men, that met the criteria for an Axis II diagnosis of avoidant personality disorder (301.82).

Ms. F reported that she had experienced depression and anxiety since early childhood, and that these symptoms had worsened during the last year, with the addition of panic attacks. During this period she had changed careers and had experienced the death of her mother after a lingering illness. Ms. F worked in a professional field that had required graduate education and enjoyed her work, though it was demanding of her time and energy and was not well paid. She was forced to share an apartment with a roommate due to financial considerations and experienced this relationship as a constant source of irritation and tension. Ms. F had not had any previous experience in psychotherapy. Her internist had recommended that she consider making use of psychiatric medication in addition to psychotherapy, but she had not followed up on this recommendation.

Ms. F was the youngest of several children and had been academically talented. Her mother was described as passive, depressed, and demanding of much of Ms. F's time and attention. Ms. F reported that her mother seemed concerned only about Ms. F's professional successes and had little interest in Ms. F's social life, hobbies, or other interests. She stated that she had been involved in her mother's care during mother's illness, and that she herself had not "felt much" about mother's death at the time or during the ensuing period. Her father was described as a distant man who "never had much to say to or about his children." He had been a shadowy figure during his wife's illness and after her death, had offered little in the way of support to Ms. F, and rarely called or visited her.

In the initial assessment of this patient at Tier 1 (behavior and social interactions), the most prominent issues were her avoidant behaviors and interpersonal anxiety that led to the lack of supportive and satisfying friendships, and of the intimate heterosexual relationship that she desired. Tier 2 phenomena (cognitive and social spheres) included preoccupation and overconcern with the minutiae of her work, which provoked intrusive thoughts of being unable to cope with her responsibilities and of losing her job. This pattern of thinking evoked considerable conscious anxiety and periodic experiences of panic. At a more unconscious level (Tier 3, which includes unconscious phenomena, mental representations, and character traits), Ms. F seemed to be afflicted with an image of herself as unlovable and as unworthy of love. She had a wish to please an implacable mother and unattainable father, resulting in mental representations of others as demanding, impossible to please, and selfishly unconcerned. Deeply felt but disavowed pools of anger, resentment, loss, grief, and deprivation were evoked by these representations of self and others.

Ms. F's familial and professional relationships also were involved in the evocation and reinforcement of these problems. Her coworkers, siblings, and father relied on her "to fill in all of the gaps," which she always did, fearing a loss of their already unreliable esteem and interest were she not to do so. Her overt anxiety, rigidly avoidant interpersonal style, and disavowed anger and resentment kept other people at a distance and limited their ability to sympathize with her plight. These reactions fed into Ms. F's unconscious sense of vulnerability and her perceptions of others as unavailable, hateful, and incapable of responding to her needs. They also added to her image of herself as unloved, and to the smoldering anger and resentment that seemed to be at the foundation of her depression. These vicious circles also kept alive her unhappy and anxiety-fraught relationships with her parents.

Ms. F's therapy began, as do most psychodynamic therapies, with an exploration of the patient's present and past life, and of the unconscious motivations, conflicts, fears, and residues of past relationships that contribute to current problems. Ms. F was encouraged to talk as freely as she could; to report dreams, fantasies, and idle thoughts; and to examine her interaction with the therapist as well. The therapist listened closely, asked Ms. F questions, and occasionally offered interpretations of the unconscious processes to which Ms. F's communications might be alluding.

These standard psychodynamic methods, however, were supplemented by integrative work at Tiers 1 and 2. The therapist targeted those behavioral, cognitive, experiential, and interpersonal variables that might benefit from integrative intervention. As we have stated several times, these integrative efforts always were considered with at least a dual purpose: of assisting Ms. F to change an ineffective, problematic issue in Tiers 1 and 2 as well as for their potential to resolve unconscious conflict and to change ways of experiencing herself and other people at Tier 3.

Two central types of integrative work in Tiers 1 and 2 were used during Ms. F's therapy. The first was employed during the early weeks of the therapy, when it became obvious how weighed down Ms. F was by her insistence on "filling in the gaps" left by those people in her life who shirked important responsibilities, knowing that Ms. F would take over. These internal demands, which manifested themselves in the form of thoughts such as, "I should be able to do more without complaining," or, "If I don't take over here, they'll be angry" (Tier 2), were modified by standard cognitive techniques of recording one's thoughts, evaluating the evidence for them, and refuting or modifying that way of thinking based on this examination. Changing these thoughts was seen as advantageous and important by the therapist for several reasons. First, change in this way of thinking by Ms. F ob-

viously would reduce her experience of being overwhelmed, as always being behind in things, and would lessen her anxiety and make her less prone to panic. Second, this reduction in suffering might stabilize a rather shaky therapeutic relationship in which Ms. F had been having some difficulty letting go of her transferential reactions to the therapist, as she experienced him as a parent who expected her to meet everyone else's needs. Third, it had become clear that the pain and preoccupation caused by these deeply familiar and ingrained thoughts and behavioral patterns had become defenses against the anger, resentment, and neediness that they continued to evoke. In the sessions, these issues had become resistances that precluded any exploration of such psychodynamic meanings and origins.

This integrative intervention accomplished much. Ms. F became less anxious and prone to panic as she learned to "stop filling in." At the same time, she achieved important insight into her history and its transference manifestation in the therapy. This technique helped her to experience her therapist as someone who wanted her to take on less and to get more out of life and therefore enabled Ms. F to make a crucial discrimination between her transference and her real experience of the therapist. As she saw, in a deeply felt way, how she had come to perceive the therapist as someone from her past, she began to explore the ways in which these transference perceptions influenced her relationships outside therapy, specifically with regard to the frequency with which she cast potential friends and lovers in the role of her hurtful siblings and parents. Finally, as her need "to fill in" became less pressing and less frequent, Ms. F was able to relax her resistance against exploring these issues. Her new understanding of her unconscious fear of being unlovable, and of the resulting self-hatred that this self-perception had generated, allowed Ms. F the chance to reevaluate those mental representations. In addition, as she more frequently took the chance of saying no, she learned that her worst fears of abandonment sometimes were not confirmed. It is impossible to determine how much of Ms. F's transference was based solely on her expectations as a function of historical factors and how much on the experience of the active therapist in the relationship. Had the therapist been more silent, the same issues probably would have arisen but would have been treated as a deficit rather than an active way of experiencing a long-wished-for and previously absent nurturance by the therapist.

These new experiences helped her free herself from many of the interpersonal vicious circles that had fueled her anger and resentment and allowed her to find a few new friends and to begin to go out on dates. These new experiences had an impact on her at all three tiers. New and more assertive behavior was accepted and therefore tacitly reinforced by new friends. Her progress in modulating her conscious fears and concerns about "filling in" also were supported. And, at the psychodynamic level, these new relationships gradually helped Ms. F to integrate the anger, sadness, and resentment that she had disavowed through most of her life. As a result, her anxiety, panic and depression gradually abated.

As Ms. F's therapy continued, her dreams and the contents of her conversation in sessions began to coalesce around the death of her mother and the unresolved grief connected with that loss. Psychodynamic work did not seem helpful. Ms. F noted that she had attained a much greater intellectual appreciation of the effects of her unresolved grief but that she could not feel much about this event or its aftermath. Attempts to analyze her defenses against her grief led nowhere but to frustration and dejection.

This impasse indicated that an integrative shift might be helpful. The therapist suggested an experiential, Gestalt-therapy-influenced exercise in which Ms. F imagined herself in conversation with her mother as they sat together in the therapist's office. Ms. F hesitantly, and with considerable

embarrassment began this dialogue but soon fell into the dialogue more naturally. After a couple of sessions she found herself experiencing and expressing the sadness, fear, anger, and guilt that she had disavowed since her mother's death.

In addition to these important changes, some other gains accrued from this integrative intervention. These changes were of immediate conscious benefit to the patient, and they also aided the psychodynamic work of the therapy. Ms. F found that her painful dialogue with her mother had led to a new sense of confidence and more acceptance of her own needs, wishes, and anger. She decided that she would give more weight to relationships with people who were open to knowing about her feelings, positive and negative, and began to describe herself as "throwing her weight around a little" with her siblings and with her father on his rare visits. She also reported that the therapist's active interest in helping her to grieve, and his ability to tolerate and to empathize with the feelings that she had contacted during the Gestalt exercise, had been helpful in allowing her to test, challenge, and modify the negative view of emotional intimacy that she long had held.

Ms. F's therapy lasted about 20 months and was conducted on a once-weekly basis. Approximately 65–75% of the sessions might be identified as psychodynamically oriented exploration, whereas the remaining time was spent working in the active, integrative way described previously. Ms. F decided to end therapy after this period because she felt she had come as far as she could and needed a break to consolidate her gains and all that she had learned. She had been free from any major depressive episodes and from panic attacks for over 6 months. Her ongoing level of anxiety had improved, though she noted that it was her hope that she would have more anxiety-free hours and days in the future. Her relationship with her roommate had improved to the point that they had developed a casual friendship, occasionally sharing a meal or going to a movie together, and Ms. F's level of irritation and tension about sharing her home had diminished. She had made a couple of other female friends and was hopeful that her relationship with one of these women could become a closer and enduring friendship. She continued to date and to feel guardedly optimistic about marrying, though she had not yet established the serious intimate relationship with a man that she wanted.

CURRENT AND FUTURE TRENDS

The integrative therapies constitute a heterogeneous group of approaches and, as such, future trends must be considered in a differentiated way. First, we make some general comments that pertain to all the integrative therapies and then we consider trends that are more specific to different approaches to psychotherapy integration.

The first general comment pertains to the paucity of supportive research, a problem that certainly is not restricted to the integrative therapies. As reviewed earlier, some approaches do have research support (e.g., Linehan, 1987) and some rely on research for the specifics of intervention (e.g., Beutler et al., 2002). However, the majority of the integrative therapies do not have much, if any, support, and this clearly is an area for future development. There is awareness in the integrative community both of the research that has been produced and of this need (Glass, Arnkoff, & Rodriguez, 1998), and we hope that the future will provide more documentation of effectiveness.

It is important to recognize the breadth of research efforts that are possible. Efficacy research, with its emphasis on randomized assignment of cases to the therapy of interest and to control groups, is not a promising design because the nature of integration includes the ongoing innovation that makes the required manualization of treatment

difficult to achieve. Effectiveness research, which studies therapy as it is practiced in the field, is more likely to be suitable to the integrative therapies because they are less rigid in their approach to specific interventions and thus would be difficult to standardize, as is required by efficacy research. This concern probably is true of most therapies, but it is particularly problematic for the integrative therapies. Finally, we hope that most integrative therapists would view themselves as local clinical scientists (Stricker & Trierweiler, 1995; Trierweiler & Stricker, 1998) and would adopt a scientific attitude toward the work being done in their consulting rooms. The local clinical scientist is typified by a scientific attitude toward psychotherapy, the maintenance of a reflective and self-critical attitude, the application of general research data where available, and the quest for confirmatory data for individual cases wherever possible.

Psychotherapy integration is "a growth industry" because it captures what most therapists actually do rather than what they were trained to do. There are many indications of its growth. For example, SEPI, home to many integrative therapists, has increased in size substantially over the years. SEPI's *Journal of Psychotherapy Integration* has now been in existence for more than a decade. Important compilations of developments in psychotherapy now routinely include chapters on psychotherapy integration. For example, a recent four-volume handbook of psychotherapy devoted an entire volume to integrative/eclectic approaches (Lebow, 2002).

It is likely that theory will play an increasing role in the development of the integrative therapies. For example, the well-documented observation of the critical role of common factors may lead to a development of a theory of common factors (e.g., Arkowitz, 1992). Regarding technical eclecticism, those approaches that have a theoretical underpinning guiding the eclecticism (e.g., Beutler et al., 2002) are likely to prove more appealing than those guided ac-

therapy. In G. Stricker & J. R. Gold (Eds.), *Comprehensive handbook of psychotherapy integration* (pp. 87–100). New York: Plenum Press.

Safran, J. D., & Messer, S. B. (1997). Psychotherapy integration: A postmodern critique. *Clinical Psychology: Science and Practice, 4,* 140–152.

Safran, J. D., & Segal, Z. (1990). *Interpersonal process in cognitive therapy.* New York: Basic Books.

Sears, R. R. (1944). Experimental analysis of psychoanalytic phenomena. In J. Hunt (Ed.), *Personality and the behavior disorders* (pp. 191–206). New York: Ronald Press.

Shapiro, D., & Firth-Cozens, J. (1990). Two year follow-up of the Sheffield Psychotherapy Project. *British Journal of Psychotherapy, 151,* 790–799.

Sollod, R. N. (1993). Integrating spiritual healing approaches and techniques into psychotherapy. In G. Stricker & J. R. Gold (Eds.), *Comprehensive handbook of psychotherapy integration* (pp. 237–248). New York: Plenum Press.

Stricker, G. (1994). Reflections on psychotherapy integration. *Clinical Psychology: Science and Practice, 1,* 3–12.

Stricker, G. (in press). Using homework in psychodynamic psychotherapy. *Journal of Psychotherapy Integration.*

Stricker, G., & Gold, J. R. (Eds.). (1993). *Comprehensive handbook of psychotherapy integration.* New York: Plenum Press.

Stricker, G., & Gold, J. R. (1996). An assimilative model for psychodynamically oriented integrative psychotherapy. *Clinical Psychology: Science and Practice, 3,* 47–58.

Stricker, G., & Gold, J. (2002). An assimilative approach to integrative psychodynamic psychotherapy. In J. Lebow (Ed.), *Comprehensive handbook of psychotherapy: Vol. 4. Integrative–eclectic* (pp. 295–316). New York: Wiley.

Stricker, G., & Trierweiler, S. J. (1995). The local clinical scientist: A bridge between science and practice. *American Psychologist, 50,* 995–1002.

Tobin, D. (1995). Integrative psychotherapy for bulimic patients with comorbid personality disorders. *Journal of Psychotherapy Integration, 5,* 245–264.

Trierweiler, S. J., & Stricker, G. (1998). *The scientific practice of professional psychology.* New York: Plenum Press.

Wachtel. P. L. (1977). *Psychoanalysis and behavior therapy: Toward an integration.* New York: Basic Books.

Wachtel. P. L. (1989). *The poverty of affluence.* New York: Free Press.

Wachtel, P. L. (1997). *Psychoanalysis, behavior therapy, and the representational world.* Washington, DC: American Psychological Association.

Weinberger, J. (1993). Common factors in psychotherapy. In G. Stricker & J. R. Gold (Eds.), *Comprehensive handbook of psychotherapy integration* (pp. 43–58). New York: Plenum Press.

Westen, D. (1988). Transference and information processing. *Clinical Psychology Review, 8,* 161–179.

Wolfe, B. (1992). Integrative therapy of the anxiety disorders. In J. C. Norcross, & M. R. Goldfried (Eds.), *Handbook of psychotherapy integration* (pp. 373–401). New York: Basic Books.

Wolfe, B. E. (2001). A message to assimilative integrationists: It's time to become accommodative integrationists: A commentary. *Journal of Psychotherapy Integration, 11,* 123–131.

Zapparoli, G., & Gislon, M. (1999). Betrayal and paranoia: The psychotherapist's function as an intermediary. *Journal of Psychotherapy Integration, 9,* 185–198.

10

Brief Psychotherapies

MICHAEL F. HOYT

I think the development of psychiatric skill consists in very considerable measure of doing a lot with very little—making a rather precise move which has a high probability of achieving what you're attempting to achieve, with a minimum of time and words.
—HARRY STACK SULLIVAN (1954, p. 224)

We first consider some general principles of brief therapy and then turn our attention to several approaches that have been developed specifically to address issues of length of treatment: (1) brief psychodynamic therapy; (2) brief redecision therapy; and (3) brief Ericksonian, strategic, and solution-focused therapy. Although these various models emerged from different treatment traditions, they all focus on the idea of increasing efficiency and raise important theoretical and technical questions about therapeutic epistemology, putative mechanisms of change, and power and authority and the roles of the therapist and patient. Before turning to specifics, let us first consider what different brief therapies have in common.

THE CONCEPT OF BRIEF THERAPY

When a therapist and patient endeavor to get from Point A (the problem that led to therapy) to Point B (the resolution that ends therapy) via a direct, parsimonious, and effi-

cient route, we say that they are deliberately engaging in *brief therapy*. The approach is intended to be quick and helpful, nothing extraneous, no beating around the bush. Another closely related term is "time-limited therapy," which explicitly emphasizes the temporal boundedness of the treatment. Synonymous with brief therapy is the phrase "planned short-term therapy," meaning literally a "deliberately concise remedy/restoration/improvement." As Bloom (1992) has written: "The word planned is important; these works describe short-term treatment that is intended to accomplish a set of therapeutic objectives within a sharply limited time frame" (p. 3). This is how de Shazer (1991a) describes it:

> "Brief therapy" simply means therapy that takes as few sessions as possible, not even one more than is necessary. . . ."Brief therapy" is a relative term, typically meaning: (a) fewer sessions than standard, and/ or (b) a shorter period of time from intake to termination, and/or (c) a lower number of sessions and a lower frequency of sessions from start to finish. (pp. ix–x)

"Brevity" and "shortness" are watchwards signaling efficiency, the contrast being the more intentionally protracted course of traditional long-term (usually psychodynamic) therapy. Actually, most therapy is *de facto* brief, by default or design, meaning a few sessions, weeks to months. As Budman and Gurman (1988) and others (Bloom, 1992; Garfield, 1986; Koss & Butcher, 1986; Messer & Warren, 1995) have noted, numerous studies have reported the average length of treatment to be three to eight sessions. The modal or most common length of treatment is actually only one session. Even with this "briefest of brief" duration, many successful outcomes are reported (Bloom, 1981, 1992; Hoyt, 1994d, 2000a; Hoyt, Rosenbaum, & Talmon, 1992; Rosenbaum, Hoyt, & Talmon, 1990; Talmon, 1990, 1993).

Various authors have offered different definitions of what constitutes brief therapy. Some have emphasized a number of sessions, such as "5–10," "12," or "up to 20"; some have emphasized certain types of problems they attempt to address, while others have focused more on the idea of the passage of time being a contextual pressure (Hoyt, 1990). Budman and Gurman (1988), for example, eschew a specific number of sessions in their definition, instead referring to deliberate or planned brief therapy as "time sensitive" or "time effective" treatment. Setting a specific number of sessions may at times be helpful, however, to provide structuring (Wells, 1982) or to deliberately stimulate a termination process (Hoyt, 1979; Mann, 1973). Attention to temporal parameters is important as Parkinson's law ("Work expands or contracts to fit the allotted time") may operate in psychotherapy (Appelbaum, 1975). Generally, the focus should be on making the most of each session. Focused intentionality is the key. Make everything count; do not be wasteful. Get to it.

Planned or intentional brief therapy is predicated on the belief and expectation that change can occur *in the moment,* particularly if theoretical ability, practical skill, and interest in efficacy are brought to bear. The work is not superficial or simply technique oriented; it is precise and beneficial, often yielding enduring long-term benefits as well as more immediate gains. Indeed, brief therapists recognize that what really counts is what happens *after* the session, and thus need to see its impact (outcome: change and durability) before assessing the "goodness" of a session (Hoyt, 2000a).

Koss and Butcher (1986; see also Koss & Shiang, 1994) have concluded from their major review of the research literature on psychotherapy outcome that brief and long-term methods are equally effective, and that brief methods are more cost-effective. Many comparative research studies may actually underestimate the effectiveness of planned brief therapy, because so few of the therapists in the original studies were specifically oriented or trained in brief therapy methods (Hoyt & Austad, 1992; Koss, Butcher, & Strupp, 1986; Messer & Warren, 1995). Although one can ignore these findings or argue that brief therapy and long-term therapy have different goals, the equivalence of outcomes is compelling.

Why not try a short-term approach first? This is consistent with the advice of Wolberg (1965, p. 140): "The best strategy, in my opinion, is to assume that every patient, irrespective of diagnosis, will respond to short-term treatment unless he proves himself refractory to it. . . . If this fails, he can always then resort to prolonged therapy." This is similar to the position expressed by the psychoanalyst Basch (1995):

> I believe that one cannot decide arbitrarily, on the basis of either symptoms or character structure, that a patient will not benefit from brief therapy. Indeed, it is my position that all patients who are not psychotic or suicidal should be thought of as candidates for brief psychotherapy until proven otherwise. (p. xi)

Writing from their multimodal cognitive-behavioral perspective, Lazarus and Fay (1990) also make clear their observation:

Some long-term therapy is not only inefficient (taking longer than necessary because it
was insufficiently focused or precise), but
even detrimental because of the reinforcement of pathological self-concepts. One of
the great advantages of the short-term focus
is that if the therapy doesn't work, it will be
apparent much sooner. . . . In this regard, to
paraphrase an old saying, effective treatment
depends far less on the hours you put in, than
on what you put into those hours. (pp. 39–40)

And even if longer-term therapies sometimes do produce results that may be preferable, the question remains "Who will pay
for such extended treatments?" Most patients want more efficient help. Given the
social and professional imperative to provide psychological services to the wide
range of persons who might need and benefit from mental health care, the thrust of
the accumulated data seems clear. However,
before we turn to some of the specific ways
that effective brief psychotherapies endeav-
or to translate complicated understanding
into methods likely to yield results sooner
rather than later, let us consider some of the
overarching principles that guide the practice of brief therapy.

BASIC BELIEFS THAT CAN PROMOTE OR IMPEDE EFFECTIVE BRIEF THERAPY

The fundamental assumption of all forms of
deliberate brief therapy is an attitude and
expectation—supported by various theories, methodologies, and findings—that significant and beneficial changes can be
brought about relatively quickly. The brief
therapist recognizes that there is no time
but the present. Historical review may yield
some clues about how the patient is "stuck"
and what may be needed to get "unstuck"
(Hoyt, 1990), but whatever the therapist's
particular theoretical orientation, primary
effort is directed at helping the patient recognize options in the present that can result
in enhanced coping, new learning, growth,

and other beneficial changes. Yapko (1990)
has noted three factors that determine
whether a patient will benefit from brief
therapy interventions: (1) the person's primary temporal orientation (toward past,
present, or future); (2) the general value giv-
en to "change," whether he or she is more
invested in maintaining tradition or seeking
change; and (3) the patient's belief system
about what constitutes a complete therapeutic experience.

It is this fundamental assumption—that
with skillful facilitation, useful changes can
be set into motion relatively quickly, and
that patients can then maintain and often
expand the benefits on their own—that underlies the "universal elements" or "common ingredients" of brief treatment that
have been synthesized by various authors
(Bloom, 1992; Budman & Gurman, 1988;
Friedman & Fanger, 1991; Hoyt, 1995a,
2000b; Hoyt & Austad, 1992; Koss &
Butcher, 1986; Wells & Phelps, 1990). As
Budman, Friedman, and Hoyt (1992) have
written, the most frequently cited generic
components of brief treatment are:

1. Rapid and generally positive working alliance between therapist and patient.
2. Focality, the clear specification of
achievable treatment results and goals.
3. Clear definition of patient and therapist
responsibilities, with a relatively high
level of therapist activity and patient participation.
4. Emphasis on the patient's strengths,
competencies, and adaptive capacities.
5. Expectation of change, the belief that
improvement is within the patient's (immediate) grasp.
6. Here-and-now (and next) orientation,
the primary focus being on current
functioning and patterns in thinking,
feeling, and behaving—and their alternatives.
7. Time sensitivity, making the most of
each session as well as the idea of intermittent treatment replacing the notion
of a once-and-for-all definitive "cure."

This set of defining characteristics is reflected in the comparison of the dominant values of long-term and short-term treatment presented in Table 10.1.[1]

Many of these same value differences can also be detected in the "resistances" or contrary attitudes some therapists hold about brief or short-term therapy (Hoyt, 1985a, 1990, 1991; see also Messer & Warren, 1995, pp. 43–49):

1. *The belief that "more is better,"* often held despite the lack of evidence justifying the greater expense of long-term or open-ended treatment (Bloom 1992; Budman & Gurman, 1988; Koss & Butcher, 1986).

2. *The myth of the "pure gold" of analysis* (to use Freud's [1919] term for idealized insight and interpretation) and the faulty assumption that change and growth necessarily require "deep" examination and that anything else is dismissable as "superficial"

or "merely palliative." While making clear his preference for orthodox analysis, Freud (1919) acknowledged the value of combining techniques to produce a more effective therapeutic instrument. It should also be noted that in his last great clinical paper, "Analysis Terminable and Interminable," Freud (1937) seemed to regret the "interminable" nature of pure analysis.

3. *Belief in the inappropriateness of greater therapist activity,* including the need to be selectively focused, confrontative, directive, and risk taking.

4. *The confusion of patients' and therapists' interests,* the tendency of therapists to seek and treat perfectionistically putative "complexes" and "underlying personality issues" rather than attend directly to patients' complaints and stated treatment goals. Most patients seek therapy because of a specific problem and want the most succinct help available.

TABLE 10.1. Comparative Dominant Values of the Long-Term and Short-Term Therapist

Long-term therapist	Short-term therapist
1. Seeks change in basic character.	Prefers pragmatism, parsimony, and least radical intervention; does not believe in the notion of "cure."
2. Believes that significant change is unlikely in everyday life.	Maintains an adult developmental perspective from which significant psychological change is viewed as inevitable.
3. Sees presenting problems as reflecting more basic pathology.	Emphasizes patients' strengths and resources.
4. Wants to "be there" as patient makes significant changes.	Accepts that many changes will occur "after therapy."
5. Sees therapy as having a "timeless" quality.	Does not accept the timelessness of some models of therapy.
6. Unconsciously recognizes the fiscal convenience of long-term patients.	Fiscal issues often muted, either by the nature of the practice or the organizational structure.
7. Views therapy as almost always benign and useful.	Views therapy as sometimes useful and sometimes harmful.
8. Sees therapy as being the most important part of the patient's life.	Sees being in the world as more important than being in therapy.
9. Views therapist as responsible only for treating a given patient.	Views therapist as having responsibility for treatment of a population.

Note. From Budman and Gurman (1988, p. 11). Copyright 1988 by The Guilford Press. Reprinted by permission.

5. *Financial pressures,* the temptation to hold on to that which is profitable and dependable, as well as other incentives such as the pleasures of intimate conversation and the lure of vicariously living through an extended relationship.

6. *Countertransference and termination problems,* including the need to be needed and difficulties saying good-bye. The term "countertransference" is used here in the specific sense, following Freud (1910, 1915), of meaning a reaction or counter to the patient's transference (e.g., the therapist has difficulty letting go because the patient presents as needy and guilt evoking). In other instances, it may be more the therapist's own transference (unconscious agenda), not the patient's "pull," that is the source of termination difficulties.

7. *Psychological reactance,* the interesting response of valuing something more if you cannot have it (Brehm, 1966). Being told that one has to treat a patient with brief therapy (e.g., because of insurance restrictions or simply because that is what the patient wants) may trigger resentment and the thought, "No one is going to tell me what to do. I'm a professional." The fact is, however, that restrictions such as patients' willingness and ability to pay, insurance limits, and clinic policies regarding possible length of treatment do get imposed. There is also the social responsibility to provide needed services to the many rather than many services to the privileged few (Hoyt 1985b, 2000b; Hoyt & Austad, 1992). Given these necessities, we may have to treat more people briefly, even if it helps them!

The foregoing notwithstanding, there are certainly times when short-term therapy usually will not be adequate and appropriate—including severe psychiatric disorders, instances when a longer process is required for the patient to make desired changes, or when ongoing support is required to maintain a tenuous psychosocial adjustment— although the basic attitudes of making the most of each session, accessing strengths and

resources, and taking as few sessions as possible will still be valuable. Indeed, if the needs of more than a handful of patients are to be served, the skillful application of brief therapy methods whenever possible will be necessary to make longer-term treatments available for those who truly need them.

To summarize this section, it appears that there are essentially three factors that tend to determine the length of treatment:

1. The theoretical orientation of the therapist, whether his or her beliefs and working assumptions align the therapist more with the list of dominant values in the left- or righthand column in Table 10.1.
2. Money—how much and for how long the patient can afford to pay.
3. The patient's problems, situation, personality, psychopathology, expectations, and capacities.

WHY DO PATIENTS COME TO THERAPY?

Most patients come to therapy because they hope that working with a psychotherapist will soon relieve some state of unhappiness, distress, or dysfunction that has become so troublesome that professional consultation appears preferable to continuing the status quo.[2] The person feels that something timely has to be done because, as the old adage has it, "If you don't change directions, you'll wind up where you're heading." As Budman and Gurman (1988) have articulated, there are five common answers to the question, "Why now does a patient come for treatment?"—five interrelated themes or foci that can often be addressed productively in brief therapy:

1. *Loss,* including bereavement and divorce, as well as other losses such as certain changes in social status, health problems, and betrayals of trust and confidence.
2. *Developmental dysynchronies,* life-cycle transitions or passages for which the pa-

tient is not well prepared and which thus present problems of adjustment (e.g., adolescent emancipation, marriage, starting a family, the empty-nest syndrome, and retirement).

3. *Interpersonal conflicts,* problems with significant others such as spouse, children, authority figures, coworkers, and friends.

4. *Specific symptoms,* such as depression, anxiety, or sexual dysfunctions.

5. *Personality issues,* characterological issues that come to the fore if the patient makes them the focus of therapy and/or if they impede within- or between-session work to the extent that they require direct attention for therapy to be successful.

Although brief psychodynamic therapists require careful assessment for patient suitability (discussed later) and some brief multimodal therapists (see Lazarus, 1997, 1989) do an initial comprehensive symptom assessment, most brief therapists generally do not consider assessment to be a separate process to be completed before beginning treatment but, rather, see the two as inextricably intertwined. The questions one asks help to co-create the reality in which therapist and patient work, and the patient's responses to trial interventions provide useful information about what is likely to be beneficial. It is helpful to keep in mind the idea that the word "diagnosis" comes from Greek and Latin words (*via gnosis*) meaning "the way of knowing," and this is just what a good functional diagnosis should do: provide information that illuminates a path (Hoyt, 1989). Pathology-oriented nosology may contain some important information, but it is seldom enough. Consider, for example, the five axes of the fourth edition, text revision of *Diagnostic and Statistical Manual of Mental Disorders* (DSM-IV-TR; American Psychiatric Association, 2000):

I. Clinical Disorders and Other Conditions That May Be a Focus of Clinical Attention

II. Personality Disorders and Mental Retardation

III. General Medical Conditions

IV. Psychosocial and Environmental Problems

V. Global Assessment of Functioning, usually expressed by a numerical index.

Important data may be summarized in the DSM-IV-TR (and may be especially useful for communicating with insurance companies and clinical researchers as well as for differentially diagnosing whether medication is likely to be of help), but reviewing the axes also reveals a potentially discouraging orientation toward "disease" and "sickness." As Barten (1971) notes, "Our training predisposes us to describe areas of illness rather than areas of health, and this illness orientation can make the prognosis of a great many people appear rather bleak" (p. 8). Similarly, de Shazer and Weakland comment that "It's not a mental health industry; it's a mental illness industry" (quoted in Hoyt, 1994c, p. 20). Consider what the five DSM-IV-TR axes tell us about a person:

I. What's wrong with the patient now

II. What's been wrong with the patient for a long time

III. What's wrong with the patient's body

IV. What's wrong with the patient's social situation

V. What's the patient's overall level of dysfunction or maladaption

Data such as these, including information about potential suicidality and alcohol and substance abuse, can be vital, but we also need to focus on the patient's strengths and capacities, his or her beliefs, resources, and motivations for treatment to proceed successfully.

A therapist wanting to do effective brief treatment will need to accomplish a number of tasks early on with a patient:

1. Make contact and establish rapport.
2. Define the purpose of the meeting.
3. Orient and instruct the patient on how to use therapy.
4. Create an opportunity for the patient to express thoughts, feelings, and behavior.
5. Assess the patient's problems, strengths, motivations, goals, and expectations.
6. Establish realistic (specific and obtainable) treatment goals.
7. Make initial treatment interventions, assess effects, and adjust accordingly.
8. Assign tasks or "homework" as appropriate.
9. Attend to such business matters as future appointments and fees.

It is important in the first session to engage the patient and to introduce some novelty. As will be seen in the cases presented here, as well as those reported in *The First Session in Brief Therapy* (Budman, Hoyt, & Friedman, 1992), in virtually all successful brief therapies something new happens in the first meeting. More of the same (behavior, outlook, defense, etc.) does not produce change. Whether it is conceptualized as an intrapsychic compromise between an impulse and an anxiety, a "game people play," or a self-perpetuating maladaptive interpersonal pattern, a symptom is an attempted solution to a problem that does not work or that engenders unwanted results (Edelstien, 1990; Fisch, Weakland, & Segal, 1982; Yapko, 1992). Effective therapy involves breaking such a pattern, doing something different. The novelty may come by seeing oneself and one's situation differently, by practicing a new way of transacting with others, by experiencing unacknowledged feelings, by utilizing strengths and abilities that were overlooked previously or newly learned. Whatever the means, the brief therapist looks for ways to start or amplify the patient's movement in the desired direction as soon as possible.

Attending carefully to the early identification of specific, achievable goals promotes effective brief work (Cade & O'Hanlon,

1993; de Shazer, 1985, 1988, 1991b; Goulding & Goulding, 1979; Haley, 1977, 1989; O'Hanlon & Weiner-Davis, 1989). Operational definitions contribute to treatment accountability, counter the temptation to diffuse/confuse/refuse focality, and help to assure that genuinely obtainable results are not replaced with vague or unrealistic "missions impossible" or "therapeutic perfectionism" (Malan, 1976). Questions such as the following help to focus treatment and involve the patient:

- What problem are you here to solve?
- If you work hard and make some changes, how will you be functioning differently?
- What are the smallest changes you could make that would tell that you are heading in the right direction?
- At those times when the problem is not so bad or is absent, what are you doing?
- What will tell us we're done?
- How will we know when to stop meeting like this?
- How might therapy help, and how long do you expect it to take?

Treatment revolves around what the patient wants to accomplish plus the answers to three interrelated transtechnical, heuristic questions (Hoyt, 1990, 1995a, 2000b):

1. How is the patient "stuck" (what is the problem or pathology)?
2. What does the patient need to get "unstuck?" (Sometimes detected by identifying what they are doing differently at times when they are not "stuck.")
3. How can I, as therapist, facilitate or provide what is needed?

The good brief (or any) therapist needs to be multitheoretical, able to conceptualize and reckon from a variety of perspectives lest patients be forced into the Procrustean bed of a pet theory or technique or be dismissed and blamed for being resistant, unmotivated, or ego deficient. As the saying

goes, "If all one has is a hammer, everything begins to look like a nail." How you look helps determine what you will see, and what you see helps determine what you will do (Hoyt, 1994b, 2000b). The importance of having "an array of observing positions" has been well described by Gustafson (1986; see also White & Epston, 1990), who identifies four key paradigms in tracing the history of attempts to answer the question of how patients get stuck and unstuck:

> Psychoanalysis sees the hidden demands of the animal in us. The analysis of character sees the "constant attitude" which protects the animal from without. Interpersonal interviewing sees the interactions which tie us into trouble with other people. Systemic interviewing sees these interactions in the service of stable social relations. (p. 6)

The therapist wishing to be parsimonious (brief and effective) may need to choose which conceptualization(s) will allow for the best chance of a change-producing intervention. Should the approach be toward revealing the intrapsychic domain of warded-off feelings, modifying the patient's typical way of viewing and meeting the world, altering the social skills with which the patient interacts, or changing the rules of the labyrinthine games that ensnare patients into maintaining the status quo? Or what else? And how to do so? Education and skill instruction? Cognitive-behavioral techniques? Psychodynamic interpretations? Solution-focused questions? Systemic interviewing and strategic interventions? Hypnosis? Commonsense appeals or wise exhortations? The brief therapist asks: *What would be likely to work with this patient and this therapist in this context at this time?*

INTERLUDE: A BRIEF HISTORY OF BRIEF THERAPY

People have been having problems and getting help since time immemorial, although the history of psychotherapy as a practice and a profession is considered to have begun in earnest only about 100 years ago (Freedheim, 1992; Zeig, 1987). Sigmund Freud, usually thought of as the founder of psychoanalysis, was also the father of brief therapy. Reading his early cases (Breuer & Freud, 1893–1895), one finds him working actively with patients and treating them in days, weeks, and months rather than years. Psychoanalysis was also a research instrument, however, and treatment became longer and longer as the early pioneers became fascinated with the psychological phenomena that would emerge (such as Oedipal fantasies and transference neuroses) if the therapist remained a relatively inactive and neutral "blank" screen while the patient freely associated. An early effort to experiment with more active methods in treatment was made by Ferenczi and Rank (1925), but some of their methods were questionable and the time for revisionism was not right because psychoanalysis was still struggling to establish itself. At the end of his life, Freud (1937) expressed his frustration about the limited therapeutic benefits of psychoanalysis and called for the development of new methods based on the psychoanalytic understanding of transference, resistance, and unconscious material.

World War II intervened, with many consequences for the practice of brief (and other) psychotherapy. Prior to the war, psychological treatment usually had been a long-term luxury of the privileged and had fallen under the purview of the psychoanalytic and psychiatric–medical establishment. There were so many soldiers needing services, however, that (1) psychologists and clinical social workers were finally recognized as bona fide psychotherapy providers rather than being relegated to their respective "auxiliary" roles as psychometric testers and home visitors; (2) group therapy was greatly expanded as a treatment of choice (and necessity) rather than being an isolated and rare specialty; (3) the Veterans Administration (VA) medical system emerged as a training ground for mental health professionals; and, most salient to our present topic, (4) interest was spurred in treatment methods that would help soldiers quickly reduce symptoms and return to function either in the combat zones or back in civilian life. Psychoanalytic theory continued to predominate, but "reality factors" were becoming increasingly influential—harbingers of what is today called "accountability" (Cummings, 2000; Hoyt, 1995a; Johnson, 1995; VandenBos, Cummings, & DeLeon, 1992).

In 1946, Alexander and French published *Psychoanalytic Therapy: Principles and Applications.* The book was (and is) extraordinary, revisiting and updating many of the ideas of Ferenczi and Rank (1925) regarding the use of greater therapist activity and suggesting that the length and frequency of sessions might be varied, both from case to case and within the same patient's treatment, to avoid excessive dependency in the patient that prolonged therapy and to bring about what Alexander and French referred to as a "corrective emotional experience." Many successful brief therapies were reported. Still, the politics of psychoanalysis were not yet ripe for change and it remained for two leading psychoanalytic figures of the time, Bibring (1954) and Gill (1954), to publish their seminal papers about modifying the parameters of treatment and to call it psychoanalytically *oriented* therapy (and not psychoanalysis) before attempts at psychodynamic modifications were recognized as legitimate by the mainstream.

By the early 1950s, a number of workers were exploring what could be done using psychodynamic principles in more active and shorter treatment. In London, Balint, Ornstein, and Balint (1972) and Malan (1963, 1976) were developing "focal psychotherapy"; in Boston, Sifneos (1972) was beginning to experiment with "short-term anxiety-provoking psychotherapy"; and in New York, Wolberg (1965) was investigating various ways of shortening the length of treatment, including using hypnotherapy to work through patients' resistance more

quickly. At the same time, several other important figures were becoming disenchanted with psychoanalysis and began to originate other, more active methods for bringing about psychological change more rapidly. Perls, Heiferline, and Goodman (1951) began to develop the theory and techniques of Gestalt therapy; Wolpe (1958), Wolpe and Lazarus (1966), and Lazarus (1976) were developing behavior therapy; Ellis (1962, 1992; see also Beck, 1976; Meichenbaum, 1977) began to develop rational-emotive therapy, the first systematic form of what is now called "cognitive therapy"; and Berne (1961, 1972) began to develop transactional analysis. In Palo Alto, California, the innovative psychiatrist and pioneering family therapist Don Jackson founded the Mental Research Institute. A number of publications started calling professional attention to the expanding field of brief therapy, including important books by Malan (1963), Wolberg (1965), Bellak and Small (1965), Parad (1965), Barten (1971), and Lewin (1970). Concurrently, the psychiatrist Milton Erickson (1980) was still working in relative obscurity in Phoenix, Arizona, but his uniquely creative uses of hypnosis and strategic interventions to capitalize on patients' existing capacities would soon be recognized (especially with the 1973 publication of Jay Haley's *Uncommon Therapy: The Psychiatric Techniques of Milton H. Erickson, M.D.*) and contributed greatly both to the emerging family therapy movement and to various schools of strategic and systemic therapy.

Writing about the expanding spectrum of the brief therapies, Barten (1971) underscored the convergence of a number of historical developments, including a growing professional commitment to providing appropriate mental health services to all segments of the community, an increasing shift from psychoanalysis to more ego-oriented techniques and a recognition of the value of limited therapeutic goals, diversification of the roles of mental health professionals, long overdue recognition of the special needs of the disadvantaged, and increased consumer demand for economically feasible services. The community mental health movement of the 1960s and the federal Health Maintenance Organization (HMO) Act of 1973 gave further mandate to brief treatment. Strategic therapists were guided by Haley (1963, 1973, 1977), Madanes (1981, 1984), and the work of the Mental Research Institute of Palo Alto (Fisch et al., 1982; Watzlawick, Beavin, & Jackson, 1967; Watzlawick, Weakland, & Fisch, 1974) and the Brief Family Therapy Center of Milwaukee (de Shazer, 1982, 1985, 1988), while psychodynamicists wanting to work more concisely drew special inspiration from the work of Sifneos (1972), Mann (1973), Malan (1963, 1976), and Davanloo (1978, 1980). In 1988, a conference titled "Brief Therapy: Myths, Methods and Metaphors," sponsored by the Milton H. Erickson Foundation, was held in San Francisco, with several thousand mental health professionals attending (Zeig & Gilligan, 1990); several such conferences have been held since (see Zeig, 2002a).

The recent enormous acceleration in various forms of managed mental health care—which by 1992 covered approximately 100 million Americans, and by year 2000 covered approximately 160 million Americans—has given further impetus to the development and expansion of various forms of brief therapy. As Haley (2001) has written, "With nothing to restrain the length of therapy, there would not be a theory of dosage. . . . The prediction that therapy would get longer and longer was undone by adventurous therapists willing to use common sense, and the insurance companies guiding us all to shorter and cheaper jobs" (pp. 13–14). (Wells and Phelps [1990] characterize this emerging trend as "Survival of the Shortest.") However, although various managed care organizations, insurance companies, HMOs, clinics, counseling services, and consumers all desire, and often require, brief treatment to the extent that it provides less expensive treatments, it is important not to conflate the terms "brief

therapy" and "managed care" (Hoyt, 2001b). As I have written elsewhere (Hoyt, 1995a, 2000b), there are numerous ethical and practical problems with the way some managed care organizations go about their business, including undertreatment of some patients. Although brief therapy principles (such as having clear goals, spending more time looking forward rather than backward, and emphasizing client strengths and resources) can be useful with those persons requiring longer or ongoing care (see Duncan, Hubble, & Miller, 1997; Kreider, 1998; Rowan & O'Hanlon, 1998; Yapko, 1990), it should be noted that brief therapy models were not developed to serve managed care. As Steve de Shazer, the co-originator of solution-focused therapy, has remarked, "We are not a response to managed care. We've been doing brief therapy for 30 years. We developed this a long time before managed care was even somebody's bad idea" (quoted in Short, 1997, p. 18). Similarly, Michael White (1997), the co-originator of narrative therapy, has commented, "We all have good reason to be concerned about . . . developments in delivery service that are being increasingly dictated by the economics of the 'free' marketplace, not by what might be in the best interests of persons according to criteria that are important to them" (p. vi). Haley (quoted in Yapko, 2001) sees both positives and negatives:

> I think we should send all the managed care people to social work school! *Something* should be done with them, because to have business people determining how therapy should be done, and for how many sessions, seems bizarre. But, with all the years that have been spent studying therapy, I think that a managed care system could have some positive things about it, too. I think many therapists have no idea how to do therapy—they just sit there in therapy and listen to someone for months or more. Now, therapists have to know how to formulate a problem, make an intervention, and then they have to check their results—or their results will be checked for them. So, some ideas of managed care are good. But, at the

same time, when you have businessmen deciding on treatment they'll choose what is cheapest, and what is most profitable, and that may be hiring the cheapest therapists who may be the most inadequate. (p. 200)

THE STRUCTURE OF BRIEF THERAPY

While we have already emphasized the importance of the first session in brief therapy as a prelude to considering some specific approaches, it will be helpful to gain an orienting perspective on the overall structure of treatment, the issues and tasks associated with the early, middle, and later stages of psychotherapeutic work. Brief psychotherapy (as well as other, more prolonged or open-ended treatments) can be conceptualized as having a structure of five sequenced phases. In actual practice, of course, the phases blend into one another rather than being discretely organized. The structure tends to be epigenetic or pyramidal; that is, each phase builds on the prior phase, so that successful work in one is a precondition for the next (e.g., the patient electing treatment and the therapist applying selection criteria and accepting the patient precedes forming a working alliance, which precedes focusing and making a contract, which precedes termination, which precedes continuing work and following through).

As noted elsewhere (Gustafson, 1986; Hoyt, 1995a; Hoyt & Miller, 2000), there is often an interesting parallel between the process of each individual session and the structure of the overall course of treatment: Like the idea of ontogeny recapitulating phylogeny, each session and each therapy involves connecting, working, and closing. Often, there is also a parallel process wherein brief therapy students/trainees repeat in sequence with their supervisors some of the same issues that are concurrently occurring between the students and their patients (Dasberg & Winokur, 1984; Frances & Clarkin, 1981b; Hoyt, 1991).

The questions one asks, beginning with the first, do much to set the theme and temporal orientation of each session and the overall treatment (Goulding & Goulding, 1979; Hoyt, 1990; Kaiser, 1965). Asking "What's better?" moves the focus more toward strengths and competencies, whereas asking "What's wrong?" invites *problem talk* rather than *solution talk* (de Shazer, 1988; Furman & Ahola, 1992). Similarly, if one asks, for example, "How have things gone?" the direction is largely toward reviewing the *past*. If one instead asks, "What are you experiencing?" or "What are you willing to change today?" the direction is more *present* centered. Asking "What do you need to discuss to do well next week?" or "How will you be different when the problem is solved?" points to the *future*.

As seen in Figure 10.1, each phase of treatment has its special issues:

1. *Pre: Election and selection.* Even before the first session occurs, change often begins with the recognition of a problem and the decision to seek therapy (Weiner-Davis, de Shazer, & Gingerich, 1987). Can the therapist capitalize on this? How? What may need to happen before change is possible? Is the patient ready, and what will circumstances permit? Is the patient a willing customer, an unwilling complainant, or simply a visitor (de Shazer, 1988)? Looked at from a somewhat different perspective, we can recognize the importance of the patient's stage of change: Is the patient in the precontemplation, contemplation, planning, action, or maintenance stage (Hoyt & Miller, 2000; Prochaska, DiClemente, & Norcross, 1992)? It is also good to remember that there are some patients—spontaneous improvers, nonresponders, and negative therapeutic reactors—for whom "no treatment" may be the prescription of choice (Frances & Clarkin, 1981a).

2. *Early.* As already discussed, key issues involve forming a working alliance; assessing patients' strengths, weaknesses, and motivations; finding a psychological focus, es-

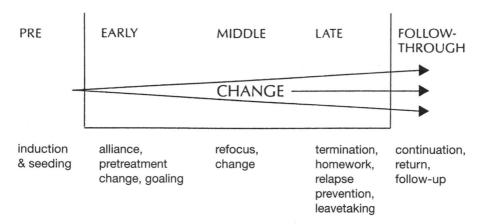

FIGURE 10.1. The temporal structure of brief therapy. From Hoyt (2000a, p. 218). Copyright 2002 by Taylor & Francis. Reprinted by permission.

tablishing achievable goals, and forming a treatment plan and contract; introducing novelty and getting the patient actively involved in treatment; and attending to business matters. No mean feat!

3. *Middle phase.* This is the "working through" stage, meaning staying on task, doing homework, and applying the lessons of therapy in real life, as well as possibly increasing insight into the original and present-day sources of problems. Maintenance and possible refinement of a central theme/focus/goal occur here.

4. *Late phase.* This includes termination and possible mourning: possible arousal of underlying separation–individuation issues in both patient and therapist, with possible return of symptoms and temptations to avoid ending; the need to subtract the therapist from the successful equation (Gustafson, 1986); maintaining gains, goal attainment assessment, possible homework or tasks, continuing change, and avoiding possible backsliding or "self-sabotage"; relapse prevention; inviting a follow-up or "check-in" appointment with the possibility of later return to treatment; and leavetaking. Careful attention is paid to ending not too soon but not later than necessary. (Hoyt, 2000a).

5. *Follow-through.* This includes continuation of psychological work and change be-

yond the formal ending of therapist–patient contact. Internalization of favorable aspects of the treatment occur here. In short-term therapy, much more than in longer treatments, change processes may be started or amplified without being completely worked through during the course of formal treatment. This is consistent with the distinction between treatment goals and life goals (Ticho, 1972), the former involving getting "unstuck" and better equipped to deal with whatever life presents down the road. There is also, of course, the possibility of intermittent, episodic, serial, or distributed therapy (Bennett, 1983, 1984; Budman, 1990; Cummings & Sayama, 1995; Hoyt, 1990, 2000b)—the patient can return later for additional treatment as needed.

SOME SPECIFIC MODELS OF BRIEF THERAPY

There are various models or "schools" of brief therapy (see Bloom, 1992; Budman, 1981; Budman, Hoyt, & Friedman, 1992; Carlson & Sperry, 2000; Gustafson, 1986; Wells & Giannetti, 1990, 1993; Zeig & Gilligan, 1990). Although each case is different and the skillful application of psychological principles is part of what makes therapy an interesting and artful endeavor, there are broad general guidelines in theory and practice that distinguish different forms of brief treatment. We highlight and illustrate a few of them here, but the reader should keep in mind three important caveats: (1) no summary or case presentation can do more than suggest a few broad brushstrokes—by necessity, more has been omitted than included under each rubric, and therefore in each section there are basic references cited to guide those wishing to get started on a fuller study of a particular approach; (2) most therapy is eclectic and integrative, drawing ideas and methods from a range of sources rather than adhering to one particular theory; and (3) as Milton Erickson said, "Each person is a unique individual. Hence, psychotherapy should be formulated to meet the uniqueness of the individual's needs, rather than tailoring the person to fit the Procrustean bed of a hypothetical theory of human behavior" (quoted in Zeig & Gilligan, 1990, p. xix).

Short-Term Psychodynamic Psychotherapies

Beginning with Freud, numerous theoreticians and clinicians have applied the psychoanalytic concepts of the unconscious, resistance, and transference to brief forms of treatment. Indeed, many of Freud's cases were "brief," just a few sessions lasting weeks or months. Building on the principles described in Freud's (1914) paper, "Remembering, Repeating, and Working Through," various short-term dynamic methods have been developed to bring the patient to a greater awareness of his or her maladaptive defenses, warded-off feelings, and counterproductive relationship patterns. As many reviewers have noted (see Crits-Cristoph & Barber, 1991; Levenson & Butler, 1999; Malan, 1976; Messer & Warren, 1995), the emphasis in all of the various short-term dynamic psychotherapies has been on increased therapist activity within a limited, central focus. There has been a gen-

eral recognition that relative inactivity on the part of the therapist in the face of increasing resistance leads to prolonged and diffuse treatment. Hence, Malan (1980), in an allusion to Freud's (1919) paper "Turnings in the Way of Psychoanalysis," refers to Freud's technique of free association as "a wrong turning" that leads to "doubtful therapeutic effectiveness" (pp. 13–14). Brief dynamic therapists endeavor to promote change within a focalized area of conflict via an admixture of de-repression and affective release, corrective emotional experience and internalization of a benign therapist–patient relationship, relearning, and application of the patient's will.

Let us sketch a few of the main short-term psychodynamic approaches in terms of their central characteristics of focus, primary techniques and length of treatment and then consider a case vignette.

1. *Short-term anxiety-provoking psychotherapy* (Sifneos, 1987, 1992). This approach is primarily for carefully selected patients with Oedipal conflicts. Anxiety-provoking confrontations and transference interpretations are made by a teacher/therapist endeavoring to produce emotional relearning. Length of treatment varies but is typically about 6 to 15 sessions.

2. *Short-term dynamic psychotherapy* (Malan, 1963, 1976). This method also focuses on issues of Oedipal conflict and loss, with research evidence indicating a positive correlation between therapy outcome and the therapist emphasizing interpretive links between transference and past (i.e., parents) relationship issues as well as between outcome and the therapist emphasizing issues of termination and loss. Treatment is typically 30 to 40 sessions.

3. *Short-term intensive dynamic psychotherapy* (Davanloo, 1978, 1980, 1991; McCullough-Vaillant, 1997). The therapist functions as a "relentless healer," vigorously confronting and interpreting defenses until there is an "unlocking of the unconscious" and a breakthrough into true feelings. The

focus is broad, with strong emphasis on characterological defenses as they are manifested within the basic psychoanalytic "triangle of conflict" (impulse-feeling/anxiety/defense) and "triangle of person" (transference/current significant persons/past significant persons), with special attention directed toward an experience in the transference. As McCullough (2000) has written: "The core maladaptive conflict can be thought of as an affect phobia (i.e., fear of one's own emotional responses because of conflictual feelings associated with them). The treatment can be conceptualized as an exposure (to conflicted feelings) and response prevention (of defensive avoidance) to achieve desensitization of the feared but adaptive affects" (p. 130). Treatment length generally varies from 5 to 40 sessions, with progress expected to be evident early on.

4. *Stress response therapy and microanalysis* (Horowitz et al., 1984). The focus is on the patient's "states of mind," "self-schemas," "role-relationship models," and information-processing styles (couched in an explicitly cognitive language) to help the patient rework and emotionally master a recent stress event (such as the death of a loved one). Patients typically alternate between "intrusive–repetitive" and "denial–numbing" phases as they work through their stress response, usually over the course of 12 sessions.

5. *Time-limited dynamic psychotherapy* (Levenson, 1995; Strupp & Binder, 1984). A "cyclical maladaptive pattern" is identified and interpreted, involving acts of self, expectations of others, acts of others, and self-introjects. The therapist is empathic, appreciating the pull of countertransference as an opportunity to provide insight and a corrective emotional experience. Research on this method consistently indicates that "the quality of the therapeutic relationship, established early in the interaction, proved to be an important predictor of outcome. In particular, therapy tended to be successful if by the third session the patient felt accepted, understood, and liked by the therapist"

(Binder & Strupp, 1991, p. 157). Treatment is usually 25 sessions.

6. *Time-limited psychotherapy* (Mann, 1973; Mann & Goldman, 1982; Rasmussen & Messon, 1986). A firm 12-session treatment framework is established with an emphasis on the patient's sense of self and his or her present and "chronically endured pain." The preset termination date focuses conscious and unconscious attention on the passage of time, creating a context in which the empathic therapist helps the patient look at and master underlying separation issues that become manifest in terms of themes of unresolved mourning, activity versus passivity, independence versus dependence, and adequate versus diminished self-esteem.

Messer and Warren (1995), in their comprehensive review of various models of brief psychodynamic therapy, characterize the first three of the foregoing approaches (Sifneos, Malan, Davanloo) as "the drive/structural model"; the next two approaches (Horowitz, and Strupp and Binder) as "the relational model" (in which they also include the work of Luborsky & Crits-Christoph [1990] and of Weiss, Sampson, & Mt. Zion Psychotherapy Research Group, 1986]); and the last approach (Mann) as "an integrative psychoanalytic model." As Messer and Warren note, "The techniques employed by the drive/structuralist therapists, especially Davanloo and Sifneos, include direct confrontation of patients' defenses, which requires a rather bald show of therapist authority and assertiveness" (p. 46). Critics of these methods (e.g., Gustafson, 1986; Westen, 1986) perceive them as authoritarian. Messer and Warren note, however, the following:

> [the drive/structural therapists] would not view themselves as authoritarian so much as active, even relentless, in helping patients to face up to and wrestle with their problems. . . . They seek to help patients muster the courage to combat their self-deceptions, defenses, and

resistances in the service of exposing and re-solving what they have distorted and kept hidden from themselves and others. . . . What we seem to have here is a value dispute. The drive/structural therapists claim that challenge and confrontation in the service of the patient's becoming freer of neurotic conflict is justified. The critics contend that the putative ends do not justify the means employed because the therapists have merely imposed their view of reality on patients, thereby detracting from their autonomy. (p. 111)

What is at stake here is more than "style." "Drive/structural" model therapists consider their view to be "the truth," "not as hypothesis, metaphor, or construct, but as given—an obvious and proven fact" (Messer & Warren, 1995, p. 113). Again, Messer and Warren (1995) elaborate:

Although the source of the critics' claims may lie in the forceful and charismatic nature of the personalities involved, or in their confrontative techniques, a more fundamental consideration is the epistemological basis from which these three therapists [Sifneos, Malan, Davanloo] operate. The air of certainty with which they formulate the patient's dynamics and interpret them suggest that they embrace the correspondence concept of truth. Within this framework, knowledge of objects and events is gained through observation of things as they are, independent of the theories of the observer. The correspondence theory is wedded to realism which assumes a world and mental events that have their own nature apart from our perceptions of them. This theory of truth was once the normative one in science, and it largely constituted Freud's view as well. . . . For Freud, there was one correct fit to the puzzle of the patient's symptoms, dreams, slips, and so forth. (p. 112)

They contrast the *correspondence* theory to another perspective:

The alternative to the correspondence theory is the *coherence* theory of truth, which posits that there is more than one true description of the world. It is associated with the philosophical school of thought called idealism.

The coherence theory regards the reality of objects and events as a function of how they are experienced by observers, not as they "actually are," as realism espouses. Objects only take on meaning by virtue of the theory we invent to define them; that is, they are constructed and constituted by our beliefs and ideas. . . . In this view, one does not "unlock the unconscious," have an unadorned view of "the multifoci core neurotic structure," or the elements of the oedipal complex, nor does one achieve an apodictically accurate dynamic focus. Rather, one constructs a narrative that pulls together the pieces of personality functioning with the knowledge that other constructions are always possible. . . . Narrative coherence rather than external correspondence to an actual reality becomes the criterion of truth. (p. 113)

Brief dynamic therapists working within the relational model, as Messer and Warren (1995) note, have

an object relational view of mind, with internalized representations of self, other, and interaction as fundamental. . . . Relational views imply a concept of personality that is organized around structures of mind that are fundamentally oriented toward the object world. Relational approaches, while diverse, stand together in contrast to a more purely dynamic view of mind in which the fundamental structures of personality are drives and the defenses against their direct expression, with anxiety signaling the failure of defense structures to contain unacceptable impulses. . . . [Relational models view] psychopathology in terms of recurrent patterns of interpersonal behavior which are maladaptive. From this point of view the patient inevitably construes and constructs relationships in the context of his or her past interpersonal experience, with an emphasis on the particularly powerful shaping effects of early experience. Conflict is seen as arising in the context of interpersonal relationships as the result of conflicting wishes in relation to others. (pp. 117–119, emphasis in original)

The selection and suitability criteria for working in brief psychotherapy with patients when using a relational model are less stringent, as there is less demand on the patient, especially in terms of confrontation of resistances and defenses. Correspondingly, more weight is given to the impact of the therapist's personality characteristics and to the unique interpersonal and intersubjective field that emerges in the therapeutic relationship. There is still the basic idea of bringing to light warded-off material, but the healing value ("corrective emotional experience" to use Alexander's 1946 term) of the therapeutic relationship is seen as being of equal or greater importance. Messer and Warren (1995) highlight some of the epistemological implications of the relational model:

This understanding, as well as the diminution of the therapist's authority as the final arbiter of reality, is expressed in the idea of participant-observation. In this view. . . . the therapist is seen as inexorably involved in the interpersonal and intersubjective system of patient and therapist, and therefore is accorded no categorically distinct access to reality. The therapist is placed in the paradoxical position of observing the patient's drama, which includes the therapist, and participating in that drama in an ongoing, active way. Thus, the patient's experience always includes the characteristics of the therapist as they are construed by the patient; this is differentiated from the idea of the patient projecting onto the blank screen of the classical Freudian analyst, who can impartially observe the manifestations of the transference relationship. (p. 148)

There have been many reports of how different forms of brief psychodynamic therapy have helped people come to grips with warded-off intrapsychic and interpersonal conflicts and thus achieve greater peace of mind, happiness in relationships, success at work, and the ability to say good-bye. Although the data are not without complication, the overall direction of the findings has been summarized by Hoyt (1985b):

There has been controversy in the short-term therapy literature about patient selection, therapeutic techniques, and expected outcomes. . . . Simply stated, the "conservative" position has been that brief treatment generally is appropriate only for the mildly and recently distressed, that techniques should be supportive rather than uncovering or anxiety-producing, and that expected results are basically superficial and symptom suppressive. The "radical" position, on the other hand, is just what the name literally implies: "going to the root"; the radical view is that the skillful clinician working within an explicitly short-term treatment framework can use a full range of psychodynamic methods with a variety of neurotic patients, often achieving some genuine and lasting personality modifications as well as symptomatic relief. While there is more research to be done, the general thrust of the evidence is clear: Many patients benefit from brief, focused, psychodynamic therapy. (p. 95)

Short-term dynamic psychotherapy, of course, is not for everyone. As research suggests, it requires a reasonably functional and psychologically minded patient with a grip on reality and an ability to tolerate painful emotional material. The patient also has to be available to attend sessions regularly. It is also not a panacea, because there are many biological, social, situational, and existential factors besides intrapsychic dynamics that may require clinical attention. It is also important to remember that for psychodynamic psychotherapy to be effective, regardless of whether it is short term or more extended, insight must serve as a vehicle and not as a final destination. That is, the real question is not how far back does a problem go but how much farther will it be carried forward? As one enthusiast for intensive short-term dynamic therapy has put it:

Intrinsic in short-term therapy's technique is the appeal to the individual to take action. How to change? The answer is part and parcel of the therapy's technique: the challenge to the defenses and the focus on your buried feelings exhort you to go from a passive to an active stance, to take charge of the way you look at life and deal with your emotions. (Zois, 1992, p. 212)

The following case vignette illustrates some aspects of an integrated short-term psychodynamic approach.

The Case of the Forlorn Lover

David was a 52-year-old man who sought therapy a few months after his lover died of AIDS. On the telephone, he tensely asked whether I was prejudiced against working with homosexuals. When I answered that I was not, he said he would see me at the appointment time I had offered.

He arrived a few minutes early, neatly dressed in tie and coat, coming from his job as an office manager where he had worked for many years. He spoke slowly with great control—formal, severe, constricted—as he described his dilemma. He had never been close to anyone, he reported. He had grown up in an emotionally cold European household and had then spent many years as a monk in a religious order. Finally, he had left and eventually made his way to San Francisco. He was accepting of his sexual orientation and spent most of his offwork time among gays and lesbians because of greater compatibility and to avoid discrimination. He had adopted a lifestyle of occasional brief sexual encounters until he met Richard. It was difficult for him even to speak his late friend's name, the loss was so painful. Several times he started to choke up, would put his hand over his face, and recompose himself.

Near the end of our first session, I asked him why he had come to therapy, what did he want to accomplish? "The pain is so great I can't stand it, but damn him, he made me feel and now I don't want to go back to that cold life I had before. I'm lost." He cried a bit, then pulled himself together. He remarked that he found me kind and easy to talk with, and that he was relieved that I had directly answered his question about possible antigay prejudice because his insurance restricted whom he might be able to see. He asked if he could have an appointment to come back. When I agreed

and asked when he would like to return, he indicated that his work schedule would require a 2-week interval between sessions. We set an appointment. (This time frame would also allow him to better regulate the intensity of whatever might transpire in our meetings, I thought, but did not share this with him.)

Over the next three sessions, David gradually told me more about his relationship with Richard. The telling was slow and painful. Several times, when he felt a wave of emotion, he would either close his eyes and tremble until it passed, or he would set his jaw and actively suppress his feelings. He was grieving at a pace that seemed tolerable for him while I mostly listened and occasionally asked leading questions. His level of tension and control was remarkable. He would make sure that the sessions stopped exactly on time. When I was a few minutes late to begin, he became especially cold and distant. When I commented that he seemed "somewhat tense," he paused until he was composed and then told me that he was "furious inside." I said I was sorry for the lateness and added:

THERAPIST: It is remarkable how you are able to keep your feelings in.

PATIENT: Yes, I can eliminate someone from my emotions. I am well trained not to feel.

THERAPIST: Yes, but to do that would render me useless to you. And that wouldn't be good for you.

He looked at me and palpably reconnected.

In the next two sessions, David hesitantly revealed more details about Richard, including various complaints about his drinking and bouts of irritability. David then became increasingly unforthcoming. I asked why.

PATIENT: If I talk more about him and let myself grieve then the images and memories might fade and I will have nothing left. . . . (Silence)

THERAPIST: You're trying to hold on to him in your mind the way some people keep a room exactly like it was the day someone died. It's like a museum, as though time can be frozen. . . . But it can't.

PATIENT: Oh, God, yes, that's it. (*He cries and then recomposes himself.*)

THERAPIST: So, what are you going to do?

PATIENT: I want to go forward, but I don't know how. Oh, I do, there are other people, but I'm scared.

THERAPIST: Of what?

PATIENT: Of getting hurt again.

THERAPIST: Then go slow, when you're ready. But life is in front of you.

He continued his mourning process. He also began to experiment over the next several weeks, attending a dance club, having supper with someone, even asserting himself at his workplace and refusing to acquiesce to things he felt were unfair. He was well aware of his pattern of "stuffing" his feelings and still often did so when threatened or hurt, but with increased cognizance he also sometimes expressed himself more. He even occasionally smiled and told stories that revealed a growing tenderness in his relations with others, including a new willingness to forgive and to remain involved with people rather than "eliminating" them if they were sometimes inconsiderate or annoying. He began to exercise and lost a few "extra" pounds that he had been carrying, all in preparation for the possibility of finding a new mate.

Follow-Up and Comment. This case might best be described as "eclectic–integrative" (Messer & Warren, 1995) and falling within the "expressive–supportive" range of brief dynamic therapies (Pinsker, Rosenthal, & McCullough, 1991). Attention was paid to exploring the patient's warded-off feelings, his images of self and others, and ways his defenses and relationship patterns were repeated with the therapist. Although he was largely resistant to discussing possible connections between his family-of-origin experiences and his current functioning, he gained some insight, experienced support and a renewed connection with another (male) human being, and learned to tolerate some of the painful feelings that he had tried to stifle. As one might expect, therapy termination was not easy for David. Relinquishing the therapist reminded him of losing Richard and also meant giving up a person that he had learned to trust and felt at ease talking with, but by the 12th therapy session he felt strong enough to go forward and so stopped treatment as planned. Consistent with Mann's (1973) model, themes of unresolved mourning, activity versus passivity, and independence versus dependence were prominent throughout the therapy and especially during the explicit termination phase. Indeed, there was a countertransference "pull" to extend treatment (see Hoyt & Farrell, 1984), but I did not yield to that impulse and we ended our meeting. David largely accomplished his goals for treatment—to get through the pain and to resume moving toward people rather than retreating into isolation. I encouraged him to return to therapy as needed, and he agreed to do so.

Redecision Therapy and Transactional Analysis

Eric Berne originated the transactional analysis (TA) school of therapy (Berne, 1961, 1972) out of his desire to help patients see more quickly their own role in their personal difficulties. He had been trained as a psychoanalyst, but found the psychoanalytic process too slow and ineffective. Although TA involves a complicated and comprehensive model of human development, intrapsychic organization, and interpersonal dynamics, there are three popular and readily accessible ideas from TA with which Berne is most identified: (1) the "I'm OK, You're OK" matrix of existential positions pertaining to how one regards self and others[3]; (2) the Parent–Adult–Child conceptualization of personality ego states (the progenitor of various "Inner Child" theories); and (3) the "Games People Play" (Berne, 1964) idea of recognizing many of the ulterior motivations behind dysfunctional relationship patterns.

Combining some of the theory of TA with Gestalt techniques plus many of their own innovations, Robert and Mary Goulding (1978; M. Goulding & R. Goulding, 1979) developed what they call redecision therapy. Until then, although TA was more empowering of clients in that it emphasized choice and ego functions, it still lacked an "action" component, and it largely involved "talking about" problems. The Gouldings' unique "redecision" approach is built on the theory that as children, people often adopt certain attitudes, making key life decisions (such as "Don't feel," "Don't think," "Don't be a child," "Don't grow up," "Don't be close," "Don't be important," "Don't enjoy," "Don't be") in order to survive or adapt to perceived and often veridical parental pressures.[4] In their model of therapy, the patient reenters and reexperiences the pathogenic scene as a child, via imagery and Gestalt work, and with the encouragement and support of the therapist makes a redecision that frees the patient from the pernicious injunction that he or she had earlier accepted and internalized. Rather than working within a psychodynamic transference model, in which the therapist becomes a participant-observer "object," the patient is encouraged to do two-chair Gestalt work in which he or she "becomes" the pathogenic parent (extrojecting the introject, so to speak) and then engages in a powerful dialogue in which he or she experiences and reclaims a sense of power, self-determination, and well-being. "I'm OK and will take care of myself even if you don't think I'm OK." There is implicit the idea of state-dependent learning (and relearning), the work being conducted in the voice of the present tense in order to bring to life how the patient is carrying the

conflict. A powerful combination of affect and insight is involved, with support and behavioral anchors maintaining the gains achieved.

Robert Goulding (1989; M. Goulding & R. Goulding, 1979; see also Hoyt, 1995b; Hoyt & Goulding, 1989; Kadis, 1985) describes a thinking structure to guide work in redecision therapy. Although many important details go beyond the scope of the present discussion, it should be noted that each of the following main headings is an essential feature for making this approach brief and effective:

1. *Contact,* forming an alliance with the patient.
2. *Contract,* constructing the focus or goal of treatment in a way that can be specified and achieved.
3. *Con,* emphasizing patients' power and responsibility by confronting their efforts to disown autonomy through various ways they attempt to fool ("con") themselves and therapists into believing that others control their thoughts, feelings, and behavior or with disingenuous claims of "trying" to make changes.
4. *Chief bad feelings, thoughts, behaviors, and psychosomatics,* identifying the painful or problematic counterproductive symptoms.
5. *Chronic games, belief systems, and fantasies,* clarifying the interpersonal and intrapsychic ways symptoms are maintained.
6. *Childhood early decisions,* bringing to vivid awareness a reexperience of childhood feelings via the imaginal reliving of an early pathogenic scene, including recognition of the chief parental messages (injunctions and counterinjunctions), childhood script formation, and stroking (reinforcement) patterns.
7. *Impasse resolution,* including redecisions, ego state decontamination and reconstruction (involving the strengthening of distinctions between Parent–Adult–Child functions), reparenting, and other techniques.

8. *Maintaining the victory,* including anchoring the patient's new and healthier ways of responding, making changes in stroke (reinforcement) patterns, and forming plans for how to use the redecision in the future.

Consistent with the question Eric Berne would ask himself before each session, "What can I do to cure this patient today?" (reported in Goulding & Goulding, 1979), the Gouldings have developed Berne's concept of *contractual therapy* and ask patients, as they begin each treatment session, *"What are you willing to change today?"* In this one pithy sentence, the key elements of brief therapy all occur! Here they are, spelled out (from Hoyt, 1990, pp. 125–126):

What [specificity, target, focus]
are [active verb, present tense]
you [self as agent, intrapsychic, personal functioning]
willing [choice, responsibility, initiative]
to change [alter or be different, not just "work on" or "explore"]
today [now, in the moment]
? [inquiry, open field, therapist receptive but not insistent]

The question focuses the therapist and the patient on making rapid changes. Although the therapist plays an important role in skillfully setting the context and guiding the client, there is ever present a strong emphasis on here-and-now patient autonomy and empowerment—it is the patient who sets the contract, the patient who does the work, and the patient who reaps the benefits. The following vignette illustrates this approach, which combines the theory of injunctions with Gestalt techniques "so that the patient does a great deal of experiential work *and* has a good understanding of his place in his life script, [and] is more likely to change both his behavior and his feelings" (R. Goulding, 1983, p. 634). As Mary Goulding (1990) has written, attention to contract plus redecision helps get the important work done fast.

The Case of the Woman Who Stood Up for Herself

Maria, who was 25 years old, came to therapy complaining of "insecurity" and "low self-esteem" in her relationships with men as well as in her work performance. She needed to gather her confidence to move on in her adult life. She already had some understanding that many of her insecurities stemmed from her relationship with her verbally abusive, highly critical father. "I know he did this to me," she said, "but what can I do about it?" It appeared that she needed an experience that would separate her from her past, that would "empower" her, a shift out of the "victim" position. She "knew" her father was still living in her head ("It's an old tape"), but so what?

By the end of our first meeting she had achieved several important steps:

1. Good contact with the therapist, establishing a sense of safety and working alliance.
2. Increased awareness that her pattern of low self-esteem was a carryover from how her father had treated her.
3. A greater sense of her present role or personal autonomy; that is, she could see more clearly that she did the putdowns to herself, that the origin of her problem may have been in childhood with her father but that he was not "making" her feel bad now—she was.

As the session drew near an end, I remarked: "So what you want to do, so to speak, is to get his critical voice out of your head, right?" She agreed, and the contract was made specific: to stop putting herself down and, instead, to give herself due credit and not let others demean her.

Conditions were ripe for redecision work. At our second meeting, I reiterated the contract to make sure it was still what she wanted. Maria was then asked to give an example of a recent time when she felt lacking in confidence and self-esteem. She did, and was then asked how she felt in that situation and what she had said in her head about herself and the other person. She had felt scared, she had said to herself, "I can't do anything right," and she had said about the other person, "He is mad and doesn't like you." I then said: "You feel scared, you think you can't do anything right, and he is mad at you. How does that fit in with your childhood? What do you think of?"

Maria recalled a time when she was about 6 years old. She had spilled juice in the living room, and her father was chastising her for it. I asked her to stay with the scene, to imagine it vividly, to really get into it. "Let yourself be 6 years old again and go back there, see the room and the juice on the rug and all the details, and let yourself feel yourself being that scared 6-year-old girl." Maria paused and as she recalled and "got into" the scene, one could see her get smaller and shrink into herself.

I then said to her, "Now sit in this other chair over here [Maria changed seats], and in this chair be your father, looking at the juice on the rug and being furious." With a little prompting, Maria got into the role. I then proceeded to conduct a brief "Parent interview" (McNeel, 1976), asking the "Father" his name and occupation and asking questions to evoke "his" feelings and thoughts about the little girl who in the scene would be cowering in front of him. "He" was angry and did not like to have to clean up the mess, but as he talked more it became clear that he was not all that ferocious and that he actually did love the girl, too.

I then had Maria switch back to the 6-year-old seat and from there tell her father that she was scared and that she did not like it when he yelled at her. "I'm only a little kid and I make mistakes, but I'm not bad and you shouldn't yell at me," she spontaneously added. "Yeah," I said. "Good. That's right. Stand up and tell him again. Let him know that he's not going to hurt you, and that you're OK even if you sometimes make mistakes." The little girl stood up for herself.

When she seemed done, I said, "Good job. Notice how strong you feel. Now, as you come back to yourself in the present you'll remember whenever you need to, how it feels to stand up."

Follow-Up and Comment. The role playing had a powerful effect. Using the three questions, "How do you feel? What do you say about yourself? What do you say about the other person?" as a kind of affect bridge back to an early scene often works to rapidly access a pathogenic (perhaps screen) memory, taking a different and quicker route than waiting for a transference neurosis to fully bloom. The two-chair work then allows a reworking or redecision, a new and healthier resolution of the impasse. For this patient, this was a turning point, a casting off of the "Don't Be a Child" and "Don't Be Important" injunctions she had earlier internalized. Therapy continued for another three visits, the first two occurring weekly and the last one occurring 1 month later, as the patient made plans and applied (worked through) her "breakthrough" in a variety of current life situations. With support, reminders, and practice, she learned to discount herself less and less. Her treatment goals of enhanced confidence and self-esteem were well met and demonstrated in a variety of contexts.

Students of comparative psychotherapies may see various points of contact between redecision therapy and other approaches (see Hoyt, 1995b, 1997), depending on which set of theoretical "lenses" they prefer. As Elliott (2001; Elliott & Greenburg, 1997) has noted, two-chair enactments, which can be considered a process-directive form of experiential therapy, help treatment to be brief by involving the client as an active change agent, by emphasizing the client's own dialectical (meaning-making) processes, and by focusing on clear goals identified by the client. Psychodynamically minded clinicians will appreciate the role of "insight," the redecision process involving the making conscious of something previously out of awareness—yielding what a cognitive-behaviorist might term a "cognitive restructuring" or "schema change." The primary mechanism is not interpretation of a transference, however, but is having a new experience ("redecision") via a reenactment of an early scene guided by the therapist. An Ericksonian might notice the "hypnotic confusion technique" ("in this chair be your father") and the protherapeutic labeling of her physical experience ("stand up and tell him"). Solution-focused therapists (following de Shazer, 1985, 1988) may appreciate the redecision therapist stroking the Natural Child as the evocation and amplification of exceptions to the problem pattern. Readers acquainted with narrative therapy (White, 1995; White & Epston, 1990) may see connections between the "Parent interview" (McNeel, 1976) and "internalized other interviewing" (Epston, 1993; Tomm, Hoyt & Madigan, 1998); the Gestalt two-chair part of the redecision process can also be seen, from the narrative perspective, as an "externalization of the problem" with enhancement of the client's sense of personal autonomy. As the title of one of the Gouldings' (1978) books put it, *The Power Is in the Patient.* The client is seen as competent to resolve her own problem without having to rely upon an outside expert to explain or reveal "the truth."

In all these formulations, explanation may lead to recognition, but experience leads to change. Can one really "go back"—via role playing, imagery, or transference enactment? Of course not—there is no time but the present. But "what is important," as Mary Goulding (1997) has written, "is that the client recover from the past, real and imagined, and go on to a fulfilling life" (p. 87).

Ericksonian, Strategic, and Solution-Focused Approaches to Brief Therapy

We shall now consider a number of creative methods that, in varying ways, derive their inspiration from the life and work of the remarkably innovative psychiatrist Milton H. Erickson, who seems to have emerged sui generis as a therapeutic genius (see Haley, 1973, 1994). They all have in common the idea that the client's complaints and symptoms should be taken seriously, as the target of treatment, not just as a "symbol" or "screen" for something else (which the therapist would divine). Unlike most clinicians of his time, who felt that the therapist should not deliberately attempt to influence the patient, Erickson held that it was the therapist's responsibility to direct the client and to "make something happen" that would promote the client's treatment goals. As Betty Alice Erickson (2001) (Milton's daughter and herself a skilled clinician and teacher) has written:

We used to operate under the premise that symptom removal was unimportant and possibly somewhat dangerous. Symptoms were not only generally unimportant, but dealing with them, "curing them," could obscure the real problem, which was to be found in the character and personality of the patient. Insight into problems was necessary because problems were the result of repression. It was the therapist's job to interpret and help the patient to understand causal factors because real change could not occur without that understanding. The unconscious, the source of problems, was a place full of negative forces, hostile and aggressive. . . .

All of these "new" ways of doing therapy were not necessarily "new" with Erickson. Even Freud, the father of long-term psychoanalysis, cited some of his own cases of brief therapy with a great deal of pride. . . . However, Erickson has received a great deal of the credit for transforming the face of psychotherapy and rightfully so. He was a master of brief therapy. He knew that merely changing, not even removing but just altering, a symptom could lead to deep and long-lasting changes. He understood the unconscious was a benign influence, discounted the importance of insight as a necessary component of change, and took full responsibility for initiating change. He also not only involved family members in therapy, but he would do therapy with one to produce changes in another. But

Erickson was only a part of the creation of the radical changes that have happened in psychotherapy. (pp. 52–53)

Milton H. Erickson

Erickson (1901–1980) overcame great personal adversities (such as paralytic polio) to develop a hypnosis–based approach oriented toward growth and problem solving via utilization of whatever assets the patient might bring to therapy. Erickson's work has directly or indirectly had a tremendous influence on many schools of therapy, including hypnotherapy, family therapy, and various strategic interactional approaches. For more information, see Erickson's (1980) four-volume *Collected Papers* as well as several excellent books about his concepts and techniques, such as those by Haley (1973, 1994), Havens (1989), Lankton and Lankton (1983), O'Hanlon (1987), Zeig (1982), and Zeig and Lankton (1988); the videotapes *Milton H. Erickson, M.D.: Explorer in Hypnosis and Therapy* (Haley & Richeport-Haley, 1993) and *Celebrating Milton H. Erickson, M.D.* (Erickson Foundation, 2001) also provide nice introductions.

It is especially difficult to summarize Ericksonian strategic therapy because it is so individualistically based on the talents of particular patients and therapists—a situation that also makes systematic research quite problematic. What characterizes Ericksonian work? Lankton (1990) explains:

> The Ericksonian strategic approach is a method of working with clients emphasizing common, even unconscious natural abilities and talents. Therapy goals are built upon the intelligence and health of individuals. It works to frame change in ways that reduce resistance, reduce dependency upon therapy, bypass the need for insight, and allow clients to take full credit for changes. Most problems are not viewed as internal pathologies but as the natural result of solving developmental demands in ways that do not fully work for the people involved. The Ericksonian strategic approach is distinctive in that it is associat-

ed with certain interventions upon which it relies heavily during extramural assignments and therapy sessions. These include skill building homework, paradoxical directives, ambiguous function assignments, indirect suggestions, hypnosis, reframing, metaphors, and therapeutic binds. These are not so much interventions as characteristic parts of the therapist's interactions with clients. As such they are used to motivate clients to actively participate in changing the way they live with themselves and others. (p. 364)

Lankton (1990) goes on to underscore that the Ericksonian approach emphasizes creative reorganization of relationships rather than a resistance-stimulating focus on diagnosing pathology. Noting that clients tend to follow suggestions that are most relevant to them, he also emphasizes that strategic therapy is interested in getting patients to take action outside the therapist's office:

> It is from the learning brought by new actions and not from insight or understanding that change develops. Consequently, a client's understanding or insight about a problem is not of central importance. The matter of central importance is the client's participation in new experiences and transactions that congeal developmentally appropriate relational patterns. (p. 365)

Haley (1994) also emphasizes Erickson's strong preference for using client's positive strengths for problem-solving action rather than attempting to increase "insight" via the making of psychodynamic interpretations about painful experiences:

> Let me summarize some of the differences between Erickson and the therapists of his time. . . . He focused on a presenting problem when they did not. He sought a single-session therapy when he could, and he never argued that long-term therapy was better or deeper. He used auxilliary personnel. He was personally involved. He did not make interpretations or provide insight. Other therapists were helping people remember every miserable

moment in their past, and they considered that helping people forget was wrong. Erickson induced amnesia for present and past events. He accepted what clients offered and did not correct their ideas prematurely. He made home visits. Finally, he did not merely offer reflection, but took action and gave directives. (p. 187)

For Lankton (1990), Erickson's work has seven defining characteristics:

1. *Nonpathology-based model.* Problems are seen as part of, and a result of, attempts at adaptation; symptoms are essentially natural (but limiting) responses of unique individuals.
2. *Indirection.* This concerns itself with helping an individual or members of a family discover talents and resources, options, and answers, seemingly without the aid of the therapist.
3. *Utilization.* Whatever the patient brings to the office (understandings, behaviors, motivations) is used as part of the treatment.
4. *Action.* Clients are expected and encouraged to quickly get into actions related to desired goals—a basic ingredient of most successful brief therapies regardless of theoretical orientation (Budman, Friedman, & Hoyt, 1992).
5. *Strategic.* The therapist takes responsibility for influencing the patient and is active in setting or initiating the stages of therapy.
6. *Future orientation.* The focus is on action and experience in the present and future rather than the past.
7. *Enchantment.* Treatment engages the mind, appeals to the patient, and captures the ear of the listener.[5]

Ericksonian interventions require careful attention to the three principles of (1) proper evaluation and creative planning, (2) cultivating and ensuring patient commitment, and (3) emphasizing patient strengths and tailoring treatment to the individual (K.

Erickson, 1988). The importance of how rather than why is also emphasized by Zeig (1990, 2002b), who stresses the utility of building on positive change and the accessing of the unconscious mind as a health-seeking source of solutions. He, too, values hypnosis and the tailoring and sequencing of treatment to fit the particular patient:

> The job of the therapist in Ericksonian psychotherapy can be summarized as a five-step procedure that is conducted more simultaneously than sequentially:
>
> 1. Decide what to communicate to the patient.
> 2. Decide how to communicate it. Usually this entails being indirect, but it could be the presentation of any therapeutic maneuver.
> 3. Ascertain what the patient values (i.e., the position the patient takes).
> 4. Divide the solution into manageable steps. Each step may be initiated by a therapeutic intervention.
> 5. Present the intervention within a therapeutic sequence, tailoring the intervention to fit the patient's values. This usually entails a three-step procedure: moving in small, directed Steps; Intervening; and Following Through. This procedure has been tabbed "SIFT." (Zeig, 1990, p. 373)

An "Ericksonian" perspective can be appreciated in a wide range of interventions:

1. The indirection of a police officer asking for a cup of coffee as a way of separating a domestically disputing couple (Everstine & Everstine, 1983), or the charming Japanese folktale (retold by de Shazer, 1991b) of a villager who, unable to warn his neighbors of an impending tidal wave, sets their hillside terraces on fire so that they will rush up the mountain to battle the flames and thus inadvertently be saved from drowning.
2. The use of imagery and hypnosis to construct more useful realities (Andreas & Andreas, 1989; Bandler & Grinder,

1982; Erickson, Rossi, & Rossi, 1976; Lankton & Lankton, 1983).

3. Instructing and motivating with teaching stories and metaphoric communications (Gordon, 1978; Rosen, 1982).

4. The use of provocation to challenge and motivate patients (Farrelly & Brandsma, 1974), including a last-ditch (and successful) effort to motivate a prideful patient out of a deep funk with humiliating taunts (Haley, 1973).

5. Prescribing ordeals, symptoms, and other paradoxical maneuvers (Haley, 1984; Selvini-Palazzolli, Cecchin, Prata, & Boscolo, 1978; Weeks, 1991) to get patients to abandon undesirable behaviors.

6. Assigning ambiguous tasks (such as having a couple climb a nearby peak or visit a botantical garden) to structure a decision-making experience or elicit an unconscious understanding (Furman & Ahola, 1992; Lankton & Lankton, 1986).

7. Providing directives to circumvent and alter the conflict-generating rules that govern relationships;

8. Using a woman's existing knowledge of how to make lines and circles to teach her how to write, or using a psychiatric hospital patient's belief that he was Jesus Christ by having him do carpenter work (!), or directing an isolated woman with a "green thumb" to grow and give African violet plants to thousands of people to reconnect her to the larger community (Haley, 1994; O'Hanlon & Hexum, 1990).

The basic principle underlying all these techniques and methods is utilization. The essential paradigmatic shift is from deficits to strengths, from problems to solutions, from past to future (Fisch, 1990, 1994), using whatever the patient brings in the service of healthful change. Ericksonian epistemology is pragmatic and "emergent," the therapist and client co-creating a useful worldview (Lankton & Lankton, 1998). For Erickson, the basic problem was not so much one of pathology or defect but *rigidi-*

ty, the idea that people get "stuck" by failing to use a range of skills, competencies, and learnings that they have but are not applying. Various interventions are thus designed to get people to have experiences that put them in touch with their latent or overlooked abilities. As Erickson and colleagues (1976) said: "Patients have problems because their conscious programming has too severely limited their capacities. The solution is to help them break through the limitations of their conscious attitudes to free their unconscious potential for problem solving" (p. 18).

Even a simple and relatively direct approach can have Ericksonian elements. Remembering how little can actually be conveyed through a single case presentation (including tone, timing, and nonverbal communication), consider the following report (adapted from Hoyt, 1993b; see also Hoyt, 1995c).

The Case of the Baseball Fan

Sam was a 67-year-old man when I met him sitting in a wheelchair next to his wife in the waiting room of the HMO psychiatry department. He had been referred by his internist: "Post-stroke. Fear of falling." When I introduced myself and shook hands I could see that he was a pleasant and engaging man. He had not shaved in a few days, was casually dressed, and was wearing an Oakland A's baseball cap. His wife immediately began to talk (a lot) and quickly told me that Sam could walk but was afraid to. He had come into the building on his own, then gotten into the wheelchair. She was nice and trying to be helpful, but I sensed that it would be useful to have some time with the patient alone, so I asked: "Do you want to walk or ride to my office?" He replied: "I'll take a ride, at least this time."

As I pushed him around the corner and down the corridor, we talked baseball—about a recent trade and how the game had gone that day. His remarks showed a good knowledge of the game and an alert, up-to-date interest. I asked questions, and we connected as we talked.

At my office door I stopped and asked him to take a few steps into my office and use a regular chair, so that I would not have to move the furniture around—an indirect approach that used his natural courtesy to bypass discussion of his need for the wheelchair. He obliged. When we sat down I asked, "So, what's up?" I learned that he was a retired mechanic and printing pressman. He had suffered a stroke 3 years earlier, with a residual partial paralysis of one arm and leg. He had grown "too damn dependent" on his wife, he said, but could no longer drive and had considerable difficulty walking. "I sure miss Dr. Jarrett," he interjected, referring to his former internist who had himself retired a few years earlier. When he told me what Dr. Jarrett would have said to get him moving, I "borrowed" the good doctor's mantle of authority and replied: "Took the words right out of my mouth."

Sam went on to tell me that he wanted to go to an upcoming A's game his sons had invited him to, but he had to first overcome his great fear of falling because "I get so worried and down that I freeze up." He knew how to fall safely (protecting his head and softening the fall) but was fearful because "I'm not sure what would happen to me if I fell and no one was around. I might not be able to get back up." (By coincidence, I had the night before read my then 4-year-old son a story [Peet, 1972] about a series of animals that each gets stranded, culminating with an elephant stuck on his back until an ant he befriended rescues him with the help of an ant hoard.)

Sam was a practical man with a predicament. After ascertaining that he was not worried about safety or embarrassment, I suggested: "I'll tell you what. Let's do a little experiment. I'll be you, you be the coach, and teach me how to get up." I then proceeded to sort of throw myself on the floor in front of him. He got right into it, advising me, "No, turn the other way, get up first on three points," etc. I said, "Let's try it with

my arm not working," and held it limply against my side. For the next 8 to 10 minutes I repeatedly got down on the floor and Sam instructed me on how to get myself up again.

Back in my chair, I asked him if he wanted to "try it" there in my office or wait until he got home—an "illusion of alternatives" (Watzlawick, 1978) with the underlying implication that he would perform the action. He chose to wait until he was home but offered to show me "some exercises I can still do." I watched and then asked him to "stand and do a little walking just so I can see how you do." I opened the office door and we proceeded into the corridor. We slowly made our way up and down the hallway, with my remarking a couple of times "Good," and "Nice, better than I expected." As we went up and down the hallway I switched back to baseball, asking him about the game he was planning to attend with his sons. "Where are you going to park? Which ramp will you take?" I painted aloud a vivid picture of father and sons entering the baseball stadium as we made our way up and down the hallway a couple of times.

Back in my office he expressed concern about his wife. She was trying to be helpful but was wearing out both herself and Sam with her watchfulness. "Maybe you could talk to her, too," he asked. I said I would be glad to "when you begin to do more walking on your own so that I'll really be able to convince her to back off." He understood and agreed to practice his falling and getting up, and we playfully bargained about how many times he would do it a day, settling on twice a day to start and then three times a day until I saw him in 2 weeks.

Before leaving my office I added, "You know, I think it's really important that you go to that game with your sons if you can. I know you want to, but I think it will be even more important for them. Someday they will look back and remember going to the game with you, you know what I mean?" Sam did not know exactly how baseball was in my blood, my history of going to games with my father, but he knew I was saying something heartfelt and important. It spoke to him: "I'm sure going to give it my best."

Follow-Up and Comment. When next I saw Sam he proudly walked into my office, slowly. He had been practicing and was eagerly anticipating going to the game the next week with his sons. I then brought his wife into the session and we talked about ways she could help by doing things and ways she could help by not doing things. Two weeks later, he told me about going to the game and his plans to go to another one. He also expressed the desire for more activity, and I suggested attending an older adults therapy group (see Hoyt, 1993a) as well as some other outings with neighbors and former coworkers. He followed through on these suggestions, and I remained available if and when he might again request to meet with me.[6]

Sam's worries about falling were taken seriously. The approach here was highly pragmatic, strategies being directed toward quickly getting the patient walking. It was helpful and felt natural to temporarily reverse roles, Sam becoming the teacher/coach rather than the humbled stroke patient. This was morale restoring and opened possibilities for change. The hallway walk into the ballpark was hypnotic and future oriented. His desire for assistance in managing his wife was used to further promote treatment compliance. Part of effective brief therapy is deciding what paths not to take. Exploring Sam's concerns about failing powers and limited mortality were issues that might be worthwhile (and would be addressed in the older-adults group), but first helping Sam to regain his confidence in walking and being able to get up when he fell enhanced the quality of his life and put him in a stronger position to realistically appraise his future options. This is what Sam and his wife wanted. Being alert to and using whatever

resources are available in the service of the patient's therapeutic needs—including the therapist's own personal experiences with baseball, inverted elephants, and father–son relations—is what I take Erickson and Rossi (1979) to mean when they suggest: "To initiate this type of therapy you have to be yourself as a person. You cannot imitate somebody else, but you have to do it in your own way" (p. 276).

Strategic Therapy: Jay Haley and the Mental Research Institute

Jay Haley was studying communication with Gregory Bateson's group at the Veterans Administration in Menlo Park, California, in the early 1950s when he, John Weakland, and Gregory Bateson began to visit Erickson. (Many of their conversations are transcribed in the three-volume *Conversations with Milton H. Erickson, M.D.*, which Haley [1985] subsequently edited.) Inspired by Erickson and brilliant in his own right, Haley went on to author a number of important books about the therapeutic use of strategy and power, including *Strategies of Psychotherapy* (1963), *The Power Tactics of Jesus Christ and Other Essays* (1969), *Problem-Solving Therapy* (1977), *Leaving Home* (1980/1997), *Ordeal Therapy* (1984), and *Teaching and Learning Therapy* (1996) (see also *Changing Directives: The Strategic Therapy of Jay Haley* [Zeig, 2001]). An early member of the Mental Research Institute (MRI) in Palo Alto, California—which was founded by Don Jackson, who had consulted with the Bateson group and was one of the originators of family therapy—Haley coauthored the famous "double-bind" paper (Bateson, Jackson, Haley, & Weakland, 1956). Haley later moved to the Philadelphia Child Guidance Clinic and then cofounded (with Cloe Madanes) the Family Therapy Institute of Washington, DC. More recently, he has been based in La Jolla, California, where he continues to teach, write, and make training videotapes. Although Haley's approach covers a wide variety of clinical situations, there are certain common features:

- An interactional view—the minimum unit of consideration is two people, a symptom serving some function in their relationship
- Each clinical situation is unique, and the focus is on what the client brings in
- Therapeutic influence is seen to be inevitable, so the therapist takes responsibility for directing the action and making something useful happen
- Language is appreciated, but the focus is on observable (concrete) behavior—on what people do, more than what they say.

He makes clear his preference that the therapist take charge on the first page of *Uncommon Therapy*:

> Therapy can be called strategic if the clinician initiates what happens during therapy and designs a particular approach for each problem. When a therapist and a person with a problem encounter each other, the action that takes place is determined by both of them, but in strategic therapy the initiative is largely taken by the therapist. He must identify solvable problems, set goals, design interventions to achieve those goals, examine the responses he receives to correct his approach, and ultimately examine the outcome of his therapy to see if it has been effective. The therapist must be acutely sensitive and responsive to the patient and his social field, but how he proceeds must be determined by himself. (Haley, 1973, p. 1)

On page 1 of *Problem-Solving Therapy* (Haley, 1977), he also comes right to the point:

> The therapy approach focuses on solving a client's presenting problems within the framework of the family. The emphasis is not on a method but on approaching each problem with special techniques for the specific situation. The therapist's task is to formulate a presenting symptom clearly and to design an in-

tervention in the client's social situaton to change that presenting symptom.

Haley uses common sense and plain talk to make explicit the shift toward *solvable interactional problems* rather than putative intrapsychic complexes. Thus, Haley (1977) writes:

> This is not a therapy where relationships are changed by talking about relationships but by requiring new behavior to solve a problem. . . . (p. 27)
>
> Giving directives, or tasks, to individuals and families has several purposes. First, the main goal of therapy is to get people to behave differently and so to have different subjective experiences. Directives are a way of making those changes happen. (p. 49)

And:

> If therapy is to end properly, it must begin properly—by negotiating a solvable problem and discovering the social situation that makes the problem necessary. (Haley, 1977, p. 9)

On a recent training videotape (Haley & Richeport-Haley, 2000), while he makes clear that it is behavior, not simply language, that therapists should endeavor to change, Haley also makes clear his appreciation of the interpersonal significance of subjectivity, the pragmatic relativity of "truth":

> We used to think we were going to find out The Truth. If the person had a symptom we would explore that and the past and so on and we'd come out with the explanation that was True: 'This is why the person had that symptom.' And I think more sensible people now have theories that they don't believe are true. They don't have to be true. If you have a theory that mother and father in conflict produce the child problem, that doesn't mean it's true. It means that's the best theory you can have because you can then deal with mother and father in such a way that it'll help the kid. It gives you something to do and a triangle to

be in. But that doesn't mean it's true. Truth is something else. But you need to be free to have theories that are not necessarily true but are very helpful.

Meanwhile, intercurrent with Haley's work, at the Brief Therapy Center of the MRI, John Weakland, Richard Fisch, Paul Watzlawick and Arthur Bodin (1974) published a paper titled "Brief Therapy: Focused Problem Resolution." This was followed by two seminal books, *Change: Principles of Problem Formation and Problem Resolution* (Watzlawick et al., 1974) and *The Tactics of Change: Doing Therapy Briefly* (Fisch et al., 1982). Taking a systemic perspective, they focused on what maintained the problem that brought the patient to therapy. As Weakland and Fisch (1992) explain in a chapter entitled "Brief Therapy—MRI Style":

> The interactional view of problems implies a cybernetic rather than a linear concept of causation. Therefore, with this view, it is not the origin of a problem but its persistence that is central for understanding and treatment: What unwitting behaviors function to maintain or reinforce the problem behavior, even though this is defined as undesired or undesirable? Ironically, in our clinical experience it appears over and over that some aspect of people's attempts to control or eliminate the problem—though these attempts are usually well intentioned and seemingly logical ("common sense")—constitutes the reinforcing behavior: "The 'solution' is the problem." (p. 308)

Their treatment approach, which is generally offered as a 10-session package (although patients can finish early and keep sessions "in the bank" for possible later use), follows from this conceptualization:

> Our concept of a problem is that it is a limited behavioral issue in which someone is "stuck"—although its effects may have spread widely. Our corresponding aim is to help

clients get "unstuck" so they can get on with the daily business of life as they see fit. A problem may be solved by behavioral changes—ceasing the attempted solution—or sometimes by a reevaluation of the original focus of complaint as "no problem," just one of life's daily difficulties. . . . Such interventions mainly involve suggestions for behavioral changes in the real world outside the therapy room. Usually, however, these are not direct prescriptions but depend on reframing[7] the problem situation, avoiding argument, and utilizing the clients' own preexisting ideas about people and problems—speaking the client's "language"—so as to make different problem-handling behavior appear logical and appropriate to them. Since our aim is specific behavioral change rather than intellectual understanding (which may produce no change in actual daily behavior), we do not devote much effort to clarifying and discussing the overall interactional system to those involved. (Weakland & Fisch, 1992, p. 309)

Solution-Focused (and Solution-Oriented) Therapy

Solution-focused therapy was developed in the late 1970s and 1980s by Steve de Shazer (1985, 1888) and his colleagues (see Berg, 1994; Berg & Miller, 1992; De Jong & Berg, 1997) at the Brief Family Therapy Center (BFTC) in Milwaukee, Wisconsin. de Shazer was influenced by the work of the MRI group, which in turn had been influenced by the work of the renowned psychiatrist–hypnotherapist Milton Erickson—especially Erickson's ideas about strategic intervention and the fuller utilization of clients' submerged competencies. Whereas the MRI group focused on how clients create and resolve problems, including how efforts to solve a problem sometimes actually perpetuate the problem, de Shazer and his Milwaukee-based group took a somewhat different view. They focused instead on those times (which they called "exceptions") when the presenting problem was not present, as expressed in the title of their signal counterpaper, "Brief Therapy: Focused Solution Development" (de Shazer et al., 1986).

Initially, the solution-focused approach emerged in an inductive manner, from studying what clients and therapists did that preceded clients declaring problems "solved" (or "resolved," "dissolved," or "simply no longer problems"). It was found that this happened when clients began to engage in new and different perceptions and behaviors vis-à-vis the presenting difficulty (Hoyt & Berg, 1998). This recognition led to de Shazer's "basic rules" of solution-focused therapy:

- If it ain't broke, don't fix it.
- Once you know what works, do more of it.
- If it doesn't work, don't do it again; do something different.
  (de Shazer, cited in Hoyt, 1996b, p. 314)

The basic premise is deceptively simple: Increase what works; decrease what does not work. What are the "exceptions" to the problem? What is the patient doing differently at those times when he or she is not anxious, depressed, quarreling, and so on? What has worked before? What strengths can the patient apply? What would be a useful solution? How to construct it?

Behind these apparently simple questions is a profound paradigmatic shift: competencies, not dysfunctions, are the focus; the quest is to access latent capacities, not latent conflicts. Consistent with its nonpathologizing perspective, rather than asking "How is the client stuck?" solution-focused therapists ask, "What is the client doing when they are not stuck?" The orientation is toward the future and toward the fuller appreciation and utilization of human abilities. The approach is not just technical but when taken to heart epitomizes the belief that with skillful facilitation, people have within themselves the resources necessary to achieve their goals.

Solution-focused therapy is perhaps the best known of a variety of competency-based, collaborative, future-oriented approaches. Another well-known variant is "solution-oriented" therapy (O'Hanlon, 1999; O'Hanlon & Wilk, 1987). As the titles of a number of useful books have it: *In Search of Solutions* (O'Hanlon & Weiner-Davis, 1989) and recognizing that *Some Stories Are Better Than Others* (Hoyt, 2000b), we welcome *Clues* (de Shazer, 1988) and *Keys to Solutions in Brief Therapy* (de Shazer, 1985) since *Becoming Solution-Focused in Brief Therapy* (Walter & Peller, 1992) and *Constructing Realities* (Rosen & Kuehlwein, 1996) leads to *Putting Difference to Work* (de Shazer, 1991b), *Constructive Therapies* (Hoyt, 1994a, 1996a), *Solution Talk* (Furman & Ahola, 1992), *Therapeutic Conversations* (Gilligan & Price, 1993), and *The New Language of Change* (Friedman, 1993). These may yield *Expanding Therapeutic Possibilities* (Friedman & Fanger, 1991) and *Time-Effective Psychotherapy* (Friedman, 1997), perhaps even in *Single Session Therapy* (Talmon, 1990), that will help in *Rewriting Love Stories* (Hudson & O'Hanlon, 1992), *Resolving Sexual Abuse* (Dolan, 1991), *Divorce Busting* (Weiner-Davis, 1992), *Making Friends with Your Unconscious Mind* (Hudson, 1993), providing *Family-Based Services* (Berg, 1994), *Working with the Problem Drinker* (Berg & Miller, 1992), and *Recreating Partnership* (Ziegler & Hiller, 2001)!

Clients are assisted to develop new awarenesses—not "insights" of buried pains and sorrows but of underappreciated, overlooked, perhaps forgotten hopes, skills, and resources. The focus is on enhancing "solution sight" (Hoyt, 2002). In solution-focused therapy, there is no preset length of treatment. Appointments are usually made one at a time. de Shazer reported the average length of treatment at the Brief Family Therapy Center to be 4.7 sessions (de Shazer, 1991b, pp. 57–58); in 1996, he indicated (in Hoyt, 1996b, p. 61) that the average had dropped to 3. While the therapist–client relationship may fluctuate between customer, complainant, and visitor, the concept of resistance is vitiated by the therapist taking responsibility for finding ways to work with the client's current motivation, experience, goals, ideas, values, and worldviews. The emphasis is on *solution talk,* not *problem talk.* Table 10.2 delineates some aspects of this shift.

Therapists ask certain kinds of questions to help clients focus on and "see" solutions. Here are just a few, each of which the therapist might follow with additional questions to expand clients' "solution vision" (for an extensive listing of different types and numerous examples of each, see De Jong & Berg, 1997; Hoyt, 2002; Ziegler & Hiller, 2001):

- *The Skeleton Key Question* (to elicit information about presession change or improvement): "Between now and the next time we meet, I would like you to observe, so that you can describe to me next time, what happens in your [pick one: family, life, marriage, relationship, etc.] that you want to continue to have happen." (de Shazer, 1985, p. 137)
- *The Miracle Question* (to enchant and orient toward the positive and to identify the goal of treatment): "Suppose that one night, while you were asleep, there was a miracle and this problem was solved. How would you know? What would be different?" (de Shazer, 1988, p. 5)
- *Exceptions Questions* (to identify times the presenting problem has not been present): "When in the past might the problem have happened but didn't (or was less intense or more manageable)?"
- *Endurance (or Coping) Questions* (to acknowledge difficulties and pains while still focusing on strengths and competencies): "Given all you've been through, how have you managed to keep going as well as you have?"
- *Agency (Efficacy) Questions* (to identify clients' abilities to make a difference in the desired direction): "How did you do that?" or "How did you get that to happen?"
- *Scaling Questions* (to "measure the client's own perception, to motivate and encourage, and to elucidate goals and anything else that is important to the individual client"—Berg & de Shazer, 1993, p. 9): "On a scale from 1 to 10, 1 being absolutely no [pick one: hope, motivation, progress, etc.] and 10 being com-

TABLE 10.2. Solution-Building Vocabulary

In	Out	In	Out
Respect	Judge	Forward	Backward
Empower	Fix	Future	Past
Nurture	Control	Collaborate	Manipulate
Facilitate	Treat	Options	Conflicts
Augment	Reduce	Partner	Expert
Invite	Insist	Horizontal	Hierarchical
Appreciate	Diagnose	Possibility	Limitation
Hope	Fear	Growth	Cure
Latent	Missing	Access	Defense
Assets	Defects	Utilize	Resist
Strength	Weakness	Create	Repair
Health	Pathology	Exception	Rule
Not Yet	Never	Difference	Sameness
Expand	Shrink	Solution	Problem

Note. From Hoyt (1994b, p. 4). Copyright 1994 by The Guilford Press. Reprinted by permission.

plete [hope, motivation, etc.], what number would you give your current level of [hope, motivation, etc.]? What will tell you that your level has gone up one level?"

Let's consider some excerpts from a couple therapy case (adapted from Hoyt, 2002) to see how some of these solution-focused ideas might be applied in action.

The Case of Frank and Regina

The receptionist's intake appointment note gave the clients' names, indicated their ages (29 and 30 years, respectively) and simply read, "Four months pregnant—not getting along."

When we got into my office, I remarked: "Welcome. The purpose of our meeting is to work together to find a solution to whatever brings you here today. What's up?" They mentioned that they had known each other a couple of years, were pregnant but not married, and had gotten along pretty well until recently. They then began to bicker and argue, each accusing the other of having a "bad attitude" and not doing enough. I quickly interrupted:

THERAPIST: Wait a minute! You came here because you want things to be better, don't you? (*They both nodded affirmatively*) That's why you're here. You used to get along, so you know how to—it seems you came here because you want some help figuring out how to get back to being happy together, right?

FRANK AND REGINA: Well, yeah . . .

THERAPIST: Then let me ask you, each of you—and don't get into an argument over this—on a scale of 1 to 10, how would you say your relationship is now, where "1" is "Horrible—it sucks" and "10" is "Great—couldn't be better"?

FRANK: A 2.

REGINA: Yeah, like that—a 2.

THERAPIST: OK. That gives us some room to work. Without getting into complaining, what would it take for you to think things have moved up to a 3, or even a 4? What will each of you, and the other person, be doing differently when things are getting better?

FRANK: I don't know.

REGINA: I don't know, either.

THERAPIST: Oh. OK. Let me ask you this: Suppose tonight, while you're sleeping, a miracle happens . . . and the problems that brought you here are solved! But you're sleeping, so you don't know it . . . until you wake up. Tomorrow, when you wake up, what would be some of the things you'd notice that would tell you, "Hey, things are better"?

Regina laughed, and then Frank laughed. They then sat there, looking dumbfounded, then laughed again, together. Regina spoke first:

REGINA: We'd be getting along better, not hassling.

FRANK: Yeah, we'd talk, and she wouldn't get so mad at me.

Before the window of opportunity closed, I quickly asked: "You'd be getting along—what would you be saying and doing? How about you, Regina—what would you be doing if you and Frank were getting along? And you, Frank—how would you respond to Regina, and what would you be saying to build on the positive?"

I had been quite active, interrupting them in order to direct them toward the positive. Once they were going more in the direction they said they wanted to go, I became much less directive, although still actively eliciting details and specifics that "thickened" their positive story. I inquired about "exceptions," asking about times when they had achieved some of the togetherness they sought. Whenever they began to slip back toward arguing, I gently redirected them, but did not presume to know what details and events would make their story positive. Drawing from their recall of happier times in the past and their imagination of a positive future, they seemed to be discovering and remembering—and began using—important relationship skills they already knew. They began to see each other more beneficently, slowly shifting figure and ground, moving from problem to solution.

At the end of the session, I offered a homework suggestion: "You've come up with some very good ideas about how to make things better. Between now and when we meet in a couple of weeks—and even after that—please pay attention and notice whatever you do and whatever the other person does to make things better. It may not be perfect, but try to keep track of whatever positives you or your partner do or attempt to do. When we met, I'll ask you about what you noticed."

Over the next several sessions, we focused on ways they were working better together. In one session, Frank acknowledged that "sometimes my feelings get hurt, and then I withdraw and she gets even madder." I asked their ideas about how they could handle such tense situations better ("You know yourselves and each other better than I ever could—what do you think would work for the two of you?"). Regina and Frank both suggested alternatives, and I also proffered a few ideas. We discussed back and forth what would make sense that they would be willing to try, and they playfully rehearsed a couple of options.

Whenever they reported any success, I asked for details ("Wow! How did you do that?"). They also brought up frustrations and difficulties, of course, which we discussed. I was careful, however, to keep the focus on their goals and resourcefulness. Borrowing some of Gottman's (1994) ideas about "Finding the Glory in Your Story" and Ziegler and Hiller's (2001) ideas about "Recreating Partnership," several times I asked Frank and Regina questions ("What

are some examples of ways you have compromised successfully?" "How did you make up?" "During difficult times, what are some of the things that have told you the relationship is worth pursuing?" "What did you do differently during those times you coped constructively with your frustration?") that would help highlight whatever they were doing in the direction they wanted to go. I also suggested they consider activities (such as a fun outing) that would build on the positive.

After several sessions, when Regina rated their relationship a "9" and Frank gave it a "10," I congratulated them on their good teamwork and commented (alluding to the baby): "Since you're going to be together for at least the next couple of decades, it's nice to see that you're working on the "Frank *and* Regina Story" rather than the "Frank *or* Regina Story."

In the fifth session, our last (by their choice), we reviewed their progress and how they had achieved it. We also spent a few minutes talking about challenges that were sure to come, and how they could cope:

THERAPIST: Would it be OK if I ask you a hard question?

FRANK AND REGINA: Sure—go for it.

THERAPIST: I'm glad that you're doing so well and that you're working as partners, but imagine a time in a few months after the baby's born, and you're both tired and stressed. . . . How are you going to remember then to work as a team?

FRANK: I'm sure that will happen.

REGINA: Yeah.

THERAPIST: So, how are you going to deal with it? It could be easy to get back into fighting a lot.

FRANK AND REGINA: We'll have to remember why we're together.

THERAPIST: How will you do that?

FRANK: We know we'll have difficulties, but we also know that we can solve our problems.

REGINA: Yeah. Now when we start to have an argument, we stop and remember that we're "Frank *and* Regina," and that helps us not to get into "Me *versus* You." And sometimes we talk about what we've talked about in here—how to use what you called "Solution Talk," how we used to fight and how we know how to treat each other respectfully, and how to take a time out if we need it, and how to listen to each other, and stuff like that.

Follow-Up and Comment. "Fast-forwarding" to a solution by asking the "Miracle Question" (de Shazer, 1988) does not really create a miracle, of course. Rather, it serves to disrupt a persistent negative narrative and stimulates the imagination toward creative solutions. It shifts the discourse. Patients get enchanted by the question and, with or without prompting, draw on their own wisdom and experience to create answers that are hopeful and uniquely theirs and thus more likely to occur. Various methods can then be used to promote continued changes. In solution-focused therapy, the therapist's "prime directive" is to recognize that the "client is the expert" and to help clients better access their own expertise to solve their problems (Hoyt & Berg, 1998). Every case is considered to be unique. This "poststructural revision" (de Shazer & Berg, 1992) is a nonnormative, constructivist view that emphasizes the use of language in the social construction of reality.

EVEN ONE SESSION (OR LESS) MAY BE ENOUGH (FOR NOW)

Therapy should not be "long term" or "short term." It should be sufficient, adequate, and appropriate, "measured not by its brevity or length, but whether it is efficient and effective in aiding people with their complaints or whether it wastes time" (Fisch, 1982, p. 156). Many people solve psychological problems without professional consultation. For some others, the "light touch" of a single visit may be enough, providing experience, skills, and encouragement to help them get "unstuck" and continue in their life journey. If used appropriately, such "ultra brief" treatments can promote patients' sense of self-empowerment and autonomy (versus dependency) as well as conserve limited resources for those truly requiring longer treatments.

Considerable evidence has accumulated that single-session therapy—one visit without further contact—is de facto the modal or most common length of treatment, generally occurring 20–50% of the time. Although most traditional psychotherapy training suggests that stopping after one visit is "dropping out" or "premature termination," there exists scattered through the literature anecdotal reports by leading practitioners of varying theoretical perspectives suggesting the utility of single-session therapy (SST) with selected patients. The list of authorities reporting successful one-session treatments, beginning with Freud, reads like a *Who's Who* in the psychotherapy field: Berne, Cummings, Davanloo, de Shazer, Erickson, Goulding and Goulding, Haley, Lazarus, Mahrer, Malan, O'Hanlon, Sifneos, Shapiro, Sullivan, Whitaker, Winnicott, Wolberg, Yapko, and others (see Bloom, 1981, 1992; Hoyt, 1994d; Hoyt et al., 1992; Rosenbaum et al., 1990; Talmon, 1990, 1993; Hoyt & Talmon, 1990). There are also three more systematic studies of the effectiveness of single-session therapy.

1. Medical utilization was found to be reduced 60% over 5-year follow-up after a single session of psychotherapy in a study done at the Kaiser Permanente Health Plan (the nation's largest HMO) by Follette and Cummings (1967). A second study (Cummings & Follette, 1976; see also Mumford, Schlesinger, Glass, Patrick, & Cuerdon, 1984) found the benefits of SST still in effect after 8 years and concluded that decreased medical utilization was due to a reduction in physical symptoms related to emotional stress.

2. Significant symptom improvements years later were noted by Malan, Heath, Bacal, and Balfour (1975; see also Jacobson, 1968) in 51% of "untreated" patients who had only an intake interview (which served to increase their insight and sense of personal responsibility) conducted at the Tavistock Clinic in London, and half of those patients were also judged to have made important personality modifications.

3. Patients and therapists agreed that a single treatment visit had been sufficient in 58.6% (34 of 58) of attempted SSTs in another study conducted at Kaiser Permanente by Hoyt, Rosenbaum, and Talmon (reported in Talmon, 1990). The other patients continued meeting with their therapists. On 3- to 12-month follow-ups, 88% of the SST-only patients reported either "much improvement" or "improvement" in their presenting symptoms since the session, and 65% also reported other positive "ripple" effects, figures that were slightly (and statistically insignificantly) higher than those for the 24 patients seen more than once.

There is no single method or goal for attempting SST other than being with patients and using the skills that patient and therapist bring to the endeavor. Treatments may be as varied as the patients (and therapists) and what they come to accomplish. SSTs, like all forms of psychotherapy, can occur either by default (usually when the patient stops unilaterally) or by design (when patient and therapist mutually agree that additional sessions are not then indicated). The choice of a single session (or more, or less) should, whenever possible, be left to the patient. "Let's see what we can get done today," is much more "user friendly" and likely to succeed than the resistance-stimulating, "We're only going to meet one time." Most effective SST is thus strictly not time-limited therapy—it is open-ended, the therapist mentions the possibility of one session perhaps being enough, and the patient elects to stop after one visit.

Bloom (1981) offers some suggestions for possible SSTs that could easily apply to conducting brief therapy more generally:

1. Identify a focal problem;
2. Do not underestimate client's strengths;
3. Be prudently active;
4. Explore, then present interpretations tentatively;
5. Encourage the expression of affect;
6. Use the interview to start a problem-solving process;
7. Keep track of time;
8. Do not be overambitious;
9. Keep factual questions to a minimum;
10. Do not be overly concerned about the precipitating event;
11. Avoid detours; and
12. Do not overestimate a client's self-awareness (i.e., don't ignore what may seem obvious).

Rosenbaum and colleagues (1990) also offer some useful guidelines:

1. Expect change;
2. View each encounter as a whole, complete in itself;
3. Do not rush or try to be brilliant;
4. Emphasize abilities and strengths rather than pathology;
5. Life, not therapy, is the great teacher;
6. Focus on "pivot chords," ambiguous situations that can be reframed in therapeutic ways;
7. Big problems do not always require big solutions; and
8. Terminate in a way that allows the client to realize implications and to remember and forget usefully.

A single therapy session will not be sufficient or appropriate for many patients, of course, although the following brief examples may suggest some instances in which a single visit promoted new learnings, enhanced coping and growth, and gave the patient a chance to make a productive shift or "pivot." In each case, the patient made the choice (with the therapist's assent) to complete treatment with the one session and agreed to return for additional treatment when desired.

Case 1. An elderly gentleman made an appointment in our HMO psychiatry clinic, indicating to the receptionist that his reason for seeking services was "guilt." It turned out that his wife had died in surgery the year before. He missed her. His mourning and adjustment were disrupted by his gnawing sense of guilt. He had advocated that she undergo the high-risk surgery, he said, to help her but also "for my own selfish reasons. I wanted her well so we could travel and do the things I enjoy. If I hadn't pushed her, she'd be alive today." We had a long and poignant talk. Reviewing the facts, her medical situation and prognosis (with or without surgery), the distinction between grief and guilt, her willingness to have the surgery, and "What else do you feel guilty about?" ("I wasn't always the best husband") left him feeling somewhat relieved. We discussed some practical steps he would be taking. He had a good network of support from friends and family. I then asked him what his late wife would say, or advise, if she could somehow see how he had been feeling. "She'd tell me to snap out of it. She wanted me to be happy—that's why she had the surgery." I listened, then suggested, "Perhaps every day you could do something positive, and tell yourself 'I dedicate this to her memory.'" He thought for a bit, then smiled. "I really see things differently now." He was grateful for our talk and felt no need to return.

Case 2. A ceremony was used as part of an elaborate production to help a woman "emotionally divorce" her abusive father (see Talmon, Hoyt, & Rosenbaum, 1990, pp. 45–47, for a truncated report of the case). To help consolidate her gains and demarcate a before-and-after change of status (see White & Epston, 1990), the patient (with her husband attending) read an extraordinary autobiographical plaint, played carefully selected music, and burned her father's photograph in my office. Hypnother-

apeutic "inner child" work was also done. At the end of the session and on follow-up the patient felt considerable relief in regard to her relationship with her father, but she also continued to have other psychological problems that might have benefited from additional therapy.

Although SST is obviously not a panacea or even appropriate for everyone, clinical experience and some preliminary supporting data suggest that when given the choice, many patients elect a single treatment session and find it useful, especially if the therapist is open to this possibility and oriented toward maximizing the impact of the session.

SOME STORIES ARE BETTER THAN OTHERS

As may be recalled, we earlier quoted Messer and Warren (1995, pp. 112–113) regarding the epistemological differences between what they termed the "correspondence theory" versus the "coherence theory" of truth. Simply stated, the former posits that there is one knowable truth with which our statements or descriptions can have one-to-one correspondence; the latter posits that there are multiple truths with which our statements or descriptions can accurately and meaningfully cohere. Messer and Warren go on to name some of the paradigms that describe ways relational models especially pose problems for those wanting an absolute or unequivocal answer:

Perspectivism as a philosophy of science emphasizes the observer's point of view within a particular set of contexts. *Constructivism* implies that what is known about the object of study is inevitably a function of preexisting models, theories, and assumptions. The notion of "*narrativity*" suggests that acts of perception and of knowing are prestructured and actively mediated by intrinsic requirements of coherence and human sensibility. *Participant-observation* as a method likewise stresses the involvement of the subject in the object of study. (p. 170)

These paradigms may all be seen to be part of a larger perspective, one that is sometimes placed under the rubric of *social constructionism*, (or *postmodernism*), a view that emphasizes the use of language (or "conversation") in "meaning making" and the interpersonal construction of our knowledge of reality (see de Shazer & Berg, 1992; Gergen, 1994; Hoyt, 2000a, 2001b; Watzlawick, 1984; Neimeyer & Bridges, Chapter 8, this volume). How we make sense of our worlds—the stories we tell ourselves and each other—does much to determine what we experience, our actions, and our destinies. When clients need a better story, they often come to therapy.

As I have described in *Some Stories Are Better Than Others* (Hoyt, 2000b):

> What makes some stories better than others? Ultimately, of course, the answer must come from each individual freely, lest we impose our own values or beliefs. In general terms, stories involve a plot in which characters have experiences and employ imagination to resolve problems over time. . . . From this perspective, therapy can be understood as the purposeful development of a more functional story; "better" stories are those that bring more of what is desired and less of what is not desired. . . .
>
> Aesthetics, effects, and ethics are all important. We like stories that are well told; that are vivid and eloquent; that involve the generation and resolution of some tension; that see the protagonist[s] emerge successfully, perhaps even triumphantly. A "good" story does more than merely relate "facts"; a "good story" invigorates. (pp. 19–22)

All therapists, regardless of persuasion, use their power and authority to influence clients to change their "stories" in directions thought to be helpful. Indeed, that is why they are paid. Even therapists, such as the psychodynamic drive theorists, who may believe they are "unlocking the unconscious" and "revealing the underlying truth," are selling a story. (They may also be revealing "the truth" and "unlocking the unconscious"—at least that is their story of what they're doing.) Some therapists see themselves (their story of themselves) as experts, wielding special knowledge ("insight") and power. Others may not believe they know the one "Truth" but believe they have expert knowledge regarding what the client needs and use their power to direct situations that will lead the client to what the therapist believes is needed (e.g., an emotional catharsis, a changed sense of self, or a different family relationship pattern). Others also see themselves as having expertise, but eschew the role of expert—they see their role largely as the skillful asking of questions and the arranging of contexts to help clients to recognize their own expertise.

Messer and Warren (1995) also provide an interesting discussion of what they term "the context of visions of reality." Without being able to do justice to their thoughtful discussion in this limited space, they contrast four "visions":

1. The *romantic,* in which life is an adventure or quest in which the person as hero transcends the world of experience, achieves victory over it, and is liberated from it.

2. The *ironic,* an attitude of detachment, challenging cherished beliefs, traditions, and (romantic) illusions; like the tragic vision, it emphasizes the inherent difficulties of life; there are multiple perspectives possible, so nothing is ever really complete.

3. The *tragic,* inwardly directed, full of struggle and distrust of happy endings, acknowledging the limitations of life; the clock cannot be turned back; in this view, quiet acceptance of a certain degree of despair produces wisdom.

4. The *comic,* in which life is familiar and can be controlled; effective problem solving and outward action move things from bad to better; in this view, conflict is

largely between people and their situation, not within the people, and increased capacity to perform social roles more adequately is the desired resolution.

As Messer and Warren (1995) note, psychoanalytic and psychodynamic brief treatment approaches would seem to have the most affinity with the tragic and ironic. Strategic and systemic approaches, I would add, might be situated more in the realm of the comic and perhaps the ironic. Solution-focused (and other narrative-based) approaches may be more consistent with the romantic and comic (and perhaps ironic) vision of reality. Life has its painful and tragic moments, its funniness, its adventures, and its twists. All are inevitable, but the one(s) you most prefer—the "lenses" you like to wear (or at least are trained or accustomed to)—may do a lot to influence your preference for certain ways of "storying" rather than others. One's story about one's role as therapist—as one who uses power and authority to "treat" and "fix" patients, as an operator who directs and stages contexts, as a facilitator who asks questions to promote clients' self-healing, and so on—may also go a long way toward determining which approach(es) one resonates with and chooses to apply.

A LONG FUTURE FOR BRIEF THERAPY

Brief therapy has a long history, beginning with Freud, and it appears that it will have a long future as well. The convergence of market forces, the desire of most persons for rapid relief from psychological distress, and the development of new treatment technologies augur well for the continued ascendancy of short-term therapy. HMOs, the emergence of managed care, and the continuing debate about some form of health care reform as responses to the runaway costs of health services all suggest the further expansion of brief treatment. What is

clear is that consumers, insurers, and health care professionals are all increasingly recognizing the importance of providing psychotherapeutic services that are as efficient as possible. As Shectman (1986) has said, necessity sometimes proves to be the mother of intervention. Brief therapy methods are becoming increasingly attractive, both as treatments of choice and for their value in resource conservation.

Managed care—which may be defined as various arrangements to regulate the costs, site, and/or utilization of services (Hoyt, 1995a, 2000b)—has been estimated as covering 160 million Americans in 2000, with numbers growing rapidly each year. Short-term therapy is the backbone of managed care mental health services. Cutting across various administrative systems and specific brief therapy approaches are a series of principles that characterize what Austad and Berman (1991), Austad and Hoyt (1992), Hoyt and Austad (1992), and Hoyt (1995a) have called HMO therapy. Although brief therapy (various approaches to time-effective treatment) antedated and is not the same as managed care (a term that refers to various forms of health care delivery administration), as noted earlier, the following HMO therapy principles summarize much of what constitutes effective brief psychotherapy:

1. *Rapid setting of clearly defined goals,* with an orientation toward specific problem solving.

2. *Rapid response and crisis intervention preparedness,* so that problems are dealt with before they get entrenched or produce secondary problems.

3. *Clear definition of patient and therapist responsibilities,* including an explicit understanding (sometimes called a "contract") of the purpose, schedule, and duration of treatment. The patient is encouraged to assume much of the initiative and responsibility for the work of therapy, including carrying out "homework" tasks and implementing behavioral changes outside therapy sessions.

4. *Flexible and creative use of time,* varying the frequency, length, and timing of treatment sessions according to patient needs.

5. *Interdisciplinary cooperation,* including the use of psychopharmacology when needed to restore "restorying" capacities (Hoyt, 2000b).

6. *Use of multiple formats and modalities,* with treatments sometimes involving concurrent or sequential combinations of individual, group, and/or family therapy, as well as referrals to appropriate community resources.

7. *Intermittent treatment* and a "family practitioner" model that replaces the notion of a definitive once-and-for-all "cure" with the idea that the patient can return for "serial," "episodic," or "distributed" treatment through the life cycle (Cummings & Sayama, 1995). The therapist–patient relationship may be long term although frequently abeyant; as soon as the therapist is not needed, he or she recedes into the background of the patient's life until needed again. The brief therapist operates like a road service to help people who have gotten "stuck" (Bergman, 1985) get back "on track" (Walter & Peller, 1994). But would it not be strange if, after repairing a tire, the service person jumped into the car and rode along with the individual or insisted that individual pass by the shop every week to make sure that he or she is still going okay?

8. *Accountability and results orientation,* the evaluation of services to see if work is being accomplished in an efficient manner. *Utilization review* monitors that services are not being offered wastefully; *quality assurance* makes sure treatment goals are being met.

We can expect training in brief therapy to expand dramatically in the coming years, stimulated by both the demands of consumers for more efficient mental health services and the fiscal pressures of managed care. However, although there has been some attention paid to aspects of brief ther-

apy teaching and learning—such as potential parallel processes between therapy and training (Dasberg & Winokur, 1984; Frances & Clarkin, 1981b; Hoyt, 1991), the use of manuals (Levenson & Butler, 1999), and the impact of training on skills and attitudes (Burlingame, Fuhriman, Paul, & Ogles, 1989; Henry, Schact, Strupp, Binder, & Butler, 1993; Levenson & Burg, 1999)—there has been a dearth of high-quality training for most clinicians. A study by Levenson, Speed, and Budman (1995) of psychologists in California and Massachusetts, for example, found that although most therapists report a sizable portion of their clinical work to be short-term treatment, one-third of those doing brief therapy reported having minimal training in brief therapy techniques, and more than 25% of all brief treatment hours were being conducted by clinicians with little or no formal training in the special orientation and skills of time-sensitive therapy! A more recent survey by Levenson and Evans (2000, p. 447) indicated only some improvement:

> Almost three fifths of the responding graduate school training directors indicated that their institutions offer brief therapy training (59%). This finding may be viewed as the glass being half full or half empty, depending on one's perspective. The good news is that a majority of graduate schools offer brief therapy training; the bad news is that over 40% do not, an alarmingly high percentage considering that almost 90% of psychologists report using some brief therapy in their daily practices (Davidowitz & Levenson, 1995).

Levenson and Evans (2000, p. 447) go on to report that a majority of graduate school educators indicated their brief therapy course or supervision to be cognitive-behavioral or psychodynamic in orientation, with only about one quarter checking "eclectic–integrative" (27%), "systems–strategic" (26%), or "other" (24%). (Approximately one-fourth of the educators indicated more than one theoretical orientation.) Teachers reported the most difficult training issues to involve setting limited goals, attitudinal biases in favor of long-term therapy, and selection criteria for brief therapy. As Levenson and Evans write: "In a previous study, two parameters—defining goals and a limited focus—emerged as the *sine qua non* distinguishing brief therapy from long-term therapy (Levenson & Butler, 1999). It thus appears that what the teachers view as difficult to get across to their students is the very essence of what delineates a brief therapy" (p. 449). Even in managed care settings—such as HMOs, preferred provider organizations (PPOs), and employee assistance programs (EAPs)—there has been up to now surprisingly little attention to systematic training in brief therapy (Budman & Armstrong, 1992; Hoyt, 1991). As Levenson and Evans asked at the beginning of their article, "Are students in graduate programs and internships receiving adequate and relevant training in the modes of therapy favored by managed care companies?" (p. 446).

Combining increased attention to the study and practice of brief therapy with the fiscal imperative of the managed care movement may help satisfy consumers' preferences for effective and efficient treatments and may also help provide resources for patients who would otherwise go without to receive the benefits of professional mental health care. We can hope that greater appreciation and application of both cognitive-behavioral and psychodynamic as well as eclectic–integrative, systems–strategic, and other brief therapy approaches will be promoted, and that the recommendations offered by Levenson and Evans (2000) will be carefully heeded:

1. Graduate schools need to increase their brief therapy offerings.
2. We need training of the trainers.
3. Clinical training programs should make greater use of videotapes for teaching and supervision.
4. Internship sites should make greater use of treatment manuals, especially for

teaching inexperienced trainees the fundamentals of various brief therapies.
5. Brief therapy training cannot just focus on teaching skills and theory; it should address students' negative attitudes and biases about briefer interventions.
6. There should be more specific training in brief group therapy at the internship level.
7. The department chairs and training directors in the southern states (the region in which training in brief therapy was found to be especially scarce) should convene a meeting to develop plans to expand the availability of brief therapy training.
8. Continuing education is urged for established practitioners who feel unprepared to deal with present day clinical and economic challenges because they did not get brief therapy training during their predoctoral experience.
9. Brief therapy should not be oversold to trainees or practitioners; we should not convince them or ourselves that what may be economically or administratively necessary in a specific clinical situation is what is necessarily best for the client.

CODA

The goal of brief psychotherapy, regardless of the specific theoretical approach or technical method, is to help the patient resolve a problem, to get "unstuck" and to move on. Techniques are specific, integrated, and as eclectic as needed. Treatment is focused, the therapist appropriately active, and the patient responsible for making changes. Each session is valuable, and therapy ends as soon as possible. Good outcome, not good process, is most valued. More is not better; *better* is better. The patient carries on and can return to treatment as needed. The simple truth is that most therapy *is* brief therapy and will be increasingly so; for the sake of our patients and our profession, we should learn to practice it well.

ACKNOWLEDGMENTS

I am grateful to John Frykman, Gary Seeman, and Phillip Ziegler for their thoughtful comments.

NOTES

1. To point out the strange logic that suspects those who endeavor to help quickly, Duncan, Drewry, Hubble, Rusck, and Bruening (1992; see also Haley, 1969) have written a spoof in which Duncan confesses tongue-in-cheek his weakness for efficient treatment, so typical of those with "pragmatic personality disorder," and reports that he and his Inner Child are "in recovery" and attending daily Brief Therapy Anonymous meetings!

2. Throughout this chapter the terms "patient" and "client" are used more or less interchangeably, as they tend to be in the literature. The former term may carry more connotation of distress and a quest for relief (not necessarily in a medical model, although the implication is that of a relatively passive supplicant), whereas the latter term may seem more "egalitarian" or "businesslike" (but may deny the special quality of suffering that leads people to seek mental health services). It is important to recognize what the choice of either term may imply regarding the model of helping relationship being co-constructed by the patient/client and therapist and how these implications may impact on their subsequent work together (Hoyt, 1979, 1985a).

3. The famous "I'm OK, You're OK" phrase was actually coined by Robert Goulding in a discussion with Berne (Hoyt, 1995b).

4. As discussed in Hoyt (1989), each primary injunction tends to correlate with a specific *DSM-IV-R* "Personality Disorder" (e.g., internalizing "Don't Feel" leads to "Obsessional P.D.," "Don't Think" leads to "Histrionic P.D.," "Don't Be Important" leads to "Narcissistic P.D.," "Don't Be Close" leads to "Paranoid P.D.," etc.

5. In a more recent formulation, Lankton (2001) has identified several characteristics that define the "Ericksonian Footprint": Matching, Blending, Utilizing, Elaborating Ambiguity, Reframing, and Co-Creating Outcomes.

6. As reported in Hoyt (2000a, pp. 251–252), consistent with the principle of *intermittent therapy,* over several years I met with Sam a number of times. Eventually, he became quite ill. His wife called me from a nursing home to let me know when he was dying. He was not able to use the phone, but she put one of their sons on for us to have a talk. I was able to answer some questions, make sure the wife and son were okay, convey something of my appreciation for Sam, and let the son know how warmly his father had spoken of him. I also requested that they remember me to Sam and let them know to call if I could be of assistance. A few days later, I received a message from Sam's wife that Sam was dead. I called her and wrote a condolence letter and subsequently met with her and her sons.

7. Watzlawick and colleagues (1974) explain what they call "the gentle art of reframing":

   To reframe, then, means to change the conceptual and/or emotional setting or viewpoint in relation to which a situation is experienced and to place it in another frame which fits the "facts" of the same concrete situation equally well or even better, and thereby changes its entire meaning. The mechanism involved here is not immediately obvious, especially if we bear in mind that there is change while the situation itself may remain quite unchanged and, indeed, even unchangeable. What turns out to be changed as a result of reframing is the meaning attributed to the situation, and therefore its consequences, but not its concrete facts—or, as the philosopher Epictetus expressed it as early as the first century A.D., "It is not the things themselves which trouble us, but the opinions that we have about these things." (p. 95)

SUGGESTIONS FOR FURTHER READING

Bloom, B. L. (1992). *Planned short-term psychotherapy.* Boston: Allyn & Bacon.—An encyclopedia of brief therapy approaches, each summarized and concisely illustrated in a few pages.

Budman, S. H., & Gurman, A. S. (1988). *Theory and practice of brief therapy.* New York: Guilford Press.—Overview of various methods integrated into an interpersonal–developmental–existential framework.

Budman, S. H., Hoyt, M. F., & Friedman, S. (Eds.). (1992). *The first session in brief therapy.* New York: Guilford Press.—A unique collection of chapters by various master practitioners of brief therapy in which, after short theoretical descriptions, the reader gets to look over each therapist's shoulder and see how he or she works in ways that characterize the beginning steps of effective treatment within each particular approach.

Carlson, J., & Sperry, L. (2000). (Eds.). *Brief therapy with individuals and couples.* Phoenix, AZ: Zeig, Tucker & Theisen.—Compendium of excellent chapters presenting practical strategies from many different theoretical perspectives.

de Shazer, S. (1988). *Clues: Investigating solutions in brief therapy.* New York: Norton.—Elegantly precise examination of the things that therapist and client do during a session that lead to discovering "what works" and a solution.

Fisch, R., Weakland, J. H., & Segal, L. (1982). *The tactics of change: Doing therapy briefly.* San Francisco: Jossey-Bass.—The major exposition of the highly influential strategic–interactional approach developed at the Mental Research Institute of Palo Alto, California.

Haley, J. (1973). *Uncommon therapy: The psychiatric techniques of Milton H. Erickson, M.D.* New York: Norton.—A fascinating introduction to the work of the genius who spawned many schools of strategic interventions, family therapy, and hypnotherapy.

Hoyt, M. F. (1995). *Brief therapy and managed care: Readings for contemporary practice.* San Francisco: Jossey-Bass.—Key information on methods and models of brief therapy, especially as they pertain to the evolving requirements of insurance coverage and possible health care reform.

Hoyt, M. F. (2000). *Some stories are better than others: Doing what works in brief therapy and managed care.* Philadelphia: Brunner/Mazel.—Brief treatment viewed through social constructionist lenses, with numerous examples and metaphors drawn from clinical practice as well as poetry, sports, and the movies; plus critical perspectives on the promises and problems of managed care.

O'Hanlon, W. H., & Weiner-Davis, M. (1989). *In search of solutions: A new direction in psychotherapy.* New York: Norton.—Illuminating discussions of assumptions and strategies supporting the trend toward emphasizing strengths and solutions rather than problems and pathology.

Zeig, J. K., & Gilligan, S. G. (Eds.). (1990). *Brief therapy: Myths, methods, and metaphors.* New York: Brunner/Mazel.—The proceedings of the historic 1988 San Francisco conference, containing the keynote addresses and major papers given by many presenters of various theoretical persuasions.

REFERENCES

Alexander, F., & French, T. M. (1946). *Psychoanalytic therapy: Principles and applications.* New York: Ronald Press.

American Psychiatric Association. (2000). *Diagnostic and statistical manual of mental disorders* (4th ed., text rev.). Washington, DC: Author.

Andreas, C., & Andreas, S. (1989). *Heart of the mind.* Moab, UT: Real People Press.

Appelbaum, S. A. (1975). Parkinson's law in psychotherapy. *International Journal of Psychoanalytic Psychotherapy, 4,* 426–436.

Austad, C. S., & Berman, W. H. (Eds.). (1991). *Psychotherapy in managed health care.* Washington, DC: American Psychological Association.

Austad, C. S., & Hoyt, M. F. (1992). The managed care movement and the future of psychotherapy. *Psychotherapy, 29,* 109–118.

Balint, M., Ornstein, P. H., & Balint, E. (1972). *Focal psychotherapy.* London: Tavistock.

Bandler, R., & Grinder, J. (1982). *Reframing.* Moab, UT: Real People Press.

Barten, H. H. (Ed.). (1971). *Brief therapies.* New York: Behavioral Publications.

Basch, M. F. (1995). *Doing therapy briefly.* New York: Basic Books.

Bateson, G., Jackson, D. D., Haley, J., & Weakland, J. H. (1956). Toward a theory of schizophrenia. *Behavioral Science, 1,* 251–264.

Beck, A. T. (1976). *Cognitive therapy and the emo-*

tional disorders. New York: International University Press.

Bellak, L., & Small, L. (1965). *Emergency therapy and brief psychotherapy.* Philadelphia: Grune & Stratton.

Bennett, M. J. (1983). Focal psychotherapy—terminable and interminable. *American Journal of Psychotherapy, 37,* 365–375.

Bennett, M. J. (1984). Brief psychotherapy and adult development. *Psychotherapy, 21,* 171–177.

Berenbaum, H. (1969). Massed time-limit psychotherapy. *Psychotherapy: Theory, Research and Practice, 6,* 54–56.

Berg, I. K. (1994). *Family-based services: A solution-focused approach.* New York: Norton.

Berg, I. K., & de Shazer, S. (1993). Making numbers talk: Language in therapy. In S. Friedman (Ed.), *The new language of change: Constructive collaboration in psychotherapy* (pp. 5–24). New York: Guilford Press.

Berg, I. K., & Miller, S. D. (1992). *Working with the problem drinker.* New York: Norton.

Bergman, J. S. (1985). *Fishing for barracuda: Pragmatics of brief systemic therapy.* New York: Norton.

Berne, E. (1961). *Transactional analysis in psychotherapy.* New York: Grove Press.

Berne, E. (1964). *Games people play.* New York: Grove Press.

Berne, E. (1972). *What do you say after you say hello?* New York: Grove Press.

Bibring, E. (1954). Psychoanalysis and the dynamic psychotherapies. *Journal of the American Psychoanalytic Association, 2,* 745–770.

Binder, J. L., & Strupp, H. H. (1991). The Vanderbilt approach to time-limited dynamic psychotherapy. In P. Crits-Christoph & J. P. Barber (Eds.), *Handbook of short-term dynamic psychotherapy* (pp. 137–165). New York: Basic Books.

Bloom, B. L. (1981). Focused single-session therapy: Initial development and evaluation. In S. H. Budman (Ed.), *Forms of brief therapy* (pp. 167–216). New York: Guilford Press.

Bloom, B. L. (1992). *Planned short-term psychotherapy.* Boston: Allyn & Bacon.

Brehm, J. (1966). *A psychological theory of reactance.* New York: Appleton-Century-Crofts.

Breuer, J., & Freud, S. (1893–1895). Studies in hysteria. *Standard Edition, 2,* 1–319. London: Hogarth Press, 1955.

Budman, S. H. (Ed.). (1981). *Forms of brief therapy.* New York: Guilford Press.

Budman, S. H. (1990). The myth of termination in brief therapy: Or, it ain't over till it's over. In J. K. Zeig & S. G. Gilligan (Eds.), *Brief therapy: Myths, methods, and metaphors* (pp. 206–218). New York: Brunner/Mazel.

Budman, S. H., & Armstrong, E. (1992). Training for managed care settings: How to make it happen. *Psychotherapy, 29,* 416–421.

Budman, S. H., Friedman, S., & Hoyt, M. F. (1992). Last words on first sessions. In S. H. Budman, M. F. Hoyt, & S. Friedman (Eds.), *The first session in brief therapy* (pp. 345–358). New York: Guilford Press.

Budman, S. H., & Gurman, A. S. (1988). *Theory and practice of brief therapy.* New York: Guilford Press.

Budman, S. H., Hoyt, M. F., & Friedman, S. (Eds.). (1992). *The first session in brief therapy.* New York: Guilford Press.

Burlingame, G. M., Fuhriman, A., Paul, S., & Ogles, B. M. (1989). Implementing a time-limited therapy program: Differential effects of training and experience. *Psychotherapy, 26,* 303–312.

Cade, B., & O'Hanlon, W. H. (1993). *A brief guide to brief therapy.* New York: Norton.

Carlson, J., & Sperry, L. (Eds.). (2000). *Brief therapy with individuals and couples.* Phoenix, AZ: Zeig, Tucker & Theisen.

Crits-Cristoph, P., & Barber, J. P. (Eds.). (1991). *Handbook of short-term dynamic psychotherapy.* New York: Basic Books.

Cummings, N. A. (2000). *The collected papers of Nicholas A. Cummings. Vol. 1: The value of psychological treatment* (J. L. Thomas & J. L. Cummings, Eds.). Phoenix, AZ: Zeig, Tucker & Theisen.

Cummings, N. A., & Follette, W. T. (1976). Brief therapy and medical utilization. In H. Dörken (Ed.), *The professional psychologist today: New developments in law, health insurance, and health practice* (pp. 176–197). San Francisco: Jossey-Bass.

Cummings, N. A., & Sayama, M. (1995). *Focused psychotherapy: A casebook of brief, intermittent psychotherapy throughout the life cycle.* New York: Brunner/Mazel.

Dasberg, H., & Winokur, M. (1984). Teaching and learning short-term dynamic psychotherapy: Parallel processes. *Psychotherapy, 21,* 184–188.

Davanloo, H. (Ed.). (1978). *Basic principles and techniques in short-term dynamic psychotherapy.* New York: Spectrum.

Davanloo, H. (Ed.). (1980). *Short-term dynamic psychotherapy.* New York: Jason Aronson.

Davanloo, H. (1991). *Unlocking the unconscious: Selected papers.* West Sussex, UK: Wiley.

Davidovitz, D., & Levenson, H. (1995, August). *A national survey on practice and training in brief therapy.* Paper presented at the annual convention of the American Psychological Association, New York.

De Jong, P., & Berg, I. K. (1997). *Interviewing for solutions.* Pacific Grove, CA: Brooks Cole.

de Shazer, S. (1982). *Patterns of brief family therapy: An ecosystemic approach.* New York: Guilford Press.

de Shazer, S. (1985). *Keys to solution in brief therapy.* New York: Norton.

de Shazer, S. (1988). *Clues: Investigating solutions in brief therapy.* New York: Norton.

de Shazer, S. (1991a). Foreword. In Y. M. Dolan, *Resolving sexual abuse* (pp. ix–x). New York: Norton.

de Shazer, S. (1991b). *Putting difference to work.* New York: Norton.

de Shazer, S., & Berg, I. K. (1992). Doing therapy: A post-structural revision. *Journal of Marital and Family Therapy, 18,* 71–81.

de Shazer, S., Berg, I., Lipchik, E., Nunnally, E., Molnar, A., Gingerich, W., & Weiner-Davis, M. (1986). Brief therapy: Focused solution development. *Family Process, 25,* 207–222.

Dolan, Y. M. (1991). *Resolving sexual abuse: Solution-focused therapy and Ericksonan hypnosis for adult survivors.* New York: Norton.

Duncan, B., Drewry, S., Hubble, M., Rusck, G., & Bruening, P. (1992). Brief therapyism: A neglected addiction. *Journal of Strategic and Systemic Therapies, 10,* 32–42.

Duncan, B. L., Hubble, M. A., & Miller, S. D. (1997). *Psychotherapy with "impossible" cases: The efficient treatment of therapy veterans.* New York: Norton.

Edelstien, M. G. (1990). *Symptom analysis: A method of brief therapy.* New York: Norton.

Elliott, R. (2001). Contemporary brief experiential psychotherapy. *Clinical Psychology: Science and Practice, 8,* 38–50.

Elliott, R., & Greenburg, L. S. (1997). Multiple voices in process-experiential therapy: Dialogues between aspects of the self. *Journal of Psychotherapy Integration, 7,* 225–239.

Ellis, A. (1962). *Reason and emotion in psychotherapy.* New York: Lyle Stuart.

Ellis, A. (1992). Brief therapy: The rational-emotive method. In S. H. Budman, M. F. Hoyt, & S. Friedman (Eds.), *The first session in brief therapy* (pp. 36–58). New York: Guilford Press.

Epston, D. (1993). Internalized other questioning with couples: The New Zealand version. In S. G. Gilligan & R. Price (Eds.), *Therapeutic conversations* (pp. 183–189). New York: Norton.

Erickson, B. A. (2001). Jay Haley: A model of communication, teaching, therapy, and leading. In J. K. Zeig (Ed.), *Changing directives: The strategic therapy of Jay Haley* (pp. 45–58). Phoenix, AZ: Milton H. Erickson Foundation Press.

Erickson, K. K. (1988). One method for designing short-term intervention-oriented Ericksonian therapy. In J. K. Zeig & S. R. Lankton (Eds.), *Developing Ericksonian therapy: State of the art* (pp. 379–396). New York: Brunner/Mazel.

Erickson, M. H. (1980). *Collected papers* (Vols. 1–4) (E. Rossi, Ed.). New York: Irvington.

Erickson, M. H., & Rossi, E. (1979). *Hypnotherapy: An exploratory casebook.* New York: Irvington.

Erickson, M. H., Rossi, E., & Rossi, S. (1976). *Hypnotic realities.* New York: Irvington.

Erickson Foundation. (2001). *Celebrating Milton H. Erickson, M.D.* [Online]. Available: www.erickson-foundation.org

Everstine, D. S., & Everstine, L. (1983). *People in crisis: Strategic therapeutic interventions.* New York: Brunner/Mazel.

Farrelly, F., & Brandsma, J. (1974). *Provocative therapy.* Cupertino, CA: Meta-Publications.

Ferenczi, S., & Rank, O. (1925). *The development of psychoanalysis.* New York: Nervous and Mental Disease Publication.

Fisch, R. (1982), Erickson's impact on brief psychotherapy. In J. K. Zeig (Ed.), *Ericksonian approaches to hypnosis and psychotherapy* (pp. 155–162). New York: Brunner/Mazel.

Fisch, R. (1990). The broader implications of Milton H. Erickson's work. *Ericksonian Monographs, 7,* 1–5.

Fisch, R. (1994). Basic elements in the brief therapies. In M. F. Hoyt (Ed.), *Constructive therapies* (pp. 126–139). New York: Guilford Press.

Fisch, R., Weakland, J. H., & Segal, L. (1982). *The tactics of change: Doing therapy briefly.* San Francisco: Jossey-Bass.

Follette, W. T., & Cummings, N. A. (1967). Psychiatric services and medical utilization in a prepaid health care setting. *Medical Care, 5,* 25–35.

Frances, A., & Clarkin, J. F. (1981a). No treatment as the prescription of choice. *Archives of General Psychiatry, 38,* 542–545.

Frances, A., & Clarkin, J. F. (1981b). Parallel techniques in supervision and treatment. *Psychiatric Quarterly, 53,* 242–248.

Freedheim, D. K. (Ed.). (1992). *History of psychotherapy: A century of change.* Washington, DC: American Psychological Association.

Freud, S. (1910). The future prospects of psychoanalytic therapy. *Standard Edition, 11,* 20–74. London: Hogarth Press, 1953.

Freud, S. (1914). Remembering, repeating and working through. *Standard Edition, 12,* 145–156. London: Hogarth Press, 1953.

Freud, S. (1915). Observations on transference-love. *Standard Edition, 12,* 157–171. London: Hogarth Press, 1953.

Freud, S. (1919). Turnings in the ways of psychoanalytic therapy. *Standard Edition, 17,* 157–168. London: Hogarth Press, 1953.

Freud, S. (1937). Analysis terminable and interminable. *Standard Edition, 23,* 209–254. London: Hogarth Press, 1953.

Friedman, S. (Ed.). (1993). *The new language of change: Constructive collaboration in psychotherapy.* New York: Guilford Press.

Friedman, S. (1997). *Time-effective psychotherapy: maximizing outcomes in an era of minimized resources.* Needham Heights, MA: Allyn & Bacon.

Friedman, S., & Fanger, M. T. (1991). *Expanding therapeutic possibilities: Getting results in brief psychotherapy.* New York: Lexington Books/Macmillan.

Furman, B., & Ahola, T. (1992). *Solution talk: Hosting therapeutic conversations.* New York: Norton.

Garfield, S. L. (1986). Research on client variables in psychotherapy. In S. L. Garfield & A. E. Bergin (Eds.), *Handbook on psychotherapy and behavior change* (3rd ed., pp. 213–256). New York: Wiley.

Gergen, K. J. (1994). *Realities and relationhips: Soundings in social construction.* Cambridge, MA: Harvard University Press.

Gill, M. M. (1954). Psychoanalysis and exploratory psychotherapy. *Journal of the American Psychoanalytic Association, 2,* 771–797.

Gilligan, S., & Price, R. (Eds.). (1993). *Therapeutic conversations.* New York: Norton.

Gordon, D. (1978). *Therapeutic metaphors.* Cupertino, CA: Meta-Publications.

Gottman, J. M. (1994). *Why marriages succeed or fail . . . and how you can make yours last.* New York: Fireside/Simon & Schuster.

Goulding, M. M. (1985). *Who's been living in your head?* (rev. ed.). Watsonville, CA: WIGFT Press.

Goulding, M. M. (1990). Getting the important work done fast: Contract plus redecision. In J. K. Zeig & S. G. Gilligan (Eds.), *Brief therapy: Myths, methods, and metaphors* (pp. 303–317). New York: Brunner/Mazel.

Goulding, M. M. (1997). Childhood scenes in redecision therapy. In C. E. Lennox (Ed.), *Redecision therapy: A brief, action-oriented approach* (pp. 87–94). Northvale, NJ: Jason Aronson.

Goulding, M. M., & Goulding, R. L. (1979). *Changing lives through redecision therapy.* New York: Grove Press.

Goulding, R. L. (1983). Gestalt therapy and transactional analysis. In C. Hatcher & P. Himelstein (Eds.), *Handbook of Gestalt therapy* (pp. 615–634). New York: Jason Aronson.

Goulding, R. L. (1989). Teaching transactional analysis and redecision therapy. *Journal of Independent Social Work, 3,* 71–86.

Goulding, R. L., & Goulding, M. M. (1978). *The power is in the patient.* San Francisco: TA Press.

Gustafson, J. P. (1986). *The complex secret of brief psychotherapy.* New York: Norton.

Haley, J. (1963). *Strategies of psychotherapy.* New York: Grune & Stratton.

Haley, J. (1969). The art of psychoanalysis. In *The power tactics of Jesus Christ and other essays* (pp. 11–26). New York: Avon.

Haley, J. (1973). *Uncommon therapy: The psychiatric techniques of Milton H. Erickson, M.D.* New York: Norton.

Haley, J. (1977). *Problem-solving therapy.* San Francisco: Jossey-Bass.

Haley, J. (1984). *Ordeal therapy.* San Francisco: Jossey-Bass.

Haley, J. (Ed.). (1985). *Conversations with Milton*

H. Erickson, M.D. (Vols. 1–3). New York: Triangle Press.

Haley, J. (1989). *The first therapy session: How to interview clients and identify problems successfully* [Audiotape]. San Francisco: Jossey-Bass.

Haley, J. (1994). Typically Erickson. In *Jay Haley on Milton H. Erickson* (pp. 176–199). New York: Brunner/Mazel.

Haley, J. (1996). *Teaching and learning therapy.* New York: Guilford Press.

Haley, J. (2001). The loyal opposition. In J. K. Zeig (Ed.), *Changing directives: The strategic therapy of Jay Haley* (pp. 12–26). Phoenix, AZ: Milton H. Erickson Foundation Press.

Haley, J., & Richeport-Haley, M. (1993). *Milton H. Erickson, M.D.: Explorer in hypnosis and therapy* [Videotape]. New York: Brunner/Mazel.

Haley, J., & Richeport-Haley, M. (2000). *Jay Haley on directive family therapy* [Videotape] (Part of 6-tape series, *Learning and teaching therapy with Jay Haley: A videotape series*). La Jolla, CA: Triangle Productions.

Havens, R. A. (Ed.). (1989). *The wisdom of Milton H. Erickson* (Vols. 1 & 2). New York: Paragon House.

Henry, W. P., Schacht, T. E., Strupp, H. H., Binder, J. L., & Butler, S. F. (1993). The effects of training in time-limited dynamic psychotherapy. III. Mediators of therapists' response to training. *Journal of Consulting and Clinical Psychology, 61,* 441–447.

Horowitz, M. J., Marmar, C., Krupnick, J., Wilner, N., Kaltreider, N., & Wallerstein, R. (1984). *Personality styles and brief psychotherapy.* New York: Basic Books.

Hoyt, M. F. (1979). "Patient" or "client": What's in a name? *Psychotherapy: Theory, Research and Practice, 16,* 16–17.

Hoyt, M. F. (1985a). "Shrink" or "expander": An issue in forming a therapeutic alliance. *Psychotherapy, 22,* 813–814.

Hoyt, M. F. (1985b). Therapist resistances to short-term dynamic psychotherapy. *Journal of the American Academy of Psychoanalysis, 13,* 93–112.

Hoyt, M. F. (1989). Psychodiagnosis of personality disorders. *Transactional Analysis Journal, 19,* 101–113.

Hoyt, M. F. (1990). On time in brief therapy. In R. A. Wells & V. J. Giannetti (Eds.), *Handbook of the brief psychotherapies* (pp. 115–143). New York: Plenum Press.

Hoyt, M. F. (1991). Teaching and learning short-term psychotherapy within an HMO. In C. S. Austad & W. H. Berman (Eds.), *Psychotherapy in managed health care* (pp. 98–108). Washington, DC: American Psychological Association.

Hoyt, M. F. (1993a). Group psychotherapy in an HMO. *HMO Practice, 7,* 129–132.

Hoyt, M. F. (1993b). Two cases of brief therapy in an HMO. In A. A. Wells & V. J. Giannetti (Eds.), *Casebook of brief psychotherapies* (pp. 235–248). New York: Plenum Press.

Hoyt, M. F. (Ed.). (1994a). *Constructive therapies.* New York: Guilford Press.

Hoyt, M. F. (1994b). Introduction: Competency-based future-oriented psychotherapy. In M. F. Hoyt (Ed.), *Constructive therapies* (pp. 1–10). New York: Guilford Press.

Hoyt, M. F. (1994c). On the importance of keeping it simple and taking the patient seriously: A conversation with Steve de Shazer and John Weakland. In M. F. Hoyt (Ed.), *Constructive therapies* (pp. 11–40). New York: Guilford Press.

Hoyt, M. F. (1994d). Single-session solutions. In M. F. Hoyt (Ed.), *Constructive therapies* (pp. 140–159). New York: Guilford Press.

Hoyt, M. F. (1995a). *Brief therapy and managed care: Readings for contemporary practice.* San Francisco: Jossey-Bass.

Hoyt, M. F. (1995b). Contact, contract, change, encore: A conversation with Bob Goulding. *Transactional Analysis Journal, 25*(4), 300–311.

Hoyt, M. F. (1995c). Managed care, HMOs, and the Ericksonian perspective. In M. F. Hoyt (Ed.), *Brief therapy and managed care: Readings for contemporary practice* (pp. 163–176). San Francisco: Jossey-Bass.

Hoyt, M. F. (Ed.). (1996a). *Constructive therapies, Volume 2.* New York: Guilford Press.

Hoyt, M. F. (1996b). Solution building and language games: A conversation with Steve de Shazer. In M. F. Hoyt (Ed.), *Constructive therapies* (Vol. 2, pp. 60–86). New York: Guilford Press.

Hoyt, M. F. (1997). Foreword. In C. E. Lennox (Ed.), *Redecision therapy: A brief, action-oriented approach* (pp. xiii–xix). Northvale, NJ: Jason Aronson.

Hoyt, M. F. (Ed.). (1998). *The handbook of constructive therapies.* San Francisco: Jossey-Bass.

Hoyt, M. F. (2000a). The last session in brief

therapy: How and why to say "when. " In *Some stories are better than others* (pp. 237–261). Philadelphia: Brunner/Mazel.

Hoyt, M. F. (2000b). *Some stories are better than others: Doing what works in brief therapy and managed care*. Philadelphia: Brunner/Mazel.

Hoyt, M. F. (2001a). Constructing managed care, constructing brief therapy. *American Psychologist, 56,* 763–765.

Hoyt, M. F. (2001b). *Interviews with brief therapy experts*. New York: Brunner-Routledge.

Hoyt, M. F. (2002). Solution-focused couple therapy. In A. S. Gurman & N. S. Jacobson (Eds.), *Clinical handbook of couple therapy* (3rd. ed, pp. 335–369). New York: Guilford Press.

Hoyt, M. F., & Austad, C. S. (1992). Psychotherapy in a staff-model health maintenance organization: Providing and assuring quality care in the future. *Psychotherapy, 29,* 119–129.

Hoyt, M. F., & Berg, I. K. (1998). Solution-focused couple therapy: Helping clients construct self-fulfilling realities. In F. M. Dattilio (Ed.), *Case studies in couple and family therapy: Systemic and cognitive perspectives* (pp. 203–232). New York: Guilford Press.

Hoyt, M. F., & Farrell, D. (1984). Countertransference difficulties in a time-limited psychotherapy. *International Journal of Psychoanalytic Psychotherapy, 10,* 191–203.

Hoyt, M. F., & Goulding, R. L. (1989). Resolution of a transference-countertransference impasse using Gestalt techniques in supervision. *Transactional Analysis Journal, 19,* 201–211.

Hoyt, M. F., & Miller, S. D. (2000). Stage-appropriate change-oriented brief therapy strategies. In J. Carlson & L. Sperry (Eds.), *Brief therapy with individuals and couples* (pp. 289–330). Phoenix, AZ: Zeig, Tucker & Theisen.

Hoyt, M. F., Rosenbaum, R. L., & Talmon, M. (1992). Planned single-session psychotherapy. In S. H. Budman, M. F. Hoyt, & S. Friedman (Eds.), *The first session in brief therapy* (pp. 59–86). New York: Guilford Press.

Hoyt, M. F., & Talmon, M. (1990). Single-session therapy in action: A case example. In M. Talmon, *Single-session therapy* (pp. 78–96). San Francisco: Jossey-Bass.

Hudson, P. (1993). *Making friends with your unconscious mind: The user friendly guide*. Omaha, NE: Center Press.

Hudson, P., & O'Hanlon, W. H. (1992). *Rewriting love stories: Brief marital therapy*. New York: Norton.

Jacobson, G. (1968). The briefest psychiatric encounter: Acute effects of evaluation. *Archives of General Psychiatry, 18,* 718–724.

Johnson, L. D. (1995). *Psychotherapy in the age of accountability*. New York: Norton.

Kadis, L. B. (Ed.). (1985). *Redecision therapy: Expanded perspectives*. Watsonville, CA: WIGFT Press.

Kaiser, H. (1965). The problem of responsibility in psychotherapy. In L. B. Fierman (Ed.), *Effective psychotherapy: The contribution of Hellmuth Kaiser* (pp. 1–13). New York: Free Press.

Koss, M. P., & Butcher, J. N. (1986). Research on brief psychotherapy. In A. E. Bergin & S. L. Garfield (Eds.), *Handbook of psychotherapy and behavior change* (3rd ed., pp. 627–670). New York: Wiley.

Koss, M. P., Butcher, J. N., & Strupp, H. H. (1986). Brief psychotherapy methods in clinical research. *Journal of Clinical and Consulting Psychology, 54,* 60–67.

Koss, M. P., & Shiang, J. (1994). Research on brief therapy. In A. E. Bergin & S. L. Garfield (Eds.), *Handbook of psychotherapy and behavior change* (4th ed., pp. 664–700). New York: Wiley.

Kreider, J. W. (1998). Solution-focused ideas for briefer therapy with longer-term clients. In M. F. Hoyt (Ed.), *The handbook of constructive therapies* (pp. 341–357). San Francisco: Jossey-Bass.

Lankton, S. R. (1990). Ericksonian strategic therapy. In J. K. Zeig & W. M. Munion (Eds.), *What is psychotherapy? Contemporary perspectives* (pp. 363–371). San Francisco: Jossey-Bass.

Lankton, S. R. (2001, December 6). *The basic footprint of Erickson's work*. Keynote address at eighth International Congress on Ericksonian Approaches to Hypnosis and Psychotherapy, Phoenix, AZ.

Lankton, S. R., & Lankton, C. (1983). *The answer within: A clinical framework for Ericksonian hypnotherapy*. New York: Brunner/Mazel.

Lankton, S. R., & Lankton, C. (1986). *Enchantment and intervention in family therapy*. New York: Brunner/Mazel.

Lankton, S., & Lankton, C. (1998). Ericksonian emergent epistemologies: Embracing a new paradigm. In M. F. Hoyt (Ed.), *The handbook of constructive therapies* (pp. 116–136). San Francisco: Jossey-Bass.

Lazarus, A. A. (1976). *Multimodal behavior therapy.* New York: Springer.

Lazarus, A. A. (1989). *The practice of multimodal therapy.* Baltimore: Johns Hopkins University Press.

Lazarus, A. A. (1997). *Brief but comprehensive psychotherapy: The multimodal way.* New York: Springer.

Lazurus, A. A., & Fay, A. (1990). Brief psychotherapy: Tautology or oxymoron? In J. K. Zeig & S. G. Gilligan (Eds.), *Brief therapy: Myths, methods, and metaphors* (pp. 36–51). New York: Brunner/Mazel.

Levenson, H. (1995). *Time-limited dynamic psychotherapy: A guide to clinical practice.* New York: Basic Books.

Levenson, H., & Burg, J. (1999). Training psychologists in the era of managed care. In A. J. Kent & M. Hersen (Eds.), *A psychologist's proactive guide to managed mental health care* (pp. 113–140). Hillsdale, NJ: Erlbaum.

Levenson, H., & Butler, S. F. (1999). Brief psychodynamic individual psychotherapy. In R. Hales, S. C. Yudofsky, & J. Talbot (Eds.), *American Psychiatric Press textbook of psychiatry* (pp. 1133–1156). Washington, DC: American Psychiatric Press.

Levenson, H., & Evans, S. A. (2000). The current state of brief therapy training in American Psychological Association–accredited graduate and internship programs. *Professional Psychology: Research and Practice, 31,* 446–452.

Levenson, H., Speed, J., & Budman, S. H. (1995). Therapists' experience, training, and skill in brief therapy: A bicoastal survey. *American Journal of Psychotherapy, 49,* 95–117.

Lewin, K. K. (1970). *Brief psychotherapy: Brief encounters.* St. Louis, MO: Warren H. Green.

Luborsky, L., & Crits-Christoph, P. (1990). *Understanding transference: The CCRT method.* New York: Basic Books.

Madanes, C. (1981). *Strategic family therapy.* San Francisco: Jossey-Bass.

Madanes, C. (1984). *Behind the one-way mirror.* San Francisco: Jossey-Bass.

Malan, D. H. (1963). *A study of brief psychotherapy.* London: Tavistock Press.

Malan, D. H. (1976). *The frontier of brief psychotherapy.* New York: Plenum Press.

Malan, D. H. (1980). The most important development in psychotherapy since the discovery of the unconscious. In H. Davanloo (Ed.), *Short-term dynamic psychotherapy* (pp. 13–23). New York: Jason Aronson.

Malan, D. H., Heath, E. S., Bacal, H. A., & Balfour, H. G. (1975). Psychodynamic changes in untreated neurotic patients. II. Apparently genuine improvements. *Archives of General Psychiatry, 32,* 110–126.

Mann, J. (1973). *Time-limited psychotherapy.* Cambridge, MA: Harvard University Press.

Mann, J., & Goldman, R. (1982). *A casebook in time-limited psychotherapy.* New York: McGraw-Hill.

McCullough, L. (2000). Short-term therapy for character change. In J. Carlson & L. Sperry (Eds.), *Brief therapy with individuals and couples* (pp. 127–160). Phoenix, AZ: Zeig, Tucker & Theisen.

McCullough-Vaillant, L. (1997). *Changing character: Short-term anxiety-regulating psychotherapy for restructuring defenses, affects, and attachments.* New York: Basic Books.

McNeel, J. (1976). The Parent interview. *Transactional Analysis Journal, 6,* 61–68.

Meichenaum, D. (1977). *Cognitive behavior modification.* New York: Plenum Press.

Messer, S. B., & Warren, C. S. (1995). *Models of brief psychodynamic therapy: A comparative approach.* New York: Guilford Press.

Mumford, E., Schlesinger, H., Glass, G. V., Patrick, C., & Cuerdon, B. A. (1984). A new look at evidence about reduced cost of medical utilization following mental-health treatment. *American Journal of Psychiatry, 141,* 1145–1158.

O'Hanlon, W. H. (1987). *Taproots: Underlying principles of Milton H. Erickson's therapy and hypnosis.* New York: Norton.

O'Hanlon, W. H. (1999). *Do one thing different: And other uncommonly sensible solutions to life's persistent problems.* New York: William Morrow.

O'Hanlon, W. H., & Hexum, A. L. (1990). *An uncommon casebook: The complete clinical work of Milton H. Erickson, M.D.* New York: Norton.

O'Hanlon, W. H., & Weiner-Davis, M. (1989). *In search of solutions: A new direction in psychotherapy.* New York: Norton.

O'Hanlon, W., & Wilk, J. (1987). *Shifting contexts: The generation of effective psychotherapy.* New York: Guilford Press.

Parad, H. J. (Ed.). (1965). *Crisis intervention: Selected readings.* New York: Family Service Association of America.

Peet, B. (1972). *The ant and the elephant.* Boston: Houghton Mifflin.

Perls, F. S., Hefferline, R. F., & Goodman, P. (1951). *Gestalt therapy.* New York: Julian Press.

Phillips, M. (1988). Changing early life decisions using Ericksonian hypnosis. *Ericksonian Monographs, 4,* 74–87.

Pinsker, H., Rosenthal, R., & McCullough, L. (1991). Dynamic supportive psychotherapy. In P. Crits-Christoph & J. P. Barber (Eds.), *Handbook of short-term dynamic psychotherapy* (pp. 220–247). New York: Basic Books.

Prochaska, J. O., DiClemente, C. C., & Norcross, J. C. (1992). In search of how people change. *American Psychologist, 47,* 1102–1114.

Rasmussen, A., & Messer, S. B. (1986). A comparison and critique of Mann's time-limited psychotherapy and Davanloo's short-term dynamic psychotherapy. *Bulletin of the Menninger Clinic, 50,* 163–184.

Rosen, S. (1982). *My voice will go with you: The teaching tales of Milton H. Erickson.* New York: Norton.

Rosen, H., & Kuehlwein, K. (Eds.). (1996). *Constructing realities: Meaning-making perspectives for psychotherapists.* San Francisco: Jossey-Bass.

Rosenbaum, R., Hoyt, M. F., & Talmon, M. (1990). The challenge of single-session therapies: Creating pivotal moments. In R. A. Wells & V. J. Giannetti (Eds.), *Handbook of the brief psychotherapies* (pp. 165–189). New York: Plenum Press.

Rowan, T., & O'Hanlon, W. H. (1998). *Solution-oriented therapy for chronic and severe mental illness.* New York: Wiley.

Selvini-Palazzoli, M., Cecchin, G., Prata, G., & Boscolo, L. (1978). *Paradox and counterparadox.* New York: Jason Aronson.

Shectman, F. (1986). Time and the practice of psychotherapy. *Psychotherapy, 23,* 521–525.

Short, D. (1997, Summer). Interview: Steve de Shazer and Insoo Kim Berg. *Milton H. Erickson Foundation Newsletter, 17*(2), 1, 18–20.

Sifneos, P. E. (1972). *Short-term psychotherapy and emotional crisis.* Cambridge, MA: Harvard University Press.

Sifneos, P. E. (1987). *Short-term dynamic psychotherapy: Evaluation and technique* (rev. ed.). New York: Plenum Press.

Sifneos, P. E. (1992). *Short-term anxiety-provoking psychotherapy: A treatment manual.* New York: Plenum Press.

Strupp, H. H., & Binder, J. L. (1984). *Psychotherapy in a new key: A guide to time-limited dynamic psychotherapy.* New York: Basic Books.

Sullivan, H. S. (1954). *The psychiatric interview.* New York: Norton.

Talmon, M. (1990). *Single-session therapy.* San Francisco: Jossey-Bass.

Talmon, M. (1993). *Single session solutions.* Reading, MA: Addison-Wesley.

Talmon, M., Hoyt, M. F., & Rosenbaum, R. (1990). Effective single-session therapy: Step-by-step guidelines. In M. Talmon, *Single-session therapy* (pp. 34–56). San Francisco: Jossey-Bass.

Ticho, E. A. (1972). Termination of psychoanalysis: Treatment goals, life goals. *Psychoanalytic Quarterly, 41,* 315–333.

Tomm, K., Hoyt, M. F., & Madigan, S. P. (1998). Honoring our internalized others and the ethics of caring: A conversation with Karl Tomm. In M. F. Hoyt (Ed.), *The handbook of constructive therapies* (pp. 198–218). San Francisco: Jossey-Bass.

VandenBos, G. R., Cummings, N. A., & DeLeon, P. H. (1992). A century of psychotherapy: Economic and environmental influences. In D. K. Freedheim (Ed.), *History of psychotherapy* (pp. 65–102). Washington, DC: American Psychological Association.

Walter, J. L., & Peller, J. E. (1992). *Becoming solution-focused in brief therapy.* New York: Norton.

Walter, J. L., & Peller, J. E. (1994). "On track" in solution-focused brief therapy. In M. F. Hoyt (Ed.), *Constructive therapies* (pp. 111–125). New York: Guilford Press.

Watzlawick, P. (1978). *The language of change: Elements of therapeutic communication.* New York: Norton.

Watzlawick, P. (Ed.). (1984). *The invented reality: How do we know what we believe we know? (Contributions to constructivism).* New York: Norton.

Watzlawick, P., Beavin, J. H., & Jackson, D. D. (1967). *Pragmatics of human communication: A study of interactional patterns, pathologies, and paradoxes.* New York: Norton.

Watzlawick, P., Weakland, J. H., & Fisch, R. (1974). *Change: Principles of problem formation and problem resolution.* New York: Norton.

Weakland, J. H., & Fisch, R. (1992). Brief therapy—MRI style. In S. H. Budman, M. F. Hoyt, & S. Friedman (Eds.), *The first session in brief therapy* (pp. 306–323). New York: Guilford Press.

Weakland, J. H., Fisch, R., Watzlawick, P., & Bodin, A. M. (1974). Brief therapy: Focused problem resolution. *Family Process, 13,* 141–168.

Weeks, G. R. (Ed.). (1991). *Promoting change through paradoxical therapy.* New York: Brunner/Mazel.

Weiner-Davis, M. (1992). *Divorce busting.* New York: Fireside/Simon & Schuster.

Weiner-Davis, M., de Shazer, S., & Gingerich, W. J. (1987). Building on pre-treatment change to construct the therapeutic solution: An exploratory study. *Journal of Marital and Family Therapy, 13,* 359–363.

Weiss, J., Sampson, H., & Mt. Zion Psychotherapy Research Group. (1986). *The psychoanalytic process: Theory, clinical observations, and empirical research.* New York: Guilford Press.

Wells, R. A. (1982). *Planned short-term treatment.* New York: Free Press/Macmillan.

Wells, R. A., & Giannetti, V. J. (Eds.). (1990). *Handbook of the brief psychotherapies.* New York: Plenum Press.

Wells, R. A., & Giannetti, V. J. (Eds.). (1993). *Casebook of the brief psychotherapies.* New York: Plenum Press.

Wells, R. A., & Phelps, P. A. (1990). The brief psychotherapies: A selective review. In R. A. Wells & V. J. Giannetti (Eds.), *Handbook of the brief psychotherapies* (pp. 3–26). New York: Plenum Press.

Westen, D. (1986). What changes in short-term psychodynamic psychotherapy? *Psychotherapy, 23,* 501–512.

White, M. (1995). *Re-authoring lives: Interviews and essays.* Adelaide, Australia: Dulwich Centre Publications.

White, M. (1997). *Narratives of therapists' lives.* Adelaide, Australia: Dulwich Centre Publications.

White, M., & Epston, D. (1990). *Narrative means to therapeutic ends.* New York: Norton.

Wolberg, L. R. (Ed.). (1965). *Short-term psychotherapy.* New York: Grune & Stratton.

Wolpe, J. (1958). *Psychotherapy by reciprocal inhibition.* Stanford, CA: Stanford University Press.

Wolpe, J., & Lazarus, A. A. (1966). *Behavior therapy techniques.* New York: Pergamon Press.

Yapko, M. D. (1990). Brief therapy tactics in longer-term psychotherapies. In J. K. Zeig & S. G. Gilligan (Eds.), *Brief therapy: Myths, methods, and metaphors* (pp. 185–195). New York: Brunner/Mazel.

Yapko, M. D. (1992). Therapy with direction. In S. H. Budman, M. F. Hoyt, & S. Friedman (Eds.), *The first session in brief therapy* (pp. 156–180). New York: Guilford Press.

Yapko, M. D. (2001). Jay Haley on Jay Haley. In J. K. Zeig (Ed.), *Changing directives: The strategic therapy of Jay Haley* (pp. 183–202). Phoenix, AZ: Milton H. Erickson Foundation Press.

Zeig, J. K. (Ed.). (1982). *Ericksonian approaches to hypnosis and psychotherapy.* New York: Brunner/Mazel.

Zeig, J. K. (Ed.). (1987). *The evolution of psychotherapy.* New York: Brunner/Mazel.

Zeig, J. K. (1990). Ericksonian psychotherapy. In J. K. Zeig & W. M. Munion (Eds.), *What is psychotherapy? Contemporary perspectives* (pp. 371–377). San Francisco: Jossey-Bass.

Zeig, J. K. (Ed.). (2001). *Changing directives: The strategic therapy of Jay Haley.* Phoenix, AZ: Milton H. Foundation Press.

Zeig, J. K. (Ed.). (2002a). *Brief therapy: Lasting impressions.* Phoenix, AZ: Milton H. Erickson Foundation Press.

Zeig, J. K. (2002b). Clinical heuristics. In J. K. Zeig (Ed.), *Brief therapy: Lasting impressions* (pp. 41–62). Phoenix, AZ: Milton H. Erickson Foundation Press.

Zeig, J. K., & Gilligan, S. G. (Eds.). (1990). *Brief therapy: Myths, methods, and metaphors.* New York: Brunner/Mazel.

Zeig, J. K., & Lankton, S. R. (Eds.). (1988). *Developing Ericksonian therapy: State of the art.* New York: Brunner/Mazel.

Ziegler, P., & Hiller, T. (2001). *Recreating partnership: A solution-oriented, collaborative approach to couples therapy.* New York: Norton.

Zois, C. (1992). *Think like a shrink.* New York: Warner.

11

Family Therapies

NADINE J. KASLOW
BARBARA M. DAUSCH
MARIANNE CELANO

HISTORICAL BACKGROUND

Historians, anthropologists, sociologists, and religious scholars have acknowledged the centrality of the family unit since the beginning of civilization. There is an historical precedent for community leaders to aid a family when an individual member is distressed. However, only during the past century has there been documented use of education, counseling, or therapy to help the family unit. This section traces influential activities in the development of family therapy during the past century.

The roots of family therapy date to the late 1800s and early 1900s and are found in the social work, marriage and family life education, and marriage counseling movements (Thomas, 1992). From its inception, social work has considered the family the unit of concern, and social workers have played key roles in the practice of family therapy. The marriage and family life education movement provided preventive classes for individuals, typically women, interested in learning about marriage, parenting, and family life. These students often discussed their own relationships and were offered guidance, prompting the family-life ap-

proach to change its didactic focus to a more practical approach. These early efforts at informal counseling paved the way for more formal marital counseling, conducted by professionals trained in marital counseling. Many leaders in the marriage and family-life education movement later served as pioneers of marital counseling.

Marriage counseling centers were established in the 1930s, the most notable being the Marriage Council of Philadelphia headed by Emily Mudd. Similar developments were afoot in Europe, including the establishment of the Marriage Guidance Council in Great Britain under David and Vera Mace. During the 1930s and 1940s, the field became increasingly professionalized, as evidenced by the emergence of two organizations, the National Council of Family Relations (NCFR) for family life educators and the American Association of Marriage Counselors (AAMC) for marital counselors. Both organizations remain active today, although the AAMC, renamed the American Association of Marriage and Family Therapy (AAMFT) in the 1970s, expanded its goals and redefined its membership criteria. Family therapy also has origins in clinical psychiatry, a field historically devoted to treating individuals' psychopathology from a psychodynamic perspective. Many early family theorists, who had extensive psychoanalytic training, began including family members in the treatment. This change reflected their concern that the patient's symptoms partially were maintained by dysfunctional family interactional patterns and that individual therapy was insufficient to change these patterns. The evolution of family theory also can be traced to the application of general systems and communication theories to understanding human interactions (e.g., Bateson, 1972). Many family therapy models are systemic and underscore the interrelatedness and reciprocal influences of the individual, the family, and the social system.

Early research undergirding family theories and therapy was conducted with adults with schizophrenia and their families. This research stemmed from clinicians' observations of the relation between family patterns and the behaviors of people with schizophrenia-spectrum disorder diagnoses. The seminal paper linking family communication patterns to the development of psychopathology in a family member was titled "Toward a theory of schizophrenia" (Bateson, Jackson, Haley, & Weakland, 1956). Using anthropological methods and social systems theory, these authors asserted that the essential family determinant in the development of schizophrenia was "double bind" communications, two or more contradictory messages from the same person in which a response is required by the recipient and failure to please the presenter is guaranteed. The double-bind concept has been reworked and now is considered more pertinent to the maintenance, rather than the etiology, of symptoms associated with schizophrenia. In addition to the aforementioned researchers and their colleague Virginia Satir, at the Mental Research Institute (MRI) in Palo Alto, other family therapy founders studied persons with schizophrenia and their families: (1) Theodore Lidz, at Johns Hopkins and then at Yale, and his

coworkers Fleck, Cornelison, and R. Lidz; (2) Murray Bowen, at the Menninger Clinic in Topeka and with Lyman Wynne at the National Institute of Mental Health (NIMH) in Washington, DC; (3) Ivan Boszormenyi-Nagy, at Eastern Pennsylvania Psychiatric Institute in Philadelphia; and (4) Carl Whitaker, at Emory in Atlanta and later in Madison, Wisconsin, and his colleagues in Atlanta, Thomas Malone and John Warkentin. Other leaders at this time were Bell, one of the first to conduct sessions with all family members, and Christian Midelfort, who authored the first book solely devoted to family therapy.

Simultaneous with the foregoing developments, clinicians feeling frustrated in their individual contacts with children turned their focus to the family. Nathan Ackerman, a child psychiatrist and psychoanalyst, asserted that the family was the proper unit of diagnosis and treatment. His article, "Family Diagnosis: An Approach to the Preschool Child" (Ackerman & Sobel, 1950), has been considered by some to be the founding document of the family therapy movement. Some early family research was conducted in child guidance clinics. For example, Salvador Minuchin and colleagues at the Philadelphia Child Guidance Center studied family therapy with delinquents, low-socioeconomic-status families, and psychosomatic families (Minuchin, Montalvo, Guerney, Rosman, & Schumer, 1967).

The second wave of the family therapy movement (1962–1977) began with the publication of *Family Process,* the first family therapy journal. Training centers were established throughout the country. Emphasis was placed on certification and licensure, with AAMFT recognized as the official accrediting agency for training programs. This decade witnessed the development of competing schools of thought and training models and an increasing focus on outcome studies and interactional research. The end of the second wave was marked by the establishment of the American Family Therapy Academy (AFTA) in 1977, under the leadership of Bowen. Unlike its interdisciplinary predecessors, AFTA initially was composed primarily of psychiatrist family therapists; over time, it has evolved into an interdisciplinary organization.

The most recent chapter in the history of family therapy (post–1977) encompasses a number of significant changes. First, in addition to the development of a broader range of models of family theory and therapy (Gurman & Kniskern, 1991), integrative models have been developed that borrow from various family theories and other schools of therapy or that are created as integrative approaches (e.g., Breunlin, Schwartz, & MacKune-Karrer, 1997; Feldman, 1992; Henggeler, Schoenwald, Borduin, Rowland, & Cunningham, 1998; F. W. Kaslow, 1991; Lebow, 1997; Pinsof, 1995). Second, over the past decade, there have been interorganizational efforts to develop a classification schema on relational diagnosis (F. W. Kaslow, 1996). Consistent with this, the fourth edition of *Diagnostic and Statistical Manual of Mental Disorders* (DSM-IV; American Psychiatric Association, 1994) includes a Global Assessment Scale of Relational Functioning (GARF; Group for the Advancement of Psychiatry Committee on the Family, 1996; Yingling, Miller, McDonald, & Galewaler, 1998), on which relationships can be rated on a continuum ranging from competent and optimal relationship functioning to disruptive and dysfunctional relationship functioning. In addition to attending to the development of a relational classification schema, there are efforts to develop strategies for relational assessment and intervention (e.g., F. W. Kaslow, 1996; Magnavita, 2000). Third, there has been increased emphasis on empirical verification of family therapy tenets and the efficacy of family interventions, made possible by the development of reliable and valid assessment measures and interactional coding schemata (Nurse, 1999; Snyder, Cozzi, & Mangrum, 2002) and by the increased collaboration between scientists and practitioners. The family psycholo-

gy movement, a division of the American Psychological Association (Division 43), has played a pivotal role in the refinement of family research. Most relevant to this chapter is the empirical support for the effectiveness of family therapy compared to control and alternative conditions in enhancing family interactions and decreasing symptoms (Baucom, Shoham, Mueser, Daiuto, & Stickle, 1998; Diamond, Serrano, Dickey, & Sonis, 1996; Estrada & Pinsof, 1995). Consistent with the movement within psychology toward establishing evidenced-based practices and defining effective treatments for specific, there has been progress toward establishing empirically supported family treatments (e.g., Denton, Walsh, & Daniel, 2002; Marsh, 2001). Importance has been placed on basic concepts of establishing evidence-based practices, including identifying principles that guide the application of intervention, for example, understanding the stages of therapeutic change. There is additional emphasis on tracking progress through therapy and applying research findings in family research whenever possible, such as data on expressed emotion (e.g., Miklowitz & Hooley, 1998). There is also increased emphasis on the conduct of qualitative research in family therapy (Faulkner, Klock, & Gale, 2002). Fourth, interest in prevention, particularly focused on divorce and distress, has been relatively recent (e.g., for prevention of couple distress, see Silliman, Stanley, Coffin, Markman, & Jordan, 2002); for prevention of externalizing child behaviors, see Webster-Stratton & Taylor, 2001) and has focused primarily on bolstering couples' adaptive processes (e.g., Bradbury, Fincham, & Beach, 2000). Programs focusing on the prevention of abuse have traditionally focused on stranger violence and are only more recently addressing violence within families due to the fact that a person is twice as likely to be assault by a relative (Schewe, 2002). Incorporated into abuse prevention programs are factors placing individuals at risk including sociodemographic features, individual pathology, and characteristics of relationships

(Low, Monarch, Hartman, & Markman, 2002). Fifth, ethical guidelines specifically for conducting family therapy (AAMFT, 1998) and family research (e.g., N. J. Kaslow & Gurman, 1985) have been developed, and overall there has been increased attention paid to ethics in marriage and family therapy (Marsh & Magee, 1997). Emphasis on consumer protection also is evidenced by the passage of state licensure and certification bills for the practice of marital and family therapy. Sixth, there has been a dramatic increase in the literature addressing family therapy training and supervision over the past 15 years (Liddle, Breunlin, & Schwartz, 1988). This has been true across multiple disciplines and across multiple theoretical perspectives (Todd & Storm, 1997) and has included didactic and experiential components (e.g., Helmeke & Prouty, 2001). Commonly used supervision models include videotaping, live supervision, and cotherapy dyads or teams. Seventh, the field has become more sensitive to diversity in families, with particular emphasis on ethnicity (e.g., Celano & Kaslow, 2000; N. Kaslow, Wood, & Loundy, 1998), race (e.g., McGoldrick, 1998), gender (e.g., Walters, Carter, Papp, & Silverstein, 1992), and social class (Boyd-Franklin & Bry, 2000). There is a burgeoning awareness of the necessity of conducting culturally competent and gender-sensitive family therapy (Ariel, 1999; Philpot, Brooks, Lusterman, & Nutt, 1997) and family research (see Liddle, Bray, Levant, & Santiste-ban, 2002). Eighth, there has been an increased emphasis on a biopsychosocial perpsective in conceptualizing and treating families (Sperry, 2001). This is evidenced by such trends as a greater appreciation for the need to incorporate pharmacological interventions into family interventions (e.g., Kopelowicz, Liberman, & Zarate, 2002), the burgeoning field of medical family therapy (e.g., McDaniel, Lusterman, & Philpot, 2001) and the marriage between such fields as pediatric psychology and family psychology (Kazak, Simms, & Rourke, 2002). Finally, recent years have witnessed the interna-tionalization of the field, with the development of the International Family Therapy Association (IFTA) and the International Academy of Family Psychologists (IAFP) and the publication of materials on international family therapy (e.g., F. W. Kaslow, 1982, 2000). Family therapy in the United States has been influenced increasingly by the clinical and theoretical developments throughout the world, most notably the Milan School (e.g., Boscolo, Cecchin, Hoffman, & Penn, 1987; Prata, 1990; Selvini-Palazzoli, Cirillo, Selvini, & Sorrentino, 1989).

THE CONCEPT OF THE FAMILY

Family theory has viewed the family as the primary unit of focus, departing from the traditional view that dysfunctional behavior primarily is influenced by individual characteristics, such as personality. Recently, attempts have been made to integrate individual personality development, family development, and the sociocultural context within which the individual and family are embedded (Feldman, 1992).

The nuclear family traditionally was defined as a group of people connected by blood or legal bonds that shared a residence. This definition has evolved to include groups of people perceived to be a family, united by marriage, blood, or residence sharing. Stepfamilies, cohabitating heterosexual couples and families, same-sex couples and families, foster families, adoptive families (including those with international adoptions), and commuter marriages represent variations of the modern family. Despite changes in the structure of family systems, the family's primary function continues to be mutual exchange among family members to meet the physical and emotional needs of each individual.

General systems theory, which emerged from the biological sciences, provides the theoretical underpinnings for major family therapy models. A *system* is a group of elements interacting with one another (von Bertalanffy, 1968). Paradoxically, family units continually change and advance toward greater levels of organization and functioning (anamorphosis), simultaneously self-regulating to maintain equilibrium, or *homeostasis.* The balance between change and stability enables the family to function adaptively throughout the family's and individual's life cycle.

Family systems continuously exchange information via *feedback loops,* circular patterns of responses in which there is a return flow of information within the system. *Positive feedback* increases deviation from the steady state, enabling the family to evolve to a new state. However, too much amplification of the deviation may destroy the system. For example, a fight between intimate partners simultaneously may increase intimacy and self-definition, or the fight may escalate out of control. *Negative feedback* counteracts deviations in the system to restore homeostasis. For example, a child may become symptomatic after his or her sibling becomes less overinvolved in the parental relationship.

As these examples suggest, family interactions reflect circular causality in which single events are viewed as both cause and effect and reciprocally related with no beginning or end to the causal sequence of events. According to the structural functionalism that dominated U.S. social science during the 1950s and 1960s (Parsons & Bales, 1955), families may be viewed in terms of structure and function. Structure refers to the family organization, the way in which the subsystems are arranged, and the power hierarchy or chain of command. The key structural property of the family unit is its *wholeness,* namely, the whole is greater than the sum of its parts. The family unit comprises interdependent subsystems that carry out distinctive functions to maintain themselves and sustain the system as a whole. Each individual is his or her own subsystem. Each family member belongs to several subsystems simultaneously, providing the basis for differential relationships with other family members. Subsystems can be formed by generation (e.g., parental or sibling subsystem), gender (e.g., mother–daughter dyad), interest (e.g., shared hobbies), and/or function (e.g., caregivers). The family unit also is a subsystem, as it interacts with the extended family, larger community, and outside world.

Subsystems are delineated and separated by *boundaries,* which protect the subsystem's integrity while allowing interaction between subsystems. Boundaries can be more or less permeable and adapt to the changing needs of the family system. Impairments in adaptive functioning arise if boundaries are too *rigid,* not allowing adequate communication between subsystems, or too *diffuse,* allowing too much communication with other subsystems. In an extreme form, rigid boundaries lead to disengagement, where family members are isolated from one another and function autonomously. Diffuse boundaries are associated with enmeshment, where family members are overinvolved in one another's lives. Family systems also have boundaries that regulate transactions with the outside world. An *open system* has relatively permeable boundaries, permitting interaction with the outside community without compromising the integrity of the family system. Conversely, a *closed system* has relatively rigid boundaries, minimizing contact with the outside world.

To maintain their structure, family systems have *rules,* operating principles enabling them to perform the tasks of daily living. Some rules are negotiated openly and are overt, whereas others are unspoken and covert. Healthy families have rules that are consistent, clearly stated, and fairly enforced over time yet can be adapted to the changing developmental needs of the family.

Each family member plays a number of *roles,* exhibiting a predictable set of behaviors associated with their social position.

One's family of origin, gender, and generation within the nuclear family may influence one's role behavior. Roles may include that of partner, parent, child, sibling, victim, caregiver, martyr, scapegoat, and hero. Optimally, family members' roles are negotiated to accommodate the needs of the family unit and the developmental stages of the participants, as well as to eliminate dysfunctional roles (e.g., victim). Changes in gender roles as a result of the feminist movement and women's increased presence in the workforce in recent decades, for example, have had a powerful impact on family functioning as men and women have to negotiate new interactive patterns and at-home responsibilities. According to the structural functionalist view, all behavior (e.g., roles, symptoms, and communication patterns) serves a purpose. For example, an individual's maladaptive behavior may return the family to homeostasis. Specifically, an adolescent with an eating disorder increasingly may become symptomatic following graduation, leading to greater family involvement and concern about her transition to college. The eating disorder may slow down the separation–individuation process, which the family perceives as threatening to its integrity. Although this symptom may return the family to a homeostatic state, it impedes the adolescent's individual development. However, the symptom may enable the family to receive psychotherapeutic help to cope with the family developmental crisis associated with launching a child.

Family rituals often demark important family transitions, such as beginnings, endings, separations, and unions and provide a context within which to notice and oftentimes honor these important changes. Rituals can be prescribed in an effort to intervene in family patterns and promote change by challenging the status quo and opening up new options for family members (Imber-Black, Roberts, & Whiting, 1988). Typically, carrying out a ritual runs counter to a particular way of doing something and can elucidate inherent contradictions or chaos in family members' behavior.

Family Development

Family development refers to the growth of individual family members; changes in the structure, tasks, and interactional process of the family unit over time; and the reciprocally related subcycles involving the marital/partnership–parental couple, the sib-ship, and the extended family. Passage through family life-cycle stages includes continuous and discontinuous change. Each stage qualitatively is different; developmental tasks are negotiated in new ways. Successful passage through these stages depends on the effectiveness of developmentally appropriate negotiations of tasks and stressors. A family member's symptom may reflect the family's difficulty moving from one developmental stage to the next (Haley, 1976). Interactions at any family life-cycle stage are influenced by interactions at earlier stages, and thus dysfunctional resolution at one stage increases the likelihood of further impairments in the family's functioning.

Carter and McGoldrick (1989) delineated six stages of the American *family life cycle,* a model that acknowledges the confluence of situational, developmental, and family-of-origin (historical) stressors. The first stage, between families, encompasses the unattached young adult's tasks of separation–individuation, the development of close relationships, and the establishment of an identity linked to one's educational pursuits, job, or career. The second stage, the joining of families through marriage, describes the development of the new marital dyad/romantic partnership and the realignment of relationships with one's family of origin and social support system to include the partner. In the third stage, the family with young children adjusts the marital/partnership bond to include children, incorporate parenting roles, and redefine relationships with extended family to include grandparents. In the fourth stage, the family with adolescents flexibly supports the adolescents' drive for autonomy and self-definition. The adults redirect their attention to their own personal and professional development and often become cargivers for their parents. Parents launching children and moving on characterizes the fifth stage. Parents support their young adult children's physical separation from the family, renegotiate the couple system as a more intimate dyad, develop more egalitarian relationships with their adult children, reorganize the family system to include in-laws and grandchildren, and cope with failing health and death of parents. In the sixth stage, the family in later life, the couple explores new family and social role options and addresses loss and mortality, and the adult children express their respect for their parents' wisdom and experience. Carter and McGoldrick underscore the variability in the family life cycle associated with different sociocultural contexts, characterizing distinctive features of the life cycles of low-income and professional families and families of various ethnic, racial, and religious backgrounds. For example, families migrating to a new country face changes in the nature and structure of relationships often across generations, based on the interface of their new culture with cultural patterns from their country of origin (N. J. Kaslow, Celano, & Dreelin, 1995). As such, migration represents another life-cycle phase for these families. Others have described specific variations in life cycle including those of single-parent families (Ginsberg, 2002; Miller, 1992), remarried and stepfamilies (Visher & Visher, 1996), and gay and lesbian families (James, 2002; Patterson, 2002) and the role of children in the family life cycle (Combrinck-Graham, 2001).

Normal Family Functioning

What is a normal or healthy family? The answer to this question is complex and depends on the theoretical perspective used. Family theorists differ in their views of the applicability of the construct of normality to individual family members, family units, or a combination of the two. For example, can families be considered normal if one person evidences symptoms? Conversely, can an individual be deemed as normal if he or she grows up in a dysfunctional family yet functions adaptively? Normal families may evidence (1) asymptomatic family functioning (absence of symptoms of dysfunction), (2) optimal family functioning (successful according to the values of a given conceptual paradigm), (3) average family functioning (fits a typical or prevalent pattern and falls in the normal range), and/or (4) transactional family processes (adaptation over the course of the family life cycle to a particular socioecological context) (Walsh, 1982).

Some authors (e.g., Satir & Baldwin, 1983) depict healthy families as those composed of healthy individuals. According to these authors, human beings basically are good and strive for growth. Health may be evident in several functional domains: physical, spiritual, contextual, nutritional, interactional, sensual, emotional, and intellectual. Just as the various components of each individual's functioning contribute to his or her overall sense of self, each family member's sense of self contributes to the overall level of health in the family system.

Using a systemic perspective, clinical researchers have developed schemata (e.g., Epstein, Bishop, & Baldwin, 1982; Olson, Sprenkle, & Russell, 1979) and portraits (e.g., Whitaker & Bumberry, 1988) of healthy family functioning. The pattern of characteristics indicative of healthy functioning changes across the family life cycle (Olson et al., 1983) and depends on the family's sociocultural context. Cohesion, change, and communication are the key dimensions along which family functioning is characterized. Family cohesion refers to the level of emotional bonding among family members and the commitment family members have to the unit. Optimal families are cohesive, with a clear, yet flexible structure. Generational and individual boundaries are mutually understood, allowing a sense of closeness and belonging to coexist with respect for the privacy of the individual and the subsystems. Healthy families encourage age-appropriate autonomy for all members, express a range of well-modulated positive and negative emotions, are supportive of and empathically attuned to one another, maintain a sense of humor even in the face of adversity, and are open to receiving feedback from each other. Family members share beliefs, enabling them to transcend their immediate reality and address existential concerns such as meaning/purpose of life, self-definition, and mortality. These transcendent values are transmitted across generations, thus connecting a nuclear family with its past and future and with the larger social environment. Finally, these families have a worldview that is optimistic and they are cognizant of their place in the world.

Change refers to the degree of flexibility within the system. Healthy families adapt their power structure, role relationships, and rules in response to situational and developmental demands and new information from the environment. Relatively equal power is the norm for the marital/partnership dyad. A clear power hierarchy exists between the parental subsystem and the children, and control and authority dynamics are clear to all members. The power dynamics change throughout the family life cycle, with power becoming more shared as the children mature. Standards for controlling behavior are reasonable, and there is ample opportunity for modification of these standards using skilled negotiation and problem solving. Family functions are filled such that members are not overburdened with too many roles, and there is flexibility in roles played. These families recognize when they need community assistance.

In the communication domain, healthy families communicate clearly and effectively about their feelings and practical matters. There is congruence between the content and process of the communications (*contextual clarity*) such that few double-binding messages occur. For example, a verbal expression of loving feelings is communicated in a caring tone, with physical gestures consistent with the positive feeling being expressed. This is in contrast to a double-bind communication in which a person verbalizes loving feelings in a hostile tone of voice, with minimal eye contact, and a physical distancing.

Pathological or Dysfunctional Family Functioning

Historically, psychiatric diagnoses indicating pathology have been applied to individuals. Many family theorists argue that psychiatric nomenclature is less relevant in understanding family pathology than are family interaction patterns. The gap between the psychiatric viewpoint and family systems theories is evidenced by the lack of a family classification system in DSM-IV (American Psychiatric Association, 1994), despite efforts of the Coalition on Family Diagnosis in working with the DSM-IV task forces to implement a system in DSM-IV (F. W. Kaslow, 1993, 1996). Instead, the GARF (Group for the Advancement of Psychiatry Committee on the Family, 1996) developed by members of the coalition was included in the appendix of DSM-IV. The GARF is a 1–100-point (low to high) scale, single-item measure assessing the level of functioning of a family or other relational unit. In addition, *The Handbook of Relational Diagnosis,* articulating 30 diagnostic categories, is the first attempt to formalize systemic assessment for the purpose of further research (F. W. Kaslow, 1996).

Family theorists' conceptualizations of dysfunction emphasize either the development of family classification schemata or the linking of family interaction patterns to individual psychopathology. Family researchers have developed classification schemata describing the functioning of family units from healthy/adaptive to severely dysfunctional/extreme along the previously discussed dimensions of cohesion, change, and communication (Beavers & Hampson, 1993; Olson, 2000). Severely dysfunctional families are inflexible and not adaptable; they fail to change in response to environmental or situational demands or developmental changes. They tend to be undifferentiated and to have poor boundaries, and they fail to provide an environment conducive to the healthy development of each individual and the establishment of trusting relationships. Severely dysfunctional families have a poorly defined power structure, impaired communication (e.g., inconsistent communications), difficulties with problem solving and negotiation, and a pervasively negative affective quality with minimal expressions of caring and warmth. There is, however, heterogeneity in the expression of the family pathology dependent on the family's characterization on such dimensions as cohesion, adaptability, and communication style.

Olson (2000) developed a circumplex model of family functioning, describing the family's level of adaptability and cohesion. Family adaptability describes a continuum of functioning related to the extent to which the family system is flexible and able to change its power structure, role relationships, and rules in response to situational and developmental demands. A healthy family is flexible or structured in its approach to change, whereas unhealthy families either are chaotic at one extreme of the continuum or rigid at the other extreme of the continuum in their approach to dealing with change. Family cohesion, also a continuous variable, refers to the degree of emotional bonding (separate vs. connected) family members have toward one another. An adaptive level of family cohesion is one in which family members either are separated or connected, as opposed to the extremes of the continuum (disengaged or enmeshed). A balance between adaptability and cohesion is associated with optimal family functioning and healthy individual

development, whereas extreme functioning on both dimensions characterizes dysfunctional families. Four types of dysfunctional families emerge in this classification schema: chaotically disengaged, chaotically enmeshed, rigidly disengaged, and rigidly enmeshed. Chaotically disengaged families feel disconnected from one another. Unrestricted external influences are allowed, blurred boundaries predominate, and the family's interaction is unpredictable, marked by limited and/or erratic leadership and discipline, endless negotiations, and dramatic role shifts and rule changes. Similar to chaotically disengaged families, rigidly disengaged families experience a sense of isolation within the family, with their primary bonds being with individuals outside the family system. However, rigidly disengaged families also are characterized by an authoritarian leadership style, with strict and rigidly enforced rules, limited negotiations, and stereotyped roles. Chaotically enmeshed families present as extremely close, with high loyalty demands and little tolerance for privacy, separateness, or external influences. This family overinvolvement prevails in an unpredictable and volatile family environment. Conversely, rigidly enmeshed families legislate their intense family closeness through strict rules, rigid roles, and an authoritarian leadership style (for review, see Olson, 2000). Research reveals that family type is associated with individual pathology. For example, many families with a juvenile delinquent member are chaotically enmeshed and family adaptability and cohesion distinguishes families of offenders from those of nonoffenders (Henggeler, Burr-Harris, & Borduin, 1991).

Another schema useful in characterizing healthy, midrange, and severely dysfunctional families is that of Beavers and Hampson (1993), based on research conducted at the Timberlawn Psychiatric Research Foundation in Dallas. Beavers and Hampson depicts family functioning according to level of adaptability and stylistic presentation, noting that stylistic differences are primarily relevant to dysfunctional families. Family adaptability is defined as the family's capacity to function competently in effecting change and tolerating individual differentiation. Families low on adaptability are more likely to be dysfunctional as they are inflexible and manifest poor boundaries and confused communication. Severely dysfunctional families, low on adaptability, may exhibit either a centrifugal or a centripetal stylistic presentation. Centrifugal families, similar to disengaged families, expect gratification from outside the family, predominantly trust non-family members, and experience premature demands for separation. Centripetal families seek gratification from within the family, have difficulties with separating and individuating, and are less trustful of the external environment, similar to enmeshed families (for review, see Beavers & Hampson, 1993).

Others have linked individual psychopathology with specific family interaction patterns. This research initially addressed the etiological role of aberrant family patterns (e.g., distorted communication) in the development of individual psychopathology, particularly schizophrenia (e.g., Bateson et al., 1956; Wynne, Ryckoff, Day, & Hirsch, 1958). As more has become known regarding the genetic and biological bases of major mental illnesses, such as schizophrenia spectrum disorders, it is clear that family patterns do not play an etiological role in these disorders. More recently, research has generated models emphasizing the function of family patterns in a wider range of individual psychopathology, for example, families with children who are aggressive (Patterson, Dishion, & Chamberlain, 1993).

During the past 20 years, research on family variables associated with the pathogenesis of psychopathology has addressed the temporal ordering and reciprocal influences of family process and psychopathology and the differential contributions of environment and heredity (Goldstein, Rosenfarb, Woo, & Nuechterlein, 1997). For example, individuals with schizophrenia spectrum disorders are most vulnerable to relapse if they reside in a family in which high levels of expressed emotion are reported (Leff & Vaughn, 1985). High expressed emotion refers to critical, hostile, and emotional overinvolved verbal attitudes revealed during an interview, toward the schizophrenic individual by his or her relatives; a dysfunctional affective style refers to similar patterns of behavior observed in the context of a laboratory-based interaction task. Individuals with depression and bipolar disorder in critical, hostile, and emotionally overinvolved families also have a poorer prognosis than do their counterparts in families characterized by low levels of expressed emotion and adaptive affective styles. These findings question the specificity of the association between high expressed emotion, negative affective style, and schizophrenia spectrum disorders, bipolar disorder, and depression. Although the bulk of research initially focused on families with a loved one with schizophrenia, investigators have established the relationship between family interaction patterns and individual disorders (Hooley & Gotlib, 2000), specifically, depression (Coyne, Kahn, & Gotlib, 1987), eating disorders (Hodes & le Grange, 1993), child aggression (Patterson et al., 1993) and child adjustment (Zimet & Jacob, 2001), alcoholism (Jacob & Johnson, 1999), anxiety disorders (Chambless & Steketee, 1999), and borderline personality disorders (Hooley & Hoffman, 1999). More recent research has expanded knowledge of this relationship and suggests a link between parental expressed emotion and adolescent and childhood depression (e.g., McCleary & Sanford, 2002; Rosenbaum Asarnow, Tompson, Woo, & Cantwell, 2001). Furthermore, the connection between parental expressed emotion and individual adjustment has extended into populations of individuals facing medical disorders (e.g. children with diabetes; Worrall-Davies, Owens, & Holland, 2002). Other research further substantiates the complexities of the link between parent–child interaction and the children's behavioral problems, whether psychiatric or medical (e.g., Eisenberg, Gershoff, & Fabes, 2001; Wamboldt & Wamboldt, 2000). Because the expressed–emotion concept implies that part of the problem lies in the negative attitudes and behaviors of family members, it has become controversial among family members who may feel blamed for their relative's disorder. Increasingly, these constructs have been linked to the course rather than the etiology of disorders and must be incorporated into a biopsychosocial understanding of psychological difficulties across the lifespan.

Investigators are struggling to answer the question: Why are only some family members symptomatic? An individual's symptoms depend on characteristics of the individual (e.g., biological predisposition, temperament, intelligence, and personality), interactive effects (e.g., parent–child attachment, marital/partnership satisfaction, sibling position, and dynamics), and extrafamilial influences (e.g., social support, economic status, and external stressors). Thus, an individual with considerable personal strengths and external resources can reside in a dysfunctional family yet function adaptively over time, whereas another family member may have fewer strengths and/or resources and thus may be more vulnerable to developing psychopathology. Each family member's personal characteristics influence how other family members interact with him or her. These interaction patterns in turn affect the individual's level of functioning. Furthermore, individual biological vulnerabilities also interact with these multiple levels of environmental stressors to create a complex explanation of the etiology of the manifestation of symptoms in human behavior (Reiss & Neiderhiser, 2000).

THE PROCESS OF CLINICAL ASSESSMENT

Multisystem, Multimethod Approach

A multisystem, multimethod approach, evaluating the individual, various dyads, and the family system as a whole using multiple assessment methods, is useful for assessing family dysfunction. Several family constructs are evaluated: structure, adaptability, emotions and needs, interaction and communication patterns, developmental stage of the individual and family, family of origin, sociocultural factors, and strengths and resources. Despite a growing consensus about the value of family assessment and the constructs to be examined, there is divergence regarding the significance, interrelationships, and underlying processes of these constructs. Various schools of thought place differential emphasis on assessing intrapsychic variables, behavioral functioning, and systemic patterns. Ideally, assessment is integrated into the therapeutic process, as it is cost-effective and yields a relatively rapid overview of family dynamics, useful in problem identification, treatment selection, evaluation of ongoing therapy, and determination of treatment efficacy. Snyder, Cavell, Heffere, and Mangrum (1995) propose a family assessment model based on five system levels from the individual to community across five domains including cognitive, affective, interpersonal, developmental, and control. When assessing a family, the clinician may use measures examining individual family members' cognitive or emotional functioning, and marital/partnership and family functioning. Marital and family functioning measurement tools can be divided into formal and informal self-report measures, observational data, and interactional coding schemata (for reviews, see Kerig & Lindahl, 2001; Nurse, 1999).

Self-Report Measures

Self-report measures are easy and inexpensive to administer and score and useful in assessing marital/partnership and family satisfaction. However, they do not adequately assess several key variables (e.g., family power), and they measure individual differences rather than a system and its interrelationships. Among the innumerable self-report measures of family adjustment, the most frequently used and psychometrically sound instruments include the Family Environment Scale (FES; Moos & Moos, 1981), the Family Adaptability and Cohesion Evaluation Scales (FACES; Olson et al., 1983), the McMaster Family Assessment Device (FAD; Epstein, Baldwin, & Bishop, 1983), and the Family Assessment Measure (FAM; Skinner, Steinhauer, & Santa-Barbara, 1983). The FES assesses three dimensions characterizing the family's social environment: relationship, system maintenance, and personal growth. The FACES, which is based on the circumplex model, addresses family cohesion and adaptability. The FAD assesses families according to the McMaster Model of Family Functioning along the dimensions of problem solving, communication, roles, affective responsiveness, affective involvement, and behavior control. The FAM provides a quantitative index of family strengths and weaknesses.

There are also numerous self-report measures of marital/partnership communication and intimacy, family life events, the quality of family life, parenting stress (e.g., Abidin, 1997), family conflict (e.g., Parent–Child Conflict Tactics Scale—Revised; Straus, Hamby, Finkelhor, Moore, & Runyan, 1998), and parenting attitudes, knowledge, and attachment (for overview, see Lindholm & Touliatos, 1993).

Observational Methods

Family research over the last 20 years has evolved from self-report methodology that is focused on individuals to a multimethod approach that accommodates a systems perspective and involves the integration of data gleaned from observation (Gottman & Notarius, 2002; Kerig & Lindahl, 2001). Direct observation provides information regarding the complexities of the interactional processes of which family members may or may not be conscious. Observational measurements are obtained by rating specified nonverbal and verbal interactions of given subsystems in response to a structured task completed in a standard setting. The resulting data are then reduced via a coding schema to glean meaning from the complex set of behaviors exchanged among family members. Most coding schemata assess six dimensions that hypothetically discriminate between normal and dysfunctional families: dominance, affect, communication, information exchange, conflict, and support/validation (Markman & Notarius, 1987).

There are numerous coding schemata to assess marital/partnership or family interactions from a microanalytic or macroanalytic perspective (Gottman & Notarius, 2000). A microanalytic coding schema is one that focuses on specific behaviors emitted by individuals in interactional sequences providing a detailed behavioral analysis, whereas a macroanalytic perspective focuses on larger units of behavior and offers a more global perspective. The Family Interaction Coding System (FICS; Patterson, Ray, Shaw, & Cobb, 1969), the most widely used family microanalytic coding system, provides a sequential analysis of aversive and prosocial behaviors in family interactions during a semistructured task to obtain a summary of the family's level of coerciveness. As a microanalytic coding systems, the FICS allows for careful analysis of complex interactions and the discrete behaviors of which these interactions are comprised. Despite the richness and ecological validity of the resultant data, the attainment, coding, and analysis of such data are labor intensive and costly. In a nonresearch environment, the process of family observation to inform treatment typically is informal and not standardized.

Macroanalytic coding schemata frequently are applied to observational data collected in a relatively unstructured situation. For example, the Beavers–Timberlawn Family Evaluation Scale is a clinician's global rating, on a 10-point Likert-type scale, of five dimensions (structure of the family, mythology, goal-directed negotiation, autonomy, family affect) based on the clinician's observations of the family's discussion of desired changes (Beavers & Hampson, 1993). Another example of a global coding system used in longitudinal research is the Iowa Family Interaction Rating Scales (IFIRS; Melby et al., 1998). It is designed to measure the quality of behavioral exchanges between parents and their adolescent children that are inclusive of both verbal and nonverbal behaviors, as well as affective and contextual dimensions of interactions. Aspects of behavior are rated on a 1–9 scale and based on the frequency, intensity, and proportion of behavior, where 1 represents the absence of the behavior and 9 represents a behavior that is mainly characteristic of the interaction (Melby & Conger, 2001). Macroanalytic coding schemata are more user friendly than are microanalytic schemata and capture the interactional Gestalt rather than each individual's discrete behaviors.

THE PRACTICE OF THERAPY, THE STANCE OF THE THERAPIST, CURATIVE FACTORS, AND TREATMENT APPLICABILITY

There is not one brand of family therapy. Thus, we would do a disservice to depict the practice of family therapy as homogenous. This section of the chapter focuses on some of the most widely practiced and influential schools of family therapy. There is inconsistency regarding how to categorize the various approaches; our presentation reflects one possible division. These schools are presented in a sequence organized by the extent to which they emphasize the past versus the present and intrapsychic versus interpersonal dimensions (N. Kaslow, F. W. Kaslow, & Farber, 1999). The psychodynamically informed, intergenerational, and family-of-origin approaches emphasize primarily the past. However, the psychoanalytic perspective also primarily focuses on intrapsychic issues, whereas the intergenera-

tional and family-of-origin models address both intrapsychic and interpersonal dimensions equally. The experiential–humanistic brands of family therapy occupy the middle of both spectrums, placing relatively equal emphasis on past and present, and on intrapsychic and interpersonal dimensions. Strategic, systemic, structural, cognitive-behavioral, postmodern/social constructivist, and psychoeducational approaches focus on the present and on interpersonal factors. To facilitate comparison of the various schools of thought, our presentation of each model considers the basic structure of the therapy, goals, therapeutic techniques and strategies, therapeutic process, role of the therapist, curative factors, and treatment applicability. Table 11.1 presents the major models of family therapy articulated below in detail. Bowen therapy would ordinarily be included in this list, however, as much of it is couple focused, it is covered by Gurman in Chapter 12.

For purposes of clarity, the models are delineated separately. However, because the schools of family therapy are relatively consistent in conceptualizing the role of psychotropic medications in the therapeutic process, a general comment here will suffice. Early in the family therapy movement, an individual's symptoms were viewed solely as reflections of dysfunction in the family system, and thus the use of medication for a symptomatic member was eschewed. As the field of family therapy has become more integrated into the mainstream of psychiatric practice and as more evidence has accumulated supporting the interaction of biological and environmental etiological factors for severe psychopathology, psychotropic medications have come to be viewed as a useful adjunct to family treatment. However, medication is offered to alleviate a family member's distressing symptoms rather than to make fundamental changes in either the individual or the family. The exception to this practice is found in the family psychoeducational approach, which stresses the importance of compliance with medication regi-

TABLE 11.1. Models of Family Therapy

Theory	Key proponents	Temporal focus	Focus of therapeutic change	Structure	Goals	Techniques	Stance of therapist
Psychodynamically informed	Ackerman, Framo, Slipp, Scharff, Scharff	Past	Intrapsychic issues	Long-term weekly treatment with unstructured sessions; membership varies depending on goals being addressed	Increase insight; strengthen ego functioning; develop more mature self-representation and more satisfying interpersonal relationships; increase access to "true self"; and develop a balance between strivings for autonomy and intimacy	Provision of "holding environment"; develop interpretations linking past and present; address resistances, transference, and countertransference dynamics; termination	Provides a "holding environment" in which the therapist serves as a good-enough parent and reparents the family
Intergenerational–contextual	Boszormenyi-Nagy	Primary focus on past; some focus on present	Equal attention to intrapsychic and interpersonal dynamics	Therapy is conducted by cotherapy team, usually on a long-term basis; participants are individuals, nuclear families, and/or multigenerational families	Identify and address invisible loyalties; repair strained family relationships	Facilitation of each family member's perspective (multidirected partiality); acknowledgment of defenses and resistances; encouragement to face ethical issues from which resistances derive; homework	Catalyst for change who aligns with healthy aspects of the family; therapists communicate empathy, flexibility, creativity, and compassion
Experiential–humanistic	Whitaker	Equal focus on past and present	Equal attention to intrapsychic and interpersonal dynamics	Relatively unstructured time unlimited therapy of intermediate duration, conducted by cotherapy team or therapist and consultant; sessions include family and may include index person's social support network	Increase family members' cohesion; help family facilitate members' individuation; increase creativity and spontaneity family as a unit and individual members	"Joining" with family; battles for structure and initiative; management (not interpretation) of resistance; definition of symptoms as efforts toward growth; explication of covert conflict; therapist's use of self (e.g., absurdity and "acting in")	Coaches or surrogate grandparents who suggest but do not direct change; therapists share their internal processes with the family without losing their differentiated sense of self

(continued)

TABLE 11.1. *Continued*

Theory	Key proponents	Temporal focus	Focus of therapeutic change	Structure	Goals	Techniques	Stance of therapist
Strategic	Haley, Madanes	Present	Interpersonal	Structured, brief intervention conducted by a single therapist; sessions may include whole family or one or more family members	Solve family's presenting problem by altering the interactional sequences maintaining the problem	Straight or paradoxical directives to change interactional sequences; reframing problem behaviors; homework	Powerful, authoritative, and often charismatic figure who persuades family to follow directives
Systemic	Selvini-Palazzoli, Prata, Boscolo, Cecchin, Hoffman, Papp	Present	Interpersonal	Relatively structured intervention consisting of 3–20 monthly sessions, conducted by a single therapist or cotherapy pair and observed/supervised by other members of therapy term	Goals are defined by family unless family's choices are harmful to one or more members	Circular questioning; positive connotation; rituals; counter-paradoxical interventions	Neutral and nonreactive; family is responsible for change
Structural	Minuchin, Aponte	Present	Interpersonal	Brief intervention typically conducted by a single therapist; sessions include family members who interact daily	Resolution of presenting problem by restructuring the family unit to facilitate more adaptive interactional patterns; change family's construction of reality regarding their presenting problem	Joining process; assessment of six domains of family functioning; restructuring techniques-enactments, boundary marking, unbalancing family alignments; homework	"Distant relative," often a colorful and dramatic figure who actively and authoritatively directs the treatment
Cognitive-behavioral	Alexander & Parsons, Epstein, L'Abate, Patterson	Present	Interpersonal	Relatively structured, brief timed-limited intervention conducted by a single therapist; session membership	Enhance marital or family satisfaction by changing members' cognitive processing of their own and one	Formal assessment of family members' beliefs, causal attributions, and expectancies regarding the present problem;	Teacher/consultant who teaches family members about cognitive and behavioral processes

414

Model	Key figures	Past/Present	Orientation	Format	Goals	Techniques	Therapist role
				depends on goals of treatment, but typically includes marital dyad or family	another's behavior	cognitive restructuring technique (e.g., logical analysis of distorted automatic thoughts); self-instructional training; homework; communication skill	and supervises their rehearsal of new behaviors
Postmodern/ social constructivist	Goolishian, Anderson, deShazer, Weiner-Davis, White,	Present	Interpersonal and Intrapsychic (meaning systems)	Relatively short-term treatment conducted by and individual therapist or therapy teams (one-way mirror or "reflecting team"); membership varies depending on the presenting problem; sessions include dialogues co-created by therapist and family members	Change the meaning (beliefs) surrounding presenting problem through dialogue to enable family members to discover and take action within the new meaning	Use of questioning and discussion techniques (e.g., "miracle question," "exception-finding questions," and "externalizing the problem"), directives, and homework assignments	Therapists are nonhierarchical participants that work collaboratively with family members; both therapist and family members equally bring expertise in finding solutions
Psychoeducational	Anderson, Hogarty, Reiss	Present	Interpersonal	Structured intervention conducted with individual families or with multiple family groups; frequency of sessions and duration of treatment depends on status of patient's psychiatric illness; treatment is typically conducted by two therapists	Integrate patient with psychiatric illness into the community; prevent relapse	Parallel meetings with patient and family to establish rapport, allay anxiety and discuss treatment philosophy; assessment culminating in development of treatment contract; educational workshops for family and friends of patient; homework; build problem solving and communication skills of family members	Therapists work collaboratively with patient, family and other members of treatment team; they are active in treatment process, providing advice, information, and support

415

mens for individuals with severe psychiatric disorders (McFarlane, 2002).

Many family therapists have integrated the various perspectives delineated below in a thoughtful and well-informed manner to address individual families and their unique problems (Lebow, 1997). We share with other integrationists the view that whereas the beginning of the family therapy field demanded explication of relatively distinct and diverse theoretical approaches, the current state of the field is served best by an integrative perspective. We also believe that it is essential that family therapy be gender-sensitive (Walters et al., 1992), culturally informed (Celano & Kaslow, 2000; McGoldrick, Giordano, & Pearce, 1996), and responsive to socioeconomic differences (Aponte, 1994). In this vein, new perspectives are being articulated that build on current intervention approaches, and that respect and take into consideration the diversity of human experience across gender, race, ethnicity, and sociocultural and socioeconomic contexts.

Psychodynamically Informed Family Therapy

As many family therapy pioneers were trained in the psychoanalytic tradition, psychodynamic concepts have been integral to the development of several family therapy models. However, given many family therapists' rebellion against the historically individual focus associated with the psychoanalytic tradition, continuities between psychoanalytic and family theories have been minimized. Psychodynamically informed family therapy is one of the only family models that acknowledges its ties to psychoanalytic thinking, valuing the role of the unconscious and past history in determining behavior and motivations, the necessity of insight for behavior change, and the importance of transference and countertransference dynamics.

Nathan Ackerman, the "grandfather of family therapy," is the most noted early psychoanalytically oriented family therapist. Other key figures include James Framo, Ivan Boszormenyi-Nagy, Robin Skynner, Norman Paul, and John Bell. Recently, some writers have integrated current psychoanalytic theory (e.g., object relations theory) with family systems models, referring to their work as *object relations family therapy* (Scharff, 1989; Scharff & Scharff, 1997). Object relations theory, with its basic assumption that the need for satisfying interpersonal relationships is a fundamental human motive, lends itself more readily to the understanding of family dynamics than does classical analytic theory, which emphasizes intrapsychic dynamics (Johnson, 1996). Attention to patterns of attachment in family relationships lends an understanding of the interpersonal dynamics inherent in behavior. When family members respond inappropriately to attachment behavior, such as prematurely forecasting loss within a relationship, there is a need to attend to these patterns. Therefore, psychodynamically oriented family therapists who are able to instill a sense of safety within the system enable the family to explore new ways of relating (Byng-Hall, 2001). In bridging psychodynamic tenets and systems theory, psychodynamically oriented family therapists attend to the complex interplay among each individual's unique personality and background, family interactional processes, and the sociocultural context.

Experience in one's family of origin (e.g., parents, grandparents, and siblings) provides the foundation for sense of self, internalized images of significant others (*introjects*), and expectations for intimate relationships. Symptomatic behavior represents unresolved conflicts stemming from one's family of origin, which are reenacted with one's family of creation (e.g., partner and children) (Framo, 1982). Reenactment occurs via individuals' use of projection of introjected "bad objects" (negative internalized image of one's parent[s]) onto significant others in their adult life (Framo, 1982). Interpersonal interactions unconsciously are interpreted in a fashion consistent with each member's inner object world of positive and negative introjects. Furthermore, each individual unconsciously seeks a mate who will be a willing recipient of his or her lost and split-off introjects, resulting in a collusive partnership (Framo, 1982).

A family member's symptom becomes part of a recurring, predictable, interactional pattern that ensures equilibrium for the individual but impairs the family's ability to adapt to change due to rigid, stereotypical, or rapidly shifting family roles (Ackerman, 1958). Such role distortions and the breakdown of role complementarity are associated with intrapsychic and interpersonal conflicts, often occurring simultaneously and exacerbating each other. Unresolved conflicts often result in the unconscious placement of a family member in a role in which he or she is consistently exposed to criticism and blamed for the family tension (scapegoating). Scapegoating further validates negative introjects, thus exacerbating individual symptoms and family dysfunction.

Central to object relations theory is the idea that attachment as an infant determines family members' personality development as adults; therefore, the cultivation of secure attachment is central to an individual's sense of self (Scharff, 1989). The assertion and resolution of needs over time within close family relationships leads to an individual's personality development or vulnerability to psychopathology. Understanding of attachment style and provision of a safe attachment or holding environment lends the essential information and the circumstances necessary to decipher dysfunctional patterns and address core dynamics responsible for these patterns.

Object relations family therapy is the dominant psychodynamically informed family therapy approach practiced today and thus the following comments are devoted to this approach. Another increasingly studied family approach that has its roots in the psychoanalytic tradition is emotionally focused family therapy (Johnson, 1996). Unfortunately, discussion of this approach is beyond the scope of this chapter.

Basic Structure of Therapy

Object relations family therapy is typically a long-term family treatment conducted on a weekly basis. The work is long term to address unresolved intrapsychic conflicts that are reenacted in one's current life and causing interpersonal and intrapsychic difficulties. Membership in the sessions may vary, depending on the presenting problem and the goals of each phase of the work. Membership may include one's family of origin, family of creation, intimate partner dyad, and/or the individual person. Concurrent treatments may be conducted. Therapy hours are relatively unstructured. Although the therapist is responsible for providing the external structure, the family's interactions and comments provide the internal structure.

Goal Setting

The goals of object relations family therapy are relatively similar across families with a variety of presenting problems and are implicit in the therapy rather than overtly discussed and negotiated. Goals are not specifically differentiated into intermediate- and long-term goals. These therapies attempt to help family members achieve increased insight; strengthen ego functioning; acknowledge and rework defensive projective identifications; attain more mature internal self and object representations; develop more satisfying interpersonal relationships supporting their needs for attachment, individuation, and psychological growth; and reduce interlocking pathologies among family members. The desired therapeutic outcome is for individual family members to have more access to their true selves, become more intimate with the true selves of significant others, and view others realistically rather than as projected parts of themselves. This enables the family to achieve a developmental level consistent with the needs of its members and the tasks to be addressed.

Techniques and Process of Therapy

In the initial phase of object relations family therapy, the therapist provides a frame, a *holding environment,* consisting of a specified time, space, and structure for the therapy. The therapist observes family interactions during an open-ended interview to ascertain family members' level of object relations, predominant defense mechanisms, and the relation between current interactional patterns and family-of-origin dynamics. A comprehensive history of each family member is conducted with all members present, with attention paid to family-of-origin dynamics, early experiences, presenting problems, and treatment history.

The importance of establishing a *therapeutic alliance* is underscored. Once an alliance is established, the therapist interprets conflicts, defenses, and patterns of interaction. Interpretations may address individual family member's dynamics and/or various family subsystems. Effective interpretations link an individual or family's history with current feelings, thoughts, behaviors, and interactions, permitting more adaptive family interactional patterns and intrapsychic changes. In making empathic interpretations, the therapist relies on theoretical knowledge and affective responses to each individual and the family unit.

The Fine family, an upper-middle-class Jewish family, sought treatment for their adolescent daughter's anorexic symptoms. During the therapy, it was discovered that the adolescent's eating disorder symptoms escalated when her father, a commercial pilot, was away from the family on lengthy trips. The therapist's own affective reactions to Mrs. Fine led the therapist to question whether she was depressed. It was revealed that although Mrs. Fine appeared to manage effectively, she became sad and hopeless during her husband's absences. The separations reactivated her unresolved grief regarding her father's death during her adolescence. The therapist conceptualized the daughter's symptoms as efforts to distract her mother from her depression, just as Mrs. Fine needed to care for her mother upon her father's death. This conceptualization led the therapist to empathically comment on how painful the separations were for each family member and to help the family develop ways for Mr. Fine to provide more object constancy for his wife (e.g., more frequent calls and e-mails and love notes left behind). This collaboratively designed intervention took into account Mr. Fine's employment, which necessitated separations; Mrs. Fine's vulnerability to separations; and the daughter's need to care for her mother in order for her mother to be emotionally available to her regardless of whether her father was present.

The primary treatment techniques are *interpretations of resistance, defenses, negative transference,* and family interaction patterns indicative of unresolved family-of-origin and intrapsychic conflicts. To facilitate change, external and internal resistances are addressed. For example, when a family member refuses to attend sessions, the therapist may interpret this individual's behavior as an expression of the family's shared reluctance to participate in the change process. Object relations family therapists address transference and countertransference dynamics to facilitate the therapeutic endeavor. Therapists use their own reactions to the family's behavior and interaction patterns (*objective countertransference*) to understand empathically the shared yet unspoken experiences of each family member regarding family interactional patterns (*unconscious family system of object relations*). Therapists employ their objective countertransference reactions to interpret interpersonal patterns in which one family member is induced to behave in a circumscribed and maladaptive fashion (*projective identification*).

The therapist, both covertly and overtly, attends to termination during each session and toward the end of the treatment process. Time boundaries for ending sessions and for ending the therapy course are respected, communicating the therapist's commitment to the family as a consultant to, rather than conductor of, the change process. The ending of each session raises issues of loss and separation, which need to be worked through in preparation for treatment termination. When appropriate, the therapist addresses how the family's history and present system of object relationships interfere with healthy, autonomous functioning. Overt discussions and interpretations regarding conflicts and feelings of separation and mourning precipitated by the finite nature of sessions help the family prepare for the ultimate termination of the family therapy. During the termination phase, salient conflicts are reviewed and unresolved family transferences in modified forms are reworked. There is an opportunity for mourning the loss of the therapist, who has become an important attachment figure. Technical errors occur when a safe holding environment has not been established, interpretations are poorly timed and do not attend to significant intrapsychic and interpersonal dynamics, and comments reflect unresolved countertransference issues rather than being empathically attuned to the family's affective experience.

> Mr. Williams, a 52-year-old African American accountant, remains unaware of his anger toward his mother for her overinvolvement in his marriage. He often spends time with his mother in a way that perpetuates her involvement. Rather than acknowledging his anger at his mother, Mr. Williams projects this anger onto his wife, a pediatrician, who accepts the projected anger and continually feels enraged at her mother-in-law: Thus, even when Dr. Williams and her mother-in-law have potentially enjoyable interactions, Dr. Williams creates conflict in the relationship to justify her anger. Mr. Williams continuously is disappointed in his wife for her conflictual and hostile relationship with his mother. One goal of the therapy was to enable Mr. Williams to become more cognizant of his negative feelings toward his mother. Working through these feelings helped him more appropriately separate from his mother and develop a more intimate relationship with his wife. Dr. Williams was freed to engage in more gratifying interactions with her mother-in-law. This work entailed understanding Mr. Williams's resistance to experience simultaneously positive and negative feelings toward his mother, the couples' reluctance to have a more intimate relationship, and Dr. Williams's propensity to engage in negative interactions with older women. This led Dr. Williams to examine unresolved negative feelings toward maternal objects, including her mother and overprotective grandmother. The termination phase entailed repeated efforts at addressing and integrating both partners' negative and positive feelings toward the therapist, who had come to represent a maternal figure for each of them.

Stance of the Therapist

Of utmost importance in conducting object relations family therapy is the provision of a "good enough" holding environment, where the therapist enables family members to feel safe and secure so that they can express openly their feelings and beliefs and feel more intimate with one another while maintaining a sense of self. The therapist functions as a "good enough" parent, reparenting the family by providing consistent nurturance, a secure attachment, and structure (e.g., limit setting) to enhance the development of individual members and the family unit.

Curative Factors

Therapy focuses on individuals' early family experiences, feelings about one another, and relationships. Primary mechanisms of change are interpretations of interpersonal patterns, including transference and countertransference dynamics, offered in the context of a positive working alliance and a safe holding environment. Interpretations help family members gain both historic–genetic and interactional insights into their psychological realities. Although the therapy does not directly teach more adaptive interpersonal skills, the development of these skills is believed to be an outgrowth of increased insight. Finally, effective management of affects elicited during the termination process is considered crucial to a successful outcome, as it provides an opportunity to rework unresolved separation issues related to one's family of origin. Although the curative factors of object relations family therapy have been articulated, there is minimal empirical validation of their efficacy with current research existing in the form of intensive, descriptive case studies (Gray, 2002).

There are specific techniques associated with object relations family therapy. Techniques, however, are considered secondary to the relationship between therapist and family and thus do not define the practice of object relations family therapy. Rather, the defining characteristic is the therapist's joining with the family and creating a safe holding environment within which family members rediscover each other and the lost parts of the self projected onto one another. Although most family therapies emphasize the therapeutic relationship, it is psychodynamically oriented family therapists who focus on the relationship as a curative factor and who use transference interpretations as a cornerstone of the treatment.

Given the importance of addressing countertransference dynamics, the therapist's psychological health and his or her family-of-origin dynamics influence the work between therapist and family. The therapist needs to address unresolved intrapsychic and interpersonal conflicts in supervision and personal treatment.

Treatment Applicability

Clinicians typically use object relations family therapy with high-functioning families in which none of the members is severely disturbed. These families tend to be psychologically minded, educated, and interested in gaining insight, and they possess the resources necessary to engage in long-term treatment. Some also have advocated its use with families with a schizophrenic, borderline, or narcissistic family member (for review, see Scharff, 1989). This therapeutic approach also has been practiced with families with young children, school-age children, and adolescents; families of divorce and remarriage; and families coping with trauma, loss, or death (e.g., Box, Copley, Magagna, & Smilansky, 1994; Scharff, 1989).

Intergenerational–Contextual Family Therapy

Intergenerational–contextual family therapy, associated with Boszormenyi-Nagy (Boszormenyi-Nagy, Grunebaum, & Ulrich, 1991; Boszormenyi-Nagy & Spark, 1973), is an outgrowth of psychodynamically informed family therapy. Intergenerational–contextual family therapy emphasizes intrapsychic and interpersonal dynamics and, though emphasizing the past, also focuses on the present.

Intergenerational–contextual family therapy, which is conceived within an ethical–existential framework, views the family of origin as central. Boszormenyi-Nagy and Spark's (1973) classic work, *Invisible Loyalties,* stresses concepts of legacy, loyalty, indebtedness to one's family of origin, and the profound influence of one's biological roots. Loyalties are structured expectations to which family members are committed. One's fundamental loyalty is to the maintenance of the family, not to self-differentiation. Family members maintain a ledger of *merits* (investments into relationships) and *debts* (obligations) for each relationship. This ledger changes according to family members' investments (e.g., supporting others) and withdrawals (e.g., exploiting others). When perceived injustices occur, repayment of psychological debts is expected. In addition, every family maintains a family ledger, a multigenerational accounting system of who owes what to whom. Obligations rooted in past generations covertly influence the behavior of family members in the present (*invisible loyalties*). Dysfunction results when individuals or families feel they have chronically imbalanced ledgers, which are not resolved. This diminishes the level of trust among family members, which may result in destructive entitlement or overindebtedness in family members who feel deprived or the presence of an identified patient scapegoated by the family. Thus, to understand the etiology, function, and maintenance of this individual's symptoms, one must consider the history of the problem, the family ledger, and unsettled individual accounts.

Michael Pasadeno and his second wife, Judy Brown, sought couple therapy shortly after the birth of their first child together (Jonathan). Michael had two older daughters from his prior marriage. He paid significant sums of child support to his former wife, adhered to visitation requirements, and sought additional opportunities for contact with his daughters. Although Judy developed a positive relationship with her stepdaughters, she was resentful of the financial compromises the newly formed stepfamily needed to make to meet Michael's child support obligations. Judy supported her husband's relationship with his daughters; however, she felt it diminished his developing relationship with his son and the intimacy in the marriage. In other words, Judy was angry about her husband's financial and emotional debts. She perceived she was investing more in the marriage than she was receiving. An examination of Judy's family-of-origin revealed that she had unresolved feelings of resentment toward her parents for paying more attention to her handicapped older brother than to her. This, in turn, heightened her dissatisfaction with her marriage, as she so desperately needed her husband to shower her with attention to make up for the attention she lacked in her family of origin.

Although Michael was committed to his blended family, he remained loyal to his promises to be a good provider for his first wife (invisible loyalty) and their children.

Basic Structure of Therapy

Intergenerational–contextual therapy is intensive long-term therapy for individuals and families, and may include multigenerational family sessions. A cotherapy team can conduct this work most effectively, as they provide a balanced model to the family unit, complementing one another (Boszormenyi-Nagy & Spark, 1973). The therapist maintains control of the sessions, encouraging members to openly express themselves and validating each individual's worth.

Goal Setting

The goals of intergenerational–contextual family therapy are universal and not dependent on specific family characteristics. The therapy aims to identify and address invisible or hidden loyalties within the family; recognize unsettled individual and family accounts; rebalance in actuality one's obligations (*rejunction process*) to repair ruptured or strained relationships and develop adaptive ways of relating, more trusting relationships, and an equitable balance of give and take among family members; and develop a preventive plan for current and future generations. Although symptom alleviation and the amelioration of distress are important intermediate goals, developing self-object delineation and responsible engagement within relationships (*self-validation*) are the overriding aims.

Techniques and Process of Therapy

In intergenerational–contextual family therapy, the assessment process involves creating a trusting atmosphere so that family members feel safe to express their sense of entitlement and indebtedness. One method used to develop a trusting therapeutic environment, *multidirected partiality*, refers to the therapist's acknowledgment of each individual's perspective on an issue. Having one's views acknowledged leads to an increased capacity to communicate and listen to others.

A comprehensive history is taken focusing on facts, psychology, interactional patterns, and relational ethics. The use of a three-or-more-generation genogram enables the therapist(s) to help the family ascertain the fairness and violations of fairness between family members and generations. In contrast to the other family therapists who have some of their roots in psychoanalytic theory, intergenerational–contextual family therapists conceptualize the assessment process as integral to the development of a trusting relationship with the family and the ongoing therapeutic process.

Following the assessment phase and the establishment of a treatment contract, intergenerational–contextual family therapy enters the working-through phase, where defenses and resistances are acknowledged. Transactions occurring during the family session are discussed in light of each individual's object relations. Major therapeutic techniques enhancing the working-through process include the therapists' siding with each family member to maintain multidirectional partiality, crediting each family member for his or her efforts to help the family, encouraging mutual accountability to replace mutual blame, and using the rejunction process. Issues of loss, separation, and abandonment are discussed during the termination phase. Successful termination occurs when individuals are able to face invisible loyalties within the family system and rebalance unsettled accounts.

Throughout the entire treatment process, the use of the cotherapy relationship enhances the work via empathic involvement in the family, acknowledgment of each family member's contribution, and investment in the trustworthiness of familial relationships. Although the cotherapists are catalysts for the change process, family meetings held

at home, family rituals, and occurrences among family members between sessions serve as the actual work. Homework may be assigned, including writing letters, making telephone calls, and visiting one's family of origin, to help family members develop more positive and trusting relationships. The most common resistances occur when the family remains fixated in symbiotic or distanced relationships and the regressive forces of therapy are experienced as intolerable. In such instances, therapy is rejected.

Less serious resistance is evident in families whose members find the in-depth reworking of relationships too painful and thus desire only the alleviation of the presenting problem. Although this goal is acceptable to the therapists, they do communicate their perspective that lasting change requires successful rebalancing of individual and family ledgers. As is the case with all insight-oriented therapies, common resistances that impede the exploration of relational balances include the mobilization of a variety of defense mechanisms, failure to develop new insights, and an unwillingness to be accountable. These resistances are not interpreted or bypassed. Rather, family members are encouraged to face in their real relationships the ethical issues from which their resistances derive, define their positions regarding these issues, and move toward multilateral consideration of one another's interests.

Stance of the Therapist

Intergenerational–contextual family therapy typically is conducted by cotherapists. These individuals align with the healthy aspects of the family. The cotherapy team communicates empathy, compassion, flexibility, complementarity, creativity, and a concern for family members' capacities for individuation and relatedness. The therapists are the catalysts for the work, take an active role in the process, and communicate that family members can help heal one another. They encourage the family to rebalance accounts and suggest alternative interaction patterns. However, from the outset, the therapeutic task belongs to the family and family members are held accountable for their actions. Thus, the therapist–family relationship is a mutual one.

Curative Factors

The primary curative mechanism is the development of a trusting alliance between the family and the therapists, a process that may be enhanced by pertinent self-disclosures on the part of the therapists. Reframing the presenting problem as reflecting unbalanced family ledgers and family loyalty conflicts and making invisible loyalties overt are additional mechanisms for change. Reframing paves the way to the redressing of the imbalances in the nuclear and extended family.

Family members are helped to face their distortions about significant family members by learning more about their histories. This knowledge enables them to have more compassion for other family members and thus to exonerate their parents and rebalance their relational account of debts and merits. This work frequently includes the parental and grandparental generation to rebalance in reality one's accounts. In these multigenerational sessions, feelings are openly expressed to develop a more meaningful dialogue and more positive interactions, which relieves the grandchildren of the burden of unsettled accounts passed down through the generations.

Insight into one's family-of-origin dynamics is crucial to the change and healing process in intergenerational–contextual family therapy. Insight is achieved through the process of dialogic relating induced by the therapist, not by classical interpretations. Insight is not sufficient for change; rather, lasting change entails efforts at rejunction. Enhanced relational capacities, a vital outcome of the work, are not conceived to be instrumental skills and thus are not taught by the therapist. Rather, it is assumed that

individuals benefit from rewarding interpersonal interactions that are an outgrowth of the rejunction process, and that enables them to relate in a healthier fashion.

Intergenerational–contextual family therapists assert that the most important transference distortions are between family members. Transference reactions may, however, occur between family members and therapists, with the therapists frequently seen as the parents. The therapists manage this transferential parentification process by helping family members understand and modify their relationships and underscoring the importance of family roles (e.g., parents are responsible for parenting their children). This occurs within a context of nurturance in which the therapist provides the necessary reparenting to support the rejunction process.

The therapist's personal maturity and the degree to which he or she has worked through a sense of entitlement and is conscious of family loyalties influences his or her capacity for multidirectional partiality, which in turn, affects the effectiveness of the rejunction process and thus the therapeutic endeavor. Countertransference reactions are construed as resources for deepening one's engagement in the multilateral process and thus, if well understood, can enhance the rejunction process.

> Sam, a 43-year-old competent health care professional, became emotionally overwhelmed when his couple's therapist informed him of an upcoming hiatus in the treatment for medical reasons. The patient's strong reaction harkened back to his early adolescence when his older sister was in a car accident and became comatose and his parents were preoccupied with her extended recovery and subsequent impairments. Although rationally he understood his parents' need to attend primarily to his sister, he felt emotionally abandoned and that his needs were not important. The therapist and patient realized that this particular event provided an opportunity for reparenting the patient regarding feelings of ne-

glect and sense of isolation in dealing with
the myriad affects associated with the physical problems of a loved one. Working
through the therapist's absence, by discussing openly and in a supportive relationship the feelings associated with the
therapist's illness and providing additional
supports to the patient during this time led
Sam to feel more able to discuss with his
parents that traumatic time in the life of the
family. Not only was he able to more
openly share his feelings and needs, but he
also experienced more empathy for each of
his family members' plights, which led
them to develop more mutual and trusting
relationships and enabled them to rebalance their relational "need" accounts. As a
result of this work with his family of origin, Sam and his partner, Bob, reported
more open communication in their partnership and a greater level of intimacy.

Treatment Applicability

Intergenerational–contextual family therapy
is applicable to most human problems
(Boszormenyi-Nagy et al., 1991). However,
it may be most efficacious in conjunction
with other established treatments for individual symptoms (e.g., medications for an
individual's depression or substance abuse
treatment). It is important to note, however,
that minimal empirical validation of the efficacy of this approach exists.

Experiential and Humanistic Family Therapies: Experiential Symbolic Family Therapy

An experiential–humanistic perspective, a
philosophy of growth, assumes that growth
is a natural and spontaneous process and
that pain is a natural component of such
growth. As a function of this view, experiential and humanistic family therapies conceptualize dysfunctional behavior as a failure to fulfill one's potential for personal
growth. These schools emphasize present
experiences and affects and associated
meanings attributed to these experiences. A

number of theorists have been identified
with the experiential–humanistic school of
family therapy, including Carl Whitaker
(Whitaker & Keith, 1981), Virginia Satir
(Satir & Baldwin, 1983), Fred Duhl and
Bunny Duhl (1981), Walter Kempler
(1981), and David Kantor and William Lehr
(1975). Although each of these individuals
works with families in different ways, they
share common philosophical tenets. First, all
believe that therapeutic change does not result from emotional catharsis, insight, or intellectual reflection but, rather, from the immediacy of the relationship and the process
co-created by the family and an involved
therapist. Second, they strive to behave as
real, authentic individuals in their interactions with clients, a stance that ideally promotes spontaneity as well as idiosyncratic
interventions. Finally, all emphasize choice,
free will, human capacity for self-determination, and self-fulfillment. Due to space
limitations, only Whitaker's approach is detailed. A discussion of Satir's key experiential therapeutic techniques is useful in family therapy and because many of these
techniques are couple oriented, they are
covered by Gurman in Chapter 12, "Marital
Therapies."

Experiential symbolic family therapy was
developed by Whitaker and associates, at
Emory University in Atlanta and later at the
University of Wisconsin-Madision. Whitaker's approach is atheoretical; theory is
viewed as a hindrance to clinical practice
(Whitaker, 1976). His views, however, on
the healthy or well-functioning marriage
and family and on pathological or dysfunctional marriage and family have been articulated, particularly as they influence the
therapy process (Roberto, 1991).

Basic Structure of Therapy

Symbolic experiential family therapy is
time unlimited and of intermediate duration. It is conducted at a variable frequency,
usually weekly or biweekly, with monthly
sessions in the latter phases. Sessions opti-

mally include the symptomatic family member, the nuclear family residing with the symptomatic person, the extended families, and the index person's social support network. Therapy usually is conducted by a cotherapy team or may include a therapist and a consultant.

Goal Setting

The ultimate goals of experiential symbolic family therapy apply to all dysfunctional couple and family units. The specific operationalization of these goals is developed between a couple/family and the cotherapy team, based on the unique family system and its relational patterns. Ultimate goals are to (1) increase family members' perceptions of belongingness and cohesion, (2) help the couple or family facilitate each family member's individuation and completion of developmental tasks, and (3) foster the creativity ("craziness") and spontaneity of the family unit and individual members. Mediating goals include disorganizing rigid recycling of interaction to allow for more adaptive responses, activating and allowing constructive anxieties by positively reframing symptoms as efforts toward competence, expanding the presenting problem to include each members' role in the dysfunction, encouraging and supporting new decisions, creating transgenerational boundaries, and creating a therapeutic suprasystem in which the family and cotherapy team develop a shared meaning system and intermember alliances (Roberto, 1991).

Techniques and Process of Therapy

Similar to most other therapies, experiential symbolic family therapy includes beginning, middle, and end phases. The therapy becomes less structured as treatment progresses. Out-of-session homework assignments are not typically given, with the exception of preparation for the extended family reunion. Resistances are considered inevitable in the change process and are not interpreted. Rather, they are managed with a combination of challenge, support, and humor.

During the beginning phase, therapists establish personal contact with the family (joining), using metaphors, reframing, and humor to engage the family in a relatively nonthreatening fashion (Satir & Baldwin, 1983). The battle for structure and the battle for initiative must be fought before the family trusts the cotherapy dyad enough to allow them to help the family reorganize to cure the scapegoated member and develop greater differentiation (Whitaker & Keith, 1981). The battle for structure, which begins at the initial contact, refers to a battle over ground rules regarding treatment structure, session membership, scheduling, and fees. This battle is completed when a minimum of a two-generational structure to the therapy is established, with the therapist(s) in charge and having maximal freedom to move in and out of the family system and "call the shots." The battle for structure, if successfully won, induces regression in the family, engenders an intense transference relationship, and communicates that therapy is "serious business." The battle for initiative occurs after the therapeutic structure is established, the therapeutic relationships are formed, and the family situation is delineated. The cotherapy team encourages the family to take initiative for their own growth and responsibility for life decisions. This battle is resolved when the cotherapy team establishes an existential adult-to-adult relationship with each family member, with mutual involvement in the therapeutic exchange from all participants. During this phase, information is gleaned regarding the presenting problem, families of origin, and family interactions. Symptoms are reframed as attempts to grow and the mutual responsibility of multiple parties are emphasized, thus decreasing scapegoating.

Virginia, a 27-year-old office manager, presented for therapy complaining that she had developed symptoms of bulimia nervosa after becoming involved with Cindy, her first lesbian lover. Virginia and Cindy had been living together for the past 3½ years, and reportedly had a satisfactory relationship. However, Virginia acknowledged that she became more symptomatic whenever she was angry at Cindy. The couple had never overtly discussed Virginia's bulimic symptoms and Virginia had sought help without Cindy's knowledge. After the initial evaluation session, the therapist recommended couple therapy, and Virginia adamantly refused. They agreed to meet a second time and discuss the situation. During the second session, the therapist was aware that the battle for structure had begun and must be won by the therapist if meaningful change was to occur. The therapist, therefore, articulated clearly to Virginia her view that change would not occur unless Cindy was included in the treatment. Couple sessions were begun reluctantly by both partners and a second therapist joined the treatment. Although the therapists had won the battle for structure, it became clear that the battle for initiative was now the central focus. Specifically, although both Virginia and Cindy attended sessions promptly and regularly and were responsible about paying the bill, Virginia refused to discuss her bulimia in Cindy's presence, and Cindy denied any awareness of difficulties in their relationship. The couple was not taking any responsibility for the content and process of the therapeutic encounters. The therapists attempted to make overt the covert undertones in the couple's communication. For example, one of the therapists provided the following personal anecdote: "You know, I just had the following recollection and I don't know why. I remember when I was a young child and I would become angry at my mother for trying to boss me around, I would go in my bedroom, cover my face with a pillow, and scream so that no one could hear me. When my mother would try to talk with me, I said that nothing was the matter." Such personal vignettes were coupled with other metaphors about how unexpressed anger inhibits healthy communication and efforts to grow. During the

seventh session, Virginia and Cindy reported a recent fight about "something stupid" and then slowly began exploring their disappointments in their relationship, their difficulties expressing their anger directly toward one another for fear of being rejected, and their desire for more closeness and communication. The battle for initiative was therefore under way.

In the middle phase, the family defines and actively addresses its life difficulties with the help of the cotherapists, who have become personally involved with the family. Throughout this phase, Whitaker and Keith (1981) advocate implementing techniques to facilitate change and create alternative interaction patterns that reduce scapegoating and blame of the caretaking parent. Some specific techniques used include redefining symptoms as efforts toward growth; explicating covert conflict; separating interpersonal and internal stress, and modeling fantasized alternatives to stress; the therapists' use of self, including unconscious material, absurdity, and "acting-in" (affective confrontation of family members by the therapist); involving grandparents and other extended family members in treatment; and reversing roles (for review, see Roberto, 1991).

More recently, and consistent with the experiential and humanistic approach, attention has been paid to the use of play with families during this phase of the intervention process, in a modality referred to as family play therapy (Gil, 1994). This phase of the work may yield positive results such that the family continues to work effectively in the therapy or chooses to leave therapy feeling competent to handle problems effectively. However, this process may lead to an impotence impasse in which the therapists feel that despite their best efforts, the family does not change or take responsibility for its own problems (Keith, Connell, & Connell, 2001; Whitaker & Keith, 1981). This impasse is successfully negotiated when decisions about treatment are mutually agreed on between the family and the cotherapy team.

In the end phase, the cotherapy team disentangles itself from the family and takes a more peripheral role, intervening only when necessary (e.g., when new symptoms emerge). The family observes its own functioning and takes responsibility for making decisions and solving problems. Thus, the cotherapy team and the family work as equal partners rather than as consultant and patient. This relational shift is facilitated by several techniques used by the cotherapists, including spontaneous self-disclosure, expression of grief regarding termination, and requests for feedback about the therapy. The family and the cotherapy team part with the recognition of mutual interdependence and loss. Termination is indicated when members appear self-confident and the family demonstrates that it possesses the resources to resolve problems and tolerate life stress.

Stance of the Therapist

Experiential symbolic family therapists are actively engaged in the family's interactional process yet do not direct the therapy. They listen, observe, attend to their own affective reactions, and intervene actively to change the family's functioning without focusing on the etiology of the difficulties. These therapists openly express warmth and caring for the family and use their personalities (true self) in sharing their internal processes with the family without losing their differentiated sense of self. They are like "coaches" (who observe and suggest but do not direct or change) or surrogate grandparents, roles that require structure and discipline as well as caring and personal availability. Emphasis on participant observation underscores the family's responsibility for change, even though the therapists are responsible for the interventions.

Experiential symbolic family therapy is typically conducted by a cotherapy team, which enables each therapist to perform unique functions and to interchange these functions when indicated. The cotherapy team models adaptive interpersonal relationships and provides experiential alternatives for family interactions.

Curative Factors

The basic assumption of experiential symbolic family therapy is that families change as a result of experiences, not through education or interpretation (Whitaker & Keith, 1981). Chief mechanisms for change are the experience of new relational stances with family members, the expression of strong emotions, and the challenging of current interactional patterns, all of which lead to interactional insights. Interactional insights are considered more prominent and effective than are historical insights. The therapists' own roles within their families of origin and creation affect their interactions with the family and the cotherapist. Therefore, family therapy for the therapist is strongly encouraged.

Treatment Applicability

Experiential symbolic family therapy has been used with families in which the index person presents with a range of problems, including severe forms of psychopathology (i.e., schizophrenia). However, it is particularly difficult to use this approach with families in which an individual member presents with severe personality disorders, notably antisocial or narcissistic personality disorders. In addition, in families coping with a trauma such as divorce or abuse, this treatment may be emotionally overwhelming and thus contraindicated. No treatment may be recommended when the family is dissatisfied with treatment elsewhere and when a marital/partnership dyad has completed a successful course of therapy and experiences acute difficulties. Although the proliferation of writings on symbolic experiential family therapy and individual family's subjective attestations of improvement is suggestive of this model's efficacy, empirical studies have not been presented in the literature.

Strategic Family Therapy

A number of groups of family therapists can be classified as strategic family therapists: (1) the communications school of the MRI group and later the Brief Therapy Center in Palo Alto, which initially included Gregory Bateson, Don Jackson, John Weakland, Jay Haley, and Virginia Satir and later added Paul Watzlawick, Richard Fisch, and Arthur Bodin (Bateson et al., 1956; Watzlawick, Weakland, & Fisch, 1974) (for an overview, see Weakland & Ray, 1995); and (2) Haley (1976) and Cloe Madanes's (1991) *problem-solving therapy*. Strategic therapy approaches are influenced heavily by Bateson's focus on communication processes and the strategic therapy of Milton Erickson.

Strategic approaches, which are change rather than growth oriented, view problems as maintained by maladaptive family interaction sequences, including faulty and incongruent hierarchies and malfunctioning triangles. The behavioral sequences observed in the family's attempts to solve the problem are assumed to perpetuate the presenting problem (Haley, 1976). These sequences of behavior are viewed as complex and circular, rather than linear, and therefore change within the family system is a necessary prerequisite for individual change. Problems are also conceptualized as resulting from prior unsuccessful attempts to solve a given difficulty (Watzlawick et al., 1974).

These approaches are ahistorical, emphasizing present interactions and communications rather than the past. These models attend to metacommunications (communications about communications) among family members, focusing on the covert, nonverbal messages that amplify the meaning of overt, verbal messages. The presenting problem is an analogical message, a metaphor for underlying dysfunction (Keim, 2000). For example, a couple's fighting over trivial matters may reflect their power and/or intimacy struggles. The following discussion focuses on Haley and Madanes's brand of strategic therapy, as illustrative of strategic approaches.

Basic Structure of Therapy

Strategic therapies are brief interventions, which may include the whole family or only one or two members of a family system. Sessions occur weekly or biweekly and are conducted by a single therapist. The approach is structured, as the therapist directs the questioning, gives directives, and intervenes actively.

Goal Setting

The primary goal is solving the family's presenting problem within the social context. This is accomplished by the therapist and family setting small, concrete goals related to the presenting problem. Goals are formulated as increases in positive behaviors rather than reduction of problematic behaviors, which helps the family feel motivated, as success seems possible. Additional and more long-term goals include altering the interaction sequences maintaining the problem, and helping family members resolve a crisis and progress to the next stage of the family and individual life cycle.

Thus, successful strategic therapy achieves *second-order change* (Watzlawick et al., 1974), fundamental changes in the family system's structure and functioning, rather than *first-order change,* in which superficial modifications are made that do not affect the structure of the system itself. For example, in a family with an oppositional adolescent who repeatedly demands to borrow the family car, first-order change may be evident when the parents become more lenient about allowing their son to borrow the car and the son becomes more willing to comply with parental requests. This improved state of affairs is considered first-order change when no other changes in the family structure or interaction patterns are noted. Second-order change becomes apparent when the adolescent evidences more compliant behavior in the context of age-appropriate separation from his parents, and his parents become closer to each other and thus no longer need to triangulate their son in their relationship. In such cases, the executive power hierarchy is strengthened concurrent with an increased level of intimacy within the marital/partnership subsystem. In addition, the adolescent forms more age-appropriate peer relationships and his oppositional behavior serves to define identity without engaging in self- or other-destructive behavior.

Techniques and Process of Therapy

Problem-solving therapy is a process that occurs in stages until the presenting problem is resolved and other treatment goals are achieved. The first stage encompasses the initial interview, in which the family problem and the context within which it is embedded are ascertained. This interview is divided into five stages: (1) social stage—therapist makes direct contact with each family member, makes initial hypotheses about the family, and matches the family's mood; (2) problem stage—therapist asks formal questions regarding the problem; (3) interaction stage—therapist asks family members to talk with one another about the problem and observes communication patterns; (4) goal-setting stage—therapist ascertains changes desired by the family and specifies these in behavioral terms; and (5) task-setting stage—therapist gives the family a directive, typically a homework assignment, designed to alter dysfunctional interaction sequences.

Once a family diagnosis is determined and the problem is defined, the therapist formulates a therapeutic approach consisting of an overall plan for a series of tactical interventions, labeled directives. These directives serve several functions: change the underlying interaction sequences maintaining the problem, intensify the therapeutic relationship, and gather information about the family, particularly its resistance to change. Directives may be straight or paradoxical. Straight directives, designed to elicit the family's cooperation with the therapist's request, are useful in crisis situations. Paradoxical directives are useful when the family is resistant to change, as they encourage the family to oppose the therapist.

Strategic family therapists assess and track the cycle of family interaction sequences by asking questions, break the cycle through straightforward and/or paradoxical directives, and support termination when the presenting problem has been alleviated. Techniques are relatively indirect and non-confrontational and retrospectively focus on out-of-session behavioral sequences and emphasize out-of-session directives.

Positive feedback cycles are emphasized such that the family's homeostasis is challenged in order to change the family's behavioral patterns. Key techniques to alter existing behavioral sequences include *paradox* (giving a directive to a family member that will be resisted, therefore producing change in the desired direction); *reframing* or relabeling (use language to provide new meaning to the situation such as *positive connotation* in which problem behaviors are relabeled in a positive light); *ordeals* (recommending that a family member engage in a behavior he or she dislikes but one that would improve his or her relationship with significant others); *pretending* (prescribing that a symptomatic person pretend to exhibit his or her symptom, which reclassifies the symptom as voluntary and thus alters family members reactions); *unbalancing* through creating alternative coalitions; and prescribing homework. There are many forms of paradoxical interventions, including (1) therapeutic use of *double-bind communication;* (2) *positioning,* where the therapist accepts and exaggerates what the family members are saying, underscoring the absurdity of the situation and therefore forcing them to take a different position; (3) *restraining,* where the therapist discourages change by enumerating the dangers associated with positive change; and (4) *symptom prescription,* where the therapist directs the family member to practice his or her symptom and provides a compelling rationale for the prescription.

In strategic therapies, the time-limited nature and problem-solving focus make termination a natural process (Segal, 1991). Families are ready to terminate when significant and durable improvements in the presenting problem have occurred and the family reports handling their problems without the therapist (Segal, 1991). During the termination phase, family members are given credit for their improvements yet cautioned against developing a sense of false optimism that family problems will not return. For families hesitant about terminating, termination may be framed as a break from therapy in which gains are consolidated.

Stance of the Therapist

Strategic therapists are active and present in a powerful, authoritative, and charismatic fashion and use their powers of persuasion to convince a family to follow a precise directive, whether straightforward or paradoxical (Coyne & Pepper, 1998). These therapists have been considered by some to be highly manipulative in implementing their interventions, as is the case when they recommend that a couple chronically in conflict fight at planned times during the day for a specified period. The therapist intervenes when he or she chooses rather than when the family requests participation. Strategic therapists avoid being aligned with one family faction; however, they will voluntarily take sides to overcome an impasse.

Curative Factors

Techniques are of paramount importance in effecting change in the strategic model. Curative factors include correcting the hierar-

chy by encouraging the parental subsystem to effectively and appropriately use its power, helping family members negotiate and reach agreements, and reuniting family members in an effort to heal old wounds (Madanes, 1991). Insight is not valued and interpretations, in the classical sense, are rare. Family members are not educated directly in interpersonal skills, yet the directives offered typically require the development of a more adaptive interpersonal style. Change in the index person's problem behavior is inextricably interwoven with systemic changes. Therapists who discuss strategic family therapy approaches pay little attention to the therapist's psychological health or personality.

Treatment Applicability

While strategic therapy has been applied to couples and families presenting with a wide variety of problems, specific applications are noteworthy. Haley's problem-solving therapy and the MRI group's strategic therapy approaches have documented efficacy in case studies and treatment outcome and follow-up research for schizophrenia, anorexia, substance abuse, violence, and anxiety disorders (e.g., Nardone, 1995). Madanes (1991) adapted strategic family therapy for incestuous families and developed a 16-step intervention for reparation. Although there are few methodologically sophisticated treatment process and outcome research addressing the efficacy of strategic approaches to family intervention, there is empirical support for the use of brief strategic approaches with Latino high-risk youth (Kazdin, 2002). Strategic brief therapy has been shown to integrate pertinent aspects of culture in order to prove effective for these populations (Santisteban et al., 1997; Szapocznik & Williams, 2000).

Systemic Family Therapy

Systemic family therapy was pioneered in Italy by the Milan group, originally consisting of Mara Selvini-Palazzoli and colleagues Luigi Boscolo, Gianfranco Cecchin, and Guiliana Prata (Boscolo & Bertrando, 1996; Boscolo et al., 1987; Selvini-Palazzoli, Boscolo, Cecchin, & Prata, 1978). In 1980, the group divided, with Selvini-Palazzoli and Prata focusing on research and clinical endeavors and finding a universal, invariant prescription relevant to all families. In 1985, Selvini-Palazzoli, with a separate group of research collaborators, delineated a systemic model of psychotic processes in families (Selvini-Palazzoli et al., 1989). Boscolo and Cecchin emphasized training new generations of systemic family therapists. They asserted that interventions should remain flexible, with alternative interventions tailored to the family being viewed as optimal. Systemic family therapy has been popularized in the United States by Hoffman at the Ackerman Institute and in Amherst, Massachusetts and by Papp, Silverstein, and their colleagues at the Ackerman Institute in New York. The development of systemic family therapy has been a complex and dynamic process, the evolution of which has been detailed (Campbell, Draper, & Crutchley, 1991; for review, see Mosconi, Gonzo, Sorgato, Tirelli, & Tomas, 1999). More recently, many systemic family therapists have integrated a postmodern perspective, a belief that there is no objective truth surrounding the problem or family functioning and, thus, the therapist engages in a participatory process with a family to "discover" new solutions (see "Postmodern Family Therapy," later). These systemic family therapists refer to themselves as post-Milan and incorporate new techniques and perspectives along with the original concepts set forth by the Milan group (for review, see Campbell, 1999).

Like strategic approaches, Bateson influenced systemic family therapists. The systemic model is the purest application of Bateson's *circular epistemology*. The Milan model focuses on process rather than structure. Consistent with the beliefs posited by the MRI group, the systemic approach views the family and therapist as an ecosystem in which each member affects the health of all other members over time. Thus, symptomatic behavior is perpetuated by *rule-governed transactional patterns*. The symptom keeps the family system in a homeostatic state. In accord with Bateson's cybernetic model, systemic therapists view the family as a nonlinear and complex cybernetic system, with interlocking feedback mechanisms and repetitive patterns of behavior sequences. Systemic family therapists are unified in their efforts to comprehend the meaning of *second-order cybernetics* (the cybernetics of cybernetics) and to use these understandings as a basis for practicing family therapy.

Basic Structure of Therapy

Systemic therapy is a long brief intervention conducted with all family members present. Sessions frequently are spaced at monthly intervals, allowing time for the intervention to take effect and elicit change throughout the system. Typical courses of therapy are between 3 and 20 sessions, with 10 sessions being modal. The number of sessions is agreed on in advance and adhered to rigidly. A single therapist, cotherapy pair, or other members of the therapy team providing live supervision through a one-way mirror may conduct the sessions. Observers behind the mirror enhance the objectivity of the therapist(s) working directly with the family. The therapists are responsible for structuring the process of the sessions.

Goal Setting

The therapist's goals are to create a context within which the family's belief system can be explored and change can occur. This is accomplished by the therapist maintaining a systemic view of the family and offering a new conceptualization (cognitive map) of the family's problems. However, family members determine the specific goals. Furthermore, how the family changes is considered the responsibility of its members. If the therapist does not agree with the family's goals, he or she respects the family's wishes unless the family's choices may be harmful to one or more family members (e.g., abusive behavior toward a child).

Techniques and Process of Therapy

Systemic family therapists, who incorporate a more evolutionary perspective than do their strategic counterparts, assert that problematic behaviors emerge when the family's *epistemology* (rules and conceptual framework for understanding reality) is no longer adaptive. Thus, they attempt to create an environment in which new information inviting spontaneous change is introduced to foster the family's development of an alternative epistemology. Using this framework, sessions follow a relatively standard format, including (1) the presession during which the therapists gather information for the session; (2) the session during which information is given and discussions occur allowing observation of the family's transactional patterns; (3) discussion of the session in a separate room by the therapist/cotherapy pair and behind-the-mirror observers, during which suggestions, opinions, and observations are shared, culminating in a systemic hypothesis and associated intervention; (4) rejoining the family by the therapist or cotherapy pair to offer a comment and a prescription (typically a paradoxical directive which may be offered in a form of a letter) for an outside the session task; and (5) postsession therapy team discussion of the family's reaction to the intervention and a written formulation summarizing the session.

Systemic family therapists use many techniques described in the strategic therapy section. They combine the basic principles of paradoxical intervention (Watzlawick et al., 1974) with *systemic hypotheses* (hypotheses to explain behavior that create a framework from which to ask questions

and devise interventions) and *rituals* (individualized prescription of an action or series of actions designed to alter the family's roles). A number of techniques are associated particularly with the Milan school of systemic family therapy. *Circular questioning,* in which one member is asked to comment on the interactional behaviors of two other members, is an effective diagnostic and therapeutic technique. Circular questioning addresses family members' differential perceptions and experiences of events and relationships. This enables the therapist and the family to perceive differences nonjudgmentally, to conceptualize problems systemically (e.g., what is the function of the symptom), and to intervene accordingly.

Positive connotation is a form of reframing in which the therapist labels all behavior positive because it maintains family homeostasis and cohesion. Positive connotation fosters the family's acceptance of the therapists' interventions and leads the family to question why symptomatic behavior is essential for family cohesion. Interventions, based on the hypothesized systemic formulations of family games, are made to all family members through paradoxes and the use of rituals or counterparadoxical prescriptions. *Rituals,* designed to address the conflict between unspoken (analogic) and spoken family rules, are prescriptions directing the family to change its behavior leading to modification of associated cognitive maps. *Counterparadoxical* interventions occur when the therapist places the family in a therapeutic double bind to counteract the family members' pattern of paradoxical communications. The use of counterparadoxical interventions, in which the overt communication is for the family not to change, is based on the assumption that symptomatic behavior maintains the homeostasis and thus a prescription of no change supports the homeostatic tendency of the family. Thus, rather than issuing prescriptions designed to elicit resistance, systemic therapists offer prescriptions designed to provide information about family connectedness. Taken together, these interventions uncover family games, introduce a new cognitive map, and engender the family to discover the solution to its problems via a transformation in family rules and relationships.

Because behavioral goals are not specified, it is often unclear when the therapy should be terminated. Termination typically occurs when the problem behavior is alleviated or when the family no longer perceives the behavior to be a problem. Therapist and family usually mutually agree that they have no reason to continue to meet and thus a decision to terminate is made. The therapist may recommend to the family members that they return for a review session at a later point in time.

Stance of the Therapist

Unlike strategic therapists, systemic therapists historically have taken a relatively neutral, objective, and nonreactive stance as they avoid becoming part of any family alliance or coalition. This position of neutrality, in which the therapist avoids issues of hierarchy, power, and alignments, typically allows for maximum leverage for achieving change. The therapist is free to attend to the system in its entirety and is not pulled into the family games), specific repetitive patterns of family interaction (Selvini–Palazzoli et al., 1989). Selvini–Palazzoli and colleagues (1989) have advocated that the therapist develop a relationship with each partner, openly share his or her hypotheses for what is occurring in the family system, and minimize the use of paradoxical techniques. Consistent with the cybernetics of cybernetics, the referring source and the therapy team are considered integral parts of the coevolving ecosystem, affecting each other in circular feedback loops.

Curative Factors

Systemic family therapy shares with other approaches respect and empathy for the family, a value on joining with the family, an acknowledgment of interlocking family behaviors, an awareness of the importance of offering alternative cognitive maps, and a recognition of providing an appropriate context within which to conduct the work. Mechanisms of change associated specifically with systemic family therapy include interviewing the family in a manner that permits individuals to develop new connections between events and their meanings and creating a new family meaning system that leads to the development of alternative behaviors and interaction patterns. This work does not require insight and the value of insight is minimized. Interpretations are not incorporated in this approach.

The therapist's personality is considered important in the endeavor insofar as it enables the therapist to relate attentively while simultaneously entertaining systemic hypotheses. Although it is acknowledged that the therapist's personality influences the family and the work, it is not considered central to the change process. Therapy is most efficacious when there is a good fit between the therapist and the family such that the family permits the therapist to explore and challenge its belief system and the therapist can provide feedback in a challenging, yet respectful manner.

Treatment Applicability

The Milan group's systemic approach has been used with families with a variety of severe emotional problems, most notably psychosomatic (Selvini–Palazzoli, 1974), and psychotic symptoms (Selvini–Palazzoli et al., 1978). Campbell and colleagues (1991) assert that the Milan approach is appropriate for any family whose solution to their problems has become interwoven with the family's meaning system such that alternative solutions for problem solving are limited.

Evaluations of treatment efficacy are sparse; however, one systematic outcome study comparing problem solving versus systemic family therapies found that although both interventions yielded significant symptom reduction, families completing the systemic treatment evidenced a broader systemic perspective regarding their family's functioning (Bennun, 1986). Another study found that in families referred to a child outpatient clinic, when compared with standard child outpatient treatment, families that received Milan family therapy exhibited more change among family members and required less time for treatment (Simpson, 1991). Treatment effectiveness studies include both single and comparative group outcome trials, investigations of therapeutic process, review of cases, and satisfaction surveys. Results suggest symptomatic change in the majority of cases (Carr, 1991); however, more methodologically rigorous research focusing on treatment of specific populations is needed.

Structural Family Therapy

Minuchin and colleagues (e.g., Auerswald, Montalvo, Aponte, Haley, Hoffman, and Rosman) founded the structural model of family therapy (S. Minuchin, 1974; S. Minuchin & Nichols, 1998; S. Minuchin et al., 1967), which serves as the basis for much of the family therapy conceptualized and practiced today. The model was an outgrowth of the authors' work at the Philadelphia Child Guidance Clinic, where they worked with conduct-disordered and antisocial youth and their families from a low socioeconomic status who were predominantly African American. The model continues to be used and expanded for the African American population as it incorporates a more ecostructural perspective in which the family's transactions with outside agencies and systems are the focus of concern (Boyd-Franklin & Bry, 2000; P. Minuchin, Colapinto, & Minuchin, 1998).

Structural family therapy is a theoretically based approach for intervening with children/adolescents who are the index person and their families, which incorporates structuralist conceptualizations. Adaptive and maladaptive functioning are described in terms of the organized patterns of interactions among individuals, their families, and the environment. Individual functioning is understood in light of the individual's interaction with the social context. The structural model identifies a number of basic concepts relating to the structure, communication patterns, and expression of affect, which are useful in explaining the family's organization, coping patterns, and adaptation to developmental transitions (for review, see the aforementioned books written by Minuchin and colleagues; Colapinto, 1991). Structural organization refers to relational patterns common to all families, influenced by the personal idiosyncracies of each family, adapted for addressing social tasks in a developmentally sensitive fashion within the context in which the family is embedded.

Family transactional patterns provide information about boundaries, hierarchies, alignments, and power. *Boundaries* demarcate *subsystems* and are the rules that define who participates and how in various tasks and activities (S. Minuchin, 1974). Families are *hierarchically organized,* with caregivers in the executive subsystem positioned above their children. *Alignment* refers to the joining or opposition of one member of a system to another in carrying out an operation (Aponte & Dicesare, 2000). Under the rubric of alignment are the concepts of *coalition* (a covert alliance between two family members against a third) and *alliance* (two individuals share a common interest not held by a third person). *Power,* also referred to as force, has been defined as the relative influence of each family member on the outcome of an activity (Aponte & Dicesare, 2000). The structural dimensions of boundaries and alignments depend on power for action and outcome (Aponte & Dicesare, 2000).

Dysfunctional families have impairments in boundaries, alignments, and/or power balance evidenced by the failure to adapt to stressors in a developmentally appropriate manner. Families evidence maladjustment when they rigidly and tenaciously cling to familiar interaction patterns. The nature of the family dysfunction associated with the manifestation of symptoms or problems may be categorized according to the structural dimensions of boundary, alignment, and power that are most salient. The terms "enmeshment" and "disengagement" refer to maladaptive expressions of family boundaries and reflect extreme points on a continuum of family contact. Another family pattern indicative of impairments in family boundaries has been termed the "violation of function boundaries." The classic example of this inappropriate intrusion of one family member into the domain of other family members is the case of the parental or parentified child, where the child assumes the power, authority, and responsibilities that more appropriately belong to someone in the *executive subsystem*.

Common dysfunctional family alignments include stable coalitions, detouring coalitions, and triangulation and require at least three participants. *Stable coalitions* are those in which two family members are consistently in agreement against a third person. When the two allies agree that the third person is the source of their problem (i.e., our son's bad behavior causes our relationship problems), a *detouring coalition* is formed to reduce the stress in the dyad, giving the impression of harmony.

Triangulation occurs when an opposing family member (frequently one of the parents) demands that a third person (typically a child) side with him or her against the opposing party. The third person consequently feels a split alliance, necessitating siding with one party and then the other. This process emotionally paralyzes the triangulated individual, resulting in symptomatic behavior. Dysfunctional family patterns relevant to the power dimension often are indicative of a lack of functional power, which reflects the inability of family members to use their authority to implement their assigned roles. The classic example is that of weak executive subsystem functioning, in which the parental subsystem fails to exert the force required to guide the children.

Additional structural problems that incorporate more than one of the key structural dimensions are worthy of note. *Cross-generational stable coalitions,* in which partners argue their conflict through their child, reflect problems with boundaries and alignments. Chronic cross-generational stable coalitions are commonly evident in families in which a member presents with a psychosomatic illness or a substance abuse problem (Colapinto, 1991). Families deficient on all three structural domains are underorganized, having limited coping strategies and structure that they employ rigidly yet inconsistently. In contrast, healthy families have well-defined, elaborated, flexible, and cohesive family structures that accommodate the changing functions and roles of individual family members, the various family subsystems, and the sociocultural environment (Aponte Dicesare, 2000).

Basic Structure of Therapy

The structure of this intervention approach is flexible in terms of number of therapists; which family members participate in an interview; and location, length, and frequency of interviews. Typically, however, structural family therapy is a brief intervention (5 to 7 months on average) whose primary participants are family members who interact daily. Rather than focusing predominantly on the content (what is said) of family communication, the primary focus is on verbal and nonverbal interactional processes as they reflect the family structure. A single therapist most often conducts structural family therapy, because the therapeutic techniques employed are more difficult to carry out when coordination between two therapists is required. The presence of a cotherapy dyad also makes it technically more difficult to exert maximal control over the family's transactional patterns. Although a one-way mirror may be used for purposes of family restructuring (e.g., removing the children to have them observe the caregivers interact), there rarely is a consultant behind the mirror. However, when more than one therapist is involved in a case, it is optimal for these extra therapists to serve as observers behind the mirror.

Goal Setting

Typically, the primary goal negotiated between the therapist and the family is the resolution of the presenting problem. The therapist helps the family identify common goals when possible and acknowledge conflicting goals when they exist. The family may desire resolution of the presenting problem with a focus on the index person and a lack of attention to underlying structural patterns. However, the therapist asserts that this goal can only be attained by restructuring the family unit so that more adaptive interaction patterns prevail. A second important aim of the work is to change the family's construction of reality (S. Minuchin & Fishman, 1981). In other words, the therapist helps the family develop alternative explanatory schemata for viewing the problem, which enables them to develop more adaptive family transactions.

Techniques and Process of Therapy

The structural family therapy approach entails three cyclical and overlapping stages: joining, assessing, and restructuring. Similar to other family therapists, structural family therapists join the family rapidly and in a position of leadership, which enables the therapist to develop an understanding of the family's construction of reality and structure. To facilitate the joining process, the therapist uses three procedures: maintenance (supporting the existing structure of the family or subsystem); tracking (following the content of the family's communication with minimal intervention), and mimesis (adopting the style and affective experience of the family); The therapist ini-

tially accepts the family's view of the presenting problem as the real problem and designs interventions to ameliorate the problem by changing the structure of the family system. As symptom reduction proceeds, the family may gain more confidence in the therapist's expertise and thus be more inclined to address underlying structural issues.

The assessment stage focuses on six domains of family functioning: (1) structure, boundary quality, and resonance (sensitivity to the actions of individual members and tolerance for deviation from the family norm); (2) flexibility and capacity for change; (3) interaction patterns of the spousal/intimate partnership, parental, and sibling subsystems; (4) role of index person and how his or her symptom maintains family homeostasis; (5) ecological context within which the presenting problem develops and is maintained; and (6) developmental stage of the family and its individual members. This assessment enables the therapist to develop a family map and diagnosis in which links between structural problems and current symptoms are delineated.

Cassandra, a 15-year-old Caucasian female, was referred for an evaluation after she was suspended from school for "doing crack" in the school bathroom. An evaluation was conducted with Cassandra; her older brother, George, who had recently moved into a dormitory at the local state college; and their mother, Ms. Sutton, a single parent who was employed as a salesperson. Mr. and Mrs. Sutton had divorced when the children were young, and Mr. Sutton had infrequent contact with his children. George and Ms. Sutton had been extremely close, and Ms. Sutton had often sought George's advice on how to handle Cassandra. George often took on a paternal role toward his younger sister, taking responsibility for both protecting and disciplining her. Cassandra had many friends, unlike her older brother, spending considerable time outside of the family. Since her brother had left home, Cassandra's schoolwork had deteriorated. In addition, Cassandra and her mother had become more withdrawn from one another. A structural assessment revealed the following: The Sutton family was having difficulty negotiating the developmental transition of "launching children and moving on." This difficulty was compounded by a preexisting family structure characterized by a parental child, lack of appropriate generational boundaries, a stable coalition between the mother and the son against the daughter, and a restricted capacity for change as evidenced by the mother's resistance to developing intimate relationships with adults outside the family. Cassandra's substance use in the school served a protective function for the family as it distracted Ms. Sutton from her own dysphoric affects associated with her son's departure, an experience that had reactivated her pain about her earlier marital separation and subsequent divorce.

The third phase, *restructuring,* redresses the structural difficulties noted during the assessment. For example, with enmeshed families, the goal is to increase age-appropriate separation–individuation; with disengaged families, the restructuring process entails enhancing family attachments. A number of techniques have been associated with the restructuring process. The therapist is able to observe dysfunctional patterns and intervene to facilitate structural change through the use of enactments, in which the therapist promotes the family's acting out of dysfunctional and habitual transactional patterns of relating during the session. Additional techniques include escalating stress; boundary marking; unbalancing the family alignments; assigning homework tasks; and providing support, education, and guidance (for review, see Colapinto, 1991; Vetere, 2001).

According to Minuchin, a family member's symptom is indicative of dysfunctional family patterns for managing stress. He recommends escalating stress within the family system to develop more effective interaction patterns. Strategies for escalating stress include increasing the intensity of the enactment by prolonging its occurrence, in-

troducing new variables (e.g., new family members), blocking typical patterns of relating by challenging the communication rules and structure of the family, emphasizing differences, or suggesting alternative transactions during the session that may provide a useful model for changing interactions outside the session. Spatial interventions, including rearranging the seating and removing members from the room temporarily and having them observe the interactions from behind a one-way mirror, alter the perspectives of family members regarding the interrelationships in an effort to improve interpersonal boundaries. Minuchin advocates assigning tasks to the family, both inside and outside (homework) the session. Tasks are diagnostic probes that yield valuable information about the family's openness to change and serve to change maladaptive family communication patterns and structure. Tasks may be assigned in a direct fashion, paradoxically, or in a combination of the two.

Stance of the Therapist

S. Minuchin (1974) describes the role of the therapist as that of a distant and friendly relative who takes an active and authoritative stance by asking probing and open-ended questions and giving directions and homework assignments. Consistent with Minuchin's persona, the structural family therapist is often colorful and dramatic, demands that family members accommodate to the therapist to facilitate therapeutic progress, and communicates his or her expertise in assisting the family members to mobilize their adaptive resources to facilitate change. The structural family therapist is, thus, the stage director or producer of the family drama.

Curative Factors

Emphasis is on interactions occurring in the present and the therapeutic task is one of behavior change as opposed to insight. The structural approach is more symptom oriented than the psychoanalytic schools yet less symptom focused than strategic therapies. Furthermore, the structural approach is technique oriented, incorporates a developmental perspective in understanding the association between individual/family life-stage transitions and dysfunction, conceptualizes communicational sequences or transactional patterns in terms of both cybernetic properties and organizational structure of the family, and views the family assessment process in a holistic framework taking into account the therapist's impact on the family in the data gathering process. Resistance to change is either circumvented through the use of enactments or directly challenged by escalating the stress within the family system. However, resistances to change are not typically interpreted by the therapist. Genuine change in the index person occurs only when the family structure is transformed.

The effective use of structural family therapy techniques requires both clarity of purpose and a complex balancing of a commitment to change with sensitivity to corrective feedback from the family on the part of the therapist (Colapinto, 1991). Other aspects of the therapist's psychological health and personality are not specifically highlighted. This is not surprising given that transference and countertransference dynamics are not considered integral to the curative process.

Treatment Applicability

Although designed initially for low-socioeconomic-status families, the structural approach has been applied successfully, according to results from empirically based treatment outcome studies, to a range of families evidencing a wide variety of problems and symptoms. For example, it has been applied and in some cases, shown to be effective with family conflict and where family member is exhibiting externalizing behavior disorders (e.g., Barkley, Guevre-

mont, Anastopoulos, & Fletcher, 1992), psychosomatic illnesses such as eating disorders (e.g., Fishman, 1996), and substance abuse (e.g., Frankel, 1990). In addition, this approach has been applied to multiproblem, disorganized families experiencing family violence (e.g., Gelles & Maynard, 1987) and to families in the process of divorce or rebuilding a remarried, blended, or stepfamily (Abelsohn & Saayman, 1991). Largely due to its origin with African American families, structural family therapy is widely used with culturally diverse populations (Kurtines & Szapocznik, 1996). The structural model has not developed an independent set of techniques for working with couples. Rather, the couple is a subsystem of the family, which may become a focus of the treatment process (Aponte & Dicesare, 2000; Nichols & Minuchin, 1999).

Cognitive and Behavioral Family Therapies

Behavioral family therapies are predicated on social learning theory and behavior exchange principles derived from both classical and operant conditioning approaches. Behavioral approaches to family treatment began with Liberman's (1970) *conjoint behavioral family and couples therapy* (Liberman, Mueser, & Glynn, 1988). More recent behavioral family approaches include Alexander and Parson's *functional family therapy* (Alexander, Pugh, Parsons, & Sexton, 2000), L'Abate and Weinstein's (1987) *structured enrichment for families,* and the *McMaster problem-solving model* (Epstein, 2002; Epstein et al., 1982). Behavioral techniques have been applied across a broad spectrum of family issues and individual problems and disorders—for example, parent–child interaction training (Herschell, Calzada, Eyberg, & McNeil, 2002), treatment of antisocial behavior in juveniles (e.g., Henggeler et al., 1998), and oppositional-defiant disorder and conduct disorder in young children (Webster-Stratton, 1996).

Despite differences in the specific techniques associated with the various forms of cognitive and behavioral family therapy (CBFT), all the approaches are built on a foundation of research findings from humans and animals, conducted in laboratory and natural settings and subjected to empirical scrutiny. Current advances incorporate key theoretical constructs and research findings from the areas of social psychology, cognitive psychology, sociology, and pathophysiology (Falloon, 1991). Therefore, unlike other models of family therapy that are tied in large part to charismatic leaders and their clinical and theoretical contributions, the progress of CBFT has depended primarily from collaborations between researchers and clinicians.

The philosophy and procedures for CBFT are based on the logical positivist research tradition for the scientific study of human behavior (Becvar & Becvar, 1996). That is, the conduct of CBFT is similar to a scientific experiment and includes (1) a testable, well-articulated conceptual framework; (2) hypotheses derived from, and consistent with, the conceptual model; (3) interventions that can be replicated and tested; and (4) objective measurement of treatment outcome.

The behavioral approach to the assessment and treatment of family problems reflects an expansion from the traditional individual approach to behavioral treatment based on the principles from both operant and respondent or classical conditioning as promulgated by such leaders as Pavlov, Watson, Skinner, and Bandura. According to this approach, maladaptive behavior is generated and maintained by environmental contingencies, including one's learning history. Interpersonal interactions reflect reciprocal patterns of behavior in which one person's behavior reinforces the other's behavior, and circular and potentially escalating patterns of interaction emerge.

With its emphasis on environmental, situational, and social determinants of behavior, the behavioral perspective is well suited to addressing problematic behavior in a family context. Like all behavioral therapists, behavioral family therapists attend to environmental events that precede and follow problem behaviors to determine how the behaviors have been learned and reinforced. In addition, these therapists underscore the family as a system, emphasizing the interdependent behavioral patterns between family members. Historically, behavioral approaches have not considered the role of relationship problems in the development and maintenance of the child's difficulties or the impact on the intimate partnership of the child's behavioral problems. More recently, however, behaviorally oriented family therapists have focused not only on the reciprocal influences of the child's behavior problems and the parent's relationship but also on the influence of the community (e.g., socioeconomic and cultural) on family and individual behavior (Henggeler et al., 1998).

Cognitive approaches to family therapy, outgrowths of individual cognitive therapy and rational-emotive therapy, assume that one's cognitive processing (e.g., perceptions, interpretations, evaluations, attributions, and expectancies) influences family members' behaviors, transactions, and emotional and behavioral reactions. Each family member experiences a number of external events, including other family members' behaviors, the combined effects of several members' behaviors toward him or her, and their observations of interactions among family members. As family members cognitively appraise these events, they develop cognitions regarding self, the relationship between self and family members, and interrelationships among family subsystems. In healthy families, these perceptions are positive, realistic, and open to change via direct verbal communication. In dysfunctional families, perceptions tend to be distorted.

Basic Structure of Therapy

CBFTs are relatively brief, time limited, and typically conducted by a single therapist. Membership varies from attendance by caregivers only (e.g., parent training) to the whole family, depending on the reason for referral. The therapy is relatively structured, with the structure provided by the therapist.

Goal Setting

A hallmark of CBFT approaches is the process of developing specific and measurable treatment goals. Goal setting follows a functional analysis that assesses (1) maladaptive affective and instrumental behaviors and the environmental contingencies supporting these behaviors and (2) the ways in which family members' reciprocal interactions affect their relational satisfaction. Based on the functional analysis, the therapist and family together delineate specific treatment goals. The intervention is discussed, and the therapist obtains a commitment from participants to participate in a specified treatment plan. This commitment may be formalized in a treatment contract.

Although treatment goals are tailored to the specific problems of the family, general goals of CBFT include changing maladaptive behaviors by modifying environmental contingencies, facilitating flexible behavior control, increasing positive interactions between family members, altering environmental conditions that interfere with positive interactions, teaching more adaptive behaviors, and facilitating the maintenance and generalization of newly acquired behavioral changes. In addition, CBFT aims to change the cognitive processing and behavior of each family member's such that relationship and family satisfaction is improved.

Techniques and Process of Therapy

CBFT include a diverse array of approaches and techniques (Falloon, 1991). The first descriptions were case studies of parents' implementation of behavioral interventions for their child's problem (Patterson & Brodsky, 1966). Change strategies addressed a particular target behavior elicited by one member (typically a child); the role of other family members was to eliminate the contingencies maintaining the problematic behavior and to initiate different contingencies to support more desirable behaviors that were incompatible with the deviant behavior. This behavior modification approach was further developed by Patterson and colleagues, who recognized that the nature of family interaction patterns made the implementation of operant strategies much more difficult in the home than in the laboratory (Patterson et al., 1993). Therefore, they focused their attention on ways to effectively implement behavioral assessment and intervention strategies to the home environment (Patterson & Forgatch, 1987). The CBFTs practiced today are built on the groundbreaking work of Patterson and coworkers. Examples of these approaches include parent training, functional family therapy (FFT), and multisystemic therapy (MST).

Parent Training

Parent training is an approach in which the therapist provides information and imparts skills to parents to better equip them to address their child's problematic behaviors (Breismeister & Schaefer, 1998). Therapists coach parents in new skills and ways of interacting with their child and supervise caregivers' implementation of these skills at home. Caregivers are recognized as offering unique and intimate insights into the day-to-day routines, behaviors, and emotional reactions of their child. Caregivers and therapists work together and share their expertise to help the caregivers better help the child. This short-term intervention approach is accessible, understandable, maintainable, generalizable, ecologically valid, and time- and cost-efficient. As a result, adults are likely to seek out this treatment, adhere to the protocol, and continue to apply skills learned over time. Parent training has been advocated for parent–child relationship disorders and for parents of children who manifest externalizing behavior disorders such as attention-deficit, disruptive behavior, developmental, and habit disorders (e.g., Herschell et al., 2002).

Parent training approaches for child emotional and behavioral problems can be classified under two broad categories: (1) behavior modification (Mabe, Turner, & Josephson, 2001) and (2) relationship enhancement (Guerney & Guerney, 1989). Due to space considerations, only the behavior modification interventions are discussed here. Behavior modification interventions are based on operant conditioning and social learning theory and focus on altering antecedents and consequences of children's behavior. The most commonly used behavioral modification approaches for young children include the work of Barkley (1998), Eyberg (Eyberg & Boggs, 1998), Patterson (Patterson & Forgatch, 1987), and Webster-Stratton (1996). These behavior modification interventions are the family-oriented child treatment with the most empirical support and validation (Herschell et al., 2002).

One form of parent training is Eyberg's *parent–child interaction therapy* for the parents of preschoolers with an array of psychological disturbances, most notably oppositional-defiant disorder (Eyberg & Boggs, 1998). This approach aims to teach children prosocial behavior, to decrease inappropriate behavior, and to teach parents to improve the quality of their relationship with their young child. The model includes two phases: (1) child-directed interaction (CDI), and (2) parent-directed interaction (PDI). In the CDI component, parents are taught traditional nondirective play techniques and are encouraged to use warmth, attention, and praise as incentives for the child to develop appropriate play and improved self-control. In the PDI phase, caregivers are taught to communicate clearly using age-appropriate instructions and commands, to provide positive and negative consequences following the child's obedience and disobedience, re-

spectively, and to understand how the child's social environment shapes his or her behavior. These techniques can be applied to novel situations as they arise, such that generalization of the child's enhanced self-control can occur. Empirical support for the efficacy of this model at posttreatment and follow-up has been found in a number of studies (Brestan & Eyberg, 1998).

Functional Family Therapy

Based on clearly articulated principles and strongly supported by empirical findings, Alexander and colleagues (Sexton & Alexander, 1999) developed FFT, a treatment approach that integrates learning, cognitive, and systems theories. Whereas most other behavioral intervention approaches are primarily focused on altering overt behavior, FFT also aspires to help the clients understand the role of their behavior in regulating family relationships. This is accomplished via the creation of a nonjudgmental therapeutic environment in which explanations are developed regarding the interactional purpose of all members' behavior. The development of such explanations enables family members to modify their attitudes, beliefs, expectations, and emotions and empowers them to feel more able to effect change (Sexton & Alexander, 1999).

Practitioners of FFT assume that all behavior is adaptive and serves the function of creating a certain outcome in interpersonal relationships. More specifically, behaviors are efforts to achieve one of three interpersonal outcomes: contact/closeness (merging), distance/independence (separating), or a combination of vacillation between the two (midpointing). The specific functions of behavior are not believed to be good or bad; however, the expression of behavior may be problematic. The therapist determines the interpersonal functions of each family member's behavior and the ways in which behavior is maintained by others within the family unit prior to instituting cognitive and behavioral changes in individuals and their families.

FFT proceeds in steps: assessment, therapy, and education. During the assessment, three levels of family functioning are evaluated: sequential or relational interaction patterns and processes in family life; adaptive functions of behavioral sequences of various family members; and individual behavioral, cognitive, and affective characteristics that may constrain or facilitate family change (Alexander et al., 2000). The data gleaned enable the therapist to determine the interactional sequences in which problems are embedded and the functions served by the behavioral sequences. During the therapy phase, interventions address family resistances, mobilize and motivate family members to change, and prepare the family to benefit from the educational interventions. Commonly used interventions include reattribution techniques (encourage family members to question their understanding of family interactional patterns and the presenting problem); relabeling (messages that recast roles, behaviors, and emotions perceived in negative terms by family members more positively and sensitize family members to the functional properties or interpersonal effects of each others' behaviors and emotions), and revalencing (messages that facilitate alternative understanding and affective responses that are more consistent with family members' expectations). These techniques implicitly communicate that the dissatisfied individual actually has greater control over the problematic interactional pattern than he or she recognizes, decrease blaming and scapegoating of family members, and lead to changed perceptions and lower family resistance to change (Alexander et al., 2000). In the educational component, the therapist offers a context in which the family can learn specific skills needed to initiate and maintain positive change and be more effective at problem resolution (Alexander et al., 2000). Instruction is offered in a manner consistent with the functional outcomes of family members' behav-

ior and the therapeutic reattributions that the therapist has created within the family unit. Educational interventions to promote behavior change include contingency contracting and management, modeling, systematic desensitization, time-out procedures, communication skills training, assertiveness training, and problem-solving training (Alexander et al., 2000).

FFTs are noted for their explications of strategies for developing a collaborative working alliance. Adherents use the following relationship-building skills to create the optimal environment and prepare the family for change: present as warm and empathic, integrate emotions and behavior, adopt a nonjudgmental stance, employ humor to reduce tension, and use selective self-disclosure to provide information to the family. Practitioners of this approach continually evaluate their impact on family members and calibrate their style of interaction in ways that maximize their fit with the family's functional characteristics.

Multisystemic Therapy

The development of MST occurred in the context of two movements: the system of care reforms promoted by the federal government and private foundations and consumer and family advocacy efforts (Henggeler et al., 1998). MST is compatible with the core values of the systems of care approach to enhancing and reforming mental health services for children, namely, that the systems of care should be child centered and community based.

MST is predicated on both family systems (Haley, 1976; S. Minuchin, 1974) and ecological (Bronfenbrenner, 1979) models. Ecological models hold that individuals are embedded (nested) within a complex of interconnected systems that encompass the individual, the family, and extrafamilial influences. MST attempts to redress three major weaknesses of existing family therapy approaches: (1) insufficient attention to individual characteristics and extrafamilial systems, (2) insufficient consideration of individual developmental issues, and (3) underutilization of proven intervention strategies based on nonsystemic paradigms (Henggeler et al., 1994). As such, MST assumes that the child is embedded within multiple, interrelated systems (including the peer group, school, and other extrafamilial systems), considers developmental perspectives, and asserts that certain nonsystemic strategies can improve a therapist's ability to help families change.

Based on the assumption that behavior problems are multidetermined and multidimensional, MST interventions are present focused and action oriented. The focus is on intrapersonal (e.g., cognitive) and systemic (e.g., family, peer, school, and community) factors. Interventions are flexible and individualized, addressing factors most commonly associated with the presenting problem (e.g., delinquent behavior), and can include some combination of individual, couple, family, and sibling therapy, as well as group work and consultation (schools, medical personnel, social service, and legal agencies, etc.). Part of an intervention may involve treatment sessions with a single caregiver (e.g., mother) on how to effectively monitor his or her child, or engaging a whole family surrounding how to resolve conflicts. A range of empirically based approaches are used in order to address the "overarching" goals set collaboratively by the therapist and family. MST therapists, unlike many family therapists, may focus their intervention on the school and community level, to enable a youth's extrafamilial systems to reinforce or support more adaptive behavior. Common clinical barriers (e.g., substance abuse problem in a parent or social isolation of the family) become part of treatment as the MST therapist makes a distinct effort to actively engage the family in treatment. This effort involves elucidating family and individual strengths and careful design of treatment resulting from the development of hypotheses surrounding the referral problem.

Bryant, a 15-year-old Caucasian male, who recently completed the ninth grade, was referred for MST treatment by his probation officer following his third appearance at juvenile court in 4 months for vandalism and school truancy. His difficulties were first noted in eighth grade when his academic performance began to deteriorate from mostly Bs to primarily Ds, he stopped playing soccer, and he started to socialize with a group of troublemakers, many of whom smoke marijuana and drink beer. Bryant lives with his parents, younger sister, and paternal grandmother. During sessions, the therapist helped the parents and Bryant develop a behavioral contract delineating specific behavioral expectations (e.g., daily school attendance), associated consequences for noncompliance (e.g., parents will inform probation officer, who in turn will pick up Bryant and place him in juvenile detention for the night), and associated contingencies for compliance (e.g., for each week of school attendance, Bryant's parents will deposit a small sum of money into an account toward the purchase of a car for Bryant). The expectations and consequences for truancy are clearly defined and thus allow for evaluation of their effectiveness with regard to both implementation and improvement in Bryant's school attendance. If the program appears to be implemented by the parents but Bryant does not demonstrate significant improvements in attendance, the behavioral contract will need to be renegotiated (e.g., the reinforcers may need to be changed to be more powerful and immediate). The family, the school, and Bryant were asked to keep tracking sheets regarding frequency of problem behaviors and implementation of behavioral contracts, and these were reviewed in weekly therapy meetings. If some aspect of the intervention protocol did not appear to be working over a 3-week period, the intervention strategy was changed. In addition to targeting specific problem areas, more general intervention strategies were used to teach all family members problem-solving skills, conflict resolution, and anger management. Further, the individual and family strengths were repeatedly noted and reinforced and all steps toward progress, no matter how small, were acknowledged.

During the first of a series of family–school meetings, participants worked together to identify the two most important areas of concern requiring intervention: (1) the lack of consequences at home for Bryant's failure to complete his homework and (2) the negative influence of antisocial peers in the classroom setting on Bryant's completion of schoolwork. Over the course of the next two meetings, and with decreasing involvement with the therapist, the Williamses and school officials collaboratively developed intervention strategies to target the identified problem areas. First, he would receive clearly defined consequences at home for his problematic behaviors at school, consistent with the approach enumerated above. The teachers agreed to fax the parents' daily reports about Bryant's academic behavior. A positive report would earn him a small sum of money and a negative report would require him to perform household chores for an additional 30 minutes that day. Second, Bryant's teachers agreed to rearrange classroom seating to ensure that Bryant was separated from acting-out students and placed next to positive role models.

Among MST therapists, there is no consensus regarding specific treatment decision rules (i.e., which interventions should be used and with whom) (Henggeler et al., 1994). Although this lack of clearly defined decision rules for treatment has been criticized by some (Kazdin, 1996), proponents of MST argue that there are multiple ways to achieve therapeutic change and that decisions regarding the approach should be made collaboratively between the therapist and the family. In addition, the MST program is consistent with the shift in the field from empirically supported treatments to empirically supported principles that guide intervention decisions. MST is delivered at locations convenient to the family (e.g., home, school, neighborhood and community) to minimize barriers to care and to facilitate generalizability of treatment gains

(Henggeler et al., 1998). This community-based model of service delivery has been associated with high engagement and low dropout rates, in large part due to the focus on treatment engagement and a strong commitment to collaboration and partnership with families. MST represents a total care, comprehensive, and generalist approach to treatment characterized by frequent intensive contacts with the family and 24-hour therapist availability. The MST therapist serves a variety of functions, including conducting various therapeutic modalities, consultations, and case management.

Stance of the Therapist

Those who practice CBFT function as scientists, collaborators, educators, role models, and teachers in the Socratic tradition. Therapists are typically active, directive, and present focused and provide didactic information to teach the family about the specific processes associated with the maladaptive behavior. They direct the treatment process, taking responsibility for setting the agenda, reviewing homework, and enforcing the treatment contract. The therapist can serve as a consultant to the family, as they test their perceptions and generate and rationally assess alternative hypotheses regarding individual and relational functioning. Because the approach is geared to the building of more adaptive skills (e.g., communication, assertiveness, problem solving, conflict resolution, and negotiation), the therapist serves as a teacher who supervises the families rehearsal of new behaviors. Although a collaborative working alliance is considered essential for behavior change, transference is not addressed specifically or considered important.

Curative Factors

The mechanisms of change in CBFT are related to the specific techniques used to attain treatment goals. For most families, learning new interpersonal skills (e.g., communication and conflict resolution) is curative. Reality testing also is viewed as essential for behavior change. In CBFT, the focus is on the present and insight is not viewed as central for accomplishing behavioral change. The relationship between the therapist and family members does not play a direct role in bringing about change. However, a therapist who has difficulty structuring the sessions (e.g., does not stop arguing between caregivers) or helping the family members to challenge their distorted cognitions is unlikely to be successful in effecting behavior change or improving relationship satisfaction.

Treatment Applicability

CBFTs have been applied to a broad range of problems (e.g., affective disorders, internalizing and externalizing child behavior problems, and substance abuse). There is increasing evidence for empirical validation of treatment in relation to specific treatment populations. Some examples of these include parent–child interaction therapy (e.g., Eyberg et al., 2001), FFT (e.g., Alexander et al., 2000), MST (e.g., Huey & Henggeler, 2001), and multidimensional family therapy (MDFT; Liddle et al., 2001). Additional emphasis has been placed on creating treatments that are not only efficacious in experimental settings but also effective in community or field settings (e.g., Henggeler, Lee, & Burns, 2002).

Behavioral parent training has been shown to be effective for managing disruptive behavior disorders, elimination disorders, and anxiety disorders. FFT yields an extremely low recidivism rate for juvenile delinquents whose families comply with treatment (Alexander et al., 2000). For adolescent substance users, MDFT has shown to effectively reduce adolescent alcohol use and increase prosocial behavior at school and home (Liddle et al., 2001). MST has been shown to be effective with populations of violent and juvenile offenders, sex-

ual offenders, and substance abusers, as well as families with youth that have psychiatric emergencies and families referred for child abuse and neglect (Cunningham & Henggeler, 2001; Huey & Henggeler, 2001; Schoenwald, Ward, & Henggeler, & Rowland, 2000). CBFT, in addition to other approaches, has been shown to decrease rate of relapse in adults with psychiatric disorders such as schizophrenia (Doane, Goldstein, & Miklowitz, 1986; Miklowitz, 1995) and bipolar disorder (Miklowitz & Goldstein, 1997). CBFT has proven effective for remarried families, families with older adults, addicted individuals, suicidal and depressed persons, and adults with sexual dysfunctions (for review, see Thomas, 1992).

Postmodern Family Therapy

The arrival of postmodern thought in the human sciences (Berger & Luckman, 1967; Gergen, 1985) represented a paradigm shift that disputes the notion that reality was fixed and knowledge was an obtainable entity. This view directly challenged some of family therapy's core assumptions in its belief that reality is socially constructed and knowledge is the product of language, experience, culture, and context. In contrast with Locke's (1689/1956) positivist notion that there is a definitive objective reality discovered through scientific experimentation, postmodern thought proposes the idea that individuals co-create reality through social exchange. The three core assumptions of postmodernism, often referred to as social constructivism, are that knowledge is created through communal rhetoric, reality is a by-product of relational exchange, and communication or language is a constantly constructed through social and cultural discourse (Gergen, 2001). Therefore, people's ideas about their relationships, their family, and their world exist within a constant flow of changing narratives that emerge from interactions between people (Hoffman, 1997). Whereas other family therapy approaches may rely on identifying and addressing dysfunctional family structures or conflicts, postmodern thought posits that problems are context bound and that symptoms do not have their roots in systemic dysfunction. Instead, problems are viewed as constructions as each family's social, cultural, and historic experiences influence the ways in which its members interpret and recount events and behavior. Postmodern therapy focuses on helping family members to change their story surrounding the problem by focusing on positive elements and unseen resources of a situation in order to create change. Its hallmark is a nonpathological approach in which the therapist works collaboratively with the family to generate new possibilities and construct alternative narratives (Goolishian & Anderson, 1992). Several examples of postmodern therapies include solution-focused brief therapy by de Shazer and colleagues at the Brief Therapy Center in Milwaukee (de Shazer, 1985, 1988), solution-oriented therapy as practiced by O'Hanlon and Weiner-Davis (1989), and narrative therapy by White and Epston (1990) through the Family Therapy Center in Auckland, New Zealand.

Basic Structure of Therapy

Postmodern therapies tend to be brief in nature and have been both praised for their simplicity and criticized for their lack of focus on long-term outcomes. They are typically conducted by a single therapist; however, one exception to this is a technique known as the reflecting team (H. Andersen, 1995). This approach involves the facilitation of conversation through a "two-way mirror," where there is open dialogue between the therapist, family, and a consultant team watching the therapy process through a one-way mirror and later dialoguing about issues the family has explored while the family watches them through the one-way mirror. Most postmodern approaches encourage as many family members to attend sessions, and in some cases, the thera-

pist may ask other members of the community or system that may be a part of the problem to attend any particular session. The structure of sessions is guided by questions generated by the therapist; however, the focus of these sessions is on dialogue generated by family members and there is no assumption that the views of either the therapist or any member of the family have any greater importance.

Goal Setting

Whereas the primary goal negotiated between the therapist and the family varies according to the type of postmodern therapy practiced (e.g., solution-focused vs. narrative therapy), the universal focus is to invite family members into the process of dialogue surrounding the problem and challenge the meaning surrounding the problem. Using direct (solution-focused therapy) or indirect (narrative therapy) means, the therapist focuses on the presenting concerns through this dialogue. In postmodern therapies, there is no direct effort to address family structure, roles, transference, or dysfunction.

Techniques and Process of Therapy

Several assumptions guide the process of postmodern therapies that distinguish it from other therapies. First, because the premise of postmodern thought involves the primacy of dialogue between therapist and family, the therapist is not considered "the expert" on the problem, thus empowering the family to find alternative accounts of their situation. Also, issues surrounding cultural diversity are more likely to be taken into consideration, as the family determines the nature of the collaborative dialogue by taking the lead in generating their own outcomes or solutions. In addition, the therapist may employ a range of techniques to facilitate change and is free to draw on any combination of techniques or strategies that promote change.

The primary technique for postmodern therapists involve engaging family members in dialogue about their problems and empowering members to change through becoming aware of, and accommodating to, each others' needs and belief systems. An example of a specific approach includes solution-focused therapy.

Solution-Focused Therapy

Because solution-focused therapists are less interested in the etiology of a problem and are primarily focused on uncovering solutions to problems, the process of therapy involves immediately engaging in therapeutic conversation. Through questioning, the therapist guides family members to stay away from "problem talk" (trying to understand why a problem has occurred) and instead to engage in "solution talk" (generating possible solutions that would address the problem). Primary in this process is the emphasis on language used, with the therapist facilitating this process by asking questions that guide the family member to focus on the future rather than retelling the past (de Shazer, 1991). This approach assumes that the family members know the solution to their problem through creating a new context within which the solution can be enacted. de Shazer (1988) calls this providing "skeleton keys" that enable family members to unlock the door to their problem rather than continuing to focus on why the door is locked.

Other features of solution-focused therapy include using Ericksonian directives whereby the therapist recasts the goal of a family member as if it were already achieved—for example, asking a question about what it would be like when the specific goal was achieved. Three types of questions attempt to highlight exceptions to behavior thought of as unchangeable and the inevitability of change: the miracle question, exception-finding question, and scaling question (Berg & Miller, 1992). The *miracle* question asks family members to think about a situation in which a miracle occurs in the middle of the night and upon waking, their problem is solved. It asks them to describe how they would know that the problem is resolved and what specifically would be different (de Shazer, 1991). The *exception-finding* question involves asks family members to identify situations (e.g., times and places) in which the problem does not occur. This allows family members to identify solutions to their problems based on their own successful experiences controlling these problems. The *scaling* question asks family members to rate on a 1–10 scale their problem and uses this rating to encourage its resolution through monitoring and forecasting progress. After determining a rating, the therapist may ask family members what it would take to move the rating one point up or down or reflect any changes in the rating as therapy progresses (e.g., "Last week you rated communication in your relationship a '5' and today you stated it was a '6', what is different this week?").

Jacob is a 15-year-old boy brought in by his mother due to concerns regarding depression following a recent move from out of state. Jacob lives with his grandparents and single mother who reported he has not made any friends and has been isolative, "moping around at home" since their move 2 months ago. Jacob stated that he didn't feel like himself and it was because he did not like living with his grandparents in their small house. Jacob's mother confirmed this and stated that they had lived together throughout Jacob's life, and for financial reasons, they had to move in with her parents, which had been stressful for her as well. During the first session, the therapist found out that Jacob believed he had too many rules at his grandparent's house. Jacob and his mother were complimented on seeking help when they did and noted that they appeared to be "a great team." Jacob was asked to describe what was different about past school/living situations in comparison to this one. Jacob was asked, "How have you made friends in the past? What's different about this time? How have prior living arrangements helped you to be more involved with friends and less 'mopey'?." Jacob was asked to describe how he would know when the problem was resolved, and what was happening during periods when he was not "moping around the house."

Stance of the Therapist

The stance of the postmodern-oriented therapist is that of a nonhierarchical collaborator and a creative agent working as a part of the family system in order to participate in creating meaning to shape new alternative meanings that would lead to solutions for change. According to Atwood and Seifer (1997), the first step in this process involves joining the "meaning systems" of the family, inviting members to explore these systems, challenging members to expand these systems, and, finally, validating and stabilizing the new system that supports resolution of the problem. Therefore, the therapist is responsible for setting the stage, stating the expectation for change, and eliciting active and collaborative participation, and reflecting new perspectives that support solutions (de Shazer, 1991). A necessary aspect of this process includes the therapist's stance of "not knowing," which means that the therapist is curious and impartial and takes a stance of not understanding the situation of another person. To facilitate therapy, a therapist must engage in active and responsive listening, shared inquiry into the situation, and asking questions that reflect this position of "not knowing" (H. Anderson, 1995), in contrast to the typical role of a therapist as a detached outside observer commenting on family process. The collaboration between therapist and family is reflective of the notion that there is no one objective truth but a series of ways to perceive their situation. This cooperative stance empowers family members to engage in the search for more adaptive solutions (White, 1995).

Curative Factors

The mechanisms by which postmodern therapies work involve the creation of new social narratives surrounding problems. Because the world is believed to be a result of social constructions (i.e., a set of attitudes, values, and beliefs about various situations, relationships, and events that are created through social interaction and dialogue), it is through deconstructing these ideas that individuals can create contexts in which solutions can be found. Most postmodern therapists concentrate on promoting small changes and believe that these small changes will lead to larger changes in the system. Postmodern therapies are not focused on changing long-standing behavior, personality problems, or pathologies but, instead, focus on engaging in dialogue to create more adaptive contexts. There has been little research showing the effectiveness of postmodern therapies; however, emerging data indicate preliminary support for solution-focused therapy (for review, see Gingerich & Eisengart, 2000).

Psychoeducational Family Therapy

Psychoeducational family therapy was first used with individuals with schizophrenia and their families (e.g., C. Anderson, Reiss, & Hogarty, 1986; Falloon, 2002) and in part, due to its efficacy in reducing relapse with this population (Goldstein & Miklowitz, 1995), has been adapted for use for individuals with other serious psychiatric illnesses (Keefler, 2001). Psychoeducational approaches have recently entered the mainstream family therapy field (for a review, see McFarlane, 2002) and have also been used in medical settings to help families to better cope with chronic illness (McDaniel, Hepworth, & Doherty, 1992). Family psychoeducational models are designed to remediate individual and family difficulties and enhance functioning. Specifically, family psychoeducation aims to train family members to be helpers to their loved ones (e.g., parent training for parents with disturbed children); teach family members communication, problem-solving, and conflict resolution skills; and prevent the emergence of problems in order to enhance the quality of family life. These interventions are most likely to be effective when conducted in a manner that respects the culturally influenced values and norms about the presenting problem and family dynamics (Jordan, Lewellen, & Vandiver, 1995).

Psychoeducational approaches are based on a multitude of theoretical perspectives (e.g., cognitive-behavioral, psychodynamic, humanistic, and eclectic), and some are atheoretical in orientation. Psychoeducational programs have been developed for such diverse areas of focus as parent training (Levant, 1986) and marriage and family enhancement and enrichment (L'Abate & Weinstein, 1987). In addition, the medical family therapy movement emphasizes the importance of educating the family so that its members can be informed consumers, collaborators in the treatment process, and better able to cope effectively with the demands of their loved one's illness. The following comments, however, focus on psychoeducational interventions for families with a loved one with a schizophrenia spectrum disorder.

Basic Structure of Therapy

Family psychoeducation, a structured treatment approach, can be conducted with an individual family (C. Anderson, Griffin, et al., 1986) or in a multiple family group format (McFarlane, 1991). The frequency of the sessions depends on the stage of the work and the status of the patient's psychiatric illness. The treatment may take a few years, with longer intervals between sessions during the latter phases. Some have argued that the psychoeducational family approach is not a form of family therapy but, rather, an approach to working with families with an individual with a biologically based illness.

Goal Setting

The intermediate goals are to stabilize the patient's condition, involve all family mem-

bers in the psychoeducation process, educate the family about psychotic illnesses and medications, establish a treatment team that includes family members and emphasizes continuity of care, encourage the use and development of the social support network, help the family cope with the complex burdens associated with a prolonged psychiatric disorder in a family member, and teach more adaptive family stress management often including communication and problem-solving skill training. The long-term goals are the prevention of relapse and the integration of the patient into the community. These goals are explicit and openly negotiated with all participants, a process that continues throughout the therapy. The underlying assumption of the model is that family members can be educated to create an optimal environment for their loved ones with a psychiatric illness, an environment that minimizes stresses exacerbating the patient's illness and enhances the patient's capacity for adaptive functioning.

Techniques and Process of Therapy

Both single-family and multiple-family psychoeducation approaches consist of four phases. The first phase begins at the time of the family member's first psychotic episode or subsequent relapse, typically an acute psychotic episode necessitating hospitalization or day treatment. The therapists (typically two clinicians) join with the family, rapidly forming an alliance with all relevant family members. Family meetings occur frequently and often are held without the patient to allay the family's anxiety and decrease distressing family–patient interactions. Separate meetings between the therapist and patient foster a supportive, working relationship and help the patient understand the philosophy of the approach. An assessment is undertaken entailing an evaluation of the present crisis, elicitation of family members' reactions to the patient's psychiatric disorder and the treatment system, and an examination of the family's structure, coping resources, and social support net-work. This phase culminates with the development of a contract, specifying the structure of the subsequent intervention.

The second phase consists of an educational workshop, which often occurs over the course of a day or weekend. However, some psychoeducational approaches use briefer, more ongoing educational workshops to communicate the information. Educational workshops are designed for family members and friends of the patient. Many advocate concurrent presentation of the educational material to the patient in a patient psychoeducational group format. Educational workshops are didactic, with a lecture and discussion format. Audiovisual aides are used to illustrate brain morphology, biochemistry of the disorder, medication effects and side effects, common symptoms and signs of the disorder, and guidelines for more effective management of the disorder. These guidelines presume that the patient's disability is caused by biological factors and that interpersonal and environmental stresses are key risk factors for relapse. The therapists educate the family to reduce expectations for rapid progress; use a relaxed manner of relating to the patient; reduce external stimulation in the patient's environment; set limits on the patient's disruptive, bizarre, or violent behavior; ignore symptoms that cannot be changed; use clear and simple communications; comply with the recommended treatment plan; maintain routine daily activities; avoid substance use; and ascertain warning signs suggestive of relapse. As time progresses, sessions are held less frequently, typically biweekly, and continue for at least 12 months. The clinician(s) meets with a single family, including the patient, or with the multiple families that attended the workshop together.

In the last phase, rehabilitation, the clinician and the family work together to increase the patient's level of adaptive functioning. Decisions to reduce the frequency of the sessions and, eventually, to terminate treatment are based on the patient's im-provement, the family's preference, and, in the case of multiple family psychoeducation, the group members' need for continued social support. Social support is crucial in helping families and patients maintain treatment gains.

Clinicians adhere to the following steps when conducting family psychoeducation sessions: (1) socialize with family and patient; (2) review the outcome of the task assigned in the previous meeting; (3) review the week's events, particularly those that may be characterized as stressors; (4) reframe the family's reported stressors in the context of the realities of the patient's illness, and integrate this with the guidelines presented during the educational component of the intervention; (5) educate the family in adaptive problem solving and communication skills; and (6) underscore the importance of medication compliance in the rehabilitation process.

Stance of the Therapist

The therapist creates a collaborative relationship with the patient, the family, and the other members of the treatment team. Psychoeducational family therapists are active during the sessions, providing direct advice, guidance, and information. They communicate their expertise in managing psychiatric disorders while recognizing the patient's and family's knowledge about the patient's unique psychiatric presentation and their resources to creatively solve family problems. The clinician's role differs depending on the phase of the work. During the joining phase, the therapist actively works to establish rapport with the family. In the educational phase, the therapists present themselves as teachers and experts in methods for managing psychiatric disorders and may facilitate the development of a social support network among families in the multiple family groups. During the rehabilitation phases, the therapists help the family to use problem solving and communication techniques to monitor the patient for relapse and help the patient to increase independent functioning.

Curative Factors

Because family researchers have linked specific types of family interaction (e.g., expressed emotion or attitudes that are critical, hostile, or overinvolved toward the patient) to the course of schizophrenia and bipolar disorder (e.g., Miklowitz, Simoneau, Sachs-Ericsson, Warner, & Suddath, 1996), intervention focuses on helping family members to communicate without blame, to make clear requests for behavior change, and to achieve consensus on conflict management and problem solving (McFarlane, 2002). The focus is not only on helping the family to provide a supportive environment for the patient but also on helping family members better cope with the stress of having a family member with a psychiatric disorder. Change is believed to be most durable when it occurs in the patient, the family, and the larger social support network. Change is not viewed as brought about by insight or interpretation but, rather, as brought about by increased knowledge, skills, and use of social support. Given the persistent nature of the psychiatric disorders for which this approach was developed, continuity of care is considered important and termination is not particularly stressed. Many of these families, particularly those in multiple family groups, choose to participate indefinitely.

Treatment Applicability

Psychoeducational approaches have been used most frequently with persons with schizophrenia spectrum disorder and their families (Falloon, 2002). However, more recently this approach has been used with families with an adult member with a mood disorder (e.g., Honig, 1997; Miklowitz & Hooley, 1998) or with a child with a mood disorder (Fristad, Gavazzi, & Soldano, 1998). In a related vein, this approach has been used to educate families in which a parent has a mood disorder (Beardslee, 2002). McFarlane (2002) asserts that the psychoeducational approach, similar in many respects to a behavioral approach, may be applicable to other problems, including sexual dysfunction, attention-deficit disorder, borderline personality disorder, and medical illnesses.

CONCLUSION

The evolution of family therapy over the course of the last century has been the product of several historical trends, all of which involve a fundamental focus on family and interpersonal process, structure, and interaction. Sociocultural, philosophical, economic, and scientific influences of the last quarter century have contributed to the development of a more divergent range of approaches and practices within family therapy, which has resulted in greater diversity within and among family therapies. This has broadened the concept of family intervention, which at the same time has enhanced the utility, flexibility, and adaptability of family-based treatment. Many models of family therapy originated from the unified theories of charismatic leaders yet have been integrated with other theories, adapted to account for sociocultural differences, measured using family-oriented assessment devices, held accountable for producing meaningful clinical outcomes, applied to prevention of problems, and focused on particularly significant contemporary societal problems (e.g., delinquent youth behavior). Although differences in family therapy models appear to have grown more divergent in some cases, there has been a greater move toward integrative family therapy approaches in many other instances. Family therapists have unified on a national and international level to articulate philosophies and standards of practice, supervision, and training.

Despite differences in family therapy models, the central concept unifying family theories involves the philosophy of general systems theory, which stipulates that all units of a system constantly interact and influence one another in an attempt to maintain homeostasis. A family therapist, in contrast to an individually focused therapist, not only takes into account these forces in accounting for problem behavior but actively engages these forces to create change. Differences in family therapy models not only involve the therapists' conceptualization of problem behavior (e.g., whether problems are a result of family structure or function) but focus on distinct methods of interacting that will lead to therapeutic change (e.g., collaborators vs. directive facilitators). As family therapies continue to evolve and be applied to contemporary problems and settings, the integration of various perspectives offered through these distinct approaches will continue to advance the work of family therapists.

SUGGESTIONS FOR FURTHER READING

Baucom, D. H., Shoham, V., Mueser, K. T., Daiuto, A. D., & Stickle, T. R. (1998). Empirically supported couple and family interventions for marital distress and adult mental health problems. *Journal of Consulting and Clinical Psychology, 66,* 53–85.—This article examines the efficacy, effectiveness, and clinical significance of empirically supported couple and family interventions for marital distress and adult psychiatric disorders such as anxiety disorders, depression, schizophrenia, and alcoholism. The authors discuss different theoretical approaches to treating individual adult disorders as well as different ways of including a partner or family in individual treatment.

Breunlin, D. C., Schwartz, R. C., & MacKune-Karrer, B. (1997). *Metaframeworks: Transcending the models of family therapy.* San Francisco: Jossey-Bass.—The authors present their metaframeworks approach to family therapy, highlighting the ways in which this approach extends and transcends existing models of family therapy. Guidelines and examples illustrate how the authors' treatment strategies can be applied to a wide range of clients and clinical problems.

Estrada, A. U., & Pinsof, W. M. (1995). The effectiveness of family therapies for selected behavioral disorders of childhood. *Journal of Marital and Family Therapy, 21,* 403–440.—This articles reviews the effectiveness of family therapies for selected childhood behavioral disorders, including internalizing, externalizing, and pervasive developmental disorders.

Johnson, S., & Lebow, J. (2000). The "coming of age" of couple therapy: A decade review. *Journal of Marital and Family Therapy, 26,* 23–38.—This article reviews significant developments in couple therapy over the last decade, including the increased emphasis on the role of emotion, the greater recognition of couple violence, and the move toward integration across treatment models.

Liddle, H. A., Santisteban, D. A., Levant, R. F., & Bray, J. H. (Eds.). (2002). *Family psychology: Science-based interventions.* Washington, DC: American Psychological Association.—This edited volume gives a historical overview of family intervention and presents empirically based therapy techniques and research strategies. The book is intended for students, therapists, and researchers committed to linking research and practice in family psychology.

Marsh, D. T. (2001). *A family focused approach to serious mental illness: Empirically supported interventions.* Sarasota, FL: Professional Resource Press.—This book is a practical guide for clinicians who work with families of patients with serious mental illness, including schizophrenia, bipolar disorder, or major depression. The authors discuss family consultation, family support and advocacy groups, family education, and family psychoeducation and psychotherapy.

McDaniel, S. H., Lusterman, D.-D., & Philpot, C. L. (Eds.). (2001). *Casebook for integrating family therapy: An ecosystemic approach.* Washington, DC: American Psychological Association.—In this companion volume to Mikesell and colleagues' *Integrating Family Therapy* (1995), family therapists present cases that illustrate integration across schools and modalities of therapy as well as a consideration of the multiple systems in which the family is embedded. The case material describes critical decisions about interventions in detail, including solutions to therapeutic impasses.

Mikesell, R. H., Lusterman, D.-D., & McDaniel, S. H. (Eds.). (1995). *Integrating family therapy: Handbook of family psychology and systems theory.* Washington, DC: American Psychological Association.—This landmark volume integrates family psychology and systems theory to examine the ways in which therapists produce family change in the context of other systems, such as school, work, medical, or social systems. Each chapter provides case material to illustrate how to apply an integrated model of family therapy.

REFERENCES

Abelsohn, D., & Saayman, G. S. (1991). Adolescent adjustment to parental divorce: An investigation from the perspective of basic dimensions of structural family therapy theory. *Family Process, 30,* 177–191.

Abidin, R. R. (1997). Parenting Stress Index: A measure of the parent–child system. In C. P. Zalaquett & R. J. Wood (Eds.), *Evaluating stress: A book of resources* (pp. 277–291). Lanham, MD: Scarecrow Press.

Ackerman, N. (1958). *The psychodynamics of family life.* New York: Basic Books.

Ackerman, N., & Sobel, R. (1950). Family diagnosis: An approach to the preschool child. *American Journal of Orthopsychiatry, 20,* 744–753.

Alexander, J. F. Pugh, C., Parsons, B., & Sexton, T. L. (Eds.). (2000). *Functional family therapy.* Golden, CO: Venture.

American Association for Marriage and Family Therapy. (1998). *Code of ethics.* Washington, DC: Author.

American Psychiatric Association. (1994). *Diagnostic and statistical manual of mental disorders* (4th ed.). Washington, DC: Author.

Anderson, C. M., Griffin, S., Rossi, A., Pagonis, I., Holder, D. P., & Treiber, R. (1986). A comparative study of the impact of education versus process groups for families of patients with affective disorders. *Family Process, 25,* 185–206.

Anderson, C. M., Reiss, D. J., & Hogarty, G. E. (1986). *Schizophrenia and the family: A practitioner's guide to psychoeducation and management.* New York: Guilford Press.

Anderson, H. D. (1995). Collaborative language systems: Toward a postmodern therapy. In R. H. Mikesell, D. D. Lusterman, & S. H. McDaniel (Eds.), *Integrating family therapy: Handbook of family psychology and systems theory* (pp. 27–44). Washington, DC: American Psychological Association.

Aponte, H. J. (1994). *Bread and spirit: Therapy with the new poor.* New York: Norton.

Aponte, H. J., & DiCesare, E. J. (2000). Structural theory. In F. M. Dattilio & L. J. Bevilacqua (Eds.), *Comparative treatments for relationship dysfunction* (pp. 45–57). New York: Springer.

Ariel, S. (1999). *Culturally competent family therapy: A general model.* Westport, CT: Praeger.

Atwood, J. D., & Seifer, M. (1997). Extramarital affairs and constructed meanings: A social constructionist therapeutic approach. *American Journal of Family Therapy, 25,* 55–75.

Barkley, R. A. (1998). *Attention-deficit hyperactivity disorder: A handbook for diagnosis and treatment* (2nd ed.). New York: Guilford Press.

Barkley, R. A., Guevremont, D. C, Anastopoulos, A. D., & Fletcher, K. E. (1992). A comparison of three family therapy programs for treating family conflicts in adolescents with attention-deficit hyperactivity disorder. *Journal of Consulting and Clinical Psychology, 60,* 450–462.

Bateson, G. (1972). *Steps to an ecology of mind: Collected essays in anthropology, psychiatry, evolution, and epistemology.* New York: Ballantine Books.

Bateson, G., Jackson, D. D., Haley, J. E., & Weakland, J. (1956). Toward a theory of schizophrenia. *Behavioral Science, 1,* 251–264.

Baucom, D. H., Shoham, V., Mueser, K. T., Daiuto, A. D., & Stickle, T. R. (1998). Empirically supported couple and family interventions for marital distress and adult mental health problems. *Journal of Consulting and Clinical Psychology, 66,* 53–85.

Beardslee, W. R. (2002). *Out of the darkened room: When a parent is depressed: Protecting the children and strengthening the family.* Boston: Little, Brown.

Beavers, W. R., & Hampson, B. B. (1993). Measuring family competence: The Beavers systems model. In F. Walsh (Ed.), *Normal family processes* (2nd ed., pp. 73–103). New York: Guilford Press.

Becvar, D. S., & Becvar, R. J. (1996). *Family therapy: A systemic integration* (3rd ed.). Boston: Allyn & Bacon.

Bennun, I. (1986). Evaluating family therapy: A comparison of the Milan and problem solving approaches. *Journal of Family Therapy, 8,* 235–242.

Berg, I. K., & Miller, S. D. (1992). *Working with the problem drinker: A solution-focused approach.* New York: Norton.

Berger, P. L., & Luckman, T. (1967). *The social construction of reality: A treatise in the sociology of knowledge.* New York: Anchor Books.

Boscolo, L., & Bertrando, P. (1996). *Systemic therapy with individuals.* London, UK: Karnac.

Boscolo, L., Cecchin, G., Hoffman, L., & Penn, P. (1987). *Milan systemic family therapy: Conversations in theory and practice.* New York: Basic Books.

Boszormenyi-Nagy, I., Grunebaum, J., & Ulrich, D. (1991). Contextual therapy. In A. S. Gurman & D. P. Kniskern (Eds.), *Handbook of family therapy* (Vol. 2, pp. 200–238). New York: Brunner/Mazel.

Boszormenyi-Nagy, I., & Spark, G. (1973). *Invisible loyalties.* New York: Harper & Row.

Boyd-Franklin, N., & Bry, B. H. (2000). *Reaching out in family therapy: Home-based, school, and community interventions.* New York: Guilford Press.

Box, S., Copley, B., Magagna, J., & Smilansky, E. M. (Eds.). (1994). *Crisis at adolescence: Object relations therapy with the family.* Northvale, NJ: Jason Aronson.

Bradbury, T. N. Fincham, F. D., & Beach, S. R. (2000). Research on the nature and determinants of marital satisfaction: A decade in review. *Journal of Marriage and the Family, 62,* 964–980.

Breismeister, J. M., & Schaefer, C. E. (1998). *Handbook of parent training: Parents as co-therapists for children's behaviors* (2nd ed., pp. 549). New York: Wiley.

Brestan, E. V., & Eyberg, S. M. (1998). Effective psychosocial treatments of conduct-disordered children and adolescents: 29 years, 82 studies, and 5,272 kids. *Journal of Clinical Child Psychology, 27,* 180–189.

Breunlin, D. C., Schwartz, R. C, & MacKune-Karrer, B. (1997). *Metaframeworks: Transcending the models of family therapy.* San Francisco: Jossey-Bass.

Bronfenbrenner, U. (1979). Contexts of child rearing: Problems and prospects. *American Psychologist, 34,* 844–850.

Byng-Hall, J. (2001). Attachment as a base for family and couple therapy. *Child Psychology and Psychiatry Review, 6,* 31–36.

Campbell, D. (1999). Family therapy and beyond: Where is the Milan systemic approach today? *Child Psychology and Psychiatry Review, 4,* 76–84.

Campbell, D., Draper, R., & Crutchley, E. (1991). The Milan systemic approach to family therapy. In A. S. Gurman & D. P. Kniskern (Eds.), *Handbook of family therapy* (Vol. 2, pp. 325–362). New York: Brunner/Mazel.

Carr, A. (1991). Milan systemic family therapy: A review of ten empirical investigations. *Journal of Family Therapy, 13,* 237–263.

Carter, E., & McGoldrick, M. (1989). *The changing family life cycle: A framework* (2nd ed.). New York: Gardner.

Celano, M. P., & Kaslow, N. J. (2000). Culturally competent family interventions: Review and case illustrations. *American Journal of Family Therapy, 28,* 217–227.

Chambless, D. L., & Steketee, G. (1999). Expressed emotion and behavior therapy outcome: A prospective study with obsessive–compulsive and agoraphobic outpatients. *Journal of Consulting and Clinical Psychology, 67,* 658–665.

Colapinto, J. (1991). Structural family therapy. In A. S. Gurman & D. P. Kniskern (Eds.), *Handbook of family therapy* (Vol. 2, pp. 417–443). New York: Brunner/Mazel.

Combrinck-Graham, L. (2001). Children in family in communities. *Child and Adolescent Psychiatric Clinics of North America, 10,* 613–624.

Coyne, J. C., Kahn, J., & Gotlib, I. H. (1987). Depression. In T. Jacob (Ed.), *Family interaction and psychopathology: Theories, methods, and findings* (pp. 509–534). New York: Plenum Press.

Coyne, J. C., & Pepper, C. M. (1998). The therapeutic alliance in brief strategic therapy. In J. D. Safran & J. C. Muran (Eds.), *The therapeutic alliance in brief psychotherapy.* (pp. 147–169). Washington, DC: American Psychological Association.

Cunningham, P. B., & Henggeler, S. W. (2001). Implementation of an empirically based drug and violence prevention and intervention program in public school settings. *Journal of Child Clinical Psychology, 30,* 221–232.

Denton, W. H., Walsh, S. R., & Daniel, S.S. (2002). Evidence-based practice in family therapy: Adolescent depression as an example. *Journal of Marital and Family Therapy, 28,* 39–46.

de Shazer, S. (1985). *Keys to solution in brief therapy.* New York: Norton.

de Shazer, S. (1988). *Clues: Investigating solutions in brief therapy.* New York: Norton.

de Shazer, S. (1991). *Putting differences to work.* New York: Norton.

Diamond, G. S., Serrano, A. C., Dickey, M., & Sonis, W. A. (1996). Current status of family-based outcome and process research. *Journal of the American Academy of Child and Adolescent Psychiatry, 35,* 6–16.

Doane, J. A., Goldstein, M. J., & Miklowitz, D. J. (1986). The impact of individual and family treatment on the affective climate of families of schizophrenics. *British Journal of Psychiatry, 148,* 279–287.

Duhl, B. S., & Duhl, F. J. (1981). Integrative family therapy. In A. S. Gurman & D. P. Kniskern (Eds.), *Handbook of family therapy* (pp. 483–516). New York: Brunner/Mazel.

Eisenberg, N. Gershoff, E. T., & Fabes, R. A. (2001). Mother's emotional expressivity and children's behavior problems and social competence: Mediation through children's regulation. *Developmental Psychology, 37,* 475–490.

Epstein, N. (2002). Couple and family therapy. In M. A. Reinecke & M. R. Davison (Eds.), *Comparative treatments of depression* (pp. 358–396). New York: Springer.

Epstein, N., Baldwin, L., & Bishop, S. (1983). The McMaster Family Assessment Device. *Journal of Marital and Family Therapy, 9,* 171–180.

Epstein, N., Bishop, D. S., & Baldwin, L. M. (1982). McMaster model of family functioning: A view of the normal family. In F. Walsh (Ed.), *Normal family processes* (pp. 115–141). New York: Guilford Press.

Estrada, A. U., & Pinsof, W. M. (1995). The effectiveness of family therapies for selected behavioral disorders of childhood. *Journal of Marital and Family Therapy, 21,* 403–440.

Eyberg, S. M., & Boggs, S. R. (1998). Parent–child interaction therapy: A psychosocial intervention for the treatment of young conduct-disordered children. In J. M. Briesmeister & C. E. Schaefer (Eds.), *Handbook of parent training: Parents as cotherapists for children's behavior problems* (2nd ed., pp. 61–97). New York: Wiley.

Eyberg, S. M., Funderburk, B. W., Hembree-Kigin, T. L., McNeil, C. B. Querido, J. G., & Hood, K. K. (2001). Parent–child interaction therapy with behavior problem children: One and two year maintenance of treatment effects in the family. *Child and Family Behavior Therapy, 23,* 1–20.

Falloon, I. R. H. (Ed.). (1991). Behavioral family therapy, In A. S. Gurman & D. P. Kniskern (Eds.), *Handbook of family therapy* (Vol. 2, pp. 65–95). New York: Brunner/Mazel.

Falloon, I. R. H. (2002). Cognitive-behavioral family and educational interventions for schizophrenic disorders. In S. G. Hofmann & M. C. Tompson (Eds.), *Treating chronic and severe mental disorders: A handbook of empirically supported interventions* (pp. 3–17). New York: Guilford Press.

Faulkner, R. A., Klock, K., & Gale, J. E. (2002). Qualitative research in family therapy: Publication trends from 1980 to 1999. *Journal of Marital and Family Therapy, 28,* 69–74.

Feldman, L. B. (1992). *Integrating individual and family therapy.* New York: Brunner/Mazel.

Fishman, H. C. (1996). Structural family therapy. In J. Werne (Ed.), *Treating eating disorders. The Jossey-Bass library of current clinical technique* (pp. 187–215). San Francisco: Jossey-Bass.

Framo, J. L. (1982). *Explorations in marital and family therapy: Selected papers of James L. Framo.* New York: Springer.

Frankel, L. (1990). Structural family therapy for adolescent substance abusers and their families. In A. S. Friedman & S. Granick (Eds.), *Family therapy for adolescent drug abuse* (pp. 229–266). Lexington, MA: Lexington Books.

Fristad, M. A., Gavazzi, S. M., & Soldano, K. W. (1998). Multi-family psychoeducation groups for childhood mood disorders: A program description and preliminary efficacy data. *Contemporary Family Therapy, 20,* 385–402.

Gelles, R. J., & Maynard, P. E. (1987). A structural family systems approach to intervention in cases of family violence. *Family Relations: Journal of Applied Family and Child Studies, 36,* 270–275.

Gergen, K. J. (1985). The social construction movement in modern psychology. *American Psychologist, 40,* 266–275.

Gergen, K. J. (2001). Psychological science in a postmodern context. *American Psychologist, 56,* 803–813.

Gil, E. (1994). *Play in family therapy.* New York: Guilford Press.

Gingerich, W. J., & Eisengart, S. (2000) Solution-focused brief therapy: A review of the outcome research. *Family Process, 3,* 477–498.

Ginsberg, B. G. (2002). 50 wonderful ways to be a single-parent family. Oakland, CA: New Harbinger.

Goldstein, M. J., & Miklowitz, D. J. (1995). The effectiveness of psychoeducational family therapy in the treatment of schizophrenic disorders. *Journal of Marital and Family Therapy. 21,* 361–376.

Goldstein, M. J., Rosenfarb, I., Woo, S., & Nuechterlein, K. (1997). Transactional processes which can function as risk or protective factors in the family treatment of schizophrenia. In H. D. Brenner & W. Boeker (Eds.), *Towards a comprehensive therapy for schizophrenia* (pp. 147–157). Kirkland, WA: Hogrefe & Huber.

Goolishian, H. A., & Anderson, H. (1992). From family to systemic therapy and beyond. In A. Z. Schwartzberg & A. H. Esman (Eds.), *International annals of adolescent psychiatry,* (Vol. 2, pp. 160–173). Chicago: University of Chicago Press.

Gottman, J. M., & Notarius, C. I. (2000). Decade review: Observing marital interaction. *Journal of Marriage and the Family. 62,* 927–947.

Gottman, J. M., & Notarius, C. I. (2002). Marital research in the 20th century and a research agenda for the 21st century. *Family Process, 41,* 159–197.

Gray, S. H. (2002). Evidence-based psychotherapeutics. *Journal of the American Academy of Psychoanalysis, 30,* 3–16.

Group for the Advancement of Psychiatry Committee on the Family. (1996). Global Assessment of Relational Functioning Scale (GARF): I. Background and rationale. *Family Process, 35,* 155–172.

Guerney, L., & Guerney, B. (1989). Child Relationship Enhancement: Family therapy and parent education. *Person-Centered Review, 4,* 344–357.

Gurman, A. S., & Kniskern, D. P. (Eds.). (1991). *Handbook of family therapy* (Vol. 2). New York: Brunner/Mazel.

Haley, J. (1976). *Problem-solving therapy.* San Francisco: Jossey-Bass.

Helmeke, K. B., & Prouty, A. M. (2001). Do we really understand?: An experiential exercise for training family therapists. *Journal of Marital and Family Therapy, 27,* 535–544.

Henggeler, S. W., Burr-Harris, A. W., & Borduin, C. M. (1991). Use of the family adaptability and cohesion evaluation scales in child clinical research. *Journal of Abnormal Child Psychology, 19,* 53–63.

Henggeler, S. W., Lee, T., & Burns, J. A. (2002). What happens after the innovation is identified? *Clinical Psychology-Science and Practice, 9,* 191–194.

Henggeler, S. W., Schoenwald, S. K., Borduin, C. M., Rowland, M. D., & Cunningham, P. B. (1998). *Multisystemic treatment of antisocial behavior in children and adolescents.* New York: Guilford Press.

Herschell, A. D., Calzada, E. J., Eyberg, S. M., & McNeil, C. B. (2002). Parent–child interaction therapy: New directions in research. *Cognitive and Behavioral Practice, 9,* 9–15.

Hodes, M., & le Grange, D. (1993). Expressed emotion in the investigation of eating disorders: A review. *International Journal of Eating Disorders, 13,* 279–288.

Hoffman, L. (1997). Postmodernism and family therapy. In J. K. Zeig, (Ed.), *The evolution of psychotherapy: The third conference* (pp. 337–348). Philadelphia: Brunner/Mazel.

Honig, A. (1997). Psychoeducation and family intervention. In A. Honig & H. M. van Praag (Eds.), *Depression: Neurobiological, psychopathological and therapeutic advances* (Vol. 3, pp. 537–550). New York: Wiley.

Hooley, J. M., & Gotlib, I. H. (2000). A diathesis-stress conceptualization of expressed emotion and clinical outcome. *Applied and Preventive Psychology, 9,* 135–151.

Hooley, J. M., & Hoffman, P. D. (1999). Expressed emotion and clinical outcome in borderline personality disorder. *American Journal of Psychiatry, 156,* 1557–1562.

Huey, S. J., & Henggeler, S. W. (2001). Effective

community interventions for antisocial and delinquent adolescents. In J. N. Hughes, A. M. La Grecca, & J. C. Conoley (Eds.), *Handbook of psychological services for children and adolescents* (pp. 301–322). New York: Oxford University Press.

Imber-Black, E., Roberts, J., & Whiting, R. A. (Eds.). (1988). *Rituals in families and family therapy.* New York: Norton.

Jacob, T., & Johnson, S. L. (1999). Family influences on alcohol and substance abuse. In P. J. Ott, R. E. Tarter, & R. T. Ammerman (Eds.), *Sourcebook on substance abuse: Etiology, epidemiology, assessment, and treatment* (pp. 166–174). Boston: Allyn & Bacon.

James, S. E. (2002). Clinical themes in gay- and lesbian-parented adoptive families. *Clinical Child Psychology and Psychiatry, 7,* 475–486.

Johnson, S. M. (1996). *The practice of emotionally focused marital therapy: Creating connection.* New York: Brunner/Mazel.

Jordan, C., Lewellen, A., & Vandiver, V. (1995). Psychoeducation for minority families: A social work perspective. *International Journal of Mental Health, 23,* 27–43.

Kantor, D., & Lehr, W. (1975). *Inside the family: Toward a theory of family process.* San Francisco: Jossey-Bass.

Kaslow, F. W. (Ed.). (1982). *The international book of family therapy.* New York: Brunner/Mazel.

Kaslow, F. W. (1991). The art and science of family psychology: Retrospective and perspective. *American Psychologist, 46,* 621–626.

Kaslow, F. W. (1993). Relational diagnosis: Past, present and future. *American Journal of Family Therapy. 21,* 195–204.

Kaslow, F. W. (Ed.). (1996). *Handbook of relational diagnosis and dysfunctional family patterns.* New York: Wiley.

Kaslow, F. W. (2000). History of family therapy: Evolution outside of the U.S.A. *Journal of Family Psychotherapy, 11,* 1–35.

Kaslow, N. J., Celano, M. P., & Dreelin, E. D. (1995). A cultural perspective on family theory and therapy. *Psychiatric Clinics of North America, 18,* 621–633.

Kaslow, N. J., & Gurman, A. S. (1985). Ethical considerations in family therapy research. *Counseling and Values, 30,* 47–61.

Kaslow, N. J., Kaslow, F. W., & Farber, E. W. (1999). Theories and techniques of marital and family therapy. In M. B. Sussman & S. K. Steinmetz (Eds.), *Handbook of marriage and the family* (2nd ed., pp. 767–792). New York: Plenum Press.

Kaslow, N. J., Wood, K. A., & Loundy, M. R. (1998). A cultural perspective on families across the life-cycle: Patterns, assessment, and intervention. In A. S. Bellack & M. Hersen (Eds.), *Comprehensive clinical psychology* (pp. 173–205). New York: Pergamon Press.

Kazak, A. E., Simms, S., & Rourke, M. T. (2002). Family systems practice in pediatric psychology. *Journal of Pediatric Psychology, 27,* 133–143.

Kazdin, A. E. (1996). Combined and multimodal treatments in child and adolescent psychotherapy: Issues, challenges, and research directions. *Clinical Psychology Science and Practice, 3,* 69–100.

Kazdin, A. E. (2002). Psychosocial treatments for conduct disorder in children and adolescents. In P. E. Nathan & J. M. Gorman (Eds.), *A guide to treatments that work* (2nd ed., pp. 57–85). London: Oxford University Press.

Keefler, J. (2001). The psychoeducational model and case management: The role of marital and family therapy in the treatment of the chronically mentally ill. In M. M. MacFarlane (Ed.), *Family therapy and mental health: Innovations in theory and practice* (pp. 185–213). Binghamton, NY: Haworth Clinical Practice Press.

Keim, J. (2000). Strategic therapy. In F. M. Dattilio & L. J. Bevilacqua (Eds.), *Comparative treatments for relationship dysfunction* (pp. 58–78). New York: Springer.

Keith, D. V., Connell, G. M., & Connell, L. C. (2001). *Defiance in the family: Finding hope in therapy.* Philadelphia: Brunner-Routledge.

Kempler, W. (1981). *Experiential psychotherapy within families.* New York: Brunner/Mazel.

Kerig, P., & Lindahl, K. (Eds.). (2001). *Family observational coding systems: Resources for systemic research.* Mahwah, NJ: Erlbaum.

Kopelowicz, A., Liberman, R. P., & Zarate, R. (2002). Psychosocial treatments for schizophrenia. In P. E. Nathan & J. M. Gorman (Eds.), *A guide to treatments that work* (2nd ed., pp. 201–228). London: Oxford University Press.

Kurtines, W. M., & Szapocznik, J. (1996). Family interaction patterns: Structural family therapy in contexts of cultural diversity. In E. D. Hibbs & P. S. Jensen (Eds.), *Psychosocial treatments for child and adolescent disorders: Empirically based strategies for clinical practice* (pp. 671–697). Washington, DC: American Psychological Association.

L'Abate, L., & Weinstein, S. E. (1987). *Structured enrichment programs for couples and families.* New York: Brunner/Mazel.

Lebow, J. (1997). The integrative revolution in couple and family therapy. *Family Process, 36,* 1–17.

Leff, J., & Vaughn, C. (1985). *Expressed emotion in families: Its significance for mental illness.* New York: Guilford Press.

Levant, R. F. (1986). *Psychoeducational approaches to family therapy and counseling.* New York: Springer.

Liberman, R. (1970). Behavioral approaches to family and couple therapy. *American Journal of Orthopsychiatry, 40,* 106–118.

Liberman, R. P., Mueser, K., & Glynn, S. (1988). Modular behavioral strategies. In I. R. H. Falloon (Ed.), *Handbook of behavioral family therapy* (pp. 27–50). New York: Guilford Press.

Liddle, H. A., Bray, J. H., Levant, R. F., & Santisteban, D. A. (2002). Family psychology intervention science: An emerging area of science and practice. In H. A. Liddle, D. A. Santisteban, R. Levant & J. Bray (Eds.), *Family psychology: Science-based interventions* (pp. 3–15). Washington, DC: American Psychological Association.

Liddle, H. A., Bruenlin, D. C., & Schwartz, R. C. (Eds.). (1988). *Handbook of family therapy training and supervision.* New York: Guilford Press.

Liddle, H. A., Dakof, G. A., Parker, K., Diamond, G. S., Barrett, K., & Tejeda, M. (2001). Multidimensional family therapy for adolescent drug abuse: Results of a randomized clinical trial. *American Journal of Drug and Alcohol Abuse. 27,* 651–688.

Lindholm, B. W., & Touliatos, J. (1993). Measurement trends in family research. *Psychological Reports, 72,* 1265–1266.

Lock, J. (2002). Treating adolescents with eating disorders in the family context: Empirical and theoretical considerations. *Child and Adolescent Psychiatric Clinics of North America, 11,* 331–342.

Locke, J. (1956). *An essay concerning human under-*standing. Chicago: Henry Regnery. (Original work published 1689)

Low, S. M., Monarch, N. D., Hartman, S., & Markman, H. (2002). Recent therapeutic advances in the prevention of domestic violence. In P. A. Schewe (Ed.), *Preventing violence in relationships: Interventions across the life span* (pp. 197–221). Washington, DC: American Psychological Association.

Mabe, P. A., Turner, M. K., & Josephson, A. M. (2001). Parent management training. *Child and Adolescent Psychiatric Clinics of North America, 10,* 451–464.

Madanes, C. (1991). Strategic family therapy. In A. S. Gurman & D. P. Kniskern (Eds.), *Handbook of family therapy* (Vol. 2, pp. 396–416). New York: Brunner/Mazel.

Magnavita, J. J. (2000). *Relational therapy for personality disorders.* New York: Wiley.

Markman, H. J., & Notarius, C. I. (1987). Coding marital and family interaction: Current status. In T. Jacob (Ed.), *Family interaction and psychopathology: Theories, methods, and findings* (pp. 329–390). New York: Plenum Press.

Marsh, D. T. (2001). *A family focused approach to serious mental illness: Empirically supported interventions.* Sarasota, FL: Professional Resource Press.

Marsh, D. T., & Magee, R. D. (Eds.). (1997). *Ethical and legal issues in professional practice with families.* New York: Wiley.

McCleary, L., & Sanford, M. (2002). Parental expressed emotion in depressed adolescents: Prediction of clinical course and relationship to co-morbid disorders and social functioning. *Journal of Child Psychology and Psychiatry and Allied Disciplines, 43,* 587–595.

McDaniel, S. H., Hepworth, J., & Doherty, W. J. (1992). *Medical family therapy: A biopsychosocial approach to families with health problems.* New York: Basic Books.

McDaniel, S. H., Lusterman, D.-D., & Philpot, C. L. (Eds.). (2001). *Casebook for integrating family therapy: An ecosystemic approach.* Washington, DC: American Psychological Association.

McFarlane, W. R. (1991). Family psychoeducational treatment. In A. S. Gurman & D. P. Kniskern (Eds.), *Handbook of family therapy* (Vol. 2, pp. 363–395). New York: Brunner/Mazel.

McFarlane, W. R. (2002). *Multifamily groups in the*

treatment of severe psychiatric disorders. New York: Guilford Press.

McGoldrick, M. (Ed.). (1998). *Re-visioning family therapy: Race, culture, and gender in clinical practice*. Metuchen: Family Institute of New Jersey.

McGoldrick, M., Giordano, J., & Pearce, J. K. (Eds.). (1996). *Ethnicity and family therapy* (2nd ed.). New York: Guilford Press.

Melby, J., & Conger, R. D. (2001). The Iowa Family Interaction Rating Scales: Instrument Summary. In P. Kerig & K. Lindahl (Eds.), *Family observational coding systems: Resources for systemic research* (pp. 33–58). Mahwah, NJ: Erlbaum.

Melby, J., Conger, R., Book, R., Rueter, M., Lucy, L., Repinski, D., Rogers, S., Rogers, B., & Scaramella, L. (1998). *The Iowa Family Interaction Rating Scales*. Ames, IA: Institute for Social and Behavioral Research.

Mikesell, R. H., Lusterman, D.-D., & McDaniel, S. H. (Eds.), *Integrating family therapy: Handbook of family psychology and systems theory*. Washington, DC: American Psychological Association.

Miklowitz, D. J. (1995). The evolution of family-based psychopathology. In R. H. Mikesell, D.-D. Lusterman, & S. H. McDaniel (Eds.), *Integrating family therapy: Handbook of family psychology and systems theory* (pp. 183–197). Washington, DC: American Psychological Association.

Miklowitz, D. J., & Goldstein, M. J. (1997). *Bipolar disorder: A family-focused treatment approach*. New York: Guilford Press.

Miklowitz, D. J., & Hooley, J. M. (1998). Developing family psychoeducational treatments for patients with bipolar and other severe psychiatric disorders: A pathway from basic research to clinical trials. *Journal of Marital and Family Therapy, 4,* 419–435.

Miklowitz, D. J., Simoneau, T. L., Sachs-Ericsson, N., Warner, R., & Suddath, R. (1996). Family risk indicators in the course of bipolar affective disorder. In C. Mundt & M. J. Goldstein (Eds.), *Interpersonal factors in the origin and course of affective disorders* (pp. 204–217). London: Gaskell/Royal College of Psychiatrists.

Miller, N. (1992). *Single parents by choice: A growing trend in family life*. New York: Insight Books.

Minuchin, P., Colapinto, J., & Minuchin, S. (1998). *Working with families of the poor*. New York: Guilford Press.

Minuchin, S. (1974). *Families and family therapy*. Cambridge, MA: Harvard University Press.

Minuchin, S., & Fishman, H. C. (1981). *Family therapy techniques*. Cambridge, MA: Harvard University Press.

Minuchin, S., Montalvo, B., Guerney, B., Rosman, B., & Schumer, F. (1967). *Families of the slums*. New York: Basic Books.

Minuchin, S., & Nichols, M. P. (1998). Structural family therapy. In F. M. Dattilio (Ed.), *Case studies in couple and family therapy: Systemic and cognitive perspectives* (pp. 108–131). New York: Guilford Press.

Moos, R. H., & Moos, B. S. (1981). *Family Environment Scale manual*. Palo Alto, CA: Consulting Psychologists Press.

Mosconi, A., Gonzo, M., Sorgato, R., Tirelli, M., & Tomas, M. (1999). From counterparadox and the Milan Model to therapeutic conversation and the Milan Systemic approach: Origin and development of the Milan Center for Family Therapy. In U. P. Gielen & A. L. Comunian (Eds.), *International approaches to the family and family therapy* (pp. 9–42). Padua, Italy: Unipress.

Nardone, G. (1995). Brief strategic therapy of phobic disorders: A model of therapy and evaluation research. In J. H. Weakland & W. A. Ray (Eds.), *Propagations: Thirty years of influence from the Mental Research Institute* (pp. 91–106). New York: Haworth Press.

Nichols, M. P., & Minuchin, S. (1999). Short-term structural family therapy with couples. J. M. Donovan (Ed.), *Short-term couple therapy* (pp. 124–143). New York: Guilford Press.

Nurse, A. R. (Ed.). (1999). *Family assessment: Effective uses of personality tests with couples and families*. New York: Wiley.

O'Hanlon, W. H., & Weiner-Davis, M. (1989). *In search of solutions: A new direction in psychotherapy*. New York: Norton.

Olson, D. H. (2000). Circumplex model of marital and family systems. *Journal of Family Therapy. 22,* 144–167.

Olson, D. H., McCubbin, H. I., Barnes, H., Larsen, A., Muxen, M., & Wilson, M. (1983). *Families: What makes them work*. Beverly Hills, CA: Sage.

Olson, D., Sprenkle, D., & Russell, C. (1979). Circumplex model of marital and family systems: Cohesion and adaptability dimensions, family types, and clinical applications. *Family Process, 18,* 3–28.

Parsons, T., & Bales, R. F. (1955). *Family socialization and interaction process.* Glencoe, IL: Free Press.

Patterson, C. (2002). Lesbian and gay parenthood. In M. H. Bornstein (Ed.), *Handbook of parenting. Vol. 3: Being and becoming a parent* (2nd ed., pp. 317–338). Mahwah, NJ: Erlbaum.

Patterson, G. R., & Brodsky, G. A. (1966). A behaviour modification programme for a child with multiple problem behaviours. *Journal of Child Psychology and Psychiatry, 7,* 277–295.

Patterson, G. R, Dishion, T. J., & Chamberlain, P. (1993). Outcomes and methodological issues relating to treatment of antisocial children. In T. R. Giles, (Ed.), *Handbook of effective psychotherapy* (pp. 43–88). New York: Plenum Press.

Patterson, G. R., & Forgatch, M. S. (1987). *Parents and adolescents living together: The basics* (Vol. I). Eugene, OR: Castalia.

Patterson, G. R., Ray, R. S., Shaw, D. A., & Cobb, J. A. (1969). *Manual for coding of family interactions* (rev. ed.). New York: Microfiche.

Philpot, C. L., Brooks, G., Lusterman, D.-D., & Nutt, R. (Eds.). (1997). *Bridging separate gender worlds.* Washington, DC: American Psychological Association.

Pinsof, W. M. (1995). *Integrative problem-centered therapy: A synthesis of family, individual, and biological therapies.* New York: Basic Books.

Prata, G. (1990). *A systemic harpoon into family games: Preventive interventions in therapy.* New York: Brunner/Mazel.

Reiss, D., & Neiderhiser, J. M. (2000). The interplay of genetic influences and social processes in developmental theory: Specific mechanisms are coming into view, *Development and Psychopathology, 12,* 357–374.

Roberto, L. G. (1991). Symbolic–experiential family therapy. In A. S. Gurman & D. P. Kniskern (Eds.), *Handbook of family therapy* (Vol. 2, pp. 444–476). New York: Brunner/Mazel.

Rosenbaum Asarmow, J., Tompson, M., Woo, S., & Cantwell, D. P. (2001). Is expressed emotion a specific risk factor for depression or a nonspecific correlate of psychopathology? *Journal of Abnormal Child Psychology, 29,* 573–583.

Santisteban, D. A., Coatsworth, J. D., Perez-Vidal, A., Mitrani, V., Jean-Gilles, M., & Szapocznik, J. (1997). Brief structural/strategic family therapy with African American and Hispanic high-risk youth. *Journal of Community Psychology, 25,* 453–471.

Satir, V., & Baldwin, M. (1983). *Satir step by step: A guide to creating change in families.* Palo Alto, CA: Science & Behavior Books.

Scharff, J. S. (Ed.). (1989). *Foundations of object relations family therapy.* Northvale, NJ: Jason Aronson.

Scharff, J. S., & Scharff, D. E. (1997). Object relations couple therapy. *American Journal of Psychotherapy, 51,* 141–173.

Schewe, P. A. (Ed.). (2002). *Preventing violence in relationships: Interventions across the life span.* Washington, DC: American Psychological Association.

Schoenwald, S. K., Ward, D. M., Henggeler, S. W., & Rowland, M. D. (2000). Multisystemic therapy versus hospitalization for crisis stabilization for youth: Placement outcomes 4 months postreferral. *Mental Health Services Research, 2,* 3–12.

Segal, L. (1991). Brief therapy: The MRI approach. In A. S. Gurman & D. P. Kniskern (Eds.), *Handbook of family therapy* (Vol. 2, pp. 171–199). New York: Brunner/Mazel.

Selvini-Palazzoli, M. (1974). *Self starvation.* London: Human Context Books.

Selvini-Palazzoli, M., Boscolo, L., Cecchin, G., & Prata, G. (1978). *Paradox and counterparadox.* Northvale, NJ: Jason Aronson.

Selvini-Palazzoli, M., Cirillo, S., Selvini, M., & Sorrentino, A. M. (1989). *Family games: General models of psychotic processes in the family.* New York: Norton.

Sexton, T. L., & Alexander, J. F. (1999). *Functional family therapy: Principles of clinical intervention, assessment, and implementation.* Henderson, NV: FFT.

Silliman, B., Stanley, S. M. Coffin, W. Markman, H. J., & Jordan, P. L. (2002). Preventive interventions for couples. In H. A. Liddle, D. A. Santisteban, R. F. Levant, & J. H. Bray (Eds.), *Family psychology: Science-based interventions* (pp. 69–87). Washington DC: American Psychological Association.

Simpson, L. (1991). The comparative efficacy of Milan family therapy for disturbed children and their families. *Journal of Family Therapy, 13,* 267–284.

Skinner, H. A., Steinhauer, P. D., & Santa-Barbara, J. (1983). The family assessment measure. Canadian *Journal of Community Mental Health, 2,* 91–105.

Snyder, D. K., Cavell, T. A., Heffere, R. W., & Mangrum, L. F. (1995). Marital and family assessment: A multifaceted, multilevel approach. In R. H. Mikesell, D.-D. Lusterman, & S. H. McDaniel (Eds.), *Integrating family therapy: Handbook of family psychology and systems theory* (pp. 163–182). Washington, DC: American Psychological Association.

Snyder, D. K., Cozzi, J. J., & Mangrum, L. F. (2002). Conceptual issues in assessing couples and families. In H. A. Liddle, D. A. Santisteban, R. F. Levant, & J. H. Bray (Eds.), *Family psychology: Science-based interventions* (pp. 69–87). Washington DC: American Psychological Association.

Sperry, L. (Ed.). (2001). *Integrative and biopsychosocial therapy: Maximizing treatment outcomes with individuals and couples.* Alexandria, VA: American Counseling Association.

Straus, M. A., Hamby, S. L., Finkelhor, D., Moore, D. W., & Runyan, D. (1998). Identification of child maltreatment with the Parent–Child Conflict Tactics Scales: Development and psychometric data for a national sample of American parents. *Child Abuse and Neglect, 22,* 249–270.

Szapocznik, J., & Williams, R. A. (2000). Brief Strategic Family Therapy: Twenty-five years of interplay among theory, research and practice in adolescent behavior problems and drug abuse. *Clinical Child and Family Psychology Review, 3,* 117–134.

Thomas, M. B. (1992). *An introduction to marital and family therapy: Counseling toward healthier family systems across the lifespan.* New York: Macmillan.

Todd, T. C., & Storm, C. L. (1997). *The complete systemic supervisor: Context, philosophy, and pragmatics.* Needham Heights, MA: Allyn & Bacon.

Vetere, A. (2001). Structural family therapy. *Child Psychology and Psychiatry Review, 6,* 133–139.

Visher, E. B., & Visher, J. S. (1996). *Therapy with stepfamilies.* New York: Brunner/Mazel.

von Bertalanffy, L. (1968). *General systems theory: Foundations, development, applications* (rev. ed.). New York: George Braziller.

Walsh, F. (Ed.). (1982). *Normal family processes.* New York: Guilford Press.

Walters, M., Carter, B., Papp, P., & Silverstein, O. (1992). *The invisible web: Gender patterns in family relationships.* New York: Guilford Press.

Wamboldt, M. Z., & Wamboldt, F. S. (2000). Role of the family in the onset and outcome of childhood disorders: Selected research findings. *Journal of the American Academy of Child and Adolescent Psychiatry, 39,* 1212–1219.

Watzlawick, P., Weakland, J., & Fisch, R. (1974). *Change: Principles of problem formation and problem resolution.* New York: Norton.

Weakland, J. H., & Ray, W. A. (Eds.). (1995). *Propagations: Thirty years of influence from the Mental Research Institute.* New York: Haworth Press.

Webster-Stratton, C. H. (1996). Early intervention with videotape modeling: Programs for families of children with oppositional defiant disorder or conduct disorder. In E. D. Hibbs & P. S. Jensen (Eds.), *Psychosocial treatments for child and adolescent disorders: Empirically based strategies for clinical practice* (pp. 435–474). Washington, DC: American Psychological Association.

Webster-Stratton, C., & Taylor, T. (2001). Nipping early risk factors in the bud: Preventing substance abuse, delinquency, and violence in adolescence through interventions targeted at young children (0 to 8 yrs). *Prevention Science, 2,* 165–192.

Whitaker, C. (1976). The hindrance of theory in clinical work. In P. J. Guerin Jr. (Ed.), *Family therapy: Theory and practice* (pp. 154–164). New York: Gardner Press.

Whitaker, C. A., & Bumberry, W. M. (1988). *Dancing with the family: A symbolic–experiential approach.* New York: Brunner/Mazel.

Whitaker, C. A., & Keith, D. V. (1981). Symbolic-experiential family therapy. In A. S. Gurman & D. P. Kniskern (Eds.), *Handbook of family therapy* (pp. 187–225). New York: Brunner/Mazel.

White, M. (1995). *Re-authoring lives: Interviews and essays.* Adelaide, South Australia: Dulwich Centre Publications.

White, M., & Epston, D. (1990). *Narrative means to therapeutic ends.* Adelaide, South Australia: Dulwich Centre Publications.

Worrall-Davies, A., Owens, D., & Holland, P.

(2002). The effect of parental expressed emotion on glycaemic control in children with type 1 diabetes: Parental expressed emotion and glycaemic control in children. *Journal of Psychosomatic Research, 52,* 107–113.

Wynne, L. C., Ryckoff, I. M., Day, J., & Hirsch, S. I. (1958). Pseudomutuality in the family relationships of schizophrenics. *Psychiatry, 21,* 205–220.

Yingling, L. C., Miller, W. E., McDonald, A. L., & Galewaler, S. T. (Eds.) (1998). *GARF assessment sourcebook: Using the DSM-IV Global Assessment of Relational Functioning.* Washington, DC: Brunner/Mazel.

Zimet, D. M., & Jacob, T. (2001). Influences of marital conflict on child adjustment: Review of theory and research. *Clinical Child and Family Psychology Review, 4,* 319–335.

12

Marital Therapies

ALAN S. GURMAN

Most therapists are about as poorly prepared for marital therapy as most spouses are for marriage.
—JAMES PROCHASKA (1978, p. 1)

HISTORICAL BACKGROUND

Prochaska's harsh assessment of the preparedness of psychotherapists to work with couples probably needs to be more muted now, 25 years later. Today, for example, there is an official Division of Family Psychology within the American Psychological Association, and exposure to at least the basics of marital therapy theory and practice is much more common in clinical training programs in psychology, psychiatry, and social work, the traditional mental health professions. Marriage and family therapy graduate students, of course, are routinely exposed to the concepts of couple therapy (Broderick & Schrader, 1991), but they comprise a small proportion of neophyte psychotherapists entering the practice of psychotherapy annually. As noted in Chapter 1, marital therapy has become commonplace in the general practice of psychotherapy by clinicians of all professional disciplines.

What Is Marital Therapy?

Psychotherapy aimed at improving some aspects of a couple's relationship can be, and often is, provided as an aspect of individual and family therapy treatment formats. For practical purposes, however, it seems reasonable to consider couple therapy as involving the presence of both relationship partners and not to include clinical methods in which the focus or emphasis is on child or adolescent problems or parent–child interaction. Although it has been debated (e.g., Gurman & Kniskern, 1986; Gurman, Kniskern, & Pinsof, 1986; Wells & Giannetti, 1986a, 1986b) whether individual treatment of couple problems is as helpful as joint treatment, I have argued that "therapeutic intents are not the same as therapeutic events" (Gurman & Kniskern, 1979, p. 5), and I consider couple-focused individual therapy, even with a "systemic twist" (Gurman & Fraenkel, 2002, p. 202), to be individual, not couple, therapy.

This chapter, then, focuses on marital therapy in the sense in which that term is usually used—that is, in reference to "conjoint therapy," a term coined by Don Jackson (1959), a Sullivanian-trained psychiatric pioneer of family therapy, and popularized by the charismatic Virginia Satir (1964). Although all psychotherapists who regularly treat couples inevitably practice some sort of "divorce therapy" (Rice & Rice, 1985), these practices do not constitute a therapeutic form, entity, or "school" of treatment that is distinct from the major couple therapy approaches and are, therefore, not addressed in this chapter. Likewise, sex therapy, a domain of obvious relevance to marital therapists, has generally not intersected with the world of marital and family therapy (Gurman & Fraenkel, 2002), and its principles and practices (McCarthy, 2002) are not considered. Finally, both primary and secondary preventive couple intervention programs have expanded rapidly recently (Bradbury & Fincham, 1990; Fraenkel, Markman & Stanley, 1997) but are not typically employed by remedially oriented clinicians.

Relationship to Family Therapy

Nathan Ackerman, the unofficial founder of family therapy, once identified "the therapy of marital disorders as the core approach to family change" (Ackerman, 1970, p. 124). Despite this early assertion, and the fact that family and couple therapy traditionally "draw from the same body of concepts and techniques" (Fraenkel, 1997, p. 380), the field of family therapy (see Kaslow, Dausch, & Celano, Chapter 11, this volume) has largely failed to embrace the practice of couple therapy as central to its identity and, in fact, has usually placed it in quite a marginalized conceptual and professional position (Gurman & Fraenkel, 2002). This marginalized position is almost universally reflected in the most influential textbooks of family therapy, which typically devote only a small fraction of their pages to marital therapy. Such marginalization occurs despite the fact that surveys repeatedly show that couple problems exceed whole-family problems in the practices of family therapists and family psychologists (Doherty & Simmons, 1996; Rait, 1988; Simmons & Doherty, 1995). As we shall see, influential contemporary approaches to couple therapy

have been derived at least as much from clinical extensions of social learning theory/behavior therapy, psychodynamic theory, and humanistic/experiential theory as from family systems theory and general systems theory, the conceptual soils in which dominant family therapy approaches were planted and have grown.

"Couples" and "Marriages"

The term "couple therapy" has recently come to replace the historically more familiar term "marital therapy" because of its emphasis on the bond between two people, without the associated judgmental tone of social value implied by the traditional term. In the therapy world, the terms are usually used interchangeably. Whether therapeutic methods operate similarly with "marriages" and with "couple" relationships in which there is commitment but no legal bond is unknown but is assumed here. Although there are philosophical advantages to the term "couple therapy," the more familiar term "marital therapy" is used here and is intended to refer to all couples in long-term, committed relationships.

Why Is Marital Therapy Important?

Significant cultural changes in the last half century have had an enormous impact on marriage and the expectations and experiences of those who marry or enter other long-term committed relationships. Reforms in divorce law (e.g., no-fault divorces), more liberal attitudes about sexual expression, the increased availability of contraception, and the growth of the economic and political power of women have all increased the expectations and requirements of marriage to go well beyond maintaining economic viability and assuring procreation. For most couples nowadays, marriage is also expected to be the primary source of adult intimacy, support, and companionship and a facilitative context for personal growth. At the same time, the "limits of human pair-bonding" (Pinsof, 2002, p. 135) are increasingly clear, and the transformations of marital expectations have led the "shift from death to divorce" as the primary terminator of marriage (Pinsof, 2002, p. 139). With changing expectations not only of marriage itself but also of the permanence of marriage, the public health importance of the "health" of marriage has understandably increased. Whether through actual divorce or chronic conflict and distress, the breakdown of marital relationships exacts enormous costs.

Recurrent marital conflict and divorce are associated with a wide variety of problems in both adults and children. Divorce and marital problems are among the most stressful conditions people face (Bloom, Asher, & White, 1978). Partners in troubled relationships are more likely to suffer from anxiety, depression and suicidality, and substance abuse and from both acute and chronic medical problems and disabilities such as impaired immunological functioning and high blood pressure and health risk behaviors such as susceptibility to sexually transmitted diseases and accident-proneness (Burman & Margolin, 1992). Moreover, the children of distressed marriages are more likely to suffer from anxiety, depression, conduct problems, and impaired physical health (Gottman, 1994).

Why Do Couples Seek Therapy?

Although physical and psychological health are affected by marital satisfaction and health, there are more common reasons why couples seek, or are referred for, conjoint therapy. These concerns usually involve relational matters such as emotional disengagement and waning commitment, power struggles, problem solving and communication difficulties, jealousy and extramarital involvements, value and role conflicts, sexual dissatisfaction, and abuse and violence (Geiss & O'Leary, 1981; Whisman, Dixon, & Johnson, 1997). Generally, couples seek therapy because of threats to the security and stability of their relationships with the most significant attachment figures of adult life (Johnson & Denton, 2002).

Functional versus Dysfunctional Relationships: The Topography of Marital Functioning

Given the variety of theoretical approaches to marital therapy to be discussed in this chapter, it is hardly surprising that therapists of different theoretical orientations define the core problems of the couples they treat quite differently. These range from whatever the couple presents as their problem to relationship skill deficits to maladaptive ways of thinking and restrictive narratives about relationships to problems of self-esteem to unsuccessful handling of normal life-cycle transitions to unconscious displacement onto the partner of conflicts with one's family of origin to the inhibited expression of normal adult needs to the fear of abandonment and isolation. These varying views of relationship difficulties lead to a wide range of clinical interventions that may be classified as focusing on behavior patterns, belief systems, and historical and wider contextual factors (Carr, 2000). The most influential of these treatment models are the focus of this chapter.

Despite these varied views of what constitutes the core of marital difficulties, in recent years marital therapists of different orientations have sought a clinically meaningful description and understanding of functional versus dysfunctional intimate relationships that rests on a solid research base (Lebow, 1999). The overwhelming majority of research in this area has come from cognitive (Baucom, Epstein, & Rankin, 1995) and behavioral (Christensen, Jacobson, & Babcock, 1995) investigators and empirically oriented social psychological investigators, especially Gottman (1979, 1999). Quite remarkably, and perhaps uniquely in the world of psychotherapy, the major findings coming from this body of research have been uniformly praised by and incorporated into the treatment models of a wide array of marital therapists ranging from eclectic to cognitive-behavioral and behavioral to humanistic and experiential and even to psychodynamic, transgenerational, and feminist (Gurman, 2002). Clearly, these findings, taken as a whole, provide a theoretically and clinically rich and credible description of the typical form and shape of healthy and unhealthy marital interactions. Therapists of different orientations will "make sense" of such findings in their own ways and will complement such findings with observations about functional versus dysfunctional marriages that are specific to their own perspectives. Because these data have been so widely recognized as relevant to clinical practice, I summarize the overall pattern of these findings.

From the perspective of both describing the markers of marital satisfaction and predicting the long-term stability of marriages, satisfied (functional, happy) couples, compared to dissatisfied (dysfunctional, unhappy) couples, show the following: (1) higher rates of pleasing behavior (defined subjectively) and lower rates of displeasing behavior; (2) lower probability of reciprocating negative behavior ("If you're nasty to me, I'll be nasty to you"); and (3) better communication skills (e.g., expressive skills such as the use of "I" statements, positive rather than aversive requests for behavior change [e.g., threats]), better receptive skills (e.g., empathic reflecting), and problem-solving skills (e.g., clarifying a discussion topic, staying on focus, not expressing negative inferences about one's partner [e.g., hidden motivations], focusing on solutions by brainstorming, taking responsibility for one's own views, and not blaming one's partner for the problem).

Poor communication and problem solving are characterized by (3a) "harsh start-ups" (usually, by wives) of problem-focused conversations (e.g., "Hey, what's up with your damned sloppiness around here!") and poor ability to repair ruptures in the couple's exchanges (e.g., by the use of humor and shows of affection or interest). Moreover, these interactions are marked by a heightened focus on affect rather than problem solving and are often accompanied by negative physiological arousal (especially in men) combined with the aroused partner's difficulty in soothing himself. Typically, this emerging pattern culminates in the rapid escalation of two-way aversive experiences, thus setting up the couple for developing a chronic pattern of emotional disengagement and withdrawal by a familiar process, in effect, of escape/avoidance conditioning. In addition, conflictual couples (3b) tend to become deadlocked over inherently unresolvable differences known as "perpetual problems" (e.g., core personality or value differences) but to mistakenly deal with these differences as though they were resolvable, thereby inevitably leading to feelings of frustration, disaffection and resentment. Finally, unhappy couples (4) try to influence each other by using misguided approaches characterized by pain control (e.g., providing emotionally painful consequences to a partner's undesired behavior via criticism, contempt, stonewalling, and/or defensiveness) rather than by mutual reciprocity.

In addition, in the cognitive realm, unhappy couples (5) show "negative attributional biases" in the form of disregarding both the presence of positive partner behavior and even increases in desired partner behavior. They see negative partner behavior as reflecting permanent characteristics and seeing positive partner behavior as reflecting temporary states. In unhappy couples, negative events have longer-lasting negative effects than they do in happy couples. Unhappy couples tend to blame each other for their couple problems while taking little responsibility for them, and they tend to make faulty attributions about their partners' motivations and intentions. They also tend to engage in cognitive distortions such as all-or-nothing thinking, overgeneralization, jumping to conclusions, and catastrophizing and magnification. Finally, unhappy couples are more likely than happy couples to have more unrealistic expectations of both marriage-in-general and of their actual partner.

A Brief History of Marital Therapy

Gurman and Fraenkel (2002) have presented a comprehensive historical account of the evolving theory and practice of marital therapy, describing four conceptually distinctive phases in this history. The first phase, "Atheoretical Marriage Counseling Formation," lasted from approximately 1930 to 1963. This period began with the opening of marriage counseling centers in several U.S. cities and in Great Britain and culminated in the first legal recognition of the marriage counseling profession in California (1963). The sole national professional organization in the field in this period was the American Association of *Marriage* Counselors, which changed its name first to the American Association of Marriage *and Family* Counselors, and finally, in 1978, to the American Association for Marriage and Family *Therapy*. These nominal changes reflected significant political accommodation to, and attempts to merge with the emerging and clearly more powerful field of family therapy (Broderick & Schrader, 1991).

Marriage counseling was a service-oriented profession, composed in large measure of obstetricians, gynecologists, clergy, social workers, and family life educators. Their clinical work, which did not regularly use conjoint therapy until well into the 1970s, focused on adjustment to culturally dominant marital roles and advice and information giving about practical aspects of married life, including sexuality and parenting. Marriage counselors did not work with couples in severe conflict, or with significant individual psychopathology and changed their "counseling" moniker to "therapy" to be more widely accepted among the traditional mental health professions. Unfortunately, this first historical phase did not produce any influential clinical theorists, and was appropriately characterized by Manus (1966) as a "technique in search of a theory" (p. 449).

Marital therapy's second phase (1931–1966), "Psychoanalytic Experimentation," began with bold challenges by such psychiatrists as Mittelman (1948) and Oberndorf (1934) to the conservative dominant psychoanalytic tradition against the inclusion of analysands' relatives in treatment. Noticing the apparent "interlocking neuroses" of married partners in psychoanalysis, and the inconsistencies in the stories told by partners in separate analyses to the same psychoanalyst, such innovators gradually experimented with different combinations and sequences of working with both partners, including some work with the conjoint approach (Greene, 1965). Even as the conjoint approach to couple therapy within psychoanalytic circles became more commonplace late in this period (Sager, 1966), the treatment focus remained largely on the partners as individuals, not on their jointly constructed dyadic system, and on the patient–therapist transference (Sager, 1967). Psychoanalytic marital therapists had not yet recognized "the healing power within couples' own relationships" (Gurman & Fraenkel, 2002, p. 208). Just at the time at which a more systemic awareness was emerging within this approach (e.g., Dicks, 1967; Sager, 1976), the conceptual cutting edge of psychoanalytic marital therapy was significantly dulled by the rapidly accelerating family therapy movement, which overwhelmingly disavowed most psychoanalytic/psychodynamic principles (Kaslow et al., Chapter 11, this volume; Nichols & Schwartz, 1998) in favor of a more mechanistic "black box" understanding of human behavior. Psychoanalytically oriented marital therapy, with rare exceptions (e.g., Framo, 1965) went underground but has resurfaced in important ways during marital therapy's recent and current phase of development (see "Object Relations Marital Therapy" section).

In marital therapy's third phase

(1963–1985), "Family Therapy Incorporation," there were a few influential voices within the family therapy field who had a major impact on marital therapy from the "family systems" perspective. Don Jackson of the Mental Research Institute (MRI) in California, Jay Haley, also of the MRI and, later, the famous Philadelphia Child Guidance Clinic, and his own Family Therapy Institute of Washington, DC, who exemplified the "system purists" (Beels & Ferber, 1969), and Murray Bowen at the Menninger Clinic, then at the National Institute of Mental Health, and later at Georgetown University, showed little or no interest in, and at times even disdain for, the psychology of the individual, unconscious motivation, and anything that smacked of the theories of mainstream psychoanalysis and psychiatry. Jackson (1959, 1965), a founder of the MRI Interactional Approach, contributed the seminal concepts of "family homeostasis" and the "marital quid pro quo," Haley (1963), a pioneer in the Strategic approach, emphasized the interpersonal functions of symptoms and the power and control dimensions of couple relationships, and Bowen (1978) created the first multigenerational family and marital therapy approach, well known for its concepts of "differentiation of self" and therapist "detriangulation." Although none of these influential perspectives ever resulted in a discernible "school" of marital therapy, the central concepts in each of them have trickled down to and permeated the thinking and practices of most psychotherapists who regularly treat couples.

The one major family therapy figure in this period who was not a "system purist" was, not insignificantly, woman and social worker Virginia Satir. Satir's (1964) classic *Conjoint Family Therapy* exuded a humanistic and experiential sensitivity and emphasis that was hard to find in most family therapy quarters during this period. Satir emphasized patients' self-esteem and both individual and relationship growth and, given the dominant trends in current marital

therapy practice (see "Experiential–Humanistic Approaches" section), has probably had the most enduring effects on marital therapy of all the important family therapy pioneers.

Marital therapy's current phase, "Refinement, Extension, Diversification, and Integration" (1986–present), has been marked by continual and significant modification of marital therapy theory, research and practice. The "Refinement" component of this phase has centered primarily on three particular treatment models: behavioral marital therapy (BMT), emotionally focused couple therapy (EFT), and insight-oriented marital therapy (IOMT). BMT has evolved through four distinct phases, beginning with the "simple behavior exchange phase," emphasizing couples' contracted trading of desired behavior (e.g., Stuart, 1969), to a "skills training phase," which emphasizes teaching couples communication and problem-solving skills (e.g., Jacobson & Margolin, 1979), to an "acceptance phase," balancing the earlier focus on behavior change with a new interest in enhancing partners' abilities to accept inevitable and unresolvable perpetual difficulties (Christensen et al., 1995), to the most recent "self-regulation phase," with a balanced emphasis on helping partners change their own behavior (both private and public) as well as that of their partners (e.g., Halford, Sanders, & Behrens, 1994). EFT (Greenberg & Johnson, 1986; Johnson & Greenberg, 1995) has reacquainted the marital field with the humanistic/experiential psychotherapy tradition (see Bohart, Chapter 4, this volume), and has singlehandedly exposed clinicians to the marital relevance of attachment theory (Bowlby, 1988). EFT has also accumulated a record of strong empirical support (Johnson, Hunsley, Greensberg, & Schindler, 1999). IOMT (Snyder, 1999), also an empirically supported approach, draws heavily on psychodynamic object relations theory (Dicks, 1967; see also Curtis & Hirsch, Chapter 3, this volume), interpersonal role theory (Anchin & Kiesler, 1982), and social learning theory, with a developmental emphasis. IOMT has made significant contributions to a renewed emphasis on insight in marital therapy, along with related recent advances in the development of object relations methods (e.g., Catherall, 1992; Scharf & Bagnini, 2002).

Marital therapy's recent "Extension" has seen a dramatic shift from marriage counseling's exclusive attention to minimally troubled, "normal" couples, to couples with partners suffering with significant psychiatric disorders, such as depression, bipolar illness, anxiety disorders, alcoholism, and violence (Gurman & Jacobson, 2002). Marital therapy's recent "Diversification" refers to its increasing attention to multiculturalism (i.e., recognizing the role of ethnicity, race, social class, religion, and sexual orientation in marital relationships and marital therapy) (e.g., Hardy & Laszloffy, 2002). "Diversification" also includes incorporation of feminist social values, especially regarding salient couple issues such as gender, power, and intimacy (Goldner, 1985). Finally, marital therapy's "Integration" refers to the revision of clinical theory and practice in the movement toward theoretical and technical integration (Gurman, 2002; Pinsof, 1995; Segraves, 1982; Weeks, 1989) with the most common integrative approaches emphasizing combinations of behavioral and psychodynamic concepts and methods.

Common Characteristics of Marital Therapy

Modern approaches to marital therapy include important concepts from *general systems theory* (the study of the relationship between and among interacting components of a system that exists over time), *cybernetics* (the study of the regulatory mechanisms that operate in systems via feedback loops), and *family development theory* (the study of how families, couples and their individual members adapt to change while maintaining their systemic integrity over time). In addition, extant models of marital therapy

have been significantly influenced, to varying degrees, by psychodynamic (especially object relations) theory, humanistic theory, and cognitive and social learning theory (see Gurman, 1978, for an extensive comparative analysis of the psychoanalytic, behavioral, and systems theory perspectives), as well as more recent perspectives provided by feminism, multiculturalism, and postmodernism (Gurman & Fraenkel, 2002).

Despite this seemingly dizzying array of significant influences on the theory and practice of marital therapy, a number of central characteristics are held in common by almost all currently influential approaches to conjoint treatment. Gurman (2001) has identified the dominant attitudes and value systems of marital (and family) therapists that differentiate them from traditional individual psychotherapists, as well as four central technical factors common to most models of marital therapy. Most marital therapists value (1) clinical parsimony and efficiency, (2) the adoption of a developmental perspective on clinical problems along with attention to current problems, (3) a balanced awareness of patients' strengths and weaknesses, and (4) a deemphasis on the centrality of treatment in patients' lives. These common attitudes significantly overlap the core treatment attitudes of brief individual therapists (Budman & Gurman, 1988; see also Hoyt, Chapter 10, this volume), and help most marital therapy to be quite brief.

Gurman also identified four central sets of technical factors that regularly characterize marital (and brief) therapy. First, the meaning of time is manifest in three particular ways. While marital therapists generally adopt a developmental perspective on clinical problems, they see an understanding of the "timing of problems" (i.e., "Why now?") as essential to good clinical practice, but with little attention paid to traditional history taking. As Aponte (1992) stated, "A therapist targets the residuals of the past in a (couple's) experience of the present" (p. 326). In addition, most marital therapists do not expend a great deal of effort in formal assessment, and thus the "timing of intervention" usually seems quite early by traditional psychotherapy standards, with active, change-oriented interventions often occurring in the first session or two. Moreover, the "timing of termination" in most marital therapy is typically handled rather differently from the ending of traditional individual psychotherapy in that it is uncommon for marital therapists to devote much time to a "working through" phase of treatment. Couples in therapy rarely find termination to be as jarring an event as do patients in individual therapy, in part because the intensity of the patient–therapist relationship in couple therapy is usually less than in individual therapy.

Second, the clear establishment of a treatment focus is essential to most marital therapists (Donovan, 1999). Many marital therapists emphasize the couple's presenting problems, some even limit their work to these problems, and all marital therapists respect them. Marital therapists typically show minimal interest in a couple's general patterns of interaction and tend to emphasize the patterns that center around the presenting problems, that is, the system's "problem-maintenance structures" (Pinsof, 1995).

Third, marital therapists tend to be eclectic, if not truly integrative, in their use of techniques (Rait, 1988), to be ecumenical in the use of techniques that address cognitive, behavioral, and affective domains of patients' experience, and, increasingly, to address both the "inner" and "outer" person. Moreover, marital therapists of varying therapeutic persuasions regularly use out-of-session "homework" tasks in an effort to provoke change that is supported in the natural environment.

Fourth, the therapist–patient relationship in most marital therapy is seen as far less pivotal to the outcome of treatment than in most individual therapy because the central healing relationship is the relationship between the marital partners. Moreover, the usual brevity of marital therapy tends to mitigate the development of an intense transference to the therapist. In contrast to much traditional individual psychotherapy, the classical "corrective emotional experience" is to be found within the couple-as-the-patient.

THE PRACTICE OF THERAPY

Psychotherapists of every theoretical orientation work with couples. Although their methods probably overlap more than proponents of particular approaches might wish or assert, there are nonetheless a number of discernibly different models of marital therapy, varying in their conceptualization of both the nature of problematic relationships and useful ways to alleviate marital conflict. Here, I describe the conceptual and technical attributes of the marital therapy approaches that seem to have had the greatest influence on training and clinical practice, ranging from early but enduring contributions such as Bowenian, psychodynamic, structural, strategic, and Satirian to more recent approaches such as behavioral, emotionally focused, integrative, and postmodern. These models are presented more or less in the order in which they initially appeared in the field, with correct temporal sequencing at times compromised for the sake of presenting philosophically similar approaches in tandem.

Transgenerational Approaches

There are four particularly influential multigenerational approaches to family therapy (Roberto-Forman, 2002): Bowen family systems therapy (Bowen, 1978), object relations therapy (Scharff & Bagnini, 2002), symbolic–experiential therapy (Whitaker & Keith, 1981), and contextual therapy (Boszormenyi-Nagy & Ulrich, 1981). Roberto-Forman (2002) provides a comprehensive comparative analysis of these approaches. Of these, Bowen family system therapy and object relations therapy have developed the clearest models of marital functioning and the treatment of marital disharmony and have had the greatest enduring impact on clinical training and practice.

Bowen Family Systems Therapy

The father of transgenerational approaches, Murray Bowen created a conceptual approach referred to as Bowen family systems therapy (BFST) that has outlived his own passing in 1990 and a body of clinical theory that pervades clinical practice, even among therapists who do not consider themselves "Bowenites." His transgenerational thinking, most prominently set forth in *Family Therapy in Clinical Practice* (Bowen, 1978), originated in the 1950s in research at the National Institute of Marital Health, while he was working to understand the role of family-of-origin interaction patterns in the development of schizophrenia (Broderick & Schrader, 1991; Guerin, 1976), ultimately focusing on the quality of the parental marriage in patients with this disorder. Papero (1995) has noted that "Bowen family systems theory . . . is not primarily a theory about marriage" (p. 11). Still, Bowen (1976) emphasized that "practically, the two spouses are usually the only ones who are important enough to the rest of the family and who have the motivation and dedication for this kind of [therapeutic] effort" (p. 392). Thus, working with the marital couple was Bowen's preferred therapy format, even when the presenting problem was not marital conflict but, rather, the symptom of one partner, or even of a child.

The central Bowen construct is *differentiation of self* and its opposite, *fusion*. Differentiation refers to a person's ability to distinguish between the *feeling process* and the *intellectual process,* or cognition. Differentiation is twofold: within self and from others. The latter requires the former. Differentiation is equivalent to psychological health and a precondition for relational (e.g., marital) health. Differentiation allows internal direction, autonomy, and thus the possibility of intimacy. Poor differentiation is associated with defensiveness, externalization, and discrediting of one's partner. Such fusion is reflected in a couple or family's *emotional stuck-togetherness* or *undifferentiated family-ego mass.*

Bowen believed that people choose partners at the same level of differentiation, a notion shared with object relations theorists (e.g., Skynner, 1976). In BFST, people seek partners who repeat early familial experience and experience-of-self, who show complementary overt behavior styles, and who expect their mates to make up for their own developmental failures. The expression of such fusion can take four forms: emotional distance (*emotional cutoff*), marital conflict, one spouse's symptoms, or the scapegoating of a child (*family projection process*). Conflict ensues when the anxiety level of one or both partners rises, whether because of external factors or factors internal to the relationship. In such circumstances, partners almost inevitably and intuitively recruit a third factor (e.g., an affair, a political cause, or a symptom) to stabilize the unsteady dyad (*triangulation*). But for Bowen, marital conflict points not only to problems in the dyad but more prominently to problems in the larger family systems of the partners—that is, their families of origin (*multigenerational transmission process*). Dysfunctional marriages bespeak undifferentiation not only within the partners but also from their families of origin.

Bowen's two other central concepts, *sibling position* and *emotional process in society* (or *societal regression*), are less central to the everyday practice of BFST.

Basic Structure of Therapy. BFST is carried out with both marital partners by a solo therapist. Although often presented as a long-term treatment project, BFST also may be conducted effectively on a short-term basis (Guerin, Fay, Fogarty, & Kautto, 1999), and with varying intervals between sessions. The therapist is active and structuring, providing a consistent style of engagement over time and across couples.

Goal Setting. The therapeutic focus in BFST is on modifying the "recursive, repetitive, chronic cycling of symptoms between marital partners and key extended family members" (Roberto-Forman, 2002, p. 120), accomplished by increasing each partner's differentiation both within self and from one's family of origin, resulting in greater "tolerance for individual differences and expression" (Roberto-Forman, 2002, p. 119). Anxiety reduction within each partner usually is sought before experimenting with direct interactions with partners' families of origin.

Techniques and Process of Therapy. Bowen's (1978) central guiding principle for therapeutic change is that "conflict between two people will resolve *automatically* if both remain in emotional contact with a third person who can relate actively to both without taking sides with either" (p. 177, emphasis added). The techniques of BFST derive directly from the approach's theory of dysfunction, and therapeutic techniques within BFST flow directly from the required stance of the therapist.

The Bowen marital therapist assumes a role of "coach" rather than healer. The therapist actively controls the flow of the session. His overriding process aim is to keep sessions calm. To this end, partners are usually encouraged to communicate through the therapist rather than to each other. Little interest is shown in the couple's immediate interaction, and relationship skills are not taught directly. The therapist is generally quite cerebral and intellectual, regulating his own emotional reactivity, without judging the marital partners. More important than any highly specific therapeutic techniques is the therapist's capacity to consistently stay in a position of *detriangulation* (emotionally neutral) vis-à-vis the couple often expressed as taking "I-positions" and avoiding side

taking. Defining "I-positions" is assumed to force the partners to relate to each other in a similar fashion.

The BFST clinician's capacity for maintaining objectivity and his knowledge of (Bowenian) family systems principles provide the central force for therapeutic change. Unlike most other therapeutic approaches, BFST calls on the therapist to actively, directly, and didactically *teach about the functioning of emotional systems.* BFST asserts that marital partners cannot achieve higher levels of differentiation than their therapist has achieved, and his deep understanding of the functioning of emotional systems is essential in this process. Therapy sessions always include a good deal of attention to *defining and clarifying the relationship between the spouses,* which emphasizes isolating "the more prominent stimulus–response mechanisms and teaching the spouses to be observers" (Bowen, 1976, p. 262). In this effort, the therapist asks each partner about his or her reactivity, feelings, and thoughts about the partner's behavior and expressions. The overriding goal, as Papero (1995) notes, is for partners "to talk and think about the process between them, not to enact it" (p. 21). Thus, through consistent defining and clarifying activities, the therapist helps each partner become more aware of his contribution to the problematic couple chain reactions. The emphasis is on changing self and managing emotional reactivity, and this is both facilitated and modeled by the therapist's consistent style of relating to each partner.

In addition to these process aspects of BFST, two other intervention methods associated with this treatment approach are prominent and common. *Family genograms* are three- (or more)-generational maps of families. Their use in BFST helps the marital partners objectively identify multigenerational family patterns and, in so doing, understand their current difficulties in a new contextual light, thus facilitating the aim of increased differentiation. Genograms visually depict core family patterns, and, in their most complex and sophisticated versions, include such wide-ranging information as family members' names, dates of birth and death, religion, geographical location, socioeconomic status, marriages and divorces, major life events (both positive and negative), cultural and ethnic identities, personality characteristics, and frequency of contact. *Family visits* to partners' families of origin are often encouraged and coached after partners have achieved at least a moderately higher level of differentiation and decreased emotional reactivity. These visits can include the goals of reconnecting with family members with whom one has had an emotional cutoff, promoting one's own differentiation by not being pulled into historically problematic patterns of relating with other family members, or merely observing existing family patterns as an aid to one's increasing objectivity.

Applicability. Although there are no *a priori* situations in which BFST would be inappropriate, as with all therapeutic approaches, there are some practical limitations for its use. First, although conjoint treatment is greatly preferred by BFST, marital partners are sometimes seen alone if therapy sessions are unmanageably volatile, or if one partner lacks sufficient motivation for this style of treatment. Roberto-Forman (2002) has noted that aspects of BFST may be experienced as quite aversive by members of those cultural/ethnic groups (e.g., Middle Eastern, Asian, and Southeast Asian) for whom examining multigenerational transmission processes may be experienced as blaming the family (especially elders) for current relationship difficulties. At the same time, BFST may be almost uniquely relevant for couples who need to develop greater differentiation associated with tensions between them that derive from cultural, ethnic, racial, and religious differences. That is, BFST is especially well positioned conceptually to help partners appreciate, reframe, and thus react differently to their differing family traditions and the meanings

associated with such traditions, rituals, and patterns.

Object Relations Marital Therapy

Object relations marital therapy (ORMT) is the variant of psychoanalytic thought that has had the most pervasive influence on the clinical theory and practice of marital therapy. Growing out of challenges to Freudian theory by British analysts, Fairbairn (1963) in particular (but also, significantly, Guntrip, 1961; Klein, 1948; Winnicott, 1960) asserted that the main drive in human experience is to be connected with a "mothering" (nurturant, responsive) person, not to struggle with sexual and aggressive impulses, as Freudians believed.

Although this point of view may seem self-evident in the modern world of psychotherapy, developmental psychology, and the like, such was not always the case. Indeed, the first psychoanalytic forays into the marital realm were cautious and tentative (Gurman & Fraenkel, 2002). In the 1930s, a small number of psychoanalysts were growing impatient with the ineffectiveness and inefficiency of treating analysands with primary marital complaints. Therapist contact with analysands' relatives was, of course, forbidden in psychoanalytic circles, so the move of those like Mittelman (1948) to seeing partners together was politically and professionally daring and dangerous. It was not until the mid–1960s that analytically oriented marital therapists were seeing couples conjointly on a regular basis. Bernard Greene's (1965) classic textbook, *The Psychotherapies of Marital Disharmony,* summarized the extant theories (mostly psychodynamic) of marital therapy in that decade. Even as conjoint therapy became more common, it remained oriented toward the two individuals. As Clifford Sager (1967), the most influential analytic marriage therapist of the 1960s and 1970s wrote, "I am not primarily involved in treating marital disharmony, which is a symptom, but rather in treating the two individuals in the marriage (p. 185). Therapy emphasized the interpretation of defenses, the use of free association and dream analysis, catharsis, and the like. The transference was still the major focus of the therapist's attention.

Because of its inherently marginalized position in the broader family therapy field, psychoanalytically oriented marital therapy receded from visibility during family therapy's "golden age" (Nichols & Schwartz, 1998, p. 9), roughly from 1975–1985, although some important contributions came forth in this period (e.g., Framo, 1976, 1981; Paul & Paul, 1975). Psychodynamic marital therapy reemerged in the 1980s, partly because of growing interest in integrative models of treatment (see "Integrative Approaches" section), partly because of the "self in the system" (Nichols, 1987) being reawakened in the family therapy field (where it had long lay dormant), and partly because of the creative efforts of a number of clinical theorists working independently to refine their approaches to couple problems (e.g., Bader & Pearson, 1988; Nadelson, 1978; Solomon, 1989; Willi, 1982). Jill Scharff (1995; Scharff & Bagnini, 2002; Scharff & Scharff, 1991) of the International Institute of Object Relations Therapy in Washington, DC, has made particularly valuable contributions to ORMT in recent years.

It was object relations theory, as first explicated in Henry Dicks's (1967) classic, *Marital Tensions,* that became the conceptual ground on which this theory, applied to working with troubled couples, rested. The central lesson from Dicks that led object relations therapists away from traditional psychoanalytic ideas was expressed cogently by Skynner (1980), a British family therapist, "the unconscious conflicts are already fully developed in the mutual projective system between the couple, and could be better dealt with directly rather than by the indirect methods of 'transference'" (pp. 276–277). The aim of therapy, then, was that of "getting the projections (in the marriage)

back somehow into the individual selves" (Skynner, 1976, p. 205).

In object relations theory, the core source of marital dysfunction is both partners' failure to see themselves and each other as whole persons. Conflict-laden aspects of oneself, presumably punished or aversively conditioned earlier in life, are repudiated and *split off* from conscious experience. That is these unwanted, anxiety-laden aspects of self are projected onto the mate, and often attacked in the mate, who, in turn "accepts" the projection (i.e., behaves in accordance with it). For example, a husband who was socialized to be "a real man" finds it unacceptable in himself to be "dependent" by asking for his wife's emotional support even when he is distressed. His wife, in turn, socialized not to be comfortable with her own competence, frequently asks her husband for advice on matters about which she is quite knowledgeable. He criticizes her for her "neediness," and she sulks in the face of his criticism, for which he also criticizes her as being "too sensitive." She angrily responds that the problem is not that she is "too sensitive" but that her husband is "too self-reliant" and, thus, distant from her. The marital impasse is bilaterally supported by a process of *projective identification,* further complicated by a *collusion,* an implicit, unspoken "agreement" not to talk about the unconscious agreement. Projective identification and collusion involve a sort of shared avoidance, a dyadic defense mechanism via unconscious communication, protecting each partner from unexpressed, and often not consciously experienced, fears and impulses (e.g., of merger, attack, or abandonment). Highly or chronically conflicted couples tend to see each other, consciously or unconsciously, in terms of past relationships instead of as "real contemporary people" (Raush, Barry, Hertel, & Swan, 1974). Such rigidity leads to polarized psychological roles, reducing a couple's capacity to respond effectively to new developmental circumstances and to accommodate to other necessary changes and requests for change.

Basic Structure of Therapy. ORMT is preferably conducted as a long-term experience, with sessions held once or twice a week over a 2-year period or longer (Scharff & Bagnini, 2002). ORMT can be used as the basis of a short-term approach but with more limited aims, such as crisis management. In either situation, in object relations couple therapy, little structuring of the sessions is provided by the therapist, who prefers to follow the lead of the couple.

Goal Setting. The ORMT therapist does not attempt to impose an agenda on therapy, or to emphasize highly specific therapy goals, which are believed to be too restrictive. Symptom removal, while certainly desirable, is not a priority because symptoms are seen as useful in that they allow a therapeutic focus on the defenses which produce the symptoms. The ORMT clinician's overriding goals are to help the couple reduce the maladaptive controlling power of their collusive arrangement, primarily by improving their *holding capacity* (i.e., their joint, dyadic ability to receive projections without counterprojection [e.g., to listen to the partner's feelings empathically without experiencing intolerable anxiety]) and their capacity for *containment* (i.e., the ability to experience, acknowledge, and regulate their own affective experience [e.g., to allow painful feelings and thoughts into consciousness, without the need to project them onto the mate]), thereby improving the partner's individuation and, thus, capacity for empathy, intimacy, and sexuality. When marital partners are unable to identify with each other's feelings, they are more likely to show reciprocal, and often rapidly escalating, problematic behavior.

Techniques and Process of Therapy. As noted, therapy sessions in ORMT are not actively controlled by the therapist. Rather, the therapist listens nondirectively, maintaining a simultaneous awareness of both partners' transferences toward him or her,

and of the mutually transferential projective system within the marriage. The therapist provides a clear and consistent environment to explore one's self and one's partner (*setting the frame*). He or she identifies and points out repetitive couple interaction patterns, paying particular attention to those that seem to be fueled by defensiveness. As the patient–therapist alliances deepen, the therapist is more likely to interpret partners' resistance to change, including self-exploration. The ORMT therapist prizes therapeutic neutrality with regard to the couple's choices and values and by avoiding siding with either partner. In this process, the therapist's use of self is a central technique. It is described as *negative capability* (Scharff & Bagnini, 2002), that is, the ability to not need to impose meaning and to "know," and is striven for by not doing too much in sessions (e.g., taking too much responsibility) and remaining open to one's own internal experience. This negative capability facilitates the therapist's capacity to take in the partners' transference reactions, and to experience his or her own *countertransference* as a way of understanding both the couple as a couple and each partner to the relationship (e.g., in receiving each partner's projections).

A central technical therapist activity in ORMT involves the *interpretation* of patient defenses in general, and especially defenses against intimacy. These might be expressed in the emerging session themes, silences, nonverbal behavior, and patients' expressed fantasies and dreams (about which the interpersonal meaning is emphasized). Termination is deemed appropriate when partners have developed adequate holding capacities, can relate more intimately, and so forth. The couple decides when termination should occur. Separating from the therapist is considered a significant part of the therapeutic process, and is treated as such.

Therapist's Role and Mechanisms of Change. In ORMT, the therapeutic alliance is fortified primarily by the therapist's ability to tolerate the marital partners' anxiety in an adequate *holding environment*. Although mostly nondirective, the therapist is not a traditional psychoanalytic "blank screen." While the ORMT therapist generally follows rather than leads, he or she is confrontative at times, as the mood of the session and the needs (and avoidances) of the couple require. Therapeutic change is mediated through the patient–therapist relationship and projectively distorted perceptions of both the therapist and one's partner are examined, interpreted as to both their current avoidance function and their historical origins, and reworked many times over the course of treatment. Clearly, the ORMT therapist must be skilled at maintaining appropriate affective boundaries, capable of holding a neutral stance, and composed in the face of the couple's anxiety in response to the therapist's low level of directiveness and structuring.

Applicability. Psychological mindedness is a fundamental characteristic of couples that are appropriate for ORMT, especially long-term ORMT. As Scharff and Bagnini (2002) put it, "Object relations couple therapy is indicated for couples that are interested in understanding and growth. It is not for couples whose thinking style is concrete" (p. 77). Contraindications for ORMT are common to other types of marital therapy (e.g., ongoing affairs, severe psychiatric disorder, and uncontrollable volatility in sessions). Couples who are most appropriate for ORMT are seeking personal and relational growth more than symptom resolution alone. In addition to its relevance to ordinary marital tensions, ORMT has been reported to be helpful in dealing with grief and mourning (Paul, 1967), lack of sexual intimacy (D. Scharff, 1982), and a variety of individual symptoms that predate, but are now affecting, the marriage.

Structural and Strategic Approaches

Structural and strategic approaches derive from some of the earliest and most influen-

tial models of family therapy. Although not initially developed for the treatment of marital problems, these approaches, long ago referred to as "system purist" (Beels & Ferber, 1969), have played significant roles in the training of thousands of marriage and family therapists over the last three decades, and elements of these approaches are regularly incorporated into the clinical practices of large numbers of psychotherapists who have other primary theoretical allegiances.

Structural–Strategic Marital Therapy

Structural therapy, developed by Salvador Minuchin (1974; Minuchin & Fishman, 1981), and strategic therapy, developed by Jay Haley (1976) and Cloe Madanes (1981), like BFST, involve marital therapy methods that evolved out of what were, and still are, among the most widely influential approaches to family therapy. Although structural therapy offers an important perspective on marital difficulties, little has been published on the structural approach to treating couples (cf. Aponte & DiCesare, 2000; Nichols & Minuchin, 1999), whereas such writings are much more common in the literature of strategic therapy (e.g., Haley, 1963; Madanes, 1990) and receive much more attention in the early bibles of strategic therapy, *Problem Solving Therapy* (Haley, 1976) and *Strategic Family Therapy* (Madanes, 1981), than in the classic structural texts (e.g., Minuchin, 1974). Although often and understandably presented as separate "schools" of therapy, the two approaches share not only a strong common personal lineage (e.g., a decade of collaboration and mutual professional stimulation in the late 1960s and 1970s by Haley and Minuchin at the former Philadelphia Child Guidance Clinic, which was closed in 2000) but also an overlapping and complementary set of constructs about both marital functioning and marital therapy. So natural is their fit that some theoretical and technical integrations of the two approaches have had significant and enduring impact on the field

(Stanton, 1980, 1981; Todd, 1986). Such integrated models were inevitable because, as Todd (1986) pointed out about the two approaches, it is "rare for either to be used in its pure form" (p. 72). Although strategic therapy is often seen as putting somewhat greater emphasis on clinical technique than on a theory of marriage (or the family), and structural therapy is often seen the other way around, in truth both models contribute substantially on both fronts to the current integrative practice of structural–strategic marital therapy (SSMT). The standard of practice and conceptualization in this integrated approach is reflected primarily in the work of James Keim (1999, 2000; Keim & Lappin, 2002), who sets forth an integration of Minuchin's structural therapy and Haley's Washington School of strategic therapy, developed at the Family Institute of Washington, DC, beginning in the mid–1970s.

Structural and strategic therapies are both present-oriented, emphasizing how a marriage, and the broader families and social contexts within which they operate, is organized. These approaches epitomize the maxim, "The system is its own best explanation." That is, the patterned regularities of the system as it now operates explain its behavior better than could be done by invoking any set of constructs that lie outside the system (e.g., in the at times highly inferential attributions of therapists). At the same time, these approaches have a strong interest in the developmental or *family life cycle* context in which problems arise. Their interest is not in excavating the past but understanding the meaning and place of problems in current developmental functioning of the marriage and family as a system that evolves over time. Structural–strategic therapists believe that symptoms often signal a developmental impasse in marital life. They also assert that symptoms are both systems maintained and systems maintaining. Symptoms are reinforced by ongoing interactions within the marital subsystem. Moreover, and this is a central tenet of SSMT, symp-toms serve to maintain systems (e.g., marriages) by serving a protective, homeostatic adaptive function for the relationship, especially when a couple cannot resolve, or perhaps even overtly identify, their central difficulties. Such problems serve to deflect conflict away from its real sources. For example, a wife who feels disempowered in her marriage becomes quite depressed, leading the couple's life to become increasingly organized around "her problem," but her lack of a voice in the marriage is not addressed or even identified.

In SSMT, formulations about the etiology of problems are at best secondary to consideration of how problems are maintained. To this end, SSMT clinicians are concerned with the *structure* of a marriage, including its repeating interactions over time with others (e.g., the partners' families of origin). Although the emphasis in SSMT has been more muted recently, for many years the central relational dynamic of marriage was thought to be *power* and *control*. As Haley (1963) said, "the major conflicts in marriage center in the problem of who is to tell whom what to do under what circumstances" (p. 227). For Haley, problems arose when the hierarchical structure was unclear, when there was a lack of flexibility, or when the relationship was marked by *rigid symmetry* or *complementarity*. Symptoms represented a way in which couples were organized by a dysfunctional incongruity in that the symptom bearer maintained relational power through his symptoms. Haley, in a classic article titled simply, "Marriage Therapy," also formulated his "first law of human relations" to explain the resistance to change so common in relationships, "when one individual indicates a change in relation to another, the other will respond in such a way as to diminish that change" (p. 234). In current usage, the term "marital hierarchy" refers to the "perceived balance of influence and contribution between spouses" (Keim & Lappin, 2002, p. 93) and refers to loving and caretaking, as well as authority. Couples with a symptomatic partner and couples with recurrent significant conflict usually have problems establishing and maintaining appropriate *marital boundaries*. Too much *enmeshment* (overinvolvement, e.g., anxiously attempting to direct too many aspects of the partner's life) limits individual growth, freedom of expression, and so on, whereas too much *disengagement* (being out of emotional contact, e.g., showing little awareness of or interest in nonmarital aspects of the partner's life) may lead to an inability to empathize, involvement in affairs, and so forth. Such couples also often have maladaptive *boundaries* with others outside the marriage (e.g., when excessive attention by one parent focused on a child *detours* the couple away from their tensions, or when one partner's overinvolvement with family of origin creates a problematic *cross-generational coalition*).

In general, in SSMT, the focus is more on how a couple is "stuck" than on how it is "sick," so that no marital structures are seen as inherently unhealthy. Rather, the emphasis is on whether the current structure allows the marriage to be flexible enough for its members to meet their individual needs as well as the needs of the marriage itself at its particular developmental juncture.

Basic Structure of Therapy. Therapy sessions can be held at any reasonable interval, but are usually weekly or biweekly. Conjoint sessions overwhelmingly dominate SSMT practice, but intermittently, portions of session time may be used to work with the individual marital partners, to obtain necessary information, or to resolidify a therapeutic alliance. On average, SSMT lasts about 8–10 sessions (at the Washington School), but there are no formal time limits to treatment. Therapists usually work alone in SSMT, because cotherapy often raises many issues about maintaining therapeutic focus and a consistent therapist stance (e.g., whether and when to use direct or indirect interventions).

Goal Setting. The strategic influence on SSMT tends to emphasize resolution of the

couple's presenting problem, whereas the structural influence on SSMT tends to emphasize reworking of the underlying marital/family structure which necessitated and maintained the original problem. Although there are some relatively universal goals in SSMT (e.g., increased couple intimacy, a better balance of power, and improved dealings with "third parties" to the marriage), each course of SSMT includes the creation of an explicit, couple-specific treatment contract. This contract specifies the couple's goals and describes the roles of both the therapist and each marital partner in attempting to achieve these goals.

The Washington School has developed a practical mnemonic guide, "PUSH," for mapping clinical problems. PUSH helps to plan relevant interventions (similar to behaviorists' "functional analysis"; see "Behavioral Approaches" section). Protection refers to the ways in which problems can be seen as motivated by a desire to help loved ones (this is not the same as protecting oneself), for example, by having a symptom. The Unit that is functionally relevant to problem maintenance often includes various third parties, and problem solutions are viewed interactionally, not intrapsychically. Sequence of Interaction refers to the immediate behavior surrounding a problem, and to interaction sequences that are behaviorally different but functionally similar and, thus, interconnected. Finally, Hierarchy alerts the therapist not only to aspects of the marital hierarchy but also to relevant hierarchies in the larger (primarily, but not necessarily family) social system.

Techniques and Process of Therapy. SSMT is generally brief and almost always pragmatic. The emphasis is not seeking the "truth" but on doing what works. Interpretation is offered by the therapist not to develop "insight" but to relabel the meaning, and thus the function, of behavior to induce observable change. The therapist is held more responsible for inducing change than in most other approaches to marital therapy. The overriding principle by which this happens is through the therapist's planful (hence, "strategic") interventions to interrupt, redirect, and change problem–maintaining sequences in the couple's interaction. A cornerstone of this type of therapist activity is the use of tasks and directives. In-session tasks are generally more associated with the structural influence on SSMT, and out-of-session tasks more often associated with strategic influences. Likewise, direct interventions (e.g., asking the couple to talk to each other about a specific topic and nonverbally interrupting husband's frequent interruptions of his wife) tend to be thought of as more structural, and indirect interventions (e.g., via the use of "paradoxical" interventions) as more strategic.

Two influential integrative structural–strategic approaches with couples have been proposed. The first approach, represented in the contributions of M. Duncan Stanton (1980, 1981) and Thomas Todd (1986), encouraged a sequential integration, suggesting that structurally oriented intervention generally be attempted first, followed by a more strategically flavored approach when structural intervention was not being helpful, or that strategic work be done from the outset if there were good clinical reasons to expect that a structural emphasis would not be effective (e.g., numerous previous treatment failures or a history of previous noncompliance). In truth, most structural–strategic couple work has always been an admixture of both of these two historically important clinical bodies of thought.

The most thoroughly developed structural–strategic intervention model for marital therapy is that of James Keim (1999, 2000), a former director of training at the Family Institute of Washington, DC, under Jay Haley and Cloe Madanes. His most recent presentation of this approach has been enhanced by his collaboration with Jay Lappin (Keim & Lappin, 2002), a former member of the senior training faculty at the Philadelphia Child Guidance Clinic.

A hallmark of SSMT is the use of varied *directives,* which Keim and Lappin (2002) define as "a communication by the therapist suggesting that a client experience, think, and/or behave differently" (p. 102). A wide range of directives has been associated with structural and, especially, strategic therapy (see, e.g., Keim, 1999, for a listing of 33 of the most commonly used categories of directives). Although structural–strategic therapists are very respectful of "client-inspired" directives (e.g., wife suggests a novel way for her and her husband to handle a recurrent problem), SSMT is, of course, more readily identifiable by virtue of "therapist-inspired" directives. *Therapist-inspired directives* can be direct (historically associated more with structural therapy) or indirect (historically associated more with strategic therapy) and can be focused more on in-session couple behavior (more "structural") or out-of-session behavior (more "strategic"). *Direct directives* often emphasize the structurally derived interventions of joining and restructuring. *Joining* is often misunderstood as being equivalent to empathy. Whereas joining includes empathic relatedness, that is, a sense of being connected to each marital partner, it also implies the therapist's capacity to form working alliances without being induced into the couple's dysfunctional patterns, roles, and interactions. Joining is technically referred to as *joining with the transaction,* implying the therapist's connection to the couple as a dyad as well as individuals. Joining is as much an attitude as it is a technique. As therapy progresses, joining merges into *tracking* (i.e., the use of patient language, idiom, and worldview to prepare for more change-focused intervention).

Restructuring involves a number of suboperations, the most common being enactment and unbalancing. In *enactment,* the therapist's attitude is one of preferring to deal directly with dysfunctional patterns rather than talk about them. To do so, the therapist (nonparadoxically) encourages the couple to deal with their problems in their usual ways in the session in order for the therapist to see the problem around which he wishes to shift the couple's interaction. Such enactments allow the therapist to try to substitute functional for dysfunctional behavior. Enactment may include the therapist's *boundary marking* (e.g., by overtly identifying the couple's usual patterns of overinvolvement and underinvolvement as maladaptive and encouraging new alternatives). *Unbalancing* therapist interventions are intended to challenge rigid marital hierarchies (e.g., by entering into a temporary *coalition* with one partner to empower that person or create new interactive possibilities). The structural–strategic therapist may also use *intensification* of the couple's interaction to restructure problem-maintaining behavior, for example, by emphasizing differences between enmeshed partners who fear conflict, by drawing out and developing implicit couple conflicts, and by *relabeling* (the purpose, function, or intention of) a recurrent behavior in order to shift a partner's attributions about that behavior. *Homework tasks* are a common direct SSMT intervention and when offered "structurally" are to be taken literally by the couple. They are usually meant to simultaneously challenge existing problematic structures and to increase adaptive behavior.

A common in-session restructuring technique is the Washington School's *coaching of negotiation,* a detailed, 14-step process for which the therapist provides the couple a written handout guide. Designed as a "win–win" experience, the negotiation coaching, which takes place over three or more sessions, requires specificity from the partners in requesting behavior change, the creation of a written negotiation document, a focus on the present and future, avoidance of sidetracking, speaking only for oneself, a balance between acceptance and change, and an insistence on positive endings to each negotiation encounter.

Common *indirect directives* are more defiance-based than direct directives (i.e., they assume individual and/or couple resistance

to change). These directives fall under the rubric of what are often called *paradoxical interventions.* They are "paradoxical" in that they direct the couple to continue their dysfunctional thinking or overt behavior rather than discontinuing it, the stance a psychotherapist is generally assumed to favor. When paradoxical techniques focus on cognition, they are called reframing, and when they focus on observable behavior, they are considered directives. *Reframing* means labeling a behavior in such a way as to give it a new, and usually more acceptable, meaning, as when a therapist uses *positive connotation* or *positive interpretation* (e.g., asking a couple to consider the heretofore unseen beneficial effects of a problem), or *ascribing noble intention* (e.g., attributing an acceptable motivation to an unwanted partner's behavior).

Paradoxical interventions that focus more on out-of-session behavior in SSMT often involve "prescribing the symptom," restraint, ordeals, and pretending. *Prescribing the symptom,* including *symptom scheduling,* calls for the therapist to present a "rationale" for a marital partner to intentionally "do" his clinical symptom or undesired behavior, especially if it is experienced as "involuntary," thus bringing it under more voluntary control. The therapist may also *restrain change* by warning the couple to *go slow,* noting the unacknowledged "dangers" of rapid improvement that would be worse than their present difficulties. *Therapeutic ordeals* call on the therapist to urge a marital partner to carry out behavior he strongly dislikes, but which is purported to have ultimate benefit for the couple. Finally, *pretending* calls on the therapist to (often playfully) instruct a marital partner to "pretend" to have dysfunctional behavior, be it symptomatic behavior or nonsymptomatic behavior that is aversive to his partner, and, if challenged by his mate about the authenticity of his behavior, to deny that any pretending is occurring.

Therapist's Role and Mechanisms of Change. The SSMT approach is often viewed as a grab bag of powerful and interesting techniques. In truth, common structural–strategic techniques merely operationalize a more basic SSMT way of thinking about problem maintenance and change, with the emphasis being on the social context of problems. In SSMT, change occurs by restructuring both the short and long couple sequences that constitute the problem and, in the case of a symptomatic partner, reinforce the problem. In this process, the therapist assumes much more responsibility for change and for creating a therapeutic environment that supports change than in many marital therapy approaches. The structural–strategic marital therapist must be able to "read" well the level of active influence needed by a given couple in order to change and be comfortable giving directives, both direct and indirect. This needed range of therapist styles parallels the need for the structural–strategic marital therapist to be flexible insofar as he or she can move between a challenging stance and a supportive stance, at times with great and serious intensity, at times with an ironic sense of humor.

Applicability. Because of SSMT's present and future focus, couples that insist on talking about the past may have limited success in this approach. Moreover, couples with incompatible goals may have difficulty with SSMT, insofar as SSMT calls for many therapist directives, and devising directives that are responsive to the needs of partners with different therapeutic aims can be difficult. Finally, because of SSMT's emphasis on a conjoint couple experience and collaborative enterprise, this approach may be contraindicated for separated couples that cannot be gotten to interact a good deal out of therapy sessions.

Brief Strategic Marital Therapy: The MRI Approach

Another influential approach to treating marital problems that emerged in the heyday of the family therapy movement is the brief problem-focused therapy of the Mental Research Institute (MRI) in Palo Alto, California, originally developed by John Weakland, Richard Fisch, Paul Watzlawick, and Arthur Bodin (1974), also called the "Interactional approach" (Bodin, 1981; Watzlawick & Weakland, 1974), or the "Palo Alto approach" (Shoham & Rohrbaugh, 2002). To further confuse the novice reader, the MRI approach (Segal, 1991) is also often referred to as "brief strategic therapy" (Shoham & Rohrbaugh, 2002), thus possibly leading to misidentifying this approach as synonymous with the strategic therapy of Haley and Madanes just described. Indeed, Haley was an early member of the Brief Therapy Center of the MRI where the core concepts of both approaches (plus the vastly different experiential model of Virginia Satir, to be discussed later) were generated. And these two "strategic" models often overlap in their application of central therapeutic techniques, especially those of the "paradoxical" variety discussed earlier. But they differ from each other in two reliable ways, one practical and one conceptual. While the Haley-type strategic approaches set no time limit to treatment, the MRI approach, certainly when applied at the MRI itself, and usually when applied elsewhere, sets a definite and almost universal time limit (see "Basic Structure of Therapy" section, which follows) and, indeed, is the only method of couple or family therapy to do so (Gurman, 2001).

More significant is the enormous difference between these "strategic" approaches on the matter of how they understand clinical problems and symptoms. Haley-like strategic therapists and structural–strategic therapists view problems and symptoms as serving protective functions in relationships. MRI-style therapists fundamentally reject the symptom-as-function view as invalid and relatedly have little interest in such notions as implicit couple and family processes or underlying relationship structures. Relatedly, and importantly, the MRI approach is *nonnormative;* that is, there is no effort in this approach to defining what constitutes a "normal" marriage. For MRI therapists, the form or topography of couple relationships is largely irrelevant (with obvious exceptions such as violence), so that if there is no complaint about the marriage, there is no marriage problem. In this way, the MRI approach is quite constructivist (see "Postmodern Approaches" section and Neimeyer & Bridges, Chapter 8, this volume) in that it sees problems not as "discovered" but as "constructed" (i.e., perceived and created through attribution and meaning making).

The MRI model views problems as the result of misguided efforts to solve *difficulties,* usually ordinary, everyday life difficulties that are typically either solvable by using common sense or must be accepted as inherently unsolvable (Watzlawick, Weakland, & Fisch, 1974). *Problems,* on the other hand, are patterns of ongoing, deadlocked, impasse-laden mishandling of difficulties.[1] These patterns are what Shoham and Rohrbaugh (2002) call "ironic processes" (i.e., when particular attempts to solve a problem actually make it worse—that is, when the "solution *is* the problem"). These ironic processes create *vicious cycles*—positive feedback loops between a problematic behavior and the actions taken to change the problematic behavior. The misguided actions taken in vicious cycles are *attempted solutions,* and therapy is aimed at replacing the vicious cycles with *virtuous cycles* also known as resolving the problem by doing "less of the same (attempted solution)" rather than the redundant previously unsuccessful "more of the same" approach. In the MRI approach, there are three types of problems. Type I problem-solving errors, known as *terrible simplifications,* occur when action is necessary but is not taken (i.e., a difficulty is dealt with as though it does not exist). Type II problem-solving errors constitute the *utopian syndrome,* when action is taken but is not really necessary (i.e., as in trying to change a nonexistent difficulty or

in trying to change what is unchangeable). The third maladaptive problem-solving pattern is *paradox* (i.e., when action is called for but is taken at the wrong level of change), that is, when marital partners attempt *first-order change* (when behavior changes but follows the original relationship rules [e.g., husband now does more household tasks but wife still has the responsibility of seeing to it that household tasks are being done]) when *second-order change* (basic change in relational structure or underlying assumptions) is required (e.g., husband now does more household tasks because he has a new attitude about men's and women's roles in marriage), or vice versa. A common example of the latter in marital therapy is the *be spontaneous! paradox,* in which misguided attempts to control naturally occurring behavior *is* the problem.

Basic Structure of Therapy. As noted, MRI marital therapy is usually time-limited, with a maximum of 10 sessions. If treatment ends without all 10 sessions being used, they are kept "in the bank" for the future. Treatment ends when goals are reached and change seems stable. In institutional settings, where the MRI approach often appears, behind-the-mirror peer consultants often participate in therapy, phoning in suggestions as needed. MRI therapists often begin with weekly meetings but soon move to longer intervals. It is interesting to note that the MRI approach is a point of view as much as a therapeutic method and was not created specifically for couple (or family, or individual) therapy per se. Thus, MRI therapists often meet with individuals who have marital problems. This notion of *customership* refers to who is most motivated for change. At times, to maximize *maneuverability,* the therapist may see the partners to a marriage separately, instead of, or in addition to, conjointly. This stance notwithstanding, recent research on the MRI approach in fact seems to support the common clinical view that marital therapy is more effective when both partners participate (Shoham & Rohr-baugh, 2002).

Goal Setting. The MRI approach emphasizes the solving of the presenting problem as quickly as possible. It does not seek insight, the development or enhancement of relationship skills, or personal growth. The overriding goal is the stable interdiction of maladaptive solution efforts (vicious cycles) that maintain the problem. Problems are defined in precise behavioral terms, as are relevant *problem–solution loops.* Aimed at second-order change, the therapist's intent is to correct "corrective" behavior. The historical origins of the problem are not of interest, except insofar as such a focus may clarify unfortunate attempted solutions. In setting treatment goals, the MRI therapist also pays a good deal of attention to the client's use of language and views of the problem (whether it is seen as internal vs. external, voluntary vs. involuntary, etc.). Awareness of such nuances helps the therapist plan the appropriate selection and use of change-oriented interventions.

Techniques and Process of Therapy. Before actively intervening to disrupt a problem–solution loop, the MRI marital therapist assesses previously attempted solutions that have, by definition of the fact that the couple is seeking help, failed. The overriding goal is to induce the couple, or even one member of the couple, to do "less of the same" behavior that is intended by them to solve the problem but actually reinforces it.

MRI techniques and tactics include both general and specific interventions. General interventions are relevant to work with most couples and problems and reflect the basic MRI stance of encouraging *therapeutic restraint.* By urging couples to *go slow,* the therapist anticipates and absorbs patients' natural tendencies to resist meaningful change and reduces their uneasy sense of urgency to resolve their problems. Likewise, the therapist may *caution about the dangers of improvement,* pointing out heretofore unforeseen negative consequences to positive changes. Or, the therapist may offer suggestions about *how to make the problem worse.*

Specific interventions with distressed couples emphasize the distinction between complementary and symmetrical relationship patterns. *Complementary interactions,* and prevailing marital styles, involve the maximizing of differences. In these marriages, negative behavior evokes different counterresponses from one's partner. In *symmetrical interactions,* there is a minimization of differences, and negative behavior by one partner evokes the same kind of behavior in one's mate (both partners withdraw from a fight, yelling by one leads to yelling by the other, etc.). Symmetrical relationships are often competitive relationships but are also more likely to keep conflict covert. As a result, they are less common among clinical couples.

Specific interventions, although always decided on in a tailor-made, case-by-case basis, include a number of relatively predictable motifs, used with couples who show distinguishable problematic interaction patterns. The usual problem-maintaining complementary relationship involves a variant of the well known "pursuer–distancer" or "demand–withdraw" pattern (e.g., demand–refuse, discuss–avoid, criticize–defend, accuse–deny). Thus, in a demand–refuse situation, the MRI therapist may encourage the demander to do less demanding, thus changing that partner's "solution" to the problem (e.g., of her husband's uncommunicativeness), perhaps by having her "merely" observe the partner in problem-evoking situations, without commentary or insistence on change. In cases heavy with criticism–defense behavior, the defending partner may be encouraged to do something different when criticized (e.g., acknowledge the criticizer's point of view, rather than explaining away his own behavior). Accusation–denial pairings (e.g., about dishonesty) may be helped by an MRI technique called *jamming.* The therapist asks the accusee to do the suspicion/accusation-evoking behavior randomly (e.g., talking to strangers in public or on the telephone), while the accuser is asked to see if she can figure out, on each occasion, what the accused partner was up to (e.g., was this "real" suspicious behavior or feigned behavior?). Both partners keep written notes on these exchanges, to be shared at the next therapy session. The combined effort of these interdictions is to decrease the information value of the interchanges and to introduce novel elements into an all-too-familiar interaction.

Although MRI interventions are sometimes seen as manipulative, in fact, to be effective, they require a highly refined sensitivity to patient's needs and to individual differences. Effective restraining or paradoxical interventions call for finely tuned appreciation of the *patient position,* how each partner sees himself and the marriage, and how each partner uniquely uses language to express his self-view and view of the world. The reframing of the meaning of patient behavior and potential consequences of behavior change is done not to induce insight but to induce cooperation with the therapist's directives for out-of-session behavior. Thus, any reframing that the marital partners find plausible is acceptable, without regard to its inherent "truth" value. To create such plausible reframes, the MRI therapist must be tuned into each partner's inner experience. Consistent with the overriding attitude of therapeutic restraint, positive changes in the course of therapy are met with cautious optimism.

Therapist's Role and Mechanisms of Change. As just noted, the therapist's role in MRI-style marital therapy is to induce change from the "outside" but by tuning into the partners' "insides." The therapeutic relationship, in its usual sense, is not heavily weighted as a vehicle for change. While respectfulness and empathy by the therapist are certainly essential in MRI therapy, the therapist–patient relationship is not at all seen as

healing. As Fisch, Weakland, and Segal (1982) have expressed the MRI view, "In doing therapy briefly . . . termination is not viewed as such a special event. The brevity of treatment and the problem-solving approach leave little room for 'developing a relationship' between patient and therapist; thus, there is little sense of a wrenching from treatment or a cutting the patient adrift to fend for himself" (pp. 175–176). Rather, healing or change comes about by the therapist's interruption and interdiction of ironic marital processes. In attempting to do so, it is incumbent upon the therapist not to recapitulate the couple's usual (problem-maintaining) dynamics. That is, the therapist must avoid *ironic therapeutic processes* (e.g., by not engaging in the same failed "solution" errors of either partner), thereby maintaining therapeutic maneuverability. Accomplishing this maneuverability usually leads to the therapist's *taking a one-down position* (e.g., by soft-selling an idea or suggestion) to promote cooperation with directives and receptivity to reframing.

Applicability. MRI-style marital therapy seems to be especially indicated when a couple has a specific and clear complaint, or when they seem to the therapist to be likely to engage reluctantly with more direct therapeutic interventions, or even to resist them altogether. MRI marital therapy is contraindicated for couples who are seeking personal growth and self-awareness. A potential therapist constraint in practicing MRI-style therapy is that he or she must be willing to limit therapeutic attention to what the marital partners complain about and resist the usual therapist temptation to broaden the scope of clinical inquiry.

Experiential–Humanistic Approaches

The two most influential experiential–humanistic approaches to marital therapy are the Satir model (Banmen, 2002; Satir, 1964, 1972), one of the earliest couple treatment methods, and emotionally focused couple therapy (Greenberg & Johnson, 1986, 1988; Johnson, 1996; Johnson & Greenberg, 1995), one of the most recent.

The Satir Model

Virginia Satir was the most visible and influential popularizer of marital and family therapy among both professional and lay audiences from the mid–1960s until about the mid–1970s. Despite her death in 1980, her legacy in the field remains strong (Banmen, 2002). The author of such classic books as *Conjoint Family Therapy* (Satir, 1972), Satir held a unique place among the pioneers of family therapy in that she was the only nationally and internationally influential female clinician in the field. Although the titles of most of her published works referred to family rather than marital therapy, most of her systems-oriented therapeutic contributions were about dyads, especially the marital dyad. Satir was a cofounder (in 1959) of the MRI in Palo Alto, California, and she established its first family therapy training program. She left the MRI in 1966, to become the first director of the famous personal growth center known as the Esalen Institute in California. Her increasing involvement in the "human potential movement" of such humanistic–experiential therapists as Carl Rogers and Fritz Perls pulled her outside the mainstream of systems therapy. Moreover, her contributions were undoubtedly undervalued by the "system purists" of her era, with their emphasis on family structures, boundaries, power, and, for some, therapeutic indirectness.

Satir, like psychoanalytic marriage therapists (Gurman & Fraenkel, 2002) and Bowen, believed that people choose partners with similar difficulties and degrees of selfhood. She asserted that individual psychological health required an ability to accept oneself and others, awareness of one's own needs and feelings, the ability to communicate clearly, and the ability to accept disagreement and others' points of view.

Marital problems arise, for Satir, when partners have low self-esteem, unrealistic expectations, and a lack of trust. Relatedly, symptoms in individuals "develop when the rules for operating do not fit needs for survival, growth, getting close to others . . ." (Satir, 1965, p. 122). For Satir, dysfunctional couples follow (implicit) rules that limit both individual growth as well as dyadic intimacy.

In her growth-and-wellness-oriented perspective, Satir believed that it is inherent in the individual to strive for positive growth, and thus symptoms express a block in this natural developmental process. Moreover, Satir believed that everyone possesses the potential and the resources for personal growth, and that blame is not a useful concept in relationship difficulties as the health of a marriage is always a shared responsibility.

In the Satir model, primacy is given to the functioning and experiencing of the individual as much as to the individual-in-relational context. The narrow roles people assume in dysfunctional relationships (e.g., "victim," "placator," "defiant one," and "rescuer") and the dysfunctional communication stances and styles they exhibit (e.g., "blamer" [self-righteous externalization], "placator" [unassertive, self-deprecating passivity], "the irrelevant individual" [appearing not to track central relationship patterns], and "the super-reasonable individual" [hyperintellectualized and appearing to be without feelings]) are fundamentally expressions of low self-esteem and poor self-concept, in contrast to the "congruent" individual (whose words and feelings match and for whom both self and others are taken into consideration). For Satir, self-esteem and the quality of communication existed in a circular relationship, so that poor self-esteem leads to poor communication and vice versa. Even in the midst of the black-box phase of family therapy's evolution, Satir never lost sight of what Nichols (1987) later called "the self in the system."

Basic Structure of Therapy. In the Satir model, treatment is almost always conjoint, as the overriding aim is to foster individual psychological growth through the development of healthier intimate relationships. Treatment can be of any length and frequency.

Goal Setting. The overriding goal of Satir model marital therapy is to foster greater *self-esteem* and *self-actualization,* achieved by increasing individual *congruence* and clarity of self-expression about relational needs, self-perceptions, and perceptions of one's partner; increased self-awareness; the removal of "protective masks" that shield authenticity; and the acceptance, indeed, valuing, of differences. As Satir (1965) put it, the goal was "not to maintain the relationship nor to separate the pair but to help each other to *take charge of himself*" (p. 125, emphasis added). These goals pertain whether a couple's presenting problems involve conflictual interaction or the symptoms of one partner.

Techniques and Process of Therapy. The Satir model is also known as "Family Reconstruction" (Nerin, 1986). *The family life fact chronology,* a genogram-like method for identifying and characterizing recurrent intergenerational family patterns, ideally occupies the first phase of therapy. The chronology not only allows usable family understanding to be generated but also serves to reduce partners' initial anxiety. Relatedly, the Satir model emphasizes the early development of the therapeutic alliance between the therapist and each partner, especially by the therapist's exposure of his or her own feelings, acknowledging the worthiness of each partner, and so on. The model emphasizes that trust in the therapeutic encounter is essential for individual and relational growth.

To these ends, a flexibly employed variety of interventions and experiential techniques is used. Common verbal methods include emphasizing the use of "I-statements," talking to rather than about one's partner, emphasizing people's positive motives more than their accumulated resentments, intensifying the immediacy of one's emotional self-awareness, clarifying communication, urging the direct expression of feelings, encouraging validation of one's partner, and acceptance of differences. Nonverbal methods are extremely varied in the Satir model and may even include such experiences as dance movement, massage, and other forms of *therapeutic touch* and *sculpting* (in which a partner "sculpts" significant family relationships by positioning oneself and one's partner, for example, to reflect their closeness/distance). Another important Satir model intervention is the dramaturgic method of *family reconstruction,* in which partners enact significant events from their own or their families' histories, based on information developed earlier during the family life fact chronology. The purpose of many of these "exercises" is to unlock partners from dysfunctional historical patterns learned in their families of origin.

Therapist's Role and Mechanisms of Change. In the Satir model, the therapist's roles are multiple, including prominently pointing out unspoken relationship "rules," eliciting conscious but unexpressed feelings, modeling facilitative communication, and using the therapist's self through expressions of warmth and caring. Satir saw the effective marital therapist as a sort of nurturant teacher whose aim was to help actively orchestrate corrective emotional experiences not as an intellectualizing "analyst" or a dispassionate problem solver. The therapist's central role, then, is to create a trusting environment in which self-exploratory and self-disclosing risks may be taken.

Applicability. Clinical experience would suggest that couples with partners who suffer from significant personality disorders, as well as those dealing with major psychiatric illness and violence or substance abuse, would not be appropriate for this style of therapy, which calls for a significant capacity to endure, indeed even to welcome, uncertainty and affective disclosure, and for a significant degree of trust of one's partner, even in the face of marital disharmony.

Emotionally Focused Couple Therapy

EFT, a synthesis of both experiential and systemic traditions in psychotherapy, was created by Susan Johnson and Leslie Greenberg, both Canadian psychologists (Greenberg & Johnson, 1986, 1988; Johnson, 1996; Johnson & Denton, 2002; Johnson & Greenberg, 1995). The name of this approach was chosen both as a statement of the belief in the centrality of emotion in intimate relationships and as a counterposition to the overwhelming absence of attention to emotion in the marital and family therapy field in the early 1980s.

EFT explicitly adheres to such humanistic–experiential therapy principles (cf. Bohart, Chapter 4, this volume) as the following: (1) the therapeutic alliance can itself be healing; (2) the inherent validity of the patient's experience is central to change, and is fostered by the therapist's authenticity and transparency; (3) given the opportunity to do so, people have the ability to make healthy choices; (4) the inner and outer realities of people's lives both need to be attended to; and (5) therapy can provide opportunities for corrective emotional experiences (Johnson & Denton, 2002). EFT is also explicitly linked to systems theory principles, such as the circularity of behavior and the idea of behavior being communicative. It differs from most other systemically oriented methods in its use of emotion to break maladaptive, repetitive cycles of couple interaction. Thus, we see the overall philosophical correspondence of EFT values to those of the Satir model.

More than any other concept that has set EFT apart from other approaches is the centrality of *attachment theory* in its understanding of marital tension and its creation of a therapeutic emphasis and style. EFT calls on attachment (Bowlby, 1988) as a theory of adult love, which emphasizes emotional "bonds" over "bargains" to be negotiated (Johnson, 1986) as the basics for committed relationships. EFT holds that all human beings have an innate, "wired-in" need for consistent, safe contact with responsive and caring others (i.e., an irreducible need for relational security). A healthy relationship *is* a secure *attachment bond,* one characterized by emotional accessibility and responsiveness. Such bonds create a mutual sense of safety, which, in turn, helps partners regulate their emotions effectively, deal with differences in the relationship, and communicate clearly. Research consistently has shown that relationship security predicts high levels of closeness, trust, and satisfaction (Cassidy & Shaver, 1999).

Marital disharmony is usually signaled by expressions of anger which, in the EFT model, is seen as a secondary emotion experienced and shown in reaction to some other, more vulnerable, primary emotion (e.g., sadness or fear). When such expressions do not elicit emotional responsiveness in the partner, a downward-spiraling process may be set in motion, from coercion to clinging to depression and despair. EFT views such eventual disengagement as a cumulative traumatic stressor.

Basic Structure of Therapy. There is nothing inherent in EFT to limit its duration, but most EFT lasts about 8 to 15 weekly sessions. Therapy usually begins with one or two joint sessions, followed by an individual session with each spouse to intensify the therapeutic alliance and gather other potentially relevant data on partners' relationship histories, followed by a resumption of joint sessions.

Goal Setting. EFT has two basic aims, exploring each partner's views of self and other, as organized by their immediate (in-session) affective experience, and helping partners to access previously unacknowledged (often to oneself, as well as to one's mate) feelings so that they may be expressed directly in the moment of the therapy session. These aims, of course, are fostered in the context of collaboratively addressing the particular difficulties and goals of each couple.

Techniques and Process of Therapy. The overall corrective emotional experience sought in EFT is achieved through a mixture of Gestalt and client-centered (see Bohart, Chapter 4, this volume) and general "systemic" interventions in which affective immediacy is high. The focus is on the present, and interpretation of unconscious motivation is used sparingly, if at all. Such corrective experiences, occurring through working with a therapist who feels safe to the couple, increases mutual empathy, decreases defensiveness, and leads to an increased, but not explicitly coached, capacity for problem solving. EFT therapists attempt to restructure interpersonal patterns to incorporate each partner's need for secure attachment.

The treatment model in EFT has been clearly described (e.g., Johnson & Denton, 2002; Johnson & Greenberg, 1995), especially in Johnson's (1996) *Emotionally Focused Couple Therapy.* Stage One, "Cycle Deescalation," emphasizing assessment and the deescalation of painful relational cycles, includes four steps: (1) creating a working alliance and delineating core conflict issues and themes, (2) mapping the recurring problematic interactions patterns in which the central problems appear, (3) accessing relevant and previously unacknowledged or insufficiently acknowledged feelings (especially *primary feelings*) behind each partner's behavioral contribution to the problematic cycles, and (4) reframing the meaning of problems in light of the underlying emotions and each partner's attachment needs and fears. Stage Two, "Changing Interactional Patterns," includes three steps: (1) encouraging each partner to "own" previously disowned attachment needs, (2) encouraging acceptance of each partner's emotional

experience, and (3) supporting the direct expression of other specific needs in the relationship. The final Stage Three, "Consideration and Integration," includes two steps: (1) developing new solutions to old problems and (2) reviewing the successes achieved in therapy and helping the couple generalize their experiences.

EFT therapists have identified a number of core interventions to aid the tasks of exploring and reformulating emotional experience, and restructuring marital interactions. Exploration and reformulation are addressed by (1) reflecting emotional experience, which focuses the session and builds alliances; (2) reframing in the context of the central cycles and attachment needs, which connects "undesirable" partner responses to new affect-based meanings and softens the view of one's partner; and (3) restructuring and shaping interactions via enactment and the therapist's choreographing specific new pieces of couple interaction, which increases accessibility and responsiveness.

Therapist's Role and Mechanisms of Change. EFT does not emphasize patients' increased insight, problem-solving skill, or emotional catharsis as the means to therapeutic gains. Rather, the central change mechanism invoked by EFT therapists is each partner's enhanced attunement to aspects of his or her own relationally relevant emotional experience. It is such *self-attunement* that softens anger, increases affective responsiveness, and heightens couple bonding. In these opportunities for self-attunement, the acceptance and validation of each partner by the EFT therapist is essential. The EFT therapist, then, is active and authentic and always on the alert for breaks in the therapeutic alliance, which must serve as the secure base on which new partner–partner interactions rest.

Applicability. The main contraindication to EFT is a situation in which heightened vulnerability would be inappropriate, such as domestic violence. Beyond such situations, EFT is appropriate for couples who intend to remain together. Several predictors of good treatment outcomes in EFT have been identified (Johnson & Denton, 2000), including the quality of the patient–therapist alliance (more predictive of outcome than the couple's overall initial distress level), the couple's commitment to therapy, and their sense that the tasks set forth in therapy appear relevant to them (i.e., they see their difficulties as centrally involving issues of closeness/distance or attachment). EFT requires a high level of therapist skill to evoke and contain unexpressed feelings, and a relatively high level of partner–partner trust. EFT may be especially helpful for inexpressive (usually male) partners, and it seems to be at least as helpful for lower socioeconomic status patients as for others. Moreover, EFT has been used successfully with patients with such varied clinical problems as depression and posttraumatic stress disorder (e.g., from childhood sexual abuse). Enhancing the marital bond may have particular healing value in these situations, as they both inherently involve violations or losses of attachment bonds.

Behavioral Approaches

No approaches to marital therapy have undergone change as rapidly as those falling under the general label of behavior therapy. This is a predictable evolution insofar as behavior therapies are strongly influenced by findings from ongoing research and are usually developed and sustained by theoretical developments in academic settings. Although behavioral models differ in their emphases (Chapman & Dehle, 2002), they derive from a common heritage in general clinical behavior therapy and cognitive-behavioral therapy.

Indeed, all variations of behavioral marital therapy (BMT) express the core philosophy of clinical behaviorism and applied social learning theory (Bandura, 1969; Antony & Roemer, Chapter 6, this volume), for ex-

ample, the central role of environmental events in shaping and maintaining behavior, the importance of operationally defining constructs, and the scientific testing of hypotheses and clinical interventions. Despite these shared attitudes, BMT has evolved through four rather distinct phases (Gurman & Fraenkel, 2002). The first two phases, "Old BMT" (Gurman & Fraenkel, 2002), correspond to what is usually called traditional behavioral couple therapy (Christensen et al., 1995) and include the "simple behavior exchange phase" and the "skills training phase" (Gurman & Fraenkel, 2002). The first phase was marked by Richard Stuart's (1969) classic article on what he called an "Operant–Interpersonal" approach to marital problems. The theoretical basis for understanding couple problems and intervening to help couples derived from social exchange theory (Thibaut & Kelley, 1959), which led Stuart to posit that the success of a marriage depended largely on the frequency and variety of positive behaviors that were reciprocated between partners. Treatment, then, emphasized the partner's specification (*objectification*) of desired positive changes from his or her mate, with tokens and other means of reinforcement of desired behavior change, leading to *behavioral exchanges.*

This simple, direct approach soon evolved into the skills training phase of BMT, ushered in particularly by Neil Jacobson and Gayle Margolin's (1979) groundbreaking treatment manual, *Marital Therapy: Strategies Based on Social Learning and Behavior Exchange Principles,* and Stuart's (1980) *Helping Couples Change: A Social Learning Approach to Marital Therapy.* In this phase, basic laboratory research on the differences between happy and unhappy couples blossomed, and the core intervention approaches of this period derived directly from such studies. Couples in unsatisfying relationships were found to communicate and problem-solve less effectively than unsatisfied couples, to use coercive rather than positive approaches to influence each other, and generally to engage in less positive, and more negative, behavior. The treatment emphasis in this period, then, assumed "skill deficits" among unhappy couples and included systematic training in communication and problem solving, at times following rather discrete learning modules.

Another domain of "deficits" and "excesses" attracting attention in this period was the cognitive, with an emphasis on partners' interpretations and evaluations of their own and each other's behavior (Baucom & Epstein, 1990) based on maladaptive information processing leading to problematic appraisals of relationship events and interactions. Social psychological research on attribution theory and clinical developments in individual cognitive therapy (see Reinecke & Freeman, Chapter 6, this volume) offered the conceptual foundation for these new BMT facets.

The second phase in BMT, "New BMT" (Gurman & Fraenkel, 2002), is most commonly associated with the development of "integrative behavioral couple therapy" (Christensen et al., 1995), set forth in *Integrative Couple Therapy* (Jacobson & Christensen, 1996), but includes other developments as well. The first subphase in this recent period is the "acceptance phase." Having found that the outcomes of traditional BMT were not as strong as they had at first appeared, and that many couples were primarily dealing with inherently unresolvable "perpetual problems" (e.g., personality styles, personal values, and lifestyle preferences) (Gottman, 1999), Jacobson and Andrew Christensen (Jacobson & Christensen, 1996) shifted from a skills training emphasis to an emphasis on mutual acceptance of such irreducible differences (i.e., an affective and cognitive shifts in partners' frames of reference for understanding and empathically tuning into important reasons why their mates behave as they do). The currently emerging subphase in the New BMT is the self-regulation period (Halford 1998; Halford et al., 1994), with a strong "change thyself" emphasis (i.e., an emphasis on changing one's own behavior that contributes to couple problems).

Basic Structure of Therapy

Although BMT is goal focused, it is not inherently a brief treatment. Nevertheless, BMT typically lasts about as long as most marital therapies (i.e., 8–20 sessions). Behavioral marriage therapists do differ from adherents of other approaches, however, by including comprehensive individual assessment sessions with each partner at the beginning phase of therapy, and in providing a thorough, systematic, and structured feedback session with the couple after the initial three or four meetings for the purpose of forming a treatment contract.

Goal Setting

Although BMT inherently emphasizes highly individualized treatment goals via its process of functional analysis, a variety of common goals are considered, with their choice depending on both the conceptual emphasis of the therapist (more or less skill-oriented, more or less cognitively oriented, more or less acceptance-oriented) and characteristics of the couple (severity of conflict, collaborative capacity, level of trust, etc.). Generally, behavioral exchange (BE) goals are worked on early in therapy with more compatible, flexible, and contained couples, as is often true of goals emphasizing the teaching of communication and problem-solving skills. Emotional acceptance strategies usually appear earlier in therapy with more combative, mistrustful, or disengaged couples, though elements of all these styles appear in most phases of BMT.

Functional analysis is key to BMT and is concerned not with the topography, or form, of behavior but with its effects. The goals of functional analysis are to identify behaviors, or patterns of behavior, of clinical concern and the conditions (behavioral, cognitive, affective) that maintain these patterns, to select appropriate interventions, and to monitor the progress of treatment. The function of behavior is understood by identifying the factors that control the behavior. Assessment requires a description of the problem behavior, including its frequency, the conditions under which it is more and less likely, and its consequences. BE and skill training emphases tend to focus more on the content of behavior, whereas acceptance-oriented intervention tends to focus more on the context of behavior. Moreover, in setting treatment goals, skills-oriented and BE-oriented therapists focus more on specific behavioral events, while acceptance-oriented therapists focus more on problematic relationship *themes,* what are more technically called *functional classes* or *response classes,* in which behaviors that have different forms share the same function. For example, husband works longer hours, reads the newspaper during marital conversations, increases his volunteer work, and spends many weekend hours in his garage workshop. The behaviors differ but may serve the same function (e.g., to reduce anxiety associated with closeness).

Common goals in BMT include increasing the overall positivity in the relationship, decreasing the overall negativity, teaching problem solving and communication skills; changing from negative (e.g., coercion, punishment) to positive (e.g., appreciation, acknowledgment) styles of influencing one's partner; modifying dysfunctional attitudes, assumptions, expectations and relationship standards, and attributions about one's partner; modifying emotional reactivity; and enhancing empathic attunement to foster greater mutual acceptance around inevitably unresolveable incompatibilities and differences, often involving dominant personality styles or deeply held personal values.

Techniques and Process of Therapy

BMT sessions initially unfold as they do in most marital therapies, with the couple raising an issue for discussion, one partner's recounting of a recent conflict situation, and so on. Some BMT sessions, or parts of sessions, are structured and closely directed by the therapist, such as when teaching interpersonal skills or new cognitive appraisal strategies, but most session time with most couples is more conversational, with the therapist doing as much following as leading. As noted earlier, BMT typically involves both behavior change interventions and acceptance-enhancing interventions.

"Old BMT" techniques feature BE and *communication and problem solving training* (CPST). BE asks the partners to specify behaviorally (*pinpoint*) what behaviors they would like to see increased in each other. Point-for-point ("tit for tat") exchanges are discouraged, as they imply mistrust and caution. Each partner individually commits to the therapist to make changes based on the partner's list but is not required to make any particular change from that list. The use of BE procedures requires active therapist structuring, guiding, and feedback, as does the use of CPST. Some of the central communication skills taught include, for the speaker or sender, the use of "I" statements rather than blaming "you" statements, measured honesty in the expression of feelings rather than "letting it all hang out," checking to see that the message sent or intended matches the message received, and, for the listener or receiver, paraphrasing and reflecting the speaker's expressions to maintain adequate understanding rather than interrupting or reacting defensively, validating, and empathizing with the speaker rather than discounting or trivializing the speaker's feelings.

Common targets for improved problem solving include discussing one (agreed on) topic at a time and not allowing sidetracking; identifying problems in terms of behavior rather than personality traits or character; avoiding "mind reading;" requesting positive ("more of") behavioral change rather than negative ("less of") behavioral change; emphasizing present- and future-oriented solution possibilities rather than (usually hostilely) rehashing the past; brainstorming a variety of potential behaviorally specific solutions and evaluating the pros and cons for each such possibility; implementing an agreed-on solution; and evaluating the effectiveness of the solution chosen.

Bibliotherapy guides such as Markman, Stanley, and Blumberg's (1994) *Fighting for Your Marriage* are often helpful in teaching both the principles and practices of effective couple communication and problem solving. During CPST, the therapist is actively structuring and guiding, modeling, or role playing facilitated behavior; providing feedback to the partners on their behavior; and explaining the rationale for particular behavioral principles and alternatives. Many behaviorally oriented couple therapists also use cognitive restructuring (CR) techniques, including many derived from cognitive therapy (see Reinecke & Freeman, Chapter 7, this volume) and others modified specifically for use with couples (Baucom, Epstein, & LaTaillade, 2002), for example, challenging automatic thoughts, examining the probabilities of certain outcomes, reconsidering the implicit meaning of behavior, examining the evidential basis for certain conclusions, and reframing the inferred motivation expectations of marriage in general and of one's partner in particular.

"New BMT" interventions reflect the significant modifications in theory and practice proposed by Jacobson and Christensen (1996). Whereas "Old BMT" emphasized rule-governed behavior, the newer *acceptance-oriented* approach emphasizes contingency-shaped behavior. *Rule-governed behavior* occurs in response to explicit verbal rules, with consequences determined by the degree to which behavior matches the rule, not by consequences (contingencies) occurring in the natural environment (e.g., wife watches more sports on television with husband because the therapist says the couple should spend more time together). All BE, CPST, and CR interventions involve rule-governed behavior changes. In significant contrast, *contingency-shaped behavior* is strengthened or weakened as a result of natural (here, marital) consequences. As a result, changes generated in this way (e.g., wife spends more TV sports time with husband because he is friendly and affectionate to her at those times) tend to feel more authentic (vs., "You're only doing this because the therapist said you should."). Change thus generated is likely to generalize outside the treatment context and not be under the stimulus control of the therapist. Moreover, many common marital problems cannot be meaningfully changed by rule-governed methods (e.g., spontaneity, trust, or sexual interest). The most important tactical change in New BMT, then, focuses on acceptance-oriented intervention, and the central technique used is "empathic joining around the problem," which involves the therapist's reformulation (reattribution) of the problem from behavior being seen as "bad," to behavior being seen as understandable in light of the vulnerabilities or other heretofore unexpressed factors that influence the "bad" behavior and allow the motivation (controlling consequences) to be seen in a new light by the partner. Such a shift is often achieved by helping the "offending" partner identify and express "the feeling behind the feeling" (what emotionally focused therapists call primary feelings), or the feelings behind the undesirable behavior. Such *softening* self-disclosures facilitate empathic responses and help to decrease the aversiveness of the behavior at issue and thus allow new responses by the receiving partner.

Other acceptance-oriented techniques include *unified detachment,* in which the couple is encouraged to discuss their problem in a more intellectual, descriptive manner as though the problem is an external "it" and *tolerance building* (i.e., reducing the pain caused by a partner's behavior even though the behavior may not change a great deal). Tolerance may be enhanced by pointing out possible positive (and, heretofore, not recognized) aspects of undesirable behavior (producing a cognitive shift), by practicing the undesirable behavior in the session (desensitization), by faking or pretending undesirable behavior at home (thus bringing it under voluntary control), and by increased self-care (filling more of one's own needs).

Finally, *self-control,* or self-regulation, strategies can be incorporated into BMT and usually focus on altering one's response to the partner's undesired behavior, changing one's approach to trying to gain cooperation from one's partner regarding changes and using stimulus control methods to limit and contain conflict.

Therapist's Role and Mechanisms of Change

In BMT, the therapist assumes a great deal of responsibility for the outcomes of the treatment experience, first based on a thorough and well-conceived functional analysis in the initial assessment phase and later working to ensure that the direction and topical focus of the unfolding therapy process remains thematically consistent, thus calling for an active stance. As in all marital therapies, a supportive, empathic attitude toward the marital partners is essential for developing trust and collaboration. More than in many other marital treatment approaches, however, the therapist in BMT takes on a decidedly instructional, didactic coaching role, especially when using behavioral exchange, cognitive restructuring, and communication/problem-solving methods and less so when emphasizing relational acceptance. Thus, in BMT, the therapist must be flexible enough to adopt different stances with the couple as both the overall focus of the therapy and the exigencies of the moment require.

Applicability

There are few specific contraindications to BMT, the main exceptions being spousal battering, significant substance abuse, and ongoing extramarital affairs. Both "Old BMT," especially emphasizing communication and problem solving, and "New BMT," emphasizing acceptance, have been studied empirically (Gurman & Fraenkel, 2002) and found to be helpful for general marital distress and dissatisfaction, with acceptance-based methods possibly more effective. Moreover, BMT (Old) has been found to be effective in treating depression, anxiety disorders (especially agoraphobia), and alcoholism. Some data suggest that "Old BMT" methods are more likely to be helpful to couples who are younger, egalitarian, and more emotionally engaged than couples who do not fit this description.

Integrative Approaches

Just as eclecticism is the most common theoretical orientation among individual psychotherapists (Bergin & Jensen, 1990), so it is among marital therapists (Rait, 1988). Lebow (1997) has referred to the integrative "revolution" in couple (and family) therapy and has argued that "the move to integration has become so much a part of our work that it largely goes unrecognized" (p. 1). The general value of such approaches involves enhancing the understanding of human behavior and enhancing treatment flexibility. It is generally agreed that there are three main types of psychotherapy integration (Stricker, 1994; Stricker & Gold, Chapter 9, this volume). *Technical eclecticism* calls on interventions from theoretically diverse methods and includes "prescriptive matching," that is, the use of particular techniques with particular symptoms, syndromes or personality (or relationship) types. *Theoretical integration* combines different theories, as well as their associated techniques, typically identifying one theory that dominates the others. The *common-factors approach* emphasizes therapeutic variables and processes that are presumed to be central to the effective conduct of all types of therapy. Fraenkel and Pinsof (2001) have proposed a fourth approach, *theoretical eclecticism,* which uses multiple theoretical perspectives simultaneously or sequentially, without integration, but with specified principles for relating and making decisions about when to use different theories and techniques. The most influential texts setting forth the broad range of marital therapy methods on which such integrations are based are Gurman and Jacobson's (2002; Jacobson & Gurman, 1986, 1995) *Clinical Handbook of Couple Therapy;* Paolino and McCrady's (1978) *Marriage and Marital Therapy: Psychoanalytic, Behavioral and Systems Theory Perspectives;* and Sholevar's (1981) *The Handbook of Marriage and Marital Therapy.*

Marital therapy integrations have brought together structural and strategic approaches (e.g., Keim & Lappin, 2002; Stanton, 1981; Todd, 1986) and behavior therapy and systemic approaches (e.g., Birchler & Spinks, 1980; Weiss, 1980), but the most common combination by far has been behavioral and psychodynamic (e.g., Berman, Lief, & Williams, 1981; Feldman, 1979; Gilbert & Shmulker, 1996; Gurman, 1981, 1992, 2002; Nichols, 1988; Segraves, 1982; Snyder & Schneider, 2002). In marital therapy, the great majority of systematic integrations have been of the theoretically integrative type, most often with object relations theory or some other psychodynamic theory serving as the conceptual core for understanding marital dynamics, and behavioral techniques being heavily relied on because of the paucity of techniques that are specific to psychodynamic marital therapy (Gurman, 1978). This retention of a core, or "home," theory and the concurrent incorporation of techniques originating outside the home theory typify what is called "assimilative integration" (Messer, 1992, 2001).

In marital therapy, two major integrative patterns have emerged. The first involves the combining of conjoint therapy with other treatment formats and modalities, such as individual therapy, and the second involves the combining, at theoretical or technical levels, of existing models of couple treatment. In the first category, two efforts stand out. Larry Feldman's (1985, 1992) "integrative marital therapy" attends to the behavioral, psychodynamic, systemic, and biological aspects of marital relationships. Feldman's approach emphasizes the judicious use of both individual and conjoint sessions, with sequences and balances between the two determined on a case-by-case basis. William Pinsof's (1995) "integrative problem-centered therapy" combines intervention from disparate therapies by moving from model to model according to a clearly delineated treatment planning decision tree (e.g., from present-focused approaches such as structural and cognitive-behavioral to historically focused approaches such as object relations and Bowenian).

Three integrative marital models stand out among the theoretically integrative approaches in balancing their attention to both psychodynamic and social learning perspectives. The marital interaction model of Ellen Berman and colleagues (1981), which evolved into the "Intersystem model" developed by Gerald Weeks (Weeks, 1989; Weeks & Treat, 2001) of the PENN Council for Relationships (formerly the Marriage Council of Philadelphia), brought together into a coherent framework Sager's (1976) blend of marital contract theory and object relations theory, multigenerational family systems theory, adult developmental theory, systems theory, and social learning theory. The Intersystem model addresses the interlocking individual, interactional, and intergenerational systems, and draws on a wide array of techniques.

Douglas Snyder's (1999) "affective reconstruction approach," or IOMT (Snyder & Wills, 1989), reflects one of the most sophisticated integrative marital models to date. Largely disseminated thus far through a series of studies demonstrating its long-term (4-year follow-up) effectiveness, IOMT emphasizes relational dispositions of individuals and their associated core individual intimate relational themes over time, including family of origin. IOMT promotes awareness of the common contradictions and incongruencies within people about their relational needs and expectations and attends to partners' behavior, feelings, and cognitions in both present and historical terms. IOMT provides an overarching framework for organizing therapeutic interventions and sequencing their use, and it draws on psychodynamic (mostly object relations), experiential, and cognitive and behavioral techniques. Insight, affective immediacy, and modification of partners' problematic attributions about each other, as well as indirect skill enhancement, are all valued in IOMT. The main phase of IOMT is called "affective reconstruction" and emphasizes the therapist's interpretations of dysfunctional relationship patterns in terms of their developmental origins and the connections of those earlier experiences to current fears, dilemmas, and interaction styles.

Brief Integrative Marital Therapy: An Integrative Illustration

Brief integrative marital therapy (BIMT), developed by Alan Gurman over the last two decades (Gurman, 1981, 1992, 2002), is a therapeutic approach to the treatment of the relationship difficulties of married or otherwise committed couples that attends simultaneously and systematically to both interpersonal and intrapersonal factors. BIMT's implicit values, intervention focus, and usual techniques tend to render it a relatively brief experience. BIMT rests on a foundation of general systems theory and adult developmental theory, including attachment theory, but is most pervasively influenced by applied social learning theory and object relations theory.

BIMT emphasizes the repetitive cycles of interaction between partners and how these cycles reciprocally include both intrapsychic process (conscious and unconscious) and overt behavior (i.e., how the deep structures and the surface structures of intimate relationships operate together). In BIMT, object relations theory provides the

way for mapping deep structures, as discussed earlier in the section on object relations marital therapy. Conflict is seen as arising when the implicit "rules" (unspoken agreements) of the relationship that are central to either partner's sense of self or core schema for close relationships are violated. BIMT emphasizes what Gurman (2002) calls "implicit behavior modification" (i.e., partners' unwitting reinforcement of undesired behavior in their mates and punishment of behavior that they consciously wish for). These reinforcing and punishing contingencies occur in circular relationship and can be triggered internally, between the spouses, or by external events.

The core assumption in BIMT is that couple therapy can lead to change in both interaction patterns and inner representational models of intimate relationships, and that such unconscious experiencing can be changed via direct, as well as indirect, therapeutic methods. In addition to its object relations base, BIMT relies heavily on the main attribute of clinical behavior therapy approaches, functional analysis, for a more fine-grained assessment of couple problems. Functional analysis is concerned not with the form of behavior but with its effects, that is, with the factors that maintain a problematic pattern, whether these factors be interactional, cognitive, affective, or biological. Functional analysis does not assume a priori that any particular class of events has more influence over a couple's difficulties than any other. In BIMT, behavior is behavior (is behavior), and "behavior" is construed broadly to include unconscious experience. Although the content of therapy sessions varies over time in BIMT, treatment is usually organized around a small number of dominant themes, what behavior therapists call response classes, in which the form of behavior is secondary to its relationship- and self-function, purpose, or effect.

Basic Structure of Therapy. BIMT strongly emphasizes the healing power of the couple's own relationship above and beyond the patient–therapist relationship; therefore, in BIMT, individual sessions are almost never held, except when the affective volatility of joint sessions cannot be kept within a manageable range by the couple and/or the therapist. Sessions are typically held biweekly, to allow adequate time between meetings for the couple's experimentation with new ways of relating, and most BIMT lasts 8–20 sessions. The therapist almost always begins sessions by asking, "What would you (two) like to focus on today?" The content and direction of the session is chosen by the couple, but the therapist is responsible for guiding the couple in ways that stay on the therapy's central thematic track.

Goal Setting. Given BIMT's strong functional analytic emphasis and its valuing of therapeutic brevity, the goals sought in any particular course of therapy are highly variable. Still, there are certain overriding goals across couples (i.e., more accurate self-perception, more accurate perception of one's partner, and resolution of presenting problems and of problems that emerge after the initial assessment).

Techniques and Process of Therapy

BIMT's central premise, that people's inner (including unconscious) models or schemata for close relationships can be changed by relevant changes in overt behavior and conscious thought, requires that a careful functional analysis of marital difficulties include behavioral specification of projective processes. These processes can be identified by some predictable patterns—for example, when partners fail to see aspects of each other's behavior (including positive changes) that are perceptible to a third person; when partners reinforce in each other the very behavior they complain about; when partners fail to see their own contributions to the couple problems; or when partners exaggerate differences and minimize similarities (Gurman, 2002).

To counter these collusive processes,

BIMT emphasizes inculcating systemic awareness in the couple, teaching/evoking relationship skills, and challenging dysfunctional relationship rules by actively interrupting and modifying collusive processes in session, linking individual and interactional experience, and creating therapeutic tasks. Interruption and modification of collusive processes are accomplished, for example, by *blocking interventions,* aimed at interrupting or diverting couple enactments of habitual unconscious shared avoidance agreements. Such process-oriented interventions include cognitive restructuring, self-control coaching, and "anti-collusive questioning." For example, "How do you protect each other from even worse pain?"; "Even though you often complain about 'X' in your mate, do you find that you sometimes do 'X' yourself?"; "What stops you from accepting what your mate is giving you, since it seems to be what you're asking for?"; or "What do you do to get your mate to behave in ways that, ironically, bother *you* so much?" Therapeutic tasks in BIMT involve *instigative interventions* that are goal directed and strategic, in the sense of trying to effect a particular change, in contrast to the more exploratory, process-oriented interventions described earlier. Tasks can occur both in session and out of session.

Therapist's Role and Mechanisms of Change. In BIMT, the therapist's overriding role is to facilitate the partners' experiencing of themselves and each other as whole persons, and to do so in a safe, yet challenging, environment that works against their repetitive joint avoidances, thus leading to more genuine encounters and improved communication and problem solving. The therapist closely tracks the alliances with each partner, and between himself and the couple as a couple, but focuses on the partner–partner alliance because that is viewed as the central healing relationship in BIMT. To these ends, a wide range (Gurman, 2002) of affect-eliciting, interpretive, and direct behavior change methods is used. Indeed, the familiar idea in behavior therapy of exposure to fearful stimuli is a principle that guides the therapist's choices about where, when, and how to intervene in the couple's dysfunctional process. In addition to traditional uncovering and interpretive activities, BIMT uses active methods to achieve psychodynamic goals (i.e., "surface" interventions for changing deep structures), both individual and dyadic.

Applicability. The principles and core technique options of BIMT appear to be applicable to both psychologically minded and more pragmatically oriented couples. Although interpretive activity by the therapist certainly can deepen the treatment experience, it is the therapist's understanding and tracking of the interactions between conscious and unconscious experience, and between observed and inferred relationship events, that allows for direct, practical interventions to serve object relational aims. Because BIMT does not *a priori* pay more attention to some aspects of experience over others but favors a functional analytic attitude, the possibilities for helpful intervention at multiple levels of experience, using a broad array of methods, are enhanced.

Postmodern Approaches

Most approaches to psychotherapy are based on an implicit world view and scientific philosophy inherent in *modernism,* a belief that there exists a knowable, observable, measurable, objective reality independent of how anyone perceives it, and that there are discernible laws of how that reality operates that can be discovered through scientific investigation. *Postmodernism,* which has influenced, *inter alia,* the arts, linguistics, ethology and political theory, as well as marital and family therapy, questions the possibility of knowing absolute "truth" and discovering of universal laws or principles to explain human behavior. In this way, unquestioned givens in knowledge systems are "*decon-structed*" (i.e., their assumptions are extracted and identified).

Within this postmodern cultural movement has emerged the perspective of *social constructionism,* with its central tenet that reality does not exist "out there" but rather is socially constructed (this is different from another postmodern perspective, *constructionism,* which emphasizes how people actively construct meaning and reality). Given the relativistic, contextualistic view that there is no one "truth," only multiple realities, it follows that in the therapy context, participants, including therapists, cannot be "experts" on reality but merely collaborative co-inquirers, co-investigators, or co-constructors. The antireductionistic bias in social constructivism also leads to an emphasis on unique patient experience and meanings rather than research-based descriptions of problems, "types" of relationships, and the like. Recently, postmodern, social constructivistic views have had wide-ranging impact on all areas of psychotherapy (see Neimeyer & Bridges, Chapter 8, this volume), including family and marital therapy. The most influential and visible postmodern marital therapy approaches to date have been solution-focused marital therapy, narrative couple therapy, and collaborative couple therapy.

Solution-Focused Marital Therapy

Of the three most influential postmodern approaches to marital therapy, solution-focused (also called solution-oriented) marital therapy (SFMT) has the most direct connections with more traditional methods of marital and family therapy. Indeed, the work of SFMT's creator, Steve de Shazer (1985, 1988), trained at the MRI, and that of his colleagues (e.g., Berg, 1994; Weiner-Davis, 1992) at the Brief Family Therapy Center in Milwaukee, Wisconsin, reflects many central MRI beliefs and values. Like the MRI approach discussed earlier, SFMT shows little interest in a couple's joint history or in the histories of its partners; is nonpathologizing in that it believes there is no absolute reality and, thus, ideas of "normality" are irrelevant; is more interested in how problems continue than in how they arose; deals only with the complaints patients bring to therapy, and does not investigate "underlying issues"; believes that problems are usually maintained by constraining definitions; and is pragmatic and time sensitive. In contrast to the MRI model, SFMT emphasizes solutions more than (some would say, almost to the exclusion of) problems, places more emphasis on cognitive than behavioral change, and emphasizes patients' resources as more central to good outcomes than therapists' attributes. Shoham, Rohrbaugh, and Patterson (1995) provide an excellent comparative analysis of the MRI and SFMT approaches.

For the postmodern solution-focused marital therapist, the notion that reality is constructed rather than discovered leads to a profound shift of emphasis from that of the MRI (and most other therapies, as well). Because problems are believed only to "exist in language," the therapist almost unswervingly emphasizes *solution talk* rather than *problem talk* (which, of course, includes talk about the history of the problem).

Basic Structure of Therapy. Solution-focused therapists, like MRI therapists, work with the most motivated persons (*customers*), not necessarily with *complainants* (who complain but appear unmotivated to change), although a good deal of their couple-oriented work occurs conjointly. Unlike the MRI approach, SFMT sets no fixed therapy limit, although it tends to be extremely brief, reported to be in the range of five to seven sessions on average, and the therapist and couple negotiate whether to meet again at the end of each session.

Goal Setting. The goals of SFMT are to resolve the presenting problem(s) by shifting how these problems are "languaged." Therapy aims, as Hoyt (2002) puts it, for "solution sight" rather than insight. Process goals em-

phasize eliciting patient competencies and resources, which solution-focused marital therapists believe people have within themselves and, thus, do not need coaching, therapist interpretations, or skill training.

Techniques and Process of Therapy. Although solution-focused therapy has developed a more recent interest in the therapeutic relationship as a core component of clinical change (Miller, Duncan, & Hubble, 1997), it is still largely identified with its *formula tasks* (i.e., therapist interventions that are used with everyone). In the *formula first session task* (called the *skeleton key question* because it fits all "locks"), presented at the end of the first session, the therapist asks the couple to observe, between sessions, what about their relationship they would like to continue, despite their current problems (thus, shifting attention to the positive, as well as the negative). With the *miracle question,* the therapist asks, "If a miracle happened, and your problem disappeared, how would you know? What would be different? What else would be different?" (This question defines the problem clearly, demonstrates how the problem currently gets in the way of the couple behaving in ways they would prefer to, and implies a hopeful future.) With *exceptions questions,* the therapist asks the couple to identify times at which the problem is usually not present, what happens differently at those times, and/or what the couple has done differently when the problem arises but is handled better than it usually is. (This implies that the couple already knows, but is insufficiently using, its own solutions, and that they have the capacity to make the problem not happen.)

Scaling questions are designed to emphasize solution finding and building and to motivate patients toward change. (For example, "On a scale from 1 to 10, 1 being no [hope, relationship commitment, treatment motivation, judgment of therapeutic progress, or any other issue of interest], and 10 being complete [hope, etc.], how would you rate yourself today?"). *Coping* (or endurance) *questions* focus on patient strengths and encourage hopefulness by asking, for example, "Despite these marital problems, how do you still hang in there? How do you keep things from getting even worse than they have been?" And *agency* (or *efficacy*) questions highlight patients' ability to make change happen by asking, for example, "How did you do that/make that happen/decide to do that?" Different types of solution-talk questions are more appropriate to different stages of therapy, but as a group, they are intended to clearly identify problems, the conditions under which they occur, and the probable consequences of their elimination; broaden the couple's view of the totality of their relationship, beyond just the problem; reinforce the couple's awareness of their own problem resolution capacities; and support the couple's hopefulness about the possibility of change.

Therapist's Role and Mechanisms of Change. SFMT disavows interest in such notions as "mechanisms of change," which assume an objectivist, modernist, "normal science" perspective. Ideas about "curative factors" suggest association with "the medical model," and are thus shunned. The solution-focused approach emphasizes collaborative, conversational meaning making and insists that changes in perceptions lead to changes in behavior, and that all such changes occur primarily, if not exclusively, through language. Solution-focused therapists also believe that it is not necessary to know why or how something works in therapy in order for it to be effective. The therapist's central role in this process is to facilitate conversations that take into account patients' motivations, goals, values, and so on, in order to find ways of maximizing patients' cooperation with change.

Applicability. Solution-focused marital therapists see no recurring applicability limits for their approach beyond those common to almost all methods of couple treatment (e.g., violence and major psychiatric impairment).

Narrative Couple Therapy

The therapeutic approach in the postmodern domain that has attracted the most attention in the past decade is narrative couple therapy (NCT), based on the seminal work of Michael White (White & Epston, 1990). The major contributors to NCT have been Jill Freedman and Gene Combs (1996, 2000, 2002) and Jeffrey Zimmerman and Victoria Dickerson (1996; Neal, Zimmerman, & Dickerson, 1999).

The narrative couple therapist, questioning all established diagnostic or descriptive systems, asserts that problems exist in cultural discourses and are seen as the effects of constraining discourses about self and relationships, not as their sources. The personal and shared *narratives* or *stories* about ourselves and the world that we experience do not merely influence our lives (e.g., by determining our behavior and perceptions) but *are* our lives. The types of culturally constructed narratives that are particularly relevant to marital therapy involve gender and socially constructed power. Indeed, these dimensions of relational experience are seen by NCT as important in almost all couple therapy situations, regardless of the content of couples' presenting problems. As Neal and colleagues (1999) have said, "it is useful to assume that gender (is) involved in one way or another" (p. 398), even if "the couple does not experience the operation of power that supports problems as linked to gender" (p. 399). Thus, NCT is a decidedly and intentionally political (or politicizing) experience, designed to liberate relationship partners from the restrictive, limiting, and oppressive assumptions of the larger culture, especially those involving notions of maleness and femaleness. This thematic emphasis can be, and often is, extended to matters of race, social class, and other domains of dominant cultural values and institutions. NCT typically becomes "a therapy of social justice" (Nichols & Schwartz, 1998, p. 418).

Basic Structure of Therapy. NCT does not adhere to principles of systems theory and, in fact, is individually focused. Because NCT seeks to help people change their most salient self- and world views, conjoint therapy is not required, and partners are seen alone if conditions warrant. In the conjoint format, the basic structure is that one partner explores his or her stories (*telling*) while the other listens (*witnessing*) and then comments on what has been said. These roles then switch. All the while, the therapist is active in helping partners elucidate, elaborate, and modify their stories.

Goal Setting. Goals, as usually thought of in psychotherapy, are not in the lexicon of NCT. Rather than narrowing the therapeutic focus, narrative therapists attempt to broaden it. Thus, "goals" are referred to as *projects* or *directions in life.* This is no mere hairsplitting, for in NCT the aim is to transform partners' individual and relational identities, not to "solve problems." NCT seeks to "separate the problem from the person" by constructing new individual and shared stories. It is a political endeavor, aimed at freeing people from oppressive cultural assumptions and empowering them to live out their *preferred stories.* NCT projects can last a few sessions or a few years.

Techniques and Process of Therapy. To convey to couples at the outset of therapy that the Narrative therapist is not to be seen as an "expert," the therapist *situates* him- or herself as a person in the collaboration in the first session, by inviting the couple to ask questions about the therapist to minimize power differentials. For the same reason, the therapist also requires his or her own *transparency,* often by sharing the reasoning behind his or her questions over the course of therapy.

NCT has come to be identified with a number of distinctive therapeutic techniques (or *practices*) that are quite out of the ordinary in the world of mainstream psychotherapy and couple therapy. The central therapeutic change strategy involves *externalizing conversations,* in which the aim is to linguistically separate the person from the problem, in part by tracing the sources of the values that unproductively support and reinforce the patient's *problem-saturated* or *problem-laden* stories. For example, while being helped to trace the origins of a maritally problematic view of women, a husband may be encouraged to think of the problematic view as an "it" that acts upon him but *is* not him. The therapist may attribute intentionality to the problem, again relating to the problem as a reified "it." He or she poses *effects questions* (e.g., "What effect does this problem have on your relationship?"), designed to lead the partners to perceive negative experiences of themselves and each other and their relationship as the effects, or results, of the problem, not as its cause. The therapist may also *construct problems* by giving them names (e.g., "'Distance' keeps getting in your way"). The essential NCT maxim is that the person is not the problem, but the problem is the problem, so that the couple has a "relationship" with "it" and may work to join together to oppose "it" having so much control in their lives.

The *reauthoring* of new stories with previously *subjugated narratives* (more productive alternative stories) includes a good deal of attention to *unique outcomes* (i.e., times at which the couple does not yield to the problem or behaves in ways that would not be predicted in light of their dominant problem-saturated story). Therapist questions about unique outcomes include *landscape of action questions* (about sequences of behavior involved in the unique outcome) and *landscape of consciousness questions* (about the meanings, beliefs, values, and intentions of a person that are implied by the unique outcome). *Thickening new plots* as an element of the reauthoring process involves connecting unique outcomes to the past and to an extended future story in which the partner (or relationship) is seen as more potent than the problem. As the couple's thickened stories are further established, the therapist will urge the *documentation and circulation of new stories* that involve varied methods designed to reinforce therapeutic gains and generalize them outside the therapist's office (e.g., presenting the couple a certificate to acknowledge a particular change; creating videotapes for their own use, in which they talk about how the progress they have made; writing letters to the couple designed to thicken recently discussed unique outcomes by asking them new questions; and encouraging the couple to share these documents with important people in their lives).

Therapist's Role and Mechanisms of Change. In NCT, the therapists participate not as professional experts with special knowledge but as people with the ability to foster collaborative "projects," to a significant extent, by asking questions that thicken new, adaptive alternative stories about oneself and one's relationship. In the NCT view, significant change occurs via the *performance of meaning* (i.e., the repeated enactment, especially in everyday life, of reworked new stories).

Applicability. NCT sees traditional individual or couple diagnosis as irrelevant to its work. NCT rejects the "scientistic criteria" (Freedman & Combs, 2002, p. 322) by which most therapists evaluate their work. Narrative therapists conclude for whom their approach is "applicable" not by their own criteria but by asking their couples in an ongoing way if their work together is being helpful.

Collaborative Couple Therapy

The last of our postmodern therapeutic models for working with couples is collaborative couple therapy (CCT), an approach developed over the last two decades by Daniel Wile (Wile, 1981, 1995, 2002). CCT is discernibly postmodern in its emphasis on a nonhierarchical, nonpathologizing therapist–patient relationship and a nonnormative view of individual and relational health. Quite unlike some constructivistic and other language-oriented approaches, however, CCT actively searches for the real (vs. arbitrary), accurate, and knowable experience-of-relationship and experience-of-self in distressed marital partners.

CCT is based on an integration and extension of Anderson's (1997) "collaborative" therapy and Apfelbaum's (Apfelbaum & Gill, 1989) ego-analytic approach, which emphasizes the superego over the id of traditional psychoanalysis. The central concept of the ego-analytic approach used to explain dysfunction, including relational dysfunction, is *unentitlement,* a state wherein people, because of shame or self-blame, do not feel free to express what they think and feel at a given moment, a state in which they lack adequate *self-compassion.* In close relationships, unentitlement leads to self-reinforcing, dominant (though shifting) problematic patterns, or states called *adversarial cycles,* in which partners lose the ability to appreciate each other's point of view, and/or to *withdrawn cycles,* in which partners lose the ability to engage at all. The antidote to these cycles or states is the *collaborative cycle* (or *empathic cycle*), in which the partners come to see their own and each other's (undesired) behavior as nonpathological, understandable responses to the (formerly) hidden and unexpressed realities of the relationship. In the CCT view, intimacy, the result of dominant collaborative cycles, evolves when both partners let each other in on who they are at the moment, mostly by *confiding* (rather than fixing, blaming or avoiding) their *leading-edge thoughts and feelings.* CCT asserts that mutual confiding is inherently collaboration inducing.

Basic Structure of Therapy. CCT does not preselect couples for inclusion, believing that one can only know if this approach fits a couple by trying it. There is no predetermined end point in CCT, and partners need not even have the same goal (e.g., staying together). Therapy is always conducted by a single therapist.

Goal Setting. Given CCT's view of what becomes problematic in relationships, it follows that each partner's *loss of voice* is the central treatment target to be addressed. The therapist's overriding aim is to help create compassionate couple conversations, wherein the goal is not to "solve the problem" but to *solve the moment,* that is, to help the partners recruit each other as resources to solve the overt problem (i.e., to turn moments of withdrawal or attack into moments of intimacy).

Techniques and Process of Therapy. The "single therapeutic task," as Wile (1999, p. 222) refers to it, is to help both partners develop, elaborate, and express their perspectives ("voices"). This singular task, according to Wile, simultaneously creates a therapist–patient alliance, addresses potential resistance, and exposes central fears. "Solving the moment" is repeatedly accomplished in CCT by establishing a *joint platform* (i.e., when a safe, meta-level conversation predominates regardless of the content of what the couple brings to each therapy session). This recurrent process goal, known as *reassembling the relationship on the next higher level,* involves *recovery conversations,* in which the therapist helps the couple create an empathic cycle by talking via *meta-conversation* about the adversarial or withdrawn cycle from which they have just emerged, and by helping the partners show appreciation of how the other partner's reactions really made sense (given what the other had been experiencing internally, but not voicing). In effect, in CCT, marital fights become the jumping-off point for intimate conversations.

The primary way in which the therapist facilitates such collaborative conversation is by becoming a *therapeutic advocate,* a bilateral spokesman for each of the partners by speculating aloud about what each may be thinking and feeling but not stating, including thoughts and feelings of which the partner him- or herself may not be aware (*discovering the heartfelt feeling*). The manner in which this is done very much resembles the well-known psychodrama technique of "doubling," or serving as an alter ego. This role is characteristically attended to by the therapist's repeatedly asking himself questions such as, "What is this person really experiencing right now? What is this person's unexpressed inner struggle?"

Therapist's Role and Mechanisms of Change. The therapist's role in CCT is to serve as the simultaneous expressive advocate of each marital partner. To do this effectively, the therapist must be in a collaborative/empathic mode toward each partner, thus requiring the therapist to take himself out of his own inevitable adversarial mode (e.g., feeling critical of a partner) and withdrawn mode (e.g., feeling disinterested), thus being unable to appreciate each partner's internal struggle and failing to see their maladaptive modes of relating for the unfortunate *fallback measures* they are. Change occurs as the couple more regularly can establish their own joint platform from which they can safely meta-communicate and show their inner struggles to each other rather than acting them out.

Applicability. CCT is relevant to those couples that experiment with the approach and find that it suits them. Perhaps the major contraindication to CCT involves the therapist. The back-and-forth emotional alter-ego role of the therapist requires not only superior "holding" capacity (as object relations theory would call it) on the therapist's part but also comfort with repeated intensifications of what is being left unsaid by the couple, and a high level of activity and initiative taking. Although CCT can generate affectively powerful and healing couple exchanges, it is not an approach for which all therapists are constitutionally well suited. (Interestingly, D. B. Wile, 2001, personal communication, has acknowledged that he himself uses his doubling, advocacy-oriented interventions for only about half of the time in most couple therapy sessions.)

RESEARCH SUPPORT

From the earliest to the most recent examinations of the pertinent empirical literature, marital therapy research has consistently demonstrated the efficacy of conjoint treatment (Baucom, Shoham, Meuser, Daiuto, & Stickle, 1998; Bray & Jouriles, 1995; Christensen & Heavey, 1999; Gurman, 1973; Gurman et al., 1986; Lebow & Gurman, 1995). Overall, marital therapy is associated with positive outcomes in about two-thirds of treated couples. This overall improvement rate, and the related effect sizes (the majority showing large values of .80 or greater) found for marital therapy, essentially match those found in the research literature on individual psychotherapy (Gurman & Fraenkel, 2002): In general, a randomly selected treated couple is better off at the end of therapy than about 70% of untreated couples. Moreover, every controlled, randomized clinical trial of marital therapy investigated to date has found treatment to be superior to no treatment. These studies of the efficacy of marital therapy have shown treatment effects that exceed those of individual therapy for marital problems, and almost always in brief therapies of 12–20 sessions.

Among the numerous approaches to marital therapy (Gurman & Jacobson, 2002), including but not limited to those discussed in this chapter, those with the largest accumulated research base to date are BMT (including cognitive-behavioral) and EFT. IOMT has also shown strong treatment effects that endure at long-term (4-year) follow-up. None of the more influential integrative models of marital therapy

discussed earlier have been studied empirically, but all of them draw on treatment components and principles present in models of therapy (e.g., BMT, EFT, and IOMT) that have received substantial research support. The results of research on the outcomes of marital therapies with a structural–strategic emphasis (Leff et al., 2000) and an MRI-style intervention (Goldman & Greenberg, 1992), though few in number to date, are quite supportive of the efficacy of these approaches. SFMT has not yet been formally tested in controlled studies. Some of the field's oldest treatment approaches (BFST) and newest approaches (NCT, CCT) also have not yet been investigated.

Finally, it should be noted that marital therapy has also been shown to play a significant remedial and preventive role in the treatment of depression, alcohol abuse, and anxiety disorders (Gurman & Fraenkel, 2002), disorders which have traditionally been thought to be treated appropriately only by individual psychotherapy.

CASE ILLUSTRATION

Paul and Kathy were the 48-year-old parents of three children, a 12-year-old daughter and 17-year-old twin sons. They had been referred to me as part of the discharge planning for Paul, who had been psychiatrically hospitalized for almost a week, following his intensifying depression, deteriorating general life functioning, and increased use of antianxiety medication. Paul generally functioned well, especially in his work as a "human resources" worker in a local corporation. He had had brief previous psychiatric hospitalizations, once in his mid-20s after graduating from college, feeling "aimless." The other time was almost 16 years before our meeting, when his twin sons were still infants and Kathy was "preoccupied with the boys," anxiously attentive to their "every move," and equally inattentive to her marriage. Over the preceding several months, Paul had become easily fatigued, despite still being quite athletic and still exercising regularly, generally pessimistic, irritable, and, as Kathy put it sarcastically, "clingy like a little baby." Kathy mostly saw Paul's depression as the result of his "personal inadequacies," especially not being as self-sufficient as she wished he would be and had thought he was during their courtship. During Paul's hospitalization, in discussion with hospital nursing staff, he revealed that although he had not overtly disagreed with Kathy's theory about the cause of his depression, in truth, he saw his depression as the result of a long-term pattern of distancing in his marriage. He told a nurse, "I don't dare to bring that up. Kathy's got so much to do, especially lately." It was in this context that the hospital staff referred Paul and Kathy to me.

Paul's symptoms had recurred as Kathy had become increasingly less involved in his life. The eldest of four children, Kathy had a long history of self-sacrifice, originating in her family of origin, in which she had been the proverbial "parentified child" of an alcoholic father and a passive and depression-prone mother. Although her father's alcohol problem had decreased over the previous decade, the marriage between Kathy's parents had never progressed much beyond a "pseudo-civil, and polite, but disconnected, relationship." Her parents had retired to a warmer climate 2 years earlier. Kathy's mother had hoped that she and her husband could "start over," but she had become increasingly depressed the last few months as her marital conflicts became more frequent, now that she and her husband spent much more time together. Kathy, in her familiar, but ambivalent role, had become extremely involved in her parents' difficulties, especially as her mother's confidante, and less involved in her own family's daily life. She had even flown to her parents' southern home twice to spend weekends with them, in an effort to intercede by "getting them talking to each other again." Although angry at her parents for "not being mature enough to run their own lives," Kathy almost never expressed such feelings to them, rationalizing that they had "been through enough pain already."

In addition to feeling that he had "basically lost my wife to her family," Paul, an interpersonally avoidant man (but, interestingly, not in his "human resources" job, where he believed in his competence), felt more and more isolated from meaningful relationships now that his twin sons were fully engaged in the adolescent world and were about to be off to college in a few months.

Paul was dependent on and angry at Kathy but feared voicing his concerns about their parallel lives. This dilemma was reminiscent of Paul's relationship to his father, who had essentially abandoned his family when Paul was 3 years old. His mother, a caring woman, had had to work numerous part-time, unskilled jobs to take care of her three children, of whom Paul was the youngest by 8 years. The family "story" was that Paul's father had left his family after Paul, whose birth was unplanned, put an additional level of responsibility on his father that he was unwilling to carry. In effect, Paul had always felt that it was *his own fault* that he had no real father, and, as a result, that he had caused his mother so much suffering, by virtue of his very existence. He had learned early and profoundly not to expect much in close relationships. Kathy had learned a similar lesson, albeit by a different route.

Indeed, this similarity formed an important part of the couple's initial attraction to each other, which Paul referred to as "the importance of looking out for the people you care about as much as yourself." While on the same wavelength in this way, Paul and Kathy also, and unfortunately, shared another core "value," but one that was not so adaptive. That is, conflict, at least overt conflict, was "not on either of our radar screens," as Kathy put it, as if to say that each of them was constantly watchful lest conflict might brew. Insecure in their early family attachments, both of them almost never dared to "rock the boat." There was virtually no overt conflict and little complaining. Even requests were initiated with caution. Each of them was expected to read the other's mind about what they needed in the relationship.

The central initial goal of therapy was to improve Paul's depression. To this end, the couple agreed that they would have to get "reinvolved," as Paul said, in order to have opportunities to build a more secure mutual attachment. But to do this, I told them, Kathy, who I said was overly burdened with taking care of others, had to take a big risk by extricating herself from her therapist-like role with her parents. I told her that I did not think we could move ahead therapeutically on their couple issues until this happened. I acknowledged her sense of absolute dread and guilt at the idea of letting her parents "fend for themselves." Both to relieve some of this guilt and to facilitate the couple's genuinely engaging in their therapy, I provided Kathy the names and phone numbers of family therapists in her parents' area. Moreover, to help counter Paul's sense of depressive inadequacy and enervation, I told him he needed to "use all the people skills you can muster from your HR (human resources) job to help Kathy get better at setting limits when her mother phoned her" in marital desperation. These structurally oriented out-of-session tasks gradually helped to dislodge Kathy from her ambivalent role with her parents.

Meeting on a weekly basis for the first 2 months, then meeting biweekly for a total of 17 sessions, we began to explore the blocks to couple closeness that had evolved over the years, quite apart from Kathy's dealings with her parents. Some of our work included coaching both Paul and Kathy with standard cognitive therapy methods about their maladaptive conscious and implicit beliefs about self-sufficiency, denial of their own needs, the dangers of conflict, and so on. But before such interventions had a chance of taking hold with them, more painful issues had to be addressed. Primary among these was the fear associated with closeness for each of them and, relatedly, the ways in which each

of them unconsciously reinforced the very kinds of behavior in each other that they found undesirable. For example, although Kathy would often criticize Paul's "clinginess," when he would occasionally venture out to initiate some independent social relationships, she would complain about his being too separate from her. This reaction would stimulate closeness seeking by Paul, which would usually meet with a cold reception, and so on. Similarly, when Paul would see Kathy in some distress (e.g., about her parents) and offer her support and make other efforts to be helpful, Kathy would often criticize him for "trying too hard to fix everything." On the other side of the equation, when Kathy would try to be helpful to Paul about a problem (e.g., work) in an indirect effort to get close to him, he would criticize her for "always trying to take over and run everybody's life." In these and other ways, the couple's unconsciously agreed on and carefully maintained dance of distance–regulation, in which each implicitly understood the other's anxiety about issues of closeness, abandonment, and so on, kept them at a level of contact that was unsatisfying but also not too anxiety arousing. Deviations from this overall pattern, as illustrated earlier, would raise anxiety, alternately, about being both too close and too far away, leading to behavior in the partner to counteract such states of affairs, thus "righting" the marital system to longer periods of civility, conflict avoidance, and relational deadness. In all this, of course, each of them saw little that they contributed to this unconsciously motivated pattern of distance regulation, kept in close control by predictable patterns of observable behavior.

Each of Paul's and Kathy's central fears of closeness (e.g., for Paul, closeness signals neglect and abandonment, harming others by putting burdens on them; for Kathy, closeness signals being too responsible for the other and leads to a loss of a sense of self) were explicitly identified ("exposed," to make a bad, but relevant, behavior therapy pun). My central role in this was to em-

pathize with each of them about their closeness fears, thus modeling empathy toward
each other for expressing such fears, thereby
blocking predictable "punishment" of each
other (e.g., criticism and withdrawal) for
such anxiety-arousing self-revelation in the
mate, and strengthening each partner's
"holding" capacity. In such nonblaming ways
as this, each partner was helped experientially to recognize his or her unwitting contribution to the couple's central difficulties and
the unconscious functions and purposes
served by such maladaptive behavior. That is,
overt behavior that appeared "maladaptive"
on the surface was quite adaptive (i.e., anxiety reducing) at a deeper level and maintained a tolerable, "just right" middle ground
of closeness/distance.

Beyond such empathic modeling and
coaching of holding behavior, I also frequently gave them "homework" tasks that
gently challenged them to "walk the walk,"
as well as "to talk the talk" of the therapy sessions. These tasks aimed both to provoke further changes in closeness and to reinforce the
thrust of the interpretive, exposure-oriented
experiential approaches used in our meetings (i.e., to promote generalization of the
effects of our shared therapeutic efforts).
Cognitive therapy interventions were also
used in this generalization-promoting way.
Commonly used problem-solving and communication coaching enhancement techniques were used not to "teach" "deficient"
skills but to strengthen the marital bond by
helping Paul and Kathy collaborate on life's
everyday stressors, decisions, and dilemmas,
and by helping them really listen to each
other carefully and closely and not be distracted by well-learned habits of escaping
from intimacy-promoting self-disclosure
and contact.

Over the course of our half year of work
together, Paul and Kathy were generally
successful at maintaining a new level of
connecting closely without undue fear of
emotionally catastrophic consequences. This
renewed comfort with each other, not insignificantly, strengthened Kathy's resolve to

maintain a more appropriate degree of disengagement from her parents' unending
struggles, just as setting firmer limits on
such involvement early in therapy had
helped to open up initial possibilities for
greater contact between Kathy and Paul.

CURRENT AND FUTURE TRENDS

In their millennial analytic review of the history of couple therapy, Gurman and
Fraenkel (2002) concluded that the most
telling irony in the field's evolution has been
that "despite its long history of struggles
against marginalization and professional
disempowerment, couple therapy . . . has
emerged as one of the most vibrant forces in
the entire domain of family therapy and psy-
chotherapy-in-general" (p. 248, original italics omitted). Like family therapy (see
Nichols & Schwartz, 1998), marital therapy
has been no stranger to conceptual and
philosophical ferment and challenges in its
relatively brief existence, as Gurman and
Fraenkel's account shows. The current tensions in the field, which provide opportunities for both synergistic growth and stultify-
ing rancor, depending on how the advocates
of opposing positions proceed, are familiar
and yet still significant: (1) the heightened
awareness of the need for scientific evaluation of both the effectiveness of marital therapy and the mechanisms by which positive
effects occur versus the postmodern critique
of all such endeavors; (2) the multilevel
"reinclusion of the individual" (Gurman &
Fraenkel, 2002), what Nichols (1987) called
the "self in the system," via both traditional
schools of thought (e.g., psychodynamic and
behavioral) and newer schools of thought
(e.g., narrative) versus the continuing preference by some to limit clinical intervention
to systemic patterns or other single experiential domains; (3) the assertion of marital
therapy's relevance in treating psychiatric
disorders versus the counterposing position
that such "disorders" exist only in language

and in particular reifying cultural contexts; and (4) the continuing proliferation of new "schools" of therapy versus the widespread support and encouragement of more integrative approaches.

In addition to the tensions between such perspectives, two other critical perspectives, feminism and multiculturalism, have challenged the normal assumptions and practices of the field. Along with postmodernism, feminism and multiculturalism have had the combined effect of forcing the field to recognize the diversity of experiences of couplehood for men versus women, and for people of different races, ethnicities, social classes, sexual orientations, genders, and other sources of meaning, expectation, and self-definition, and to examine the impact of relevant broader social beliefs on couples. Feminism, for example, has argued that how men and women view and carry out their roles and how they define and view problems in their relationships are connected to societal beliefs about gender, power, and intimacy. Thus, for example, basic systemic concepts such as complementarity can be seen not as inevitable couple patterns determined by the particularities of a given couple but as organized along gender lines in accordance with society's implicit and explicit expectations. That is, this perspective suggests that description is often confused with social prescription. Likewise, a multicultural perspective (e.g., Hardy & Laszloffy, 2002) on marriage and other committed relationships makes clear that norms about intimacy, sexuality, the distribution of power, parenting, and so on, vary among couples depending on their cultural identifications.

Critiques of marital therapies from these perspectives have sensitized therapists to the potential constraining and even damaging effects of a failure to recognize the reality of one's own necessarily limited perspectives and related biases that all therapists have about matters that pertain to marriage and other intimate relationships. But although such contemporary critiques of established therapeutic worldviews have provided evocative challenges that are both intellectually and, at times, affectively, stimulating, it is not yet entirely clear, or perhaps even at all clear, just how the new awarenesses that these points of view bring to the marital therapist should, and, indeed, can influence the moment-to-moment practices of everyday clinical work with couples. As Hardy and Laszloffy (2002) make clear, a multicultural perspective on couple therapy "is not a set of codified techniques or strategies . . . but rather a philosophical stance that significantly informs how one sees the world both inside and outside therapy" (p. 569). Relatedly, Rampage (2002) has stated that "how to *do* feminist therapy is much less well understood than is the critique of traditional (family and) couple therapy" (p. 535). Feminism and multiculturalism, then, are not clinical methodologies to be taught and refined. They are attitudes, perspectives, and worldviews. Whether the possession or development of such attitudes, perspectives, and worldviews enhances the efficacy and effectiveness of marital therapy has never been tested, and it remains unclear whether therapists who strive in their clinical work for social change reliably foster better treatment outcomes. Certainly, addressing concerns of this sort must rank among the most important challenges to the field of marital therapy.

NOTE

1. This distinction brings to mind John Weakland's distinction between normality as "one damned thing after another," and abnormality as "the same damned thing over and over."

SUGGESTIONS FOR FURTHER READING

Case Studies

Dattilio, F. M., & Bevilacqua, L. J. (Eds.). (2000). *Comparative treatment for relationship dysfunction.* New York: Springer.—Authors representing 16 theoretical orientations discuss their approaches to the same-couple case material.

Donovan, J. M. (Ed.). (1999). *Short-term couple therapy.* New York: Guilford Press.—Fourteen authors present their own clinical cases. Includes sections on psychodynamic, systemic, collaborative and postmodern approaches. Excellent editorial summation.

Gurman, A. S. (Ed.). (1985). *Casebook of marital therapy.* New York: Guilford Press.—Fourteen authors present in-depth case illustrations across a wider range of marital and couple problems than in most related books.

Research Reviews/Historical Reviews

Gurman, A. S., & Fraenkel, P. (2002). The history of couple therapy: A millennial review. *Family Process, 41,* 199–260.—Comprehensive and in-depth review of the theoretical and clinical history of the field. Also includes an historical account of trends in research since the inception of marital therapy.

Pinsof, W. M., & Wynne, L. C. (1995). The efficacy of marital and family therapy: An empirical overview, conclusions and recommendations. *Journal of Marital and Family Therapy, 21,* 585–614.—Integrative summation, integration and commentary on findings from the journal's state-of-the-art special issue on research on marital and family therapy.

Reference Volumes

Gurman, A. S., & Jacobson, N. S. (Eds.). (2002). *Clinical handbook of couple therapy* (3rd ed.). New York: Guilford Press.—The most widely used marital therapy textbook in the field. Discusses all influential treatment approaches, plus common clinical issues such as affairs, divorce, violence, substance abuse, and psychiatric disorders, and perspectives such as multiculturalism and feminism.

Halford, W. K., & Markman, H. J. (Eds). (1997). *Clinical handbook of marriage and couples interventions.* New York: Wiley.—Wide-ranging compendium on both the basic science of couple relationships and current treatment models.

Paolino, T. J., & McCrady, B. S. (Eds.). (1978). *Marriage and marital therapy: Psychoanalytic, behavioral and systems theory perspectives.* New York: Brunner/Mazel.—Groundbreaking textbook on the major domains of marital therapy circa 1980. Especially strong and in-depth presentations of clinical theory, plus an extensive comparative analysis of the three perspectives.

REFERENCES

Ackerman, N. W. (1970). Family psychotherapy today. *Family Process, 9,* 123–126.

Anchin, J. C., & Kiesler, D. J. (1982). *Handbook of interpersonal psychotherapy.* New York: Pergamon Press.

Anderson, H. (1997). *Conversation, language and possibilities: A postmodern approach to therapy.* New York: Basic Books.

Apfelbaum, B., & Gill, M. M. (1989). Ego analysis and the relativity of defense: The technical implications of the structural approach. *Journal of the American Psychoanalytic Association, 37,* 1071–1096.

Aponte, H. (1992). The black sheep of the family: A structural approach to brief therapy. In S. H. Budman, M. F. Hoyt, & S. Friedman (Eds.), *The first session in brief therapy* (pp. 324–341). New York: Guilford Press.

Aponte, H. S., & Di Cesare, E. J. (2000). Structural theory. In F. M. Dattilio & L. J. Bevilacqua (Eds.), *Comparative treatments for relationship dysfunction* (pp. 45–57). New York: Springer.

Bader, E., & Pearson, P. T. (1988). *In quest of the mythical mate.* New York: Brunner/Mazel.

Bandura, A. (1969). *Principles of behavior modification.* New York: Wiley.

Banmen, J. (Ed.). (2002). Satir today [Special Issue]. *Contemporary Family Therapy, 24*(1), 3–239.

Baucom, D. H., & Epstein, N. (1990). *Cognitive-behavioral marital therapy.* New York: Brunner/Mazel.

Baucom, D. H., Epstein, N., & LaTaillade, J. J. (2002). Cognitive-behavioral couple therapy. In A. S. Gurman & N. S. Jacobson (Eds.), *Clinical handbook of couple therapy* (3rd ed., pp. 26–58). New York: Guilford Press.

Baucom, D. H., Epstein, N., & Rankin, L. A. (1995). Cognitive aspects of cognitive-behavioral marital therapy. In N. S. Jacobson & A. S. Gurman (Eds.), *Clinical handbook of couple therapy* (pp. 65–90). New York: Guilford Press.

Baucom, D. H., Shoham, V., Meuser, K. T., Daiuto, A. D., & Stickle, T. R. (1998). Empirically supported couple and family interventions for marital distress and adult mental health problems. *Journal of Consulting and Clinical Psychology, 66,* 53–88.

Beels, C. C., & Ferber, A. (1969). Family therapy: A view. *Family Process, 8,* 280–318.

Berg, I. K. (1994). *Family-based services: A solution-focused approach.* New York: W. W. Norton.

Bergin, A. E., & Jensen, J. P. (1990). The meaning of eclecticism: New survey and analysis of components. *Professional Psychology, 21,* 124–130.

Berman, E. B., Lief, H., & Williams, A. (1981). A model of marital integration. In G. P. Sholevar (Ed.), *The handbook of marriage and marital therapy* (pp. 3–34). New York: Spectrum.

Birchler, G., & Spinks, S. (1980). A behavioral-systems marital and family therapy: Intervention and clinical application. *American Journal of Family Therapy, 8,* 6–28.

Bloom, B., Asher, S., & White, S. (1978). Marital disruption as a stressor: A review and analysis. *Psychological Bulletin, 85,* 867–894.

Bodin, A. M. (1981). The interactional view: Family therapy approaches of the Mental Research Institute. In A. S. Gurman & D. S. Kniskern (Eds.), *Handbook of family therapy* (pp. 267–309). New York: Brunner/Mazel.

Boszormenyi-Nagy, I., & Ulrich, D. N. (1981). Contextual family therapy. In A. S. Gurman & D. P. Kniskern (Eds.), *Handbook of family therapy* (pp. 159–225). New York: Brunner/Mazel.

Bowen, M. (1976). Principles and techniques of multiple family therapy. In P. J. Guerin, Jr. (Ed.), *Family therapy: Theory and practice* (pp. 388–404). New York: Gardner Press.

Bowen, M. (1978). *Family therapy in clinical practice.* New York: Jason Aronson.

Bowlby, J. (1988). *A secure base.* New York: Basic Books.

Bradbury, T. N., & Fincham, F. D. (1990). Preventing marital dysfunction: Review and analysis. In D. Frank, F. D. Fincham, & T. N. Bradbury (Eds.), *The psychology of marriage* (pp. 375–401). New York: Guilford Press.

Bray, J. H., & Jouriles, E. N. (1995). Treatment of marital conflict and prevention of divorce. *Journal of Marital and Family Therapy, 21,* 461–473.

Broderick, C. B., & Schrader, S. S. (1991). The history of professional marriage and family therapy. In A. S. Gurman & D. F. Kniskern (Eds.), *Handbook of family therapy* (Vol. 2, pp. 3–40). New York: Brunner/Mazel.

Budman, S. H., & Gurman, A. S. (1988). *The theory and practice of brief therapy.* New York: Guilford Press.

Burman, B., & Margolin, G. (1992). Analysis of the association between marital relationships and health problems: An interactional perspective. *Psychological Bulletin, 112,* 39–63.

Carr, A. (2000). *Family therapy: Concepts, process and practice.* Chichester, UK: Wiley.

Cassidy, J., & Shaver, P. R. (Eds.). (1999). *Handbook of attachment: Theory, research, and clinical applications.* New York: Guilford Press.

Catherall, D. R. (1992). Working with projective identification. *Family Process, 31,* 355–367.

Chapman, A. L., & Dehle, C. (2002). Bridging theory and practice: A comparative analysis of integrative behavioral couple therapy and cognitive behavioral couple therapy. *Cognitive and Behavioral Practice, 9,* 150–163.

Christensen, A., Babcock, J. C., & Jacobson, N. S. (1995). Integrative behavioral couple therapy. In N. S. Jacobson & A. S. Gurman (Eds.), *Clinical handbook of couple therapy* (2nd ed., pp. 31–64). New York: Guilford Press.

Christensen, A., & Heavey, C. L. (1999). Interventions for couples. *Annual Review of Psychology, 50,* 165–190.

de Shazer, S. (1985). *Keys to solution in brief therapy.* New York: Norton.

de Shazer, S. (1988). *Clues: Investigating solutions in brief therapy.* New York: Norton.

Dicks, H. V. (1967). *Marital tensions.* New York: Basic Books.

Doherty, W. J., & Simmons, D. S. (1996). Clinical practice patterns of marriage and family therapists: A national survey of therapists and their clients. *Journal of Marital and Family Therapy, 22,* 9–25.

Donovan, J. M. (Ed.). (1999). *Short-term couple therapy.* New York: Guilford Press.

Fairbairn, W. R. D. (1963). Synopsis of an object-relations theory of personality. *International Journal of Psychoanalysis, 44,* 224–225.

Feldman, L. B. (1979). Marital conflict and marital intimacy: An integrative psychodynamic–behavioral–systemic model. *Family Process, 18,* 69–78.

Feldman, L. B. (1985). Integrative multi-level therapy: A comprehensive interpersonal and intrapsychic approach. *Journal of Marital and Family Therapy, 11,* 357–372.

Feldman, L. B. (1992). *Integrating individual and family therapy.* New York: Brunner/Mazel.

Fisch, R., Weakland, J. H., & Segal, L. (1982). *The tactics of change: Doing therapy briefly.* San Francisco: Jossey-Bass.

Fraenkel, P. (1997). Systems approaches to couple therapy. In W. K. Halford & H. J. Markman (Eds.), *Clinical handbook of marriage and couples interventions* (pp. 379–414). New York: Wiley.

Fraenkel, P., Markman, H., & Stanley, S. (1997). The prevention approach to relationship problems. *Sexual and Marital Therapy, 12,* 249–258.

Fraenkel, P., & Pinsof, W. (2001). Teaching family-therapy-centered integration: Assimilation and beyond. *Journal of Psychotherapy Integration, 11,* 59–85.

Framo, J. L. (1965). Rationale and techniques of intensive family therapy. In I. Boszormenyi-Nagy & J. L. Framo (Eds.), *Intensive family therapy* (pp. 143–212). New York: Harper & Rowe.

Framo, J. L. (1976). Family of origin as a therapeutic resource for adults in marital and family therapy. You can and should go home again. *Family Process, 15,* 193–210.

Framo, J. L. (1981). The integration of marital therapy with sessions with family of origin. In A. S. Gurman & D. P. Kniskern (Eds.), *Handbook of family therapy* (pp. 133–158). New York: Brunner/Mazel.

Freedman, J., & Combs, G. C. (1996). *Narrative therapy: The social construction of preferred realities.* New York: Norton.

Freedman, J., & Combs, G. C. (2000). Narrative therapy with couples. In F. M. Dattilio & L. J. Bevilacqua (Eds.), *Comparative treatments for relationship dysfunction* (pp. 342–361). New York: Guilford Press.

Freedman, J. H., & Combs, G. (2002). Narrative couple therapy. In A. S. Gurman & N. S. Jacobson (Eds.), *Clinical handbook of couple therapy* (3rd ed., pp. 308–334). New York: Guilford Press.

Geiss, S. K., & O'Leary, K. D. (1981). Therapist ratings of frequency and severity of marital problems: Implications for research. *Journal of Marital and Family Therapy, 7,* 515–520.

Gilbert, M., & Shmulker, D. (1996). *Brief therapy with couples.* Chichester, UK: Wiley.

Goldman, A., & Greenberg, L. (1992). Comparison of integrated systemic and emotionally focused approaches to couple therapy. *Journal of Consulting and Clinical Psychology, 60,* 962–969.

Goldner, V. (1985). Feminism and family therapy. *Family Process, 24,* 31–47.

Gottman, J. M. (1979). *Marital interaction: Empirical investigations.* New York: Academic Press.

Gottman, J. M. (1994). *Why marriages succeed or fail.* New York: Simon & Schuster.

Gottman, J. M. (1999). *The marriage clinic: A scientifically based marital therapy.* New York: Norton.

Greenberg, L. S., & Johnson, S. M. (1986). Emotionally focused couples therapy. In N. S. Jacobson & A. S. Gurman (Eds.), *Clinical handbook of marital therapy* (pp. 253–278). New York: Guilford Press.

Greenberg, L. S., & Johnson, S. M. (1988). *Emotionally focused therapy for couples.* New York: Guilford Press.

Greene, B. L. (Ed.). (1965). *The psychotherapies of marital disharmony.* New York: Free Press.

Guerin, P. J., Jr. (1976). Family therapy: The first twenty-five years. In P. J. Guerin, Jr. (Ed.), *Family therapy and practice* (pp. 2–22). New York: Gardner Press.

Guerin P. J., Jr., Fay, L. F., Fogarty, T. F., & Kautto, J. G. (1999). Brief marital therapy: The story of the triangles. In J. M. Donovan (Ed.), *Short-term couple therapy* (pp. 103–123). New York: Guilford Press.

Guntrip, H. (1961). *Personality structure and human interaction.* London: Hogarth Press and The Institute of Psychoanalysis.

Gurman, A. S. (1973). The effects and effectiveness of marital therapy: A review of outcome research. *Family Process, 12,* 145–170.

Gurman, A. S. (1978). Contemporary marital therapies: A critique and comparative analysis of psychoanalytic, behavioral and systems theory approaches. In T. J. Paolino & B. McCrady (Eds.), *Marriage and marital therapy* (pp. 445–566). New York: Brunner/Mazel.

Gurman, A. S. (1981). Integrative marital therapy: Toward the development of an interpersonal approach. In S. H. Budman (Ed.), *Forms of brief therapy* (pp. 415–462). New York: Guilford Press.

Gurman, A. S. (1992). Integrative marital therapy: A time-sensitive model for working with couples. In S. H. Budman, M. Hoyt, & S. Friedman (Eds.), *The first session in brief therapy* (pp. 186–203). New York: Guilford Press.

Gurman, A. S. (2001). Brief therapy and family/couple therapy: An essential redundancy. *Clinical Psychology: Science and Practice, 8,* 51–65.

Gurman, A. S. (2002). Brief integrative marital therapy: A depth-behavioral approach. In A. S. Gurman & N. S. Jacobson (Eds.), *Clinical handbook of couple therapy* (3rd ed., pp. 180–220). New York: Guilford Press.

Gurman, A. S., & Fraenkel, P. (2002). The history of couple therapy: A millennial review. *Family Process, 41,* 199–260.

Gurman, A. S., & Jacobson, N. S. (Eds.). (2002). *Clinical handbook of couple therapy* (3rd ed.). New York: Guilford Press.

Gurman, A. S., & Kniskern, D. P. (1979). Marital therapy and/or family therapy: What's in a name? *AAMFT Newsletter, 10*(3), 1, 5–8.

Gurman, A. S., & Kniskern, D. P. (1986). Commentary: Individual marital therapy—Have reports of your death been somewhat exaggerated? *Family Process, 25,* 51–62.

Gurman, A. S., Kniskern, D. P., & Pinsof, W. M. (1986). Process and outcome research in family and marital therapy. In A. S. Bergin & S. L. Garfield (Eds.), *Handbook of psychotherapy and behavioral change* (3rd ed., pp. 565–624). New York: Wiley.

Haley, J. (1963). Marriage therapy. *Archives of General Psychiatry, 8,* 213–234.

Haley, J. (1976). *Problem solving therapy.* San Francisco: Jossey-Bass.

Halford, W. K. (1998). The ongoing evolution of behavioral couples therapy. *Clinical Psychology Review, 18,* 613–633.

Halford, W. K., Sanders, M. R., & Behrens, B. C. (1994). Self-regulation in behavioral couples therapy. *Behavior Therapy, 25,* 431–452.

Hardy, K. V., & Laszloffy, T. A. (2002). Couple therapy using a multicultural perspective. In A. S. Gurman & N. S. Jacobson (Eds.), *Clinical handbook of couple therapy* (3rd ed., pp. 569–593). New York: Guilford Press.

Hoyt, M. F. (2002). Solution-focused couple therapy. In A. S. Gurman & N. S. Jacobson (Eds.), *Clinical handbook of couple therapy* (3rd ed., pp. 335–369). New York: Guilford Press.

Jackson, D. D. (1959). Family interaction, family homeostasis and some implications for conjoint family psychotherapy. In J. Masserman (Ed.), *Individual and family dynamics* (pp. 122–141). New York: Grune & Stratton.

Jackson, D. D. (1965). Family rules: The marital quid pro quo. *Archives of General Psychiatry, 12,* 589–594.

Jacobson, N. S., & Christensen, A. (1996). *Integrative couple therapy: Promoting acceptance and change.* New York: Norton.

Jacobson, N. S., & Gurman, A. S. (Eds.). (1986). *Clinical handbook of marital therapy.* New York: Guilford Press.

Jacobson, N. S., & Gurman, A. S. (Eds.). (1995). *Clinical handbook of couple therapy* (2nd ed.). New York: Guilford Press.

Jacobson, N. S., & Margolin, G. (1979). *Marital therapy: Strategies based on social learning and behavior exchange principles.* New York: Brunner/Mazel.

Johnson, S. M. (1986). Bonds or bargains: Relationship paradigms and their significance for marital therapy. *Journal of Marital and Family Therapy, 12,* 259–267.

Johnson, S. M. (1996). *The practice of emotionally focused marital therapy.* New York: Brunner/Mazel.

Johnson, S. M., & Denton, W. (2002). Emotionally focused couple therapy: Creating secure connections. In A. S. Gurman & N. S. Jacobson (Eds.), *Clinical handbook of couple therapy* (3rd ed., pp. 221–250). New York: Guilford Press.

Johnson, S. M., & Greenberg, L. S. (1995). The emotionally focused approach to problems in adult attachment. In N. S. Jacobson & A. S. Gurman (Eds.), *Clinical handbook of couple therapy* (2nd ed., pp. 121–146). New York: Guilford Press.

Johnson, S. M., Hunsely, J., Greenberg, L., & Schindler, D. (1999). Emotionally focused couples therapy: Status and challenges. *Clinical Psychology: Science and Practice, 6,* 67–79.

Keim, J. (1999). Brief strategic marital therapy. In J. Donovan (Ed.), *Short-term couple therapy* (pp. 265–290). New York: Guilford Press.

Keim, J. (2000). Strategic therapy. In F. Dattilio & L. Bevilacqua (Eds.), *Comparative treatments for relationship dysfunction* (pp. 58–78). New York: Springer.

Keim, J., & Lappin, J. (2002). Structural–strategic marital therapy. In A. S. Gurman & N. S. Jacobson (Eds.), *Clinical handbook of couple therapy* (3rd ed., pp. 86–117). New York: Guilford Press.

Klein, M. (1948). *Contributions to psycho-analysis, 1921–1945.* London: Hogarth Press.

Lebow, J. L. (1997). The integrative revolution in couple and family therapy. *Family Process, 36,* 1–17.

Lebow, J. L. (1999). Building a science of couple relationships: comments on two articles by Gottman and Levenson. *Family Process, 46,* 27–57.

Lebow, J. L., & Gurman, A. S. (1995). Research assessing couple and family therapy. *Annual Review of Psychology, 46,* 27–57.

Leff, J., Vearnals, S., Brewin, C. R., Wolff, G., Alexander, B., Asen, K., Dayson, D., Jones, E., Chisholm, D., & Everitt, B. (2000). The London Depression Intervention Trial. Random/old controlled trial of antidepressants v. couple therapy in the treatment and maintenance of people with depression living with a critical partner: Clinical outcome and costs. *British Journal of Psychiatry, 177,* 95–100.

Madanes, C. (1981). *Strategic family therapy.* San Francisco: Jossey-Bass.

Madanes, C. (1990). *Sex, love, and violence: Strategies for transformation.* New York: Norton.

Manus, G. I. (1966). Marriage counseling: A technique in search of a theory. *Journal of Marriage and the Family, 28,* 449–453.

McCarthy, B. W. (2002). Sexuality, sexual dysfunction and couple therapy. In A. S. Gurman & N. S. Jacobson (Eds.), *Clinical handbook of couple therapy* (3rd ed., pp. 629–652). New York: Guilford Press.

Messer, S. B. (1992). A critical examination of belief structures in integrative and eclectic psychotherapy. In J. C. Norcross & M. R. Goldfried (Eds.), *Handbook of psychotherapy integration* (pp. 130–165). New York: Basic Books.

Messer, S. B. (Ed.). (2001). Assimilative integration [Special issue]. *Journal of Psychotherapy Integration, 11,* 1–154.

Miller, S. D., Duncan, B. L., & Hubble, M. A. (1997). *Escape from Babel: Toward a unifying language for psychotherapy practice.* New York: Norton.

Minuchin, S. (1974). *Families and family therapy.* Cambridge, MA: Harvard University Press.

Minuchin, S., & Fishman, H. C. (1981). *Family therapy techniques.* Cambridge, MA: Harvard University Press.

Mittelman, B. (1948). The concurrent analysis of married couples. *Psychiatric Quarterly, 17,* 182–197.

Nadelson, C. C. (1978). Marital therapy from a psychoanalytic perspective. In T. Paolino & B. McCrady (Eds.), *Marriage and marital therapy* (pp. 89–164). New York: Brunner/Mazel.

Neal, J. H., Zimmerman, J. L., & Dickerson, V. C. (1999). Couples, culture, and discourse: A narrative approach. In J. M. Donovan (Ed.), *Short-term couple therapy* (pp. 360–400). New York: Guilford Press.

Nerin, W. F. (1986). *Family reconstruction: Long day's journey into light.* New York: Norton.

Nichols, M. P. (1987). *The self in the system.* New York: Brunner/Mazel.

Nichols, M. P., & Minuchin, S. (1999). Short-term structural family therapy with couples. In J. M. Donovan (Ed.), *Short-term couple therapy* (pp. 124–143). New York: Guilford Press.

Nichols, M. P., & Schwartz, R. C. (1998). *Family therapy: Concepts and methods.* Boston: Allyn & Bacon.

Nichols, W. C. (1988). *Marital therapy: An integrated approach.* New York: Guilford Press.

Oberndorf, C. P. (1934). Folie á deux. *International Journal of Psychoanalysis, 15,* 14–24.

Paolino, T. J., & McCrady, B. S. (Eds.). (1978). *Marriage and marital therapy.* New York: Brunner/Mazel.

Papero, D. (1995). Bowen family systems and marriage. In N. S. Jacobson & A. S. Gurman (Eds.), *Clinical handbook of couple therapy* (2nd ed., pp. 11–30). New York: Guilford Press.

Paul, N. (1967). The role of mourning and empathy in conjoint marital therapy. In G. Zuk & I. Boszormenyi-Nagy (Eds.), *Family therapy and disturbed families* (pp. 186–205). Palo Alto, CA: Science and Behavior Books.

Paul, N., & Paul, B. (1975). *A marital puzzle.* New York: Norton.

Pinsof, W. M. (1995). *Integrative problem-centered therapy*. New York: Basic Books.

Pinsof, W. M. (2002). The death of til death do us part: The twentieth century's revelation of the limits of human pair-bonding. *Family Process, 41,* 135–157.

Prochaska, J. (1978). Twentieth century trends in marriage and marital therapy. In T. Paolino & B. McCrady (Eds.), *Marriage and marital therapy* (pp. 1–24). New York: Brunner/Mazel.

Rait, D. (1988). Survey results. *Family Therapy Networker, 12*(1), 52–56.

Rampage, C. (2002). Working with gender in couple therapy. In A. S. Gurman & N. S. Jacobson (Eds.), *Clinical handbook of couple therapy* (3rd ed., pp. 533–545). New York: Guilford Press.

Rausch, H. L., Barry, W. A., Hertel, R. K., & Swain, M. A. (1974). *Communication, conflict and marriage*. San Francisco: Jossey-Bass.

Rice, J. K., & Rice, D. G. (1985). *Living through divorce: A developmental approach to divorce therapy*. New York: Guilford Press.

Roberto-Forman, L. (2002). Transgenerational marriage therapy. In A. S. Gurman & N. S. Jacobson (Eds.), *Clinical handbook of couple therapy* (3rd ed., pp. 118–147). New York: Guilford Press.

Sager, C. J. (1966). The development of marriage therapy: An historical review. *American Journal of Orthopsychiatry, 36,* 458–467.

Sager, C. J. (1967). Transference in conjoint treatment of married couples. *Archives of General Psychiatry, 16,* 185–193.

Sager, C. J. (1976). *Marriage contracts and couple therapy*. New York: Brunner/Mazel.

Satir, V. (1964). *Conjoint family therapy*. Palo Alto, CA: Science and Behavior Books.

Satir, V. M. (1965). Conjoint marital therapy. In B. L. Greene (Ed.), *The psychotherapies of marital disharmony* (pp. 121–133). New York: Free Press.

Satir, V. (1972). *Peoplemaking*. Palo Alto, CA: Science and Behavior Books.

Scharff, D. E., & Scharff, J. S. (1991). *Object relations couple therapy*. New York: Jason Aronson.

Scharff, J. S. (1995). Psychoanalytic marital therapy. In N. S. Jacobson & A. S. Gurman (Eds.), *Clinical handbook of couple therapy* (2nd ed., pp. 164–193). New York: Guilford Press.

Scharff, J. S., & Bagnini, C. (2002). Object relations couple therapy. In A. S. Gurman & N. S. Jacobson (Eds.), *Clinical handbook of couple therapy* (3rd ed., pp. 59–85). New York: Guilford Press.

Segal, L. (1991). Brief therapy: The MRI approach. In A. S. Gurman & D. S. Kniskern (Eds.), *Handbook of family therapy* (Vol. 2, pp. 171–199). New York: Brunner/Mazel.

Segraves, R. T. (1982). *Marital therapy: A combined psychodynamic behavioral approach*. New York: Plenum Press.

Shoham, V., & Rohrbaugh, M. J. (2002). Brief strategic couple therapy. In A. S. Gurman & N. S. Jacobson (Eds.), *Clinical handbook of couple therapy* (3rd ed., pp. 5–25). New York: Guilford Press.

Shoham, V., Rohrbaugh, M. J., & Patterson, J. (1995). Problem- and solution-focused couple therapies: The MRI and Milwaukee models. In N. S. Jacobson & A. S. Gurman (Eds.), *Clinical handbook of couple therapy* (2nd ed., pp. 142–163). New York: Guilford Press.

Sholevar, G. P. (Ed.). (1981). *The handbook of marriage and marital therapy*. New York: Spectrum.

Simmons, D. S., & Doherty, W. J. (1995). Defining who we are and what we do: Clinical practice patterns of marriage and family therapists in Minnesota. *Journal of Marital and Family Therapy, 21,* 3–16.

Skynner, A. C. R. (1976). *Systems of family and marital psychotherapy*. New York: Brunner/Mazel.

Skynner, A. C. R. (1980). Recent developments in marital therapy. *Journal of Family Therapy, 2,* 271–296.

Snyder, D. K. (1999). Affective reconstruction in the context of a pluralistic approach to couple therapy. *Clinical Psychology: Science and Practice, 6,* 348–365.

Snyder, D. K., & Schneider, W. J. (2002). Affective reconstruction: A pluralistic, developmental Approach. In A. S. Gurman & N. S. Jacobson (Eds.), *Clinical handbook of couple therapy* (3rd ed., pp. 151–179). New York: Guilford Press.

Snyder, D. K., & Wills, R. M. (1989). Behavioral versus insight-oriented marital therapy: Effects on individual and interspousal functioning. *Journal of Consulting and Clinical Psychology, 57,* 39–46.

Solomon, M. (1989). *Narcissism and intimacy.* New York: Norton.

Stanton, M. D. (1980). An integrated structural/strategic approach to family therapy. *Journal of Marital and Family Therapy, 7,* 427–439.

Stanton, M. D. (1981). Marital therapy from a structural/strategic viewpoint. In G. P. Sholevar (Ed.), *The handbook of marriage and marital therapy* (pp. 303–334). New York: Spectrum.

Stricker, G. (1994). Reflections on psychotherapy integration. *Clinical Psychology: Science and Practice, 1,* 3–12.

Stuart, R. B. (1969). Operant–interpersonal treatment of marital discord. *Journal of Consulting and Clinical Psychology, 33,* 675–682.

Stuart, R. B. (1980). *Helping couples change.* New York: Guilford Press.

Thibaut, J. W., & Kelley, H. H. (1959). *The social psychology of groups.* New York: Wiley.

Todd, T. C. (1986). Structural–strategic marital therapy. In N. S. Jacobson & A. S. Gurman (Eds.), *Clinical handbook of marital therapy* (pp. 71–99). New York: Guilford Press.

Watzlawick, P., & Weakland, J. H. (Eds.). (1978). *The interactional view.* New York: Norton.

Watzlawick, P., Weakland, J. H., & Fisch, R. (1974). *Change: Principles of problem formation and problem resolution.* New York: Norton.

Weakland, J. H., & Fisch, R. (1992). Brief therapy—MRI style. In S. H. Budman, M. F. Hoyt, & S. Friedman (Eds.), *The first session in brief therapy* (pp. 306–323). New York: Guilford Press.

Weakland, J. H., Fisch, R., Watzlawick, P., & Bodin, A. (1974). Brief therapy: Focused problem resolution. *Family Process, 13,* 141–168.

Weeks, G. R. (Ed.). (1989). *Treating couples: The intersystem model of the Marriage Council of Philadelphia.* New York: Brunner/Mazel.

Weeks, G. R., & Treat, S. R. (2001). *Couples in treatment: Techniques and approaches for effective practice.* Philadelphia: Brunner-Routledge.

Weiner-Davis, M. (1992). *Divorce-busting: A revolutionary and rapid program for staying together.* New York: Simon & Schuster/Fireside.

Weiss, R. L. (1980). Strategic behavioral marital therapy: Toward a model for assessment and intervention. In J. P. Vincent (Ed.), *Advances in family intervention, assessment and theory* (Vol. 1, pp. 229–271). Greenwich, CT: JAI Press.

Wells, R. A., & Giannetti, V. J. (1986a). Individual marital therapy: A critical reappraisal. *Family Process, 25,* 43–51.

Wells, R. A., & Giannetti, V. J. (1986b). Rejoinder: Whither marital therapy? *Family Process, 25,* 62–65.

Whisman, M. A., Dixon, A. E., & Johnson, B. (1997). Therapists' perspectives of couple problems and treatment issues in couple therapy. *Journal of Family Psychology, 11,* 361–366.

White, M., & Epston, D. (1990). *Narrative means to therapeutic ends.* New York: Norton.

Wile, D. B. (1981). *Couples therapy: A nontraditional approach.* New York: Wiley.

Wile, D. B. (1995). The ego-analytic approach to couple therapy. In N. S. Jacobson & A. S. Gurman (Eds.), *Clinical handbook of couple therapy* (pp. 65–90). New York: Guilford Press.

Wile, D. B. (1999). Collaborative couple therapy. In J. M. Donovan (Ed.), *Short-term couple therapy* (pp. 201–225). New York: Guilford Press.

Wile, D. B. (2002). Collaborative couple therapy. In A. S. Gurman & N. S. Jacobson (Eds.), *Clinical handbook of couple therapy* (3rd ed., pp. 281–307). New York: Guilford Press.

Willi, J. (1982). *Couples in collusion.* Claremont, CA: Hunter House.

Winnicott, D. W. (1960). The theory of the parent-infant relationship. *International Journal of Psychoanalysis, 41,* 585–595.

Zimmerman, J. L., & Dickerson, V. C. (1996). *If problems talked: Narrative therapy in action.* New York: Guilford Press.

13

Group Psychotherapies

Robert R. Dies

Since its modest beginnings over nine decades ago, the field of group psychotherapy has demonstrated a remarkable evolution. Presently, there are approximately 20,000 articles published in hundreds of different journals and thousands of books on various aspects of group intervention. Although these figures are impressive, it is clear that they grossly underestimate the actual prevalence of group treatments because the vast majority of group psychotherapists do not contribute to the theoretical, empirical, or applied literature. It is not known how many clinicians actually conduct therapy groups regularly, but findings from a wide range of surveys of training programs, treatment facilities, and professional organizations for group psychotherapists suggest that literally tens of thousands of psychologists, psychiatrists, social workers, and other mental health practitioners, as well as millions of clients, spend portions of their time in group psychotherapy or group counseling each week (Dies, 1986, 1992a). There is widespread agreement that the foundations for group psychotherapy are multifaceted and include practical considerations, theoretical conceptualizations, and empirical documentation of effectiveness. Here we examine these foundations in historical perspective and look at the contemporary scene.

HISTORICAL BACKGROUND

Practical Foundations

Group psychotherapy was first and foremost a pragmatic approach to treatment. Historical accounts generally credit Joseph Pratt for originating group therapy in 1906 as a psychosocial intervention for tuberculosis patients who were unable to afford inpatient treatment (Shaffer & Galinsky, 1989). Pratt assembled patients into large groups and exhorted them to adopt a positive attitude toward their illness. His optimistic outlook was communicated to his participants and this enthusiasm, along with the patients' recognition that they were not alone in their suffering, apparently contributed to their sense of betterment. Other physicians and psychiatrists soon followed Pratt's initiative and within a few years the group lecture approach was extended to patients experiencing a variety of medical and psychological disorders. It was clear, however, that pragmatic issues took precedence over formal theory, with the result that the conceptual framework for what transpired in groups tended to be subsumed under a commonsense rationale emphasizing the usefulness of instruction, advice, support, and mutual identification among group members (Shaffer & Galinsky, 1989). Three practical advantages of group psychotherapy were regarded as most central at that time: expediency, cost-effectiveness, and staff efficiency.

Pratt's application of the lecture approach, for example, was based largely on the notion of *expediency,* that is, presenting information simultaneously to numerous patients who shared a common malady. However, early clinicians who adopted this psychoeducational strategy soon learned that it may not have been the passive assimilation of information delivered by an inspirational leader that was beneficial but, rather, the patients' opportunities to share with fellow sufferers the experience of their debilitating condition. This discovery influenced clinicians to become less interested in the sheer convenience of treating multiple people concurrently in favor of proper matching of patients in groups to maximize treatment effectiveness. Experience has shown that sound clinical judgment should take priority over practicality in selecting patients for groups (Dies, 1986). Thus, it has been documented that careful attention to screening, pregroup preparation, group composition, and minimizing the risks inherent in the cavalier assignment of patients to group treatments can lead to significant improvements in group functioning and therapeutic gains for individual patients (Dies, 1993; Dies & Teleska, 1985). The almost exclusive focus on convenience has been replaced by a more articulated rationale based on the unique merits of group interventions for the particular patients who have been referred for treatment.

The second pragmatic justification for the early use of group methods was based on *cost-effectiveness.* Pratt, for instance, worked with indigent patients who could not bear the expense of institutional care.

Today, the concept of cost-effectiveness has a variety of overtones that extend far beyond the initial reasons formulated by Pratt and other clinicians during his era. Now, the choice is not so much between inpatient and outpatient treatment, although that, too, is critical, but rather involves decisions among alternative treatment modalities. For the individual client, there is no question that group therapy is much more affordable than one-to-one methods, usually about one-third the cost. The current question, however, is not how much the individual is expected to pay for treatment but rather the willingness of third-party payers to subsidize a major portion of this cost. Fortunately, in the face of mounting pressures for cost containment from legislators, insurance underwriters, and even patient consumers, there is ample evidence that group psychotherapy is indeed more economical than individual treatments and generally just as effective in terms of clinical outcome (Dies, 1993). MacKenzie (1995) has demonstrated that there are considerable cost-saving benefits when mental health care systems are carefully designed to incorporate group treatments as the primary mode of service delivery.

The third practical advantage of group psychotherapy espoused by early workers in the field relates to *staff efficiency,* that is, the capacity of understaffed mental health agencies to accommodate more patients by assigning them to a group conducted by one or two therapists. At first glance, this rationale for group treatments appears to have merit, but in actuality several problems have been noted with this practice. Elsewhere, the author has suggested that many clinical settings use groups to compensate for the lack of adequately trained personnel (Dies, 1986). Patients may be informed that there is a waiting list for individual therapy but that they could join a group almost immediately. Unfortunately, this message conveys the unjustified bias that individual therapy is at a premium (implicitly because it is better) and that group psychotherapy is a secondary form of intervention. The regrettable consequence is that expectations regarding therapeutic effectiveness may diminish, thereby slowing the rate of treatment progress and hampering the group's potential. A sizable body of literature confirms the importance of positive expectations in the overall impact of psychological interventions (Yalom, 1995).

A related problem is that many agencies reserve "precious" individual therapy time for their more experienced practitioners and allow their less seasoned clinicians to conduct the group treatments. This practice is inconsistent with the degree of complexity of the therapeutic modalities. The group context is more demanding and requires more specialized training and experience; often the skills learned as an individual therapist may not transfer readily to the group psychotherapy situation (Dies, 1986). Furthermore, the level of experience and expertise of the group therapist have been shown make a significant difference in terms of treatment outcome (Dies, 1994b).

Although group psychotherapy was established, in large part, in response to a host of pragmatic issues, these advantages seem far less salient by contemporary standards. More compelling justification for group treatments can be found in both the theoretical and empirical literature.

Theoretical Foundations

As early clinicians attempted to understand the powerful curative forces operating within the group setting, they began to impose a theoretical framework on their experiences. Initially, psychoanalytic theory was most influential, and clinicians sought to transpose the concepts of individual psychoanalysis into the group context. Unfortunately, this juxtaposition was not always compatible, and many of the basic concepts and methods (e.g., free association and dream interpretation) had to be modified or sacrificed completely. Despite the need for compromise and concession, the psychoanalytic model continued to exert the primary thrust in the evolution of group treatments for many decades, and even today it remains as one of the most prominent models of group psychotherapy. At this time, however, proponents of virtually every theoretical persuasion endorse group psychotherapy as a viable and vital treatment modality (Dies, 1992a).

Contemporary theories of group therapy may be contrasted along a number of critical dimensions. Parloff (1968), for instance, differentiated theories in terms of the focus of the therapist's interventions: individual (intrapersonalists), interpersonal (transactionalists), and group-as-a-whole (integralists). Each perspective argues for the unique benefits of group treatments over other modalities. *Intrapersonalists* generally seek to resolve intrapsychic conflicts and view the group as especially effective in facilitating the interpretation of resistance and transference phenomena. Shaffer and Galinsky (1989) summarize other unique benefits of group psychotherapy from this perspective, including the opportunities for patients to (1) witness that they are not isolated and alone in experiencing problems; (2) discover personal resources for listening to and understanding others; (3) demonstrate, not just talk about, patterns of interpersonal relating; (4) gain insight into the effects of characterological style more quickly and forcefully; (5) experience the safety of expressing feelings through peer support and modeling; and (6) avoid the increasingly dependent patient–therapist relationship that can occur in individual treatment.

Parloff (1968) states that the second group of theorists, the *transactionalists,* are mainly interested in member-to-member relationships and view the group as furnishing unique opportunities for understanding individual patterns of relating to others. Kaul and Bednar (1978) cite four sources of learning that are special to group treatments for these interpersonally oriented clinicians. Thus, individual members may (1) profit due to learning based on their participation in, and evaluation of, a developing social micro-cosm; (2) gain as a result of their exchange of feedback within the group; (3) improve as a consequence of consensual validation de-rived from the group; and (4) benefit from the relatively unique opportunity to be reci-procally involved with other group members as both helpers and helpees. Similarly, Fuhri-man and Burlingame (1990), based on their extensive review of the empirical literature, conclude that the distinctive benefits from group treatments rely heavily on the pres-ence and observance of others, as well as en-gagement with fellow members within the group (e.g., vicarious learning, universality, and altruism, respectively).

Parloff's (1968) third vantage point, the *integralists,* places primary emphasis on group-as-a-whole processes. Participation in a therapy group ostensibly evokes shared unconscious conflicts or motivations around issues of dependency (especially in relationship to the authority of the leader), aggression, sexuality, and intimacy. By at-tending to such shared group concerns, the therapist is presumably able to treat each patient within the group. Theoretically, by interpreting to the group rather than to the individual, the impact of the therapist's in-terventions will be wider and more appro-priate because each patient will find most interpretations pertinent to some extent. The overall goal of treatment is to help pa-tients become more effective in the groups to which they belong on the outside. Thus, learning more adaptive and task-oriented styles in the here- and-now of group thera-py is thought to generalize to important groups in the patients' lives beyond the im-mediate treatment setting. The group is ac-knowledged to have more potential than one-to-one therapy for the stimulation of unconscious conflicts, and to be more effec-tive in providing a supportive and efficient learning environment through which to fa-cilitate the working through of these indi-vidual and shared problems.

In actual practice, the vast majority of clinicians incorporate interpretations at each level of analysis, although they vary substan-tially in their emphasis (Rutan & Stone, 2001). Nonetheless, each perspective regards the group modality as uniquely suited for the activation, exploration, and resolution of the maladaptive behavioral patterns and per-sonal distress that led patients to seek treat-ment in the first place (Dies, 1986). Of course, there are other critical dimensions that differentiate the most popular models of group intervention: therapist *style* in terms of activity level, openness, and structuring; therapist focus (e.g., past–present–future, af-fect–behavior–cognition, process–content, in-group–out-of-group); and, the *nature* of therapist verbalizations (e.g., confrontation, encouragement, and interpretation) (Rutan & Stone, 2001). Although a recent analysis of contemporary models of group psychother-apy shows that there is considerable confu-sion in the field about how to best distin-guish among the various perspectives, there is also substantial consensus that group treat-ments provide a powerful medium for ther-apeutic change (Dies, 1992b). Indeed, the theoretical justifications for group treat-ments are even more compelling than those based on simple pragmatics.

Empirical Foundations

Over five decades passed before it was pos-sible to offer sufficient research evidence to document the value of group treatments proposed by the originators of this ap-proach. The earliest reviews in the 1960s, based on the few outcome studies that had accumulated by that time, offered highly tentative conclusions about the efficacy of group interventions. Nevertheless, within the span of just a few more years it had be-come apparent from the mounting evi-dence that group treatments were indeed effective (Bednar & Lawlis, 1971). Subse-quent reviews of the empirical literature displayed even more confidence in the gen-eralization that various group formats were largely beneficial in their impact on group members (Dies, 1993; Piper & Joyce, 1996).

The issue of therapeutic efficacy for group treatments has been explored through a variety of methods. Just over two decades ago, for example, Smith, Glass, and Miller (1980) introduced a quantitative technique called meta-analysis in their comprehensive critique of psychotherapy outcome in hundreds of studies conducted across a wide range of clinical settings; meta-analysis examines average change scores on pre–post measures of improvement. These authors concluded that group psychotherapy was just as effective as individual treatments in the alleviation of psychological disorders. This observation has generally been supported in subsequent meta-analytic reviews (e.g., Fuhriman & Burlingame, 1994; McRoberts, Burlingame, & Hoag, 1998; Piper & Joyce, 1996).

Toseland and Siporin (1986) cautioned that generalizations derived from meta-analysis are based on studies using different therapeutic approaches rather than investigations making direct comparisons among the treatment modalities. That is, "average effect sizes" for studies of different one-to-one treatment approaches have been compared with other investigations examining outcome for varying forms of group intervention. Toseland and Siporin, therefore, scanned the literature for published reports in which individual and group treatments were directly contrasted. They identified 32 studies that satisfied their standards for experimental design and discovered that in 24 of these investigations, no significant differences in effectiveness were identified between the two treatment modalities. In the eight remaining studies, group psychotherapy was established as more effective than one-to-one treatment. Orlinsky and Howard (1986) arrived at the same conclusion of comparatively little differential outcome between individual and group treatments based on their systematic and thorough review of the psychosocial treatment literature; their generalization was based on a broader sampling of studies.

It is clear from these meta-analytic reviews and comprehensive surveys of the literature that group psychotherapy is indeed an effective form of treatment intervention. Although evidence relating specific group outcomes to particular patient diagnoses must be regarded as tentative, there is an increasing number of empirical reviews documenting the value of group treatments for patients suffering from depression (McDermut, Miller, & Brown, 2001), anxiety disorders (DeRubeis & Crits-Christoph, 1998), substance abuse (Velasquez, Maurer, Crouch, & DiClemente, 2001), eating disorders (Moreno, 1994), schizophrenia (Kanas, 1986), psychological trauma (Klein & Schermer, 2000), and other conditions. Moreover, a number of reviews have shown that the risk of negative outcome from group treatments is generally quite negligible (e.g., Erickson, 1987; Orlinsky & Howard, 1986).

Although group psychotherapy was initiated by Joseph Pratt and other early clinicians to address matters of convenience and expediency, there is little question that the theoretical and empirical foundations for group treatments have assumed much greater importance in contemporary practice. Once thought to be a secondary form of treatment, group interventions have now become the treatment of choice for many practitioners. Before we examine how participation in an intensive, change-oriented group can foster therapeutic growth, it may be useful to highlight general concepts of personality and psychopathology to better understand the rationale for group intervention.

THE CONCEPT OF PERSONALITY

There are a variety of conceptualizations of personality among clinicians who conduct therapy groups. Certainly, no one theoretical perspective can be said to embrace a monopoly in the field of group treatments. The traditional distinctions among psychodynamic, cognitive-behavioral, humanistic, and other viewpoints regarding the important formative, maintaining, and modifying factors that influence personality functioning are just as prevalent in the group treatment literature as they are elsewhere. Although critical dimensions for differentiating among various theories of personality have been outlined (e.g., conscious–unconscious, past–present–future, person–situation, holistic–analytic, purposive–mechanistic), it is clear that such "either–or" distinctions do not hold up under careful scrutiny (Hall & Lindzey, 1985).

Several years ago, for example, the author requested highly experienced group psychotherapists to identify the major theoretical orientations that best represent the contemporary practice of group psychotherapy, as well as the names of principal theorists aligned with each position (Dies, 1992b). The 111 senior clinicians who responded to the questionnaire furnished nearly 50 unique orientations and approximately 200 different names. Efforts to classify these responses into clear-cut theoretical positions proved to be rather challenging. Concepts used to describe models often overlapped or appeared in combination. For instance, "psychodynamic" was hyphenated with psychoanalytic, interpersonal, object relations, and group-as-a-whole approaches by varying numbers of respondents. Similarly, the names recommended as representatives of the various theoretical viewpoints were often highly inconsistent. Many of the names appeared under several categories (e.g., "psychodynamic" and "object relations" or "interpersonal" and "existential"). Although these dual identities may reflect an accurate portrayal of how the experts attempt to integrate their own perspectives, it is quite apparent that they suggest considerable confusion as well. Thus, Yalom (1995), whose book is the most widely used text for training prospective group therapists, was cited most frequently, but his name appeared under six different categories, including interpersonal, existential, psychodynamic, group-as-a-whole, object relations, and short term.

Ten models of group psychotherapy emerged as being most popular from this survey (they appear in order of endorsement): psychodynamic–psychoanalytic, group-as-a-whole, transactional analysis–Gestalt, interpersonal, cognitive-behavioral, object relations, group analysis, psychodrama, existential–humanistic, and self psychology. The conceptualizations of personality espoused by adherents of these theoretical models are highly divergent, as are their strategies for effecting therapeutic change. For example, the psychodynamic models (psychoanalytic, object relations, and self psychology approaches) stress the importance of early developmental phenomena, unconscious motivation, the role of defense mechanisms, repetition, and transference. Moreover, these clinicians adopt the position of therapeutic neutrality and strive to help patients explore individual dynamics and interpersonal transactions, making connections between manifest content and unresolved/unconscious conflicts that become activated within the treatment context but have as their foundation earlier experiences within dysfunctional family units. The principal goals of these clinicians are to foster insight and cathartic relief as means for promoting behavioral change.

In contrast, cognitive-behavioral and other action-oriented approaches (e.g., transactional analysis–Gestalt and psychodrama) emphasize basic learning processes in the formation of personality, current situational factors maintaining behavioral consistency, and the importance of the person's conscious assumptions in guiding behavioral choices. Based on the belief that "it is easier to act yourself into a new way of thinking than to think yourself into a new way of acting," these methods emphasize proactive structuring by the therapist and direct efforts to modify current dysfunctional thoughts, troublesome feelings, and maladaptive behaviors.

Finally, the interpersonal–existential theorists place considerable importance on positive growth tendencies, subjective experience, and relationships in shaping personality. In group treatment, they encourage honest expression, genuine encounter, and the role of the therapist as a transparent model of effective interpersonal functioning. Nevertheless, it is the quality of relationships established among the members that is primarily responsible for individual change.

Although dramatic differences exist in the models of personality that form the basis for the various systems of group psychotherapy, they inevitably share certain common assumptions. Thus, most theorists would agree with the definition provided by Phares (1991) that "personality is that pattern of characteristic thoughts, feelings, and behaviors that distinguishes one person from another and that persists over time and situations" (p. 4). Two aspects of this definition are central—stability of personality and that of distinctiveness.

Fundamental to the notion of stability or *consistency* is the premise that individuals who seek group psychotherapy will enter the treatment situation and display their central personality attributes, whether these are conceptualized as traits, learned habits, or unconscious drives. Although it may take some time for these cardinal features to become manifest, inevitably each person's "essence" will surface during the group interactions. The treatment setting provides a unique opportunity both to observe and to modify the stable aspects of personality that have proven to be counterproductive. In group psychotherapy, there is much less "talking about" outside interpersonal difficulties and more "living through" relationship issues within the context of treatment. The group therapy situation is less contrived than one-on-one treatment and, therefore, more likely to approximate the patient's day-to-day reality, that is, to stimulate the very conflicts that prompted the patient to seek treatment in the first place.

The group modality also has the potential to evoke uniquely powerful processes (e.g., consensual validation, shared unconscious fantasies, and multiple transferences) to effect changes in those maladaptive patterns. Sharing self-doubts, angry feelings, or inhibitions in the area of intimacy *with* a group of contemporaries is considerably different than disclosing those same feelings *to* an individual therapist who does not reciprocate. Similarly, struggling with peers to understand common interpersonal dilemmas while striving to construct facilitative group norms (e.g., learning how to express helpful feedback, giving support, and sharing time responsibly) represents a unique learning environment with characteristics not found in the one-to-one treatment setting. The correspondence of these interpersonal processes to external relationships increases the likelihood that learning will generalize beyond the immediate context of treatment.

The second feature that personality theories have in common relates to *distinctiveness* or to the idea that each person's unique or idiosyncratic features will emerge in everyday interactions. Once again, the value of group psychotherapy is that it provides a unique and powerful forum for exploring these individual differences. The group is viewed as a "social microcosm," or miniaturized society (Yalom, 1995), in which patients may not only learn a great deal about how different people think, feel, and behave in common situations but also discover how their own qualities and actions affect others through interpersonal feedback. In some sense, each patient serves as a therapist for others, not as an expert in psychopathology or group dynamics but as someone who, along with the other participants, can provide emotional support and consensual validation about interpersonal styles. In the individual treatment setting a therapist who comments, "many people feel that way," can be dismissed as someone whose job it is to be supportive or confrontational, but in the group situation it is much more difficult to minimize the shared input from multiple peers (Dies & Dies, 1993a).

As we have seen from this discussion, and from the earlier summary of empirical findings on treatment efficacy, participation in a therapy group can have highly positive effects on the amelioration of distress and on the modification of dysfunctional interpersonal patterns. Although it may seem counterintuitive that individuals who enter therapy because they cannot cope effectively in their relationships in the "real world" can be of considerable assistance to each other in the group treatment setting, that is precisely what happens. This observation that "patients can be therapists" requires an examination of basic assumptions about psychopathology and dysfunction.

PSYCHOLOGICAL HEALTH AND PATHOLOGY

Group psychotherapists do not share a common understanding about the nature of psychopathology any more than they adhere to identical models of personality. Moreover, their allegiance to group methods does not lead them to adopt perspectives different from their individual therapy colleagues' on how subjective distress or defective interpersonal patterns are developed or displayed. Depression and anxiety are still viewed as potentially unhealthy or debilitating emotional states, and exploitation of others and self-defeating lifestyles continue to be conceptualized as personality disorders.

Yet, group psychotherapists of all persuasions will definitely *search for the interpersonal* foundations or manifestations of psychopathology. If the focus is on etiology, the therapist will explore how early maladaptive relationships have contributed to the establishment of dysfunctional feelings or actions. If the emphasis is on symptomatic expression, the clinician will highlight how anguish and characterological deviance persistently undermine effective coping and the individual's sense of personal integrity. Thus, the common mind-set is to interpret maladjustment in interpersonal terms and to regard the group situation as uniquely

suited for the modification of pathological conditions.

According to psychodynamic theory, for example, "flaws in earlier developmental stages can be repaired if that stage can be recalled, relived, and affectively reexperienced correctively in the here and now" of group treatment (Rutan, 1992, p. 21). Similarly, interpersonal theorists assume that in "drawing attention to patients' interpersonal worlds, and the centrality of interaction within the group, as both a mechanism for illumination and for repair of interpersonal disturbance, a powerful modality is accessed" (Leszcz, 1992, p. 60). Finally, a cognitive-behavioral theorist might state that patients "usually give advice to each other, show how others' behavior had better be changed outside the group, and check to see if their homework suggestions are actually being carried out. Again, they normally interact with each other in the group itself, comment on each other's in-group behaviors, and give themselves practice in changing some of their dysfunctional interactions" (Ellis, 1992, pp. 77–78).

Implicit in each of these descriptions is a second common bond among group psychotherapists, and that is their faith that individual patients, in spite of their disabilities, have the *potential to contribute constructively* in creating a powerful therapeutic environment for effecting meaningful clinical change. Many patients initially fear that participation in a therapy group with other "disturbed" people might only exacerbate their own problems, but research findings clearly demonstrate that groups exert a positive influence on improved functioning for a vast majority of the participants (Dies, 1992a). This is even the case when the patients are regarded as seriously mentally ill (e.g., Kanas, 1986). Thus, individuals who are labeled "schizophrenic," "borderline," "anxiety disordered," or even "antisocial" are not completely maladjusted or incapacitated. "Psychopathology" is not an all-or-none phenomenon. The ability of patients to offer emotional support and understanding, to share painful feelings, to furnish interpersonal validation, and/or to challenge distorted ideas or inappropriate behaviors can be enormously helpful.

THE PROCESS OF CLINICAL ASSESSMENT

One purpose of assessment is to ensure adequate understanding of the patient's problems so that a proper assignment to treatment can be established. Unfortunately, clinicians have tended to rely too heavily on traditional diagnostic interviews and psychological tests that have not allowed this patient–treatment "match" to be made most effectively (Woods & Melnick, 1979). The use of broad-band instruments (e.g., MMPI-2 and Rorschach) is often too time-consuming and impractical in most treatment settings. Although there has been increased emphasis on (1) the development of interpersonal measures that predict social behavior in group situations (e.g., Keisler, 1986); (2) "rapid-fire," self-report instruments to identify appropriate targets for treatment modification (Corcoran & Fischer, 2000); as well as (3) efforts to employ "pretherapy group trials" (e.g., Mayerson, 1984; Yalom, 1995), the results are too limited to be of much practical value (Dies, 1993). In contrast, Maruish (2002) provides clinicians with concrete guidelines for how to "survive and thrive" in the era of managed behavioral health care. His text reviews useful psychological measures and offers helpful recommendations for developing test-based assessments of outcome.

Patients carrying a full range of diagnostic labels have been successfully treated with group methods, but the central issue is whether a particular treatment group is suitable for a specific patient at a given point in time. Thus, although some authors have argued that paranoid, drug-addicted, acutely psychotic, antisocial, or organically impaired individuals are poor candidates for group treatment, others have taken the opposite

stance based on their position that homogeneous groups could be designed to work effectively with such patients (Unger, 1989).

It has become evident that therapists do not actually select patients for group psychotherapy but rather *deselect* or exclude those who seem to be inappropriate. Vinogradov and Yalom (1989), for example, offer guidelines that are not based on traditional diagnostic criteria. Their standards for exclusion highlight the patient's inability to tolerate the group treatment situation, the likelihood of assuming a deviant role within the group, extreme agitation, potential noncompliance with group norms, and marked incompatibility with one or more of the other group members. Their inclusion indices consist of the capacity to perform the group task, motivation to participate in treatment, commitment to attend sessions regularly, and congruence of the patient's problems with the goals of the group. Klein (1985) also notes that patients who have circumscribed complaints, acute onset of symptoms, and a history of good premorbid adjustment will generally benefit most from treatment.

Other clinicians have explored factors contributing to premature dropouts from group therapy to identify potential factors relevant to selection. Thus, Roback and Smith (1987) chose to highlight characterological defenses that result in major interpersonal deficits: "Included in this category are problems with self-disclosure, difficulties with intimacy, generalized interpersonal distrust, excessive use of denial, and a tendency to be either verbally subdued or hostile" (p. 427). Other considerations include patients with unrealistic expectations, persons in situational crises who are too preoccupied to engage effectively in group therapeutic work, and borderline, narcissistic, schizoid, or acutely disturbed patients who are placed in group therapy prematurely (Dies & Teleska, 1985).

It is clear that assessment goes far beyond the issue of finding a proper "diagnosis," and that it includes a more comprehensive understanding of the patient's personality and preoccupations, as well as an adequate evaluation of the nature of treatment and the context in which it occurs (Piper, Joyce, McCallum, Azim, & Ogrodniczuk, 2002). Thus, although a particular depressed patient may be suitable for group therapy, it would be unwise to place this individual in a group composed predominantly of antisocial personalities. Nor would it be prudent to assign a chronically mental ill woman to a group composed of less troubled anxiety-disordered individuals. In both cases, we may have made an adequate "diagnosis" of the patient, but in neither instance is there an adequate match between the patient and the group. The depressed and schizophrenic patients might become misfits in their respective groups, have difficulty keeping pace with fellow members, and risk becoming either scapegoated or, even worse, group casualties. Furthermore, these two patients might require so much attention that the progress of the other group members would be stalled needlessly. Therefore, it would be more appropriate to find a reasonable alternative, such as individual therapy or a different treatment group.

At present, there is increased emphasis on how assessment tools may be used to augment treatment and to understand the variables that might improve the quality of service delivery. Elsewhere, the author has proposed a comprehensive model to illustrate how measures may be used during four phases of group treatment (Dies & Dies, 1993b). For example, in the *negotiation* phase, when patients are making decisions about entering treatment, assessment procedures are used to identify unrealistic expectations about group therapy, to educate patients about therapeutic factors and patient roles, to establish concrete treatment objectives, and to facilitate proper assignment to treatment options. One of the major deterrents to adequate commitment to therapy relates to patients' misunderstandings about the process. It has been shown that by addressing these misconceptions early, clini-

cians may substantially enhance their patients' involvement in the treatment process (Tinsley, Bowman, & Ray, 1988).

Group therapy may be especially intimidating for many individuals. Piper and Joyce (1996) have suggested that compared to individual therapy, patients often experience less control in a group. These authors also propose that there is a diminished sense of individuality, less understanding of events that transpire within a session, less privacy, and a lessened sense of safety within group treatments. Fear of attack, embarrassment, emotional contagion or coercion, and misgivings about actual harmful effects in the group setting may lead certain patients to avoid the very treatment that could best address their interpersonal conflicts (Subich & Coursol, 1985). The clinician who fails to understand these pervasive anxieties may lose many prospective patients who could be attracted to treatment if only they would be permitted to discuss these issues before a specific therapy was recommended.

During the *retention* phase of group psychotherapy, when there is a risk that patients will terminate prematurely, assessment tools may be used to identify treatment obstacles, to uncover continuing misunderstandings about therapy, and to strengthen the therapeutic bond through more effective dialogue (Dies & Dies, 1993b). Many of the evaluation procedures solicit feedback from patients about their perceptions of group process and the therapist's interventions. Thus, assessment is clearly not just used to diagnose symptomatology or dysfunction in patients but may also be applied to "diagnose" problems in the group system. For example, patients may complete a Group Climate Questionnaire to evaluate their perceptions of the group environment along such dimensions as engagement, conflict, and avoidance (MacKenzie, 1983). The Group Atmosphere Scale (Silbergeld, Koenig, Manderscheid, Meeker, & Hornung, 1975), the Group Environment Scale (Moos, 1986), and the Group Leader Behavior Instrument (Phipps & Zastowny,

1988) have also been used to understand group members' perceptions of important group events that may affect their participation in treatment.

There is a twofold purpose to this type of assessment. The first is a focus on the group system to identify dysfunction at that level (e.g., insufficient cohesion and excessive avoidance). The second goal is to detect particular individuals whose ratings of the group are discrepant from those of other patients, suggesting a failure to bond effectively with co-members or expressing discomfort about the level of a friction within the group. This information may allow the clinician to work more specifically with these patients to overcome the problems that interfere with alliance with the group and/or to confront obstacles that may impede the development of a more constructive group atmosphere.

In the remaining two stages of group development, *enhancement* and *evaluation,* assessment instruments are once again introduced to understand patient and treatment variables that may affect therapeutic progress (Dies & Dies, 1993b). Many clinicians have discovered that the periodic administration of self-report measures can add greatly to their understanding of their patients and group treatments, with the full cooperation of their patients and without significant investment of additional time (Dies, 1983a, 1987, 1992a).

This broadened view of assessment is spurred in part by a variety of pressures placed on clinicians to justify the nature of their therapeutic interventions and to document treatment progress and overall outcome. This renewed interest in evaluation is apparent in the proliferation of articles and books on how practitioners can incorporate instruments into their clinical work, not only to improve their objective understanding of diagnostic (Wetzler, 1989) and treatment issues (Antony & Barlow, 2001) but also to enhance the quality of their therapeutic interventions (Corcoran & Fischer, 2000; Dies & Dies, 1993b).

There is increased interest in cross-cultural and multicultural assessment (Dana, 2000), based on recommendations that psychotherapists must become more sensitive to issues of diversity in order to be more effective. Salvendy (1999) has argued, for example, that there are culturally determined contrasts in perceptions, attitudes, communication, and behavior which minority members may exhibit in group treatments. If not properly understood by the psychotherapist, such multiethnic differences may lead to serious obstacles in group development or contribute to counterproductive outcomes for individual clients. Some experts have discussed how clinicians may refine their understanding of multicultural counseling (e.g., Fischer, Jome, & Atkinson, 1998; Johnson, Torres, Coleman, & Smith, 1995), whereas other mental health professionals have published concrete guidelines for assessing multicultural competencies (e.g., Haley-Banez, Brown, & Molina, 1999; Hansen, Pepitone-Arreola-Rockwell, & Greene, 2000).

THE PRACTICE OF THERAPY

There are wide variations in the application of group psychotherapy that relate to differences in theoretical orientation, the style of the individual practitioner, and perhaps most important, the setting within which the treatment is conducted.

Basic Structure of Therapy

The once-a-week, 1½-hour session appears to be the most common group format, but the professional context will determine how this is modified. Certainly, in most private practice settings and outpatient agencies this arrangement is most likely to occur. For clinicians who work in inpatient or partial hospitalization programs, however, groups may meet several times each week and may even be scheduled daily. Institutionalized patients are also more likely to be exposed to a variety of adjunctive treatments, including recreational and occupational therapies, alternative group formats, and psychodrama, as well as drug treatments.

Historically, *combined treatments* have been shown to be more effective than single interventions (e.g., Parloff & Dies, 1977), but clinicians have differed in their views regarding how best to achieve this integration. At present, there is more attention devoted to the effective melding of treatment components to ensure that the special advantages of each method dovetail congruently with the unique strengths of the other interventions (Dies, 1992a). The once prevalent psychotherapy-versus-psychobiology schism, for instance, has diminished, and there are increased indications of complementarity in the group literature (Rodenhauser, 1989). Authors are addressing more specific interface issues (Fink, 1989) and discussing how to circumvent roadblocks preventing successful combined psychopharmacological and group treatments (Salvendy & Joffe, 1991). This type of integration appears to have generalized interdisciplinary support (Stone, Rodenhauser, & Markert, 1991).

There are signals of revived interest in the integration of other treatment modalities as well. For example, Wong (1983) observed that fewer publications on combined individual and group therapy appeared in the 1970s and 1980s than in the prior two decades, but he emphasized that subsequent publications give more attention to concrete guidelines for achieving successful synthesis (Gans, 1990; Lipsius, 1991). This observation seems valid for marital and group modalities as well (Coche & Coche, 1990).

Another structural variation in the application of group methods relates to *treatment duration*. Although concern has been expressed that brief forms of therapy may furnish only transitory or circumscribed relief for many individuals whose conflicts are long-standing and deeply ingrained (Dies, 1992a), predictions by experts in the mental health field suggest that the popularity of short-term group treatments will increase substantially in the foreseeable future; in contrast, more conventional time-extended and one-to-one approaches are expected to decline in importance (Norcross, Alford, & DeMichele, 1992). "Short term" generally refers to treatments that extend no more than 25 sessions (Dies & Dies, 1993a). Messer (2001) has demonstrated that proponents of most theoretical approaches to treatment have streamlined their intervention strategies to maximize the benefits of brief psychotherapy.

Several strands of influence encourage the widespread acceptance of brief group interventions, including (1) pressures from legislators, insurance companies, and patient consumers for safe and cost-efficient psychological treatments; (2) the promise of relatively rapid relief from painful emotional states without substantial commitment of time and money; and (3) the actual demonstration of the effectiveness of time-limited groups (Dies, 1992a). Managed care companies have been shown to favor group treatments that are time-limited and highly structured over individual psychotherapies (Taylor et al., 2001).

There is general agreement that brief forms of psychosocial treatment require the establishment of more modest goals, greater attention to task focus, prompt interventions, and more active participation on the part of the therapist (Koss & Butcher, 1986). Given the time-limited nature of treatment, clinicians are more likely to focus on symptomatic relief, improved self-esteem, reduction of interpersonal apprehensions, development of social skills and problem-solving strategies, and efforts to ensure that patients gain a basic sense of peer acceptance (Dies & Dies, 1993a). As the duration of therapy increases, more attention can be directed to conflicts that are less accessible to conscious awareness, to maladaptive behavioral patterns that are more rigidly entrenched, and to a greater understanding of the pathogenic developmental experiences that predispose patients to personal suffering and interpersonal strife.

To enhance the efficiency and effectiveness of short-term group treatments, clinicians are now inclined to compose groups more homogeneously. Groups consisting of members who share common life experiences (e.g., recent loss of a loved one, disability, transition back to the community after hospitalization, and sexual victimization) and/or similar symptoms are generally defined as homogeneous, although other considerations would include age, gender, and occupational status. Melnick and Woods (1976) concluded from their review of the literature that homogeneous groups appear to "coalesce more quickly, offer more immediate support to members, have better attendance, less conflict, and provide more rapid symptomatic relief. However, they are seen as remaining at more superficial levels of interaction and are less effective in producing more fundamental interpersonal learning" (p. 495).

These authors suggest that group composition should be guided toward furnishing an optimal balance between conditions maximizing interpersonal learning (heterogeneity) and considerations ensuring group preservation (homogeneity). They propose a support-plus-confrontation model favoring demographic similarity, avoidance of patients with high potential for becoming group misfits, and efforts to create a reasonable balance in terms of symptomatic patterns, interpersonal styles, and coping resources. Recent evidence suggests, however, that these concerns are probably most critical for longer-term groups because the active structuring inherent in abbreviated formats may serve to moderate the influence of composition to some extent (Waltman & Zimpfer, 1988).

Another factor in structuring group treatments relates to the distinction between *open-ended* and *closed* groups. Usually, open-ended groups continue indefinitely and maintain a consistent size by replacing patients as they conclude their own therapy (Yalom, 1995). The ebb and flow of membership has a significant affect on the group process, however, which can be detrimental if the therapist and patients do not address the issues productively. The loss of members, especially if the departures are premature, can undermine the integrity of the group system by raising questions about trust, commitment, and shared responsibility. Invariably, the addition of new patients serves to recycle unresolved issues such as those concerning confidentiality, competition, and conflicts over control and intimacy. On the other hand, if these dilemmas are addressed effectively, patients may gain valuable insights into how to communicate feelings honestly and directly, to cope with loss meaningfully, and to respond to awkward transitions more adaptively.

The closed-group format has been recommended as a way to circumvent the adverse consequences of rotating membership. Although closed groups are perhaps only feasible in short-term treatment, the stability of group composition is believed to facilitate cohesion and commitment and to allow patients to remain more productively focused on their individual goals because they are less likely to become sidetracked by group-level concerns prompted by the loss of old members and the addition of new ones.

It has become more common in the field of group psychotherapy for clinicians to incorporate *treatment manuals* to structure their sessions (Addis & Krasnow, 2000). Most often used with closed, short-term group formats, and with clients who share similar presenting symptoms, these manuals offer detailed guidelines for how to conduct group sessions. Despite differences in theoretical orientation (e.g., cognitive-behavioral, psychodynamic, and existential) these manuals share many common ingredients (Dies, 1994a). Thus, the basic rationale for treatment, ground rules for interaction, clarification of patient and therapist roles, and similar issues are reviewed early in treatment. Goal setting and evaluation of expectations also occur early, and sessions are then planned to ensure meaningful progress toward individually defined goals. Session-by-session plans for how to guide interaction (process) and what topics to address (content) are typically furnished to guarantee continuity across sessions. Concerted effort is made to establish a supportive climate for interaction by highlighting strategies for promoting group cohesion. Although these manuals vary in the specific skills that are addressed (e.g., active listening, self-talk, behavior-targeting, and self-reinforcement), most outline a sequence of learning involving general instruction, followed by problem identification, individual sharing and behavioral practice, and then interpersonal feedback.

Goal Setting

During the selection process, clinicians attempt to ensure that patients are viable candidates for group treatment—that is, distressed but not too agitated, impulsive, or manipulative to disrupt treatment; willing to cooperate with others; and generally compatible along important symptomatic and interpersonal dimensions. The paramount issue is that of "matching," that is, in evaluating the individual's appropriateness for group treatment (selection) and his or her compatibility with the other group members (composition). A corollary issue is that of contracting, which is designed to enhance the therapeutic "fit" by refining individual goals and teaching patients about treatment parameters (Dies, 1993).

Numerous reviews of the literature have shown that various interventions to prepare patients for psychotherapy (e.g., audio and videotapes, verbal instructions, printed materials, and interviews) have been quite productive in generating greater patient investment in treatment and fostering improved therapeutic outcomes (Mayerson, 1984; Orlinsky & Howard, 1986). These pretreatment interventions have attempted to mol-

lify negative anticipations regarding treatment while instilling positive role and outcome expectations, and by educating patients about constructive interpersonal behaviors, group developmental issues, and helpful therapeutic factors (Dies, 1993). Research shows that multiple strategies for informing patients about treatment are generally superior to single methods (Kivlighan, Corazzini, & McGovern, 1985), and that more realistic interventions (e.g., videotapes or practice sessions) are more productive (Tinsley et al., 1988).

Researchers have evaluated efforts to provide specific information to patients about role behaviors and group process. Kivlighan and his colleagues (1985), for example, demonstrated the value of teaching prospective group members about role-related behaviors such as self-disclosure, interpersonal feedback, anxiety management, and here-and-now interaction. Others have illustrated the merits of educating patients about various dimensions of group process (Yalom, 1995). Most critical, of course, given the patients' diffuse anxieties about group interventions, is the need to furnish a solid rationale for treatment in the group format. Mayerson (1984) tells patients that, the "group therapy setting is one which provides a special opportunity to interact with others so as to gain insight into one's current interactional patterns and to experiment with new ones" (p. 194). The interpersonal nature of psychopathology is emphasized, if not in its etiology at least in terms of its manifestation and resolution. Also highlighted in pregroup training are general ground rules (e.g., confidentiality and regular attendance), developmental trends, and a general description of therapeutic factors or central interpersonal processes that foster individual gain. These pretreatment interventions are designed to provide a coherent framework for understanding experiences and events within the group, and to minimize the likelihood of premature attrition and therapeutic casualties (Dies & Teleska, 1985).

Considerable attention is also given to the patients' individual goals for therapy. One facet of the assessment process described earlier in this chapter was to help patients identify specific treatment objectives. A variety of instruments may be introduced to facilitate this process, including standard symptom checklists, personality tests, and individualized target goal forms (Dies & Dies, 1993b). When patients are able to define their goals more concretely, they are much more likely to remain in treatment (Garfield, 1986) and to make meaningful strides in overcoming the problems that initially prompted them to seek the guidance of a mental health practitioner.

Based on their review of 35 years of empirical research on goal setting, Locke and Latham (2002) demonstrated that goals affect performance through four mechanisms: (1) by serving to direct attention and effort toward goal-relevant activities; (2) by providing an energizing function; (3) by affecting persistence; and (4) by leading to the arousal, discovery, and/or use of task-relevant knowledge and strategies. They found first that making a public commitment to goals (such as in group psychotherapy), "enhances commitment, presumably because it makes one's actions a matter of integrity in one's own eyes and in those of others" (p. 707), and second that interpersonal feedback further improves the person's goal attainment.

Process Aspects of Treatment

Careful selection of individual patients, proper assignment to appropriate treatment groups, and pregroup training and goal setting provide the foundation for effective group intervention. Nevertheless, the real "work" of therapy begins once the patient enters the group. How this work is accomplished is virtually impossible to sketch without a few words about the therapist's theoretical orientation and whether the group format is open or closed, brief or long term, or conducted within an inpatient or outpatient facility.

The therapist's *conceptual framework* will obviously influence the choice of leadership strategies and the target of interventions. Table 13.1, for example, summarizes some of the differences that were found in a sur-

TABLE 13.1. Leadership Issues during the Working Phase of Group Therapy

Psychodynamic	Interpersonal	Action-oriented
Important considerations		
Countertransference	Cohesiveness	Cognitive reframing
Transference	Countertransference	Facilitating feedback
Identifying underlying process	Facilitating self-disclosure	Goal setting
Resistance	Here-and-now activation	Here-and-now activation
Boundary management	Identifying underlying process	Behavioral practice
Interpretation	Transference	Role playing
Nonverbal communication	Therapist openness	Fostering generalization
Unimportant considerations		
Reinforcement methods	Agenda setting	Boundary management
Cognitive reframing	Reinforcement methods	Norm building
Fostering generalization	Cognitive reframing	Identifying underlying process
Role playing	Behavioral practice	Interpretation
Structured exercises	Fostering generalization	Process commentary
Teaching problem-solving	Interpretation	Subgroup formation
Behavioral practice	Teaching problem solving	Therapeutic factors

vey of experienced group psychotherapists representing different theoretical models (Dies, 1992b). These clinicians were requested to indicate the types of leadership issues that were important for therapists to understand during the working phases of group treatment.

Obviously, there are clear differences among the three different perspectives examined, with the action-oriented therapists (e.g., cognitive-behavioral) being distinctly different from both the interpersonal and psychodynamic group psychotherapists (see the "Important" and "Unimportant" items listed under each approach in Table 13.1). Thus, clinicians who are grounded in learning theory are more likely to embrace the centrality of such leadership strategies as cognitive reframing, facilitating behavioral practice, and role playing, and to deemphasize interpretation, exploration of underlying group themes, and boundary management. Almost the opposite is true for psychodynamic therapists who eschew the importance of action-based techniques (e.g., behavioral practice, cognitive reframing, and role playing), and highlight the merits of interpreting transference and countertransference phenomena, resistance, and latent group process. Those clinicians who favor the interpersonal approach share some of these considerations, but, as expected, they are uniquely inclined to endorse the importance of group cohesion and therapist self-disclosure. The specific implications of these differences are less important for this presentation than the simple fact that they demonstrate that generic models of group intervention do not exist.

Other structural and contextual variations also shape the nature of therapeutic practice. For example, in a *closed group* all the patients share a similar understanding of the scheduled number of sessions and have agreed to remain in treatment until that facet of the contract is fulfilled. They are aware of how much time is available to work on individual problems and are less likely to be diverted by issues relating to

premature dropouts and/or departures due to other patients completion of therapy. The stability of membership and common time frame will give the group system a greater sense of integrity. Although members will invariably progress at their own pace, there will be a more or less predictable sequence of themes revolving around such issues as engagement, differentiation, individuation, intimacy, mutuality, and, finally, dissolution of the group (MacKenzie & Livesley, 1983).

In an *open-ended* group, however, these developmental hurdles will be expressed uniquely as a function of who, when, and how members join or leave the group system. Thus, in the ongoing group there will not be a shared ending but a series of terminations that will require more individualized attention. Similarly, the addition of each new member will necessitate preparation of both the individual patient and the group system for the reactions that are likely to be stimulated by these changes. Thus, group "process" issues may demand more attention than individual "content" concerns in the open-ended group. This is not to suggest that closed groups are more effective (because an experienced group therapist can use these group events to create opportunities for individual growth) but, rather, to convey that these system-level transitions will clearly influence the clinician's decisions about leadership strategies.

Corresponding arguments could be offered for the contrasts between *short-term* and more *time-extended* treatments. We noted earlier that abbreviated treatments demand more attention to task efficiency. It is ill-advised, for example, for the therapist in the brief group setting to remain passive based on the hope that patients will readily assume responsibility for structuring the group experience or that they will promptly learn how to confront difficult relationship issues effectively, without some active guidance from the clinician. Indeed, a majority of the patients who enter treatment have volunteered because they have been unable to manage their own "interpersonal lives" without substantial discomfort or strife. If patients had the skills to negotiate the complex exchanges in creating a viable group system, they probably would not be seeking treatment. The group therapist on the other hand, has received specialized training and often has years of experience in how to promote facilitative group processes that are conducive to individual change.

There are likely to be dramatic differences in *context* between groups conducted within inpatient and outpatient facilities. Residential groups may convene more times each week, there are more likely to be disruptions due to the need for ancillary treatments, and patients will be more symptomatically disturbed. Issues of confidentiality take on new meaning because patients interact in so many other formal and informal ways within the therapeutic milieu (e.g., recreational therapy, psychodrama, and in the dining hall). More structured interventions such as social skills training and more confrontational leadership styles may be possible or even necessary. Thus, an inpatient therapist who directly challenges a particular patient's counterproductive interpersonal behaviors knows that other ward personnel are available after the group session to follow through and to comfort the distressed group member. In contrast, the private practitioner cannot trust that a supportive friend will be there to "pick up the pieces" after the patient has been placed on the therapeutic "hot seat" and then sent home. Therapists in the hospital setting may also make different decisions about how to share their own feelings in therapy because seriously disordered patients may have greater conflicts around "boundary issues" and may misinterpret the more transparent clinician's intentions in revealing personal experiences (Dies, 1983b).

Clearly, the nature of the therapist's interventions is influenced by a broad spectrum of factors. Nonetheless, there are several considerations that are reasonably common across treatment settings. Earlier in this chapter we noted that therapists vary in their focus of *intervention*—individual, interpersonal, or group-as-a-whole—as a function of their theoretical perspective. Despite these variations, most therapists will attend more to group-level (process) issues in the beginning phases of group development, switch to more individual patient concerns (content) in the "working phases" of the group, and then revert back to system-level themes as the group nears termination or as individual patients conclude their treatment.

Before group therapy can be effective there must first be a group. Simply convening six to eight patients in the same room is no guarantee that constructive interaction fostering individual improvement will transpire. Therapists must actively intervene to ensure that clients are motivated to discuss personal problems and to understand that risk taking may produce beneficial consequences. For this to happen, a *basic rationale for group treatment* must be conveyed and a *climate conducive to personal disclosure* must be established. Such group-level considerations as "culture building" and "norm setting" must be addressed (Yalom, 1995), and certain procedural and process guidelines must be instituted (e.g., confidentiality, ground rules about outside socializing, active listening, shared responsibility, and supportiveness). Initial structuring that clarifies the nature of the therapeutic task and builds supportive norms and highlights positive member interactions is generally essential (Dies, 1994a, 1994b; Dies & Dies, 1993a), and most clinicians will intervene to make these issues clear within the terminology of their own model of therapy.

Once patients have established a common framework for personalized interaction, experienced a sense of bonding with others (cohesion), and made at least a tentative commitment to the group, it is possible to shift the focus of intervention to more individualized therapeutic work. As patients share painful feelings and self-doubts, test faulty assumptions, risk new behaviors, and provide mutually supportive or constructively critical feedback, the level of group cohesiveness increases and even more intensive individual exploration is possible. This working phase may last for quite some time, depending on the nature of the therapeutic arrangement. Inevitably, certain patients will decide that their "work" is finished and that it is time to discontinue their treatment; in short-term groups this ending point is often built into the contract. When termination occurs it is generally necessary for the clinician to refocus on group-as-a-whole issues to some extent. The meaning of termination for the individual patient is obviously examined, but it is often necessary for the clinician to resume a more active role so that other members deal effectively with the emotional impact of the "loss," and that they discuss the implications for the group system as well (Dies & Dies, 1993). Although there are wide variations in how different therapists address these group developmental issues, virtually all clinicians modify their focus on individual, interpersonal, or group-level concerns as a function of transitional events that impact upon the entire system.

Another common ingredient across treatment settings is the *effort to translate problems into interpersonal concepts*. Whether the therapist is psychodynamic, cognitive-behavioral, or existential, the group is inherently interpersonal. For example, although depression can be viewed from a strictly individual or intrapsychic point of view, it is much more profitable to explore the social contexts that precipitate the negative affect or dysfunctional thoughts, the interpersonal consequences of feeling sad and gloomy (e.g., social withdrawal, irritability, and excessive dependency), and the interpersonal processes within the group that may be applied to alter the maladaptive condition (e.g., mutual support, feedback, altruism, and vicarious learning) (Dies, 1994b).

Similarly, most clinicians will accentuate the *activation of the here and now*. A basic premise is that their patients' troubling feelings and inadequate coping skills will be "replayed" within the group context in ways that parallel how they are manifest in relationships in the "outside" world. Thus, a patient who complains of being unable to trust others will display that cautious and guarded stance within the group. Another who has trouble with self-assertion will most likely assume a passive role in group interactions. The depressed patient who cannot understand why he or she continues to be rejected by friends and family will undoubtedly engage in comparable self-defeating and other-alienating behaviors within the group (e.g., pessimism, whining self-centeredness, and insensitivity to others' feelings). In each instance, it will not be necessary to furnish reports about problems that happen "out there" because they will be abundantly illustrated "in here." Moreover, the cohesive interpersonal forum that has been established within treatment will allow these dysfunctional patterns to be explored, confronted, and worked through in ways that are not feasible in routine social interactions (Yalom, 1995).

A majority of group psychotherapists will generally *think group*. For most clinicians (but not all), treatment is conducted *through* a group, not *in* a group. Group treatment is not one-on-one therapy with an audience, with members taking turns working exclusively with the clinician, but rather a complex interactive process in which the quality of relationships among members is much more critical to therapeutic gain than the nature of the therapist–patient bond; *it is the group that is the agent of change* not the therapist (Yalom, 1995). Research by Holmes and Kivlighan (2000) shows that there are unique processes that occur within group and individual treatments. These authors found, for example, that "the components of relationship-climate and other versus self-focus are more prominent in group psychotherapy, whereas emotional awareness-insight and problem definition-change are more central to the process of individual treatment" (p. 482).

Another way in which the "think group" framework is reflected is in the therapist's choice of interventions. Most clinicians attempt to maximize the therapeutic impact of their techniques by searching for common "core" issues that unite patients around the shared human dilemmas that brought them to treatment (e.g., damaged self-esteem and recurring self-defeating patterns) (Dies & Dies, 1993). Moreover, most group therapists will also weigh the impact of interventions in terms of individual needs versus benefits available to the remaining members. In rare instances (e.g., potential suicide) will the needs of the majority be sacrificed for the sake of an individual. Fortunately, this immediate decision is seldom faced because virtually every condition is pertinent to at least some of the other members, but there are times when an individual patient will be removed from a group when she or he is an obvious "misfit," or when the pathology is too acute or intrusive.

Group psychotherapists devote a significant portion of their time to ensure that the group climate is prepared for important individualized work. Thus, the group system is nurtured so that the patients' understanding of how change occurs is reasonably clear and that the emotional atmosphere is experienced as supportive (Dies, 1994a). When these conditions prevail, group members are more inclined to reveal intimate material, to attempt new behaviors, and to offer meaningful interpersonal feedback. These represent the "mediating goals" for group treatment. The "ultimate" goal, of course, is the amelioration of the distress and/or modification of the deviant interpersonal patterns that precipitated entrance into treatment.

As the principal standard bearer of the "group culture," the group leader facilitates a focus on developmental obstacles that might limit group cohesion or impede constructive interpersonal work (e.g., premature dropouts, irregular attendance, breaches in confidentiality, outside socializing, and subgrouping). This "social engineering" function highlights similarities among members, reinforces behaviors that indicate risk taking, encourages and supports members who model appropriate actions, confronts counternormative behavior, activates a here-and-now focus, and offers process commentary to illuminate undercurrents that are potentially detrimental (Yalom, 1995).

The formative stages of group development are negotiated so that members feel accepted and recognize the value of compliance with group norms without the need for rebellion or the fear of losing their individuality (MacKenzie, 1987). The various roles that members adopt are addressed to foster their constructive contribution to group development, whether they are the emotional or task-oriented members or those who represent more discrepant roles (e.g., the cautious or guarded individual who may help to elicit feelings that others are reluctant to share) (Bahrey, McCallum, & Piper, 1991; Livesley & MacKenzie, 1983).

Members will not enter therapy with a clear comprehension of how group treatments can promote individual improvement, and it may take them some time to reach this understanding. Their notions about how individuals overcome personal dilemmas and interpersonal conflicts are frequently based on faulty impressions gained from such sources as television situational comedies or popularized accounts of individual therapy depicting intensive uncovering of childhood traumas until flashes of insight are achieved and pent-up emotions are released, thereby effecting therapeutic "cure." Thus, from the patients' viewpoint, the goal is to discuss personal problems that are evident in outside relationships, many of which derive from earlier experiences (i.e., the so-called skeletons in the closet) so they must be reviewed in historical perspective. Furthermore, patients assume that it is the therapist's responsibility to intervene to promote therapeutic change through deft questioning, sage interpretations, and other techniques to guide the uncovering process. The other group members are viewed as ancillary, and their roles are generally confined to asking questions, giving advice, and sharing similar experiences. They in turn will have their opportunities for therapeutic change, as the focus rotates around the membership. Often, the expectation is that with sufficient probing and self-examination, "insight" will be gained and emotional "catharsis" will ensue (see Table 13.2).

Most therapists will have a different view of how group treatments foster individual growth. Although some discussion of outside and even historically based problems is inevitable, the vital importance of interpersonal translations, here-and-now activation, and the "group as agent of change" must be brought to light. It is the process of mutual exploration and sharing, not turn taking, advising (psychologizing), and staccato-style question-and-answering that facilitates therapeutic understanding and improvement. The complementary processes of self-disclosure and interpersonal feedback are pivotal in the pursuit of self-awareness, cognitive restructuring, insight into others, emotional relief, and behavioral change.

Strong affective expression (catharsis) may indeed lead to a sense of release, especially if the patient is met with genuine support, efforts to understand, and mutual sharing by others. The care and acceptance from co-members may foster greater self-acceptance, and "putting the feelings on the table" might permit more objective exploration and sorting through confusion, which in turn can result in increased self-understanding. Patients can be encouraged to explore the intensity of their feelings, to revise their biased assumptions, to place their reactions in a more realistic perspective, and to weigh the value of holding onto such feelings in view of how their lives have changed over the years. Patients might also explore whether there are other courses of action they might take in situations before their feelings escalate disproportionately; instead of permitting anger to mount to a sense of rage, they might learn to respond more promptly when significant others engage in behaviors that trigger dissatisfaction.

Similarly, the group can be used to allow patients to "test their interpersonal assumptions." Thus, group members might first share what they want most from others in their lives (e.g., respect, affection, and/or recognition) or how they wish to be viewed by others (e.g., as friendly, competent, and/or sincere). They can describe how they attempt to generate those reactions, in general, and then consider how that style has been evident within the group. Then the de-

TABLE 13.2. "Theories" of Change in Group Treatments

Patients' view	Therapist's view
Share an "outside" problem	Manifest problems within the group
Personal/individual	Interpersonal/interactional
Historical ("skeletons" in the closet)	Here-and-now activation
Therapist as "healer"	Group as "healer"
Question-and-answer format	Mutual exploration
Advise	Self-disclosure
"Psychologize"	Interpersonal feedback
Turn taking	Behavioral practice
Insight acquired ("aha")	Increased understanding of self/others
Cathartic relief (personal emotional release)	Corrective emotional experience (interpersonal encounter)
Symptomatic "cure"	Improved coping and symptomatic relief

sired results can be evaluated: "How have others responded?" "Have you indeed been judged as friendly or sincere?" For example, a patient who has worked "so hard" to show genuine interest in others, and thus gain their respect and admiration, may discover that in actuality fellow group members have been "turned off" by the "phony display" of concern. The very outcome she has diligently pursued has eluded her, as it probably does in many relationships, and will continue to do so until she realizes how her own actions undermine the goals she strives so earnestly to achieve. Constructive feedback from co-members may allow her to discover new ways to express herself and thereby gain interpersonal acceptance. She might even be given specific homework assignments to practice in outside situations. As a follow-up, she could be asked to share how her "outside experiments" worked and, depending on the outcome, encouraged to practice alternative behaviors within treatment. One of the essential skills of a group therapist is to assist patients in generalizing from the treatment setting to external circumstances; "inside" material is translated into outside applications, and "outside" problems are explored for their here-and-now relevance.

When group members are invited to reflect on the factors that have contributed to their improvement through group psychotherapy, they typically assign most of the credit to the quality of the relationships they established with their co-members (Dies, 1983b, 1993). The therapist's contributions to treatment outcome are generally regarded as less direct (e.g., process commentary and providing structure), or as less impactful. Although the group therapist may be supportive, his or her efforts are often not as powerful as the combined input from multiple caring peers. Similarly, clinicians may be open and self-disclosing, but they will seldom reveal at the same level of intimacy as the group members. Feedback from the therapist is usually regarded as useful but will rarely have the same influence as the feedback from a panel of peers.

Nevertheless, two aspects of the group psychotherapist's role may be unique in helping patients to accomplish their goals. The first of these has already been highlighted, and that is the clinician's task orientation. Yalom (1995) notes that only the group leader can perform this function: "Forces prevent members from fully sharing that task with the therapist. One who comments on process sets oneself apart from the other members and is viewed with suspicion as 'not one of us' " (p. 146). Given the therapists' designated responsibility to ensure that all members progress toward individually defined objectives, as well as the clinician's specialized knowledge of group dynamics, they are in the best position to manage the group system.

The second distinct role of group psychotherapists is their capacity for effective confrontation and interpretation. Beutler, Crago, and Arizmendi (1986) found that more effective therapists tend to confront and interpret patient affect more often than their less helpful counterparts. Moreover, clinicians who do not shy away from demonstrations of patients' anger promote "more realistic and goal-directed expressions of affect on the part of their clients. Indeed, evidence from many sources suggests that rousing patient affect and motivating them to confront their fears enhances both cognitive and behavioral changes" (p. 294). Because group members may be reluctant to challenge, at least initially, potentially volatile feelings and are disinclined to deliver negative feedback (Kivlighan, 1985), the group psychotherapist should shoulder this responsibility by modeling this behavior and by prompting, reinforcing, and shaping members' willingness and ability to engage in constructive confrontation (Dies, 1993).

There is considerable evidence that interpretation is a principal vehicle for therapeutic change: "Providing concepts for how to understand, explaining, clarifying, interpreting, and providing frameworks for how to change" foster significant levels of patient improvement (Lieberman, Yalom, & Miles, 1973, p. 238). Group members may provide some of this function for each other, but this contribution is more specifically within the province of the psychotherapist who has "acquired and perfected the skill over many years of professional training and experience" (Scheidlinger, 1987, p. 348).

THE THERAPEUTIC RELATIONSHIP AND THE STANCE OF THE THERAPIST

We have already noted broad variations in therapist style as a function of theoretical orientation, structure of therapy (e.g., short term or time extended and open or closed), stage of group development (e.g., more group-centered earlier and individually focused in the working phases), and context of treatment (e.g., inpatient vs. outpatient). We have also suggested certain commonalities across approaches, such as the tendencies to translate problems into interpersonal concepts and to "think group," the effort to provide both a meaningful framework and supportive environment for clinical change, and the activation of the here-and-now.

Three other issues seem important to address briefly, and these relate to the levels of activity and self-disclosure that are appropriate for clinicians within treatment, and the topic of cotherapy.

Therapist Activity

Although debates about the nature of therapist activity have a long history in the literature, the popularity of short-term group treatments has prompted a renewed interest in this topic (Dies, 1985). The pressure to move the group along at a faster pace through more proactive interventions has caused many clinicians to worry about the implications of "control" inherent in their role. Clearly, the action-oriented clinicians (see Table 13.1) who incorporate such techniques as role playing, cognitive reframing,

and selective reinforcement would favor a more active therapeutic stance. On the other hand, most psychodynamic group therapists would prefer less structure and a more reactive leadership posture focusing on the interpretation of transference and resistance phenomena (Rutan, 1992). Each clinician must decide which style feels most comfortable and productive within his or her own treatment context.

The concern about increased structure or direction by clinicians, however, seems overplayed. There is little evidence to suggest that patients will necessarily experience more active or planned interventions as controlling. Directiveness should not be equated with "manipulation," at least in the pejorative sense of that term. Indeed, active therapists who are viewed as supportive, dedicated to guiding the group's development for the sake of meaningful individual work, and open about their interventions and personal feelings about events within treatment are seldom depicted as manipulative (Dies, 1985). This is true even when their interventions are "scripted" through detailed treatment manuals. One popular example of such treatments would be represented by cognitive-behavioral group interventions (e.g., Heimberg & Becker, 2002; Riess & Dockray-Miller, 2001; White & Freeman, 2000). The literature on such approaches rarely discusses objections raised by group members about the manipulative aspects of group leadership, in large part because the manuals emphasize the vital importance of the "therapeutic alliance" and the quality of the relationships established among members.

Research has uniformly demonstrated that patients experience greater tension and feel more critical toward therapists who are viewed as inactive, aloof, distant, and judgmental. This leadership style frequently stimulates confrontations around issues of authority and perhaps may even facilitate the working through of problems in this area (Dies, 1983b); ironically, it is also felt by many patients to be manipulative.

As therapists become more actively negative in their focus, the risks of harmful effects to patients increase. Understandably, some degree of confrontation and tension-inducing challenge by the therapist may be essential for individual change, after a climate of trust has been developed within the group, but when the therapist "comes on too strong," patients may drop out of treatment prematurely or actually become therapeutic casualties (Dies, 1983b, 1994a; Dies & Teleska, 1985; Roback & Smith, 1987).

THERAPIST SELF-DISCLOSURE

Perhaps even more controversial is the issue of therapist self-disclosure (Dies, 1977). Once again, the debate revolves around the clinicians' theoretical predilections. Whereas both interpersonal and action-oriented clinicians may endorse therapist "transparency" for the modeling that such behavior represents, the psychodynamically oriented group therapists prefer a more neutral or nonopen position based on their belief in the fundamental importance of understanding transference projections.

There is no "right" perspective on this topic because therapists of all persuasions can be very effective. Although there is evidence that therapist self-disclosure does indeed foster greater openness among group members, it is also clear that there are other means to facilitate patient self-revelation (e.g., invitations for personal sharing, modeling by other members, and prompting and supporting such expression). Moreover, there is scant evidence to suggest that therapist self-disclosure contributes to more constructive change for individual members (Dies, 1983b, 1993, 1994a). Once again, group psychotherapists must decide for themselves which stance is most compatible with their own general approach. For many, that position reflects a willingness to be selectively open about feelings generated by

events within the sessions but to avoid revealing much about their personal lives. What most patients seem to want is an assurance that their therapist is "real" (i.e., can experience a range of normal feelings and reactions such as anxiety, sadness, and compassion), and that they can relate to the therapist on an emotional level.

Cotherapy

When groups are co-led, as is the case within a significant proportion of treatment settings, the issues of therapist activity and openness require a delicate balancing act between the two clinicians (Dies, 1983b). Although the cotherapists may differ or alternate naturally over the course of group development, it is important that there is reasonable harmony within the team. The literature suggests that compatibility despite dissimilarity is the key consideration, and that the capacity to model an open and positive relationship within sessions is central in maintaining an effective team. Interestingly, there is little evidence that co-led groups are any more productive than groups conducted by one therapist (Dies, 1983b, 1994a).

Whereas the notion that cotherapists can use their own relationship to "model" or demonstrate effective interpersonal behaviors, such as self-disclosure, mutual support, or conflict resolution, is quite appealing, it has never been documented through research. In fact, a recent empirical evaluation of the idea that mutual self-disclosure between the cotherapists serves to model such behavior for group members suggests that "modeling" may be largely a myth (McNary & Dies, 1993). Nevertheless, it does not negate the importance of co-leadership because other benefits for the clinicians (and indirectly the patients) may be the sharing of responsibility and the opportunities for professional growth through communication about individual patients and treatment process. Perhaps research measures have not been sensitive enough to detect the subtle co-leadership effects that are apparent in group treatments.

CURATIVE FACTORS OR MECHANISMS OF CHANGE

A majority of group psychotherapists are well aware of the principal "therapeutic factors" proposed by Yalom (1995) that have now received widespread attention in the literature (e.g., Bloch & Crouch, 1985; Fuhriman & Burlingame, 1990; MacKenzie, 1987):

1. Interpersonal input or feedback from group members
2. Catharsis or open expression of affect by patients
3. Group cohesiveness
4. Self-understanding
5. Interpersonal output or learning new social skills
6. Existential factors (e.g., acceptance of ultimate responsibility, aloneness, and freedom)
7. Universality (sense of commonality among patients)
8. Instillation of hope
9. Altruism toward others within the group
10. Family-of-origin reenactment
11. Guidance, advice, or suggestions from the therapist or co-members
12. Identification or imitative behavior among group members

The importance of these therapeutic factors varies in relationship to structural, contextual, and individual matters. For example, certain elements are most salient in the formative phases of group development (a structural matter). MacKenzie (1987) labeled these "nonspecific" morale factors, such as hope, altruism, universality, and cohesiveness, because they are mainly important in establishing a safe atmosphere in which patients can take individual risks. In high-turnover inpatient groups, short-term

outpatient therapy, and self-help groups (a contextual matter), these factors may play a central role in the overall evaluation of treatment. However, in most therapy groups for moderately distressed individuals, these factors rarely emerge as most salient in patients' judgments about outcome. Quite the contrary, the variables that appear with greatest regularity are cohesiveness, interpersonal input (feedback), catharsis, and self-understanding (Yalom, 1995). A fifth factor, interpersonal output (learning social skills), is also mentioned frequently.

There are clearly no universal mechanisms of change but rather a range of key dimensions that interact with clinical settings, diagnostic compositions, and forms of group therapy. Different patients (an individual matter) may benefit from various therapeutic ingredients within the same group (Lieberman, 1989), and the availability of multiple sources of learning within sessions may be even more important than any limited set of common dimensions (Lieberman, 1983). There appears to be a confluence of nonspecific factors (e.g., cohesiveness) working in concert with cognitive, affective, and behavioral ingredients to facilitate therapeutic gain (i.e., self-understanding, catharsis, and interpersonal learning and social skills acquisition, respectively) (Dies, 1993). There is no simple formula for treatment benefit.

The literature is consistent in showing that Yalom's (1995) therapeutic factors of family reenactment, guidance, and identification are seldom viewed as important by group members. It is not especially difficult to figure out why advice and imitation are not foremost in intensive group work, but the failure of family reenactment to appear as a nuclear therapeutic dimension runs counter to much of the writing about the importance of transference in the treatment context. Conceivably, the short-term nature of most of the groups evaluated in the literature precludes the emergence of this factor as pertinent. On the other hand, the emotional reliving of earlier family dynamics has been found to be decisive for a group of incest victims (Bonney, Randall, & Cleveland, 1986) and in a long-term group treatment context (Tschuschke & Dies, 1994). It is likely that minor variations across studies of therapeutic factors can be accounted for by virtue of the specialized nature of the treatment groups employed. For example, universality (i.e., the recognition by patients that they share many problems) was understandably unimportant for a male felony offender group (Long & Cope, 1980), whereas "existential awareness" was regarded as quite significant (MacDevitt & Sanislow, 1987).

Although most of the research on therapeutic factors looks at these dimensions from the point of view of patients who have completed treatment, the consistency of the findings lends considerable credence to their central importance.

TREAMENT APPLICABILITY AND ETHICAL CONSIDERATIONS

It should be evident at this point that "group treatments come in all shapes and sizes." A chapter could easily be filled just itemizing the various populations and contexts in which group psychotherapy can be found. Quite some time ago, the author published a compilation of reviews, that is, a simple listing of articles that integrate major bodies of *research* on various aspects of group treatments over a 15-year period (Dies, 1989). Nearly 100 review articles were summarized under headings covering surveys of process and outcome, research methodology, diagnostic groups, specialized populations, lifespan development, training, and various group formats. Undoubtedly, an update of this compendium would easily triple the number of integrative reports published in the group treatment literature. Were the thousands of theoretical and applied publications to be added to this list, it would be clear that virtually no potential

target of intervention has escaped the attention of group psychotherapists.

In the beginning of the chapter, I highlighted Pratt's work with tuberculosis patients as the earliest foundation for group work. Today, support and psychoeducational groups are employed for a wide range of medical illnesses, including heart disease and cancer, gastrointestinal conditions, neurological impairment, hypertension, asthma and chronic emphysema, and many others (e.g., Stern, 1993). Such groups have a powerful effect on the mental and physical well-being of most participants (Davison, Pennebaker, & Dickerson, 2000).

Various special populations have benefited from group treatments: men's and women's groups, gay and lesbian support groups, and similar homogeneously composed groups for family caregivers, individuals in midlife career change, displaced workers, visually impaired people, victims of incest, or children from alcoholic families, just to mention a few (Alonso & Swiller, 1993; Dies, 1992a; Seligman & Marshak, 1990). The entire age range has been covered: children (Riester & Kraft, 1986), adolescents (MacLennan & Dies, 1992), and the elderly (MacLennan, Saul, & Weiner, 1988).

The practice of group psychotherapy is international in scope. Although there may be differences in how practitioners in various countries conduct their treatments (Dies, 1993), there is no question that the popularity of group therapy is universal.

The brief clinical vignettes that follow can provide only a glimpse at this fascinating but extraordinarily complex field of practice.

CASE ILLUSTRATION

This short-term group consists of eight members who have been meeting weekly for 1 month in a community mental health facility. Their problems are varied, but most of these young adults have reported feeling quite unhappy about the quality of their relationships and with their own inability to handle interpersonal problems more effectively. Attendance has been regular and they have all shared, at least superficially, the basic reasons they sought treatment. The therapist realizes that the group members have a rudimentary understanding (through the pregroup contracting) about how group interaction fosters change but also knows that they have not truly *experienced* this awareness through their interactions with each other. The fourth session begins:

THERAPIST: Does anyone have any feelings carried over from our last session?

ANDY: No, but something happened to me that I'd like to talk about . . . (*without waiting for others*) . . . the girl I've been dating just decided that our relationship wasn't working out so she ended it . . . without even trying to talk it through!

BRENDA: What happened? [In early groups members frequently get into a question-asking mode to get "the story."]

ANDY: [He explains how his "girlfriend" just "dumped" him and refused to talk about it, so he went over to her place to confront her about how unfair she was being. Because he had always been so open about his feelings, he could not understand her refusal to offer an explanation.]

Andy receives supportive comments from others within the group, because he has indeed been very open about his feelings within the sessions, usually being the first to volunteer problems for discussion, and because the rejection did seem so unjust and insensitive. After a few minutes, however, the topic shifts to the theme of distrust; others, too, have been "burned" in relationships.

BRENDA: It's real difficult for me to trust guys, because they only seem to want one thing.

CATHY: Yeah, I know what you mean. I've avoided any serious dating for two years because I was really hurt by someone I truly cared about . . . I found out he was sleeping with my best friend while he was supposedly going with me.

DON: That stinks. Who do you hate worse . . . the guy or the friend?

CATHY: Probably both . . . it hurt a lot . . . since then I've really put up a wall so I don't get hurt again.

ELLEN: I can't trust people either . . . I'm afraid to get close to others because I'm not sure about their intentions.

For several minutes there is a general discussion about how members have erected defensive "walls" and become reluctant to take risks in relationships, and offering such comments as the following: "People can't be trusted," "You never know if they're really interested in who you are as a person," "I'm afraid to get close, because I don't want to go through all that pain again," and similar remarks focused on "people" in outside relationships. The therapist has listened because members have been interacting spontaneously but senses that this externally focused conversation may be an indirect or metaphorical communication about the members' concerns regarding trust within this relatively new group.

THERAPIST: Does any of this discussion of trust relate to what is going on in here?

ANDY: No, it's different in here . . . people really care and are interested in each other. [Others generally confirm this impression through their own comments.]

THERAPIST: [Despite the members' collusive denial, the clinician persists with the interpretation of here-and-now relevance but realizes that the first intervention was ineffective; members are reluctant to confront their distrust of each other directly]. It would certainly be understandable if you didn't fully trust each other yet, because this is only our fourth session. But I would guess that many of you are not confident that if you really revealed the pain and self-doubts that brought you here, that others would understand or be that interested. Some of you have been fairly quiet, and others have begun to share, but none of you has really gotten into qualities you don't like about yourself and want to change. Let's look at what makes it difficult to take those kinds of risks in here.

The members launch into a meaningful discussion about both group process issues and individual concerns that have contributed to their reluctance to share more completely (e.g., how the silence of some members has led others to feel judged, how some members have felt let down after their initial disclosures were ignored by others who switched the topic to their own problems, the fear of monopolizing group time or being faced with challenging questions, fears of crying and then feeling stupid or vulnerable, and similar apprehensions). The expression of these previously unverbalized feelings frees members to move into a discussion of desired "norms" around support, reciprocity, and shared responsibility. Thus, the clinician's persistent and constructive confrontation of the members' veiled preoccupation about a natural theme in the group's development served to pave the way toward greater group cohesion and increasingly intense individual work. This same group can be examined in the *tenth session* of treatment.

Once again Andy begins the session. In the prior two meetings he briefly described a relationship that seemed to be going quite smoothly. As noted in session 4, he was the lone dissenter when others described the "walls" they had constructed for self-protection. His position was that when relationships fail, you "move on . . . think of what was good and how you enjoyed each other . . . but when it ends you can't just crawl into a shell."

ANDY: I don't understand it, but Lisa seems to be pulling away from me. . . . I've

called several times, but she makes up excuses for not being able to talk. I'm really upset, because I've been so open and honest with her, and really treated her well. We were really getting close, and even slept together. It was a mutual decision, so it wasn't that I took advantage of her or anything like that. . . . (*He turns to the side, and in "macho pose" says quietly to the men, "It was special because I was her first."*)

ELLEN: (*irritated*) I don't blame her . . . I hope she dumps you just like Peggy and the others did!

FRED: And you're proud of that Andy? You probably sweet-talked her into it and she felt used afterwards.

Several of the other members express their disapproval, not only at Andy's insensitive display but also because of his seeming lack of insight into how his behavior might be contributing to his repeated failure in heterosexual relationships. The therapist seizes this opportunity to make this a here-and-now issue.

THERAPIST: Andy, how are you feeling about how the others are responding to you right now? [This intervention is just to check in with Andy before creating the opportunity for more meaningful work.]

ANDY: I don't understand why everyone is so intense . . . I guess I'm hurt by the attack. I thought people would know I was just kidding when I flexed my muscles and joked . . . I'm not that kind of person. You all know how open I am about my feelings and how hard I try to be sensitive to everyone. It was okay with Lisa . . . we talked about it first before going to bed.

THERAPIST: (*to the other members*) I have a sense that Andy doesn't really understand the strength of your reactions. Maybe it would help if we looked at what's going on in here right now. One way to understand this is that Andy is being rejected by you just like he gets "dumped" in relationships outside. What has he done in the group sessions over time to bring this rejection about?

BRENDA: Andy, it's not so much the "macho act" you did before . . . although I didn't like that either . . . but just the attitude you have about relationships . . . you always talk about how interested you are in the other person's feelings. I sure don't feel that way in here. We spend a lot of time talking about your problems and you rarely ask about ours.

ELLEN: I feel the same way . . . you usually start the sessions before any of us have a chance to get into our problems . . .

GORDON: (interrupting) . . . Yeah, and when we've tried to give you feedback about that you get real defensive. It's hard for you to take criticism.

ANDY: (flushed) . . . But I've really worked in here . . . I express my feelings and work on my problems.

CATHY: I think Gordon is right . . . when we confront you, you just give us that "but I'm such a great guy routine" about how open and honest you are.

THERAPIST: What do you think it would be like to be in a relationship with Andy?

BRENDA: (jumping in) I'd feel smothered . . . I don't want to hurt your feelings Andy, but you work too hard to be "Mr. Open" . . . like you're trying to prove how likable you are, but lately it's been pushing me away from you. It's like you're so wonderful that you never do anything wrong, but you screw up a lot!

HAL: One of the reasons I've been so quiet in here is because of you, Andy . . . it's always your feelings this and your feelings that . . . where is there room for me? The smothering that Brenda talked about really fits for me too . . . as I think about it, it feels like you're really needy and self-centered.

ELLEN: There's one more thing for me . . . and that is your attitude that if things

don't work out in a relationship, it's too bad and maybe time to move on. I'm afraid that could happen in here, too . . . like if you don't like the feedback, you'll just stop coming.

THERAPIST: Andy, people have been pretty direct in their reactions to you. I hope you can take in what they've said because it looks like there is a direct parallel between what happens in relationships and what has gone on in the group. You have been very open in here, but perhaps it hasn't given others the room they need in this group relationship. Your openness and desire to be such a nice guy has felt intrusive and pushed people away from you . . . they've gotten lost in this relationship and felt like they weren't very important to you. But Ellen's comment tells me that she, and I'm sure others, are concerned about you, and want to help, because they see you as "shooting yourself in the foot" in relationships and not understanding why women pull away from you.

Andy is distressed, but with the support of the therapist and other group members he is able to work with the feedback and gain increased awareness of how his style is counterproductive. His intense need for social acceptance is explored and he is helped to define alternative ways to earn recognition. In future sessions he will explore more openly the rather fragile sense of "self" that drives his defensiveness, the condescending attitude toward women (e.g., his use of the pejorative "girl" description and his sense of conquest at being the first), and his narcissism.

The here-and-now, interpersonal work with Andy was quite individual in its focus; frequently in groups several patients are working on a common theme together. For example, other patients may resort to different interpersonal styles as a result of their vulnerable self-esteem. Cathy who was so wounded when she discovered that her lover was sleeping with her best friend, and

Hal who remained so quiet throughout many of the sessions, may have much in common with Andy. Although the three of them approach relationships so differently, they may share a common bond that brings each of them to treatment—and that is their fundamental dissatisfaction with who they are as people. The ability to communicate with others through intensive interaction in the group setting is one of the reasons group treatments are so powerful.

CURRENT AND FUTURE TRENDS

There is little doubt that the practical, theoretical, and empirical foundations for group treatments rest on solid footing. Most experts in the field of mental health would agree that the use of group interventions will continue to expand. Thus, MacKenzie (2001) argues that "convincing evidence that the outcome results from group psychotherapy are equivalent to the same model delivered in an individual modality will drive this process" (p. 176). Similarly, Steenbarger and Budman (1996) have proposed that the escalating cost of health care within the private and public sectors has significant implications for the group psychotherapies, as group modalities offer cost-effective ways of delivering services to traditional outpatient and inpatient populations. Moreover, "Continued cost-containment pressures and increasing attention to outcome studies will fuel trends toward briefer, manualized group interventions and intensive group outpatient programs as alternatives to hospitalization" (p. 297).

Short-term and highly structured group treatments have received strong support in the empirical literature. The vast majority of studies of group psychotherapy have examined short-term interventions (fewer than 12 sessions), and when comparisons are made between structured and nonstructured group formats (e.g., support groups, self-help groups, and those without treatment manuals), the structured therapies clearly show more favorable outcomes (Dies, 1994a). Such results, coupled with pressures for cost containment, have led to a concerted effort to establish "empirically validated treatments" based on the belief that models and techniques are among the most important contributors to the success of psychotherapy (Ogles, Anderson, & Lunnen, 1999).

Ironically, the preponderance of research evidence, accumulated over decades of investigation, in both the individual and group psychotherapy literature, is not supportive of the superiority of specific techniques or particular schools of psychotherapy (Ahn & Wampold, 2001; Asay & Lambert, 1999). A wide array of intervention *strategies* (e.g., reinforcement, cognitive reframing, interpretation, and confrontation), *models* of treatment (e.g., cognitive-behavioral, interpersonal, psychodynamic), and therapeutic *modalities* (e.g., group vs. individual) have clearly proven their worth but not their supremacy. Thus, it may not be the specific techniques that are important but, rather, a more generalized provision of a coherent and meaningful framework for therapeutic change.

The search for the "holy grail," or the specific techniques, that will optimize treatment outcome will undoubtedly continue in the foreseeable future. This trend may be most apparent with "manualized" group formats, and especially those anchored in cognitive-behavioral approaches, because of their current popularity, ease of translation into manual format, and issues related to research expediency (e.g., ease of recruiting symptomatically compatible clients, with well defined targets for short-term treatment). However, the weight of years of empirical evidence, as well as the enormous complexity of group treatments (making it virtually impossible to disentangle the multitude of specific factors contributing to clinical improvement), would argue against finding the "right" combination of specific techniques to produce change.

An alternative view to the lack of differential treatment outcomes across models, methods, or modalities is based on the notion of *common factors,* that is, that the favorable results from psychotherapy are due to such factors as the healing context, the working alliance, and belief in the rationale for treatment and in the treatment itself (Ahn & Wampold, 2001). Asay and Lambert (1999) provide compelling evidence from their extensive review of the one-to-one and group treatment literature that these "nonspecific factors" account for a much greater proportion of outcome variance than any particular techniques.

Among the common factors most frequently studied are those focusing on the role of the therapeutic relationship. The results show that "the therapeutic alliance, measured at an early stage, accounts for a significant portion of variability in treatment outcomes. Moreover, the variance due to therapists within treatments is greater than the variance between treatments, lending primacy to the person of the therapist rather than to the particular treatment" (Ahn & Wampold, 2001, p. 255). Gurman and Gustafson (1976) noted long ago that the consistent link between relationship variables and outcome in individual psychotherapy does not receive the same level of support in group treatment. This is perhaps due to the greater importance of client-to-client relationship factors in the group modality (Dies, 1983b), but these, too, represent "common factors" rather than specific techniques.

In spite of their popularity, and demonstrated effectiveness in improving clinical outcome (in a generic way by furnishing structure), some controversy surrounds the extensive reliance on treatment manuals. For example, they have been criticized as "cookbooks" that oversimplify therapy process and force clinicians to apply techniques rigidly or inappropriately, and as overvaluing fidelity to the manual at the expense of intuition, empathy, and clinical sensitivity. (Najavits, Weiss, Shaw, & Dierberger, 2000). Beutler (1999) has shown that even when a sample of therapists follows the same manual, there are wide variations in the outcome effectiveness from clinician to clinician. Vakoch and Strupp (2000) echo the substantial variability in the styles of therapist, even after receiving intensive training in the use of a specific manual. These authors regard treatment manuals in individual and group interventions as a "starting point" but conclude that "the current preoccupation with manuals may have exceeded its usefulness, and further emphasis on the standardization of 'techniques' may impede, rather than further, the advancement of productive models of therapist training" (p. 314).

The current fascination with treatment manuals is expected to moderate in light of the overwhelming evidence that "nonspecific" or common factors (e.g., the therapeutic alliance and group cohesiveness) contribute so heavily to client improvement, and in light of findings documenting wide variability among therapists who are following the same script, especially when therapists who obtain particularly favorable outcomes after manualized training are "also the ones who were most likely to depart from the training guidelines and to follow their own judgments" (Beutler, 1999, p. 400). Training programs have been faulted for their failure to provide sufficient attention to brief treatments, and especially to group interventions (Fuhriman & Burlingame, 2001; Levenson & Davidovitz, 2000). In light of current demands for such treatments, it is likely that there will be renewed interest in training clinicians to appreciate the value of both active structuring within psychotherapy (i.e., furnishing a meaningful framework for change as, for example, through a treatment manual) and the critical importance of establishing a powerful therapeutic alliance through the demonstration of such personal qualities as empathy, compassion, sensitivity, support, and care (and encouraging such expression among members within a treatment group).

These qualities cannot be learned through a manual but require careful monitoring and supervision by an experienced clinician.

SUGGESTIONS FOR FURTHER READING

Brabender, V. (2002). *Introduction to group psychotherapy*. New York: Wiley.—This is a thorough introduction to the principles, practices, and theoretical models in group psychotherapy.

Dies, R. R. (1994). The therapist's role in group treatments. In H. Bernard & K. R. Mackenzie (Eds.), *Basics of group psychotherapy* (pp. 60–99). New York: Guilford Press.—This chapter provides a practical framework, with numerous clinical illustrations, for how to conduct group treatments.

Dies, R. R. (1994). Therapist variables in group psychotherapy research. In A. Fuhrman & G. M. Burlingame (Eds.), *Handbook of group psychotherapy* (pp. 114–154). New York: Wiley.—This chapter provides the foundation for leadership in group psychotherapy based on a review of empirical research.

Fuhriman, A., & Burlingame, G. M. (1994). Group psychotherapy: Research and practice. In A. Fuhrman & G. M. Burlingame (Eds.), *Handbook of group psychotherapy* (pp. 3–40). New York: Wiley.—This chapter gives the reader an excellent overview of research on group therapy.

White, J. R., & Freeman, A. S. (Eds.). (2002). *Cognitive-behavioral group therapy for specific problems and populations*. Washington, DC: American Psychological Association.—Various chapters in this excellent text furnish case illustrations of the cognitive-behavioral approach to group intervention with different disorders.

Yalom, I. D. (1995). *The theory and practice of group psychotherapy* (4th ed.). New York: Basic Books.—This superb volume is the most popular text in the field of group therapy.

REFERENCES

Addis, M. E., & Krasnow, A. D. (2000). A national survey of practicing psychologists' attitudes toward psychotherapy treatment manuals. *Journal of Consulting and Clinical Psychology, 68,* 331–339.

Ahn, H., & Wampold, B. E. (2001). Where oh where are the specific ingredients? A meta-analysis of component studies in counseling and psychotherapy. *Journal of Counseling Psychology, 48,* 251–257.

Alonso, A., & Swiller, H. I. (Eds.). (1993). *Group therapy in clinical practice*. Washington, DC: American Psychiatric Press.

Antony, M. M., & Barlow, D. H. (2001). *Handbook of assessment and treatment planning for psychological disorders*. New York: Guilford Press.

Asay, T. P., & Lambert, M. J. (1999). The empirical case for the common factors in Therapy: Quantitative findings. In M. A. Hubble, B. L. Duncan, & S. D. Miller (Eds.), *The heart and soul of change* (pp. 23–55). Washington, DC: American Psychological Association.

Bahrey, F., McCallum, M., & Piper, W. E. (1991). Emergent themes and roles in short-term loss groups. *International Journal of Group Psychotherapy, 41,* 329–345.

Bednar, R. L., & Lawlis, F. (1971). Empirical research in group psychotherapy. In A. E. Bergin & S. L. Garfield (Eds.), *Handbook of psychotherapy and behavior change* (pp. 812–838). New York: Wiley.

Beutler, L. E. (1999). Manualizing flexibility: The training of eclectic therapists. *Journal of Clinical Psychology, 55,* 399–404.

Beutler, L. E., Crago, M., & Arizmendi, T. G. (1986). Research on therapist variables in psychotherapy. In S. L. Garfield & A. E. Bergin (Eds.), *Handbook of psychotherapy and behavior change* (3rd ed., pp. 257–310). New York: Wiley.

Bloch, S., & Crouch, E. (1985). *Therapeutic factors in group psychotherapy*. Oxford, UK: Oxford University Press.

Bonney, W. C., Randall, D. A., & Cleveland, J. D. (1986). An analysis of client-perceived curative factors in a therapy group of former incest victims. *Small Group Behavior, 17,* 303–321.

Coche, J., & Coche, E. (1990). *Couples group psychotherapy: A clinical practice model*. New York: Brunner/Mazel.

Corcoran, K., & Fischer, J. (2000). *Measures for clinical practice: A sourcebook*. New York: Free Press.

Dana, R. H. (2000). *Handbook of cross-cultural and*

multicultural personality assessment. Mahwah, NJ: Erlbaum.

Davison, K. P., Pennebaker, J. W., & Dickerson, S. S. (2000). Who talks? The social psychology of illness support groups. *American Psychologist, 55,* 205–217.

DeRubeis, R. J., & Crits-Christoph, P. (1998). Empirically supported individual and group psychological treatments for adult mental disorders. *Journal of Consulting and Clinical Psychology, 66,* 37–52.

Dies, K. R., & Dies, R. R. (1993). Directive facilitation: A model for short-term group treatments, Part 2. *The Independent Practitioner, 13,* 177–184.

Dies, R. R. (1977). Group therapist transparency: A critique of theory and research. *International Journal of Group Psychotherapy, 27,* 177–200.

Dies, R. R. (1980). Group psychotherapy training. In A. K. Hess (Ed.), *Psychotherapy supervision* (pp. 337–366). New York: Wiley.

Dies, R. R. (1983a). Bridging the gap between research and practice in group psychotherapy. In R. R. Dies & K. R. MacKenzie (Eds.), *Advances in group psychotherapy: Integrating research and practice* (pp. 1–16). New York: International Universities Press.

Dies, R. R. (1983b). Clinical implications of research on leadership in short-term group psychotherapy. In R. R. Dies & K. R. MacKenzie (Eds.), *Advances in group psychotherapy: Integrating research and practice* (pp. 27–78). New York: International Universities Press.

Dies, R. R. (1985). Leadership in short-term group therapy: Manipulation or facilitation? *International Journal of Group Psychotherapy, 35,* 435–455.

Dies, R. R. (1986). Practical, theoretical, and empirical foundations for group psychotherapy. In A. J. Frances & R. E. Hales (Eds.), *The American Psychiatric Association annual review* (Vol. 5, pp. 659–567). Washington, DC: American Psychiatric Press.

Dies, R. R. (1987). Clinical application of research instruments: Editor's introduction. *International Journal of Group Psychotherapy, 37,* 31–37.

Dies, R. R. (1989). Reviews of group psychotherapy research. *International Association of Group Psychotherapy Newsletter, 7,* 8–11.

Dies, R. R. (1992a). The future of group therapy. *Psychotherapy, 29,* 58–64.

Dies, R. R. (1992b). Models of group psychotherapy: Sifting through confusion. *International Journal of Group Psychotherapy, 42,* 1–17.

Dies, R. R. (1993). Research on group psychotherapy: Overview and clinical applications. In A. Alonso & H. I. Swiller (Eds.), *Group therapy in clinical practice* (pp. 473–518). Washington, DC: American Psychiatric Press.

Dies, R. R. (1994a). Therapist variables in group psychotherapy research. In A. Fuhriman & G. M. Burlingame (Eds.), *Handbook of group psychotherapy* (pp. 114–154). New York: Wiley.

Dies, R. R. (1994b). The therapists' role in group treatments. In H. S. Bernard & K. R. MacKenzie (Eds.), *Basics of group psychotherapy* (pp. 60–99). New York: Guilford Press.

Dies, R. R., & Dies, K. R. (1993a). Directive facilitation: A model for short-term group treatments, Part 1. *The Independent Practitioner, 13,* 103–109.

Dies, R. R., & Dies, K. R. (1993b). The role of evaluation in clinical practice: An overview and group treatment illustration. *International Journal of Group Psychotherapy, 43,* 77–105.

Dies, R. R., & Teleska, P. A. (1985). Negative outcome in group psychotherapy. In D. T. Mays & C. M. Franks (Eds.), *Negative outcome in psychotherapy and what to do about it* (pp. 118–141). New York: Springer.

Ellis, A. (1992). Group rational-emotive and cognitive-behavioral therapy. *International Journal of Group Psychotherapy, 42,* 63–80.

Erickson, R. C. (1987). The question of casualties in inpatient small group psychotherapy. *Small Group Behavior, 18,* 443–458.

Fink, P. J. (1989). The marriage of psychobiology and psychotherapy: A discussion on the papers by Rodenhauser, Zazlav and Kalb. *International Journal of Group Psychotherapy, 39,* 469–474.

Fischer, A. R., Jome, L. M., & Atkinson, D. R. (1998). Reconceptualizing multicultural counseling: Universal healing conditions in a culturally specific context. *The Counseling Psychologist, 26,* 525–588.

Fuhriman, A., & Burlingame, G. M. (1990). Consistency of matter: A comparative analysis of individual and group process variables. *The Counseling Psychologist, 18,* 6–63.

Fuhriman, A., & Burlingame, G. M. (1994). Group psychotherapy: Research and practice. In A. Fuhriman & G. M. Burlingame (Eds.), *Handbook of group psychotherapy* (pp. 3–40). New York: Wiley.

Fuhriman, A., & Burlingame, G. M. (2001). Group psychotherapy training and Effectiveness. *International Journal of Group Psychotherapy, 51,* 399–416.

Gans, J. S. (1990). Broaching and exploring the question of combined group and individual therapy. *International Journal of Group Psychotherapy, 40,* 123–137.

Garfield, S. L. (1986). Research on client variables in psychotherapy. In S. L. Garfield & A. E. Bergin (Eds.), *Handbook of psychotherapy and behavior change* (3rd ed., pp. 213–256). New York: Wiley.

Gurman, A. S., & Gustafson, J. P. (1976). Patients' perceptions of the therapeutic relationship and group therapy outcome. *American Journal of Psychiatry, 133,* 1290–1294.

Haley-Banez, L., Brown, S., & Molina, B. (1999). Association for Specialists in Group Work principles for diversity-competent group workers. *Journal for Specialists in Group Work, 24,* 7–14.

Hall, C. S., & Lindzey, G. (1985). *Introduction to theories of personality.* New York: Wiley.

Hansen, N. D., Pepitone-Arreola-Rockwell, F., & Greene, A. F. (2000). Multicultural competence: Criteria and case examples. *Professional Psychology: Research Practice, 31,* 652–660.

Heimberg, R. G., & Becker, R. E. (2002). *Cognitive-behavioral group therapy for social phobia: Basic mechanisms and clinical strategies.* New York: Guilford Press.

Holmes, S. E., & Kivlighan, D. M. (2000). Comparison of therapeutic factors in group and individual treatment processes. *Journal of Counseling Psychology, 47,* 478–484.

Johnson, I. H., Torres, J. S., Coleman, V. D., & Smith, M. C. (1995). Issues and strategies in leading culturally diverse counseling groups. *Journal for Specialists in Group Work, 20,* 143–150.

Kanas, N. (1986). Group therapy with schizophrenics: A review of the controlled studies. *International Journal of Group Psychotherapy, 36,* 339–351.

Kaul, T. J., & Bednar, R. L. (1978). Conceptualizing group research: A preliminary analysis. *Small Group Behavior, 9,* 173–191.

Keisler, D. J. (1986). Interpersonal methods of diagnosis and treatment. In J. O. Cavenar (Ed.), *Psychiatry* (Vol. 1, pp. 1–23). Philadelphia: Lippincott.

Kivlighan, D. M. (1985). Feedback in group psychotherapy: Review and implications. *Small Group Behavior, 16,* 373–385.

Kivlighan, D. M., Corrazzini, J. G., & McGovern, T. V. (1985). Pregroup training. *Small Group Behavior, 16,* 500–514.

Klein, R. H. (1985). Some principles of short-term group therapy. *International Journal of Group Psychotherapy, 35,* 309–330.

Klein, R. H., & Schermer, V. L. (2000). *Group psychotherapy for psychological trauma.* New York: Guilford Press.

Koss, M. P., & Butcher, J. N. (1986). Research on brief psychotherapy. In S. L. Garfield &. A. E. Bergin (Eds.), *Handbook of psychotherapy and behavior change* (3rd ed., pp. 627–670). New York: Wiley.

Leszcz, M. (1992). The interpersonal approach to group psychotherapy. *International Journal of Group Psychotherapy, 42,* 37–62.

Levenson, H., & Davidovitz, D. (2000). Brief therapy prevalence and training: A national Survey of psychologists. *Psychotherapy, 37,* 335–340.

Lieberman, M. A. (1983). Comparative analyses of change mechanisms in groups. In R. R. Dies & K. R. MacKenzie (Eds.), *Advances in group psychotherapy: Integrating research and practice* (pp. 191–208). New York: International Universities Press.

Lieberman, M. A. (1989). Group properties and outcome: A study of group norms in self-help groups for widows and widowers. *International Journal of Group Psychotherapy, 39,* 191–208.

Lieberman, M. A., Yalom, I. D., & Miles, M. B. (1973). *Encounter groups: First facts.* New York: Basic Books.

Lipsius, S. H. (1991). Combined individual and group psychotherapy: Guidelines at the interface. *International Journal of Group Psychotherapy, 41,* 313–327.

Livesley, W. J., & MacKenzie, K. R. (1983). Social roles in psychotherapy groups. In R. R. Dies & K. R. MacKenzie (Eds.), *Advances in group psychotherapy: Integrating research and practice* (pp. 117–135). New York: International Universities Press.

Locke, E. A., & Latham, G. P. (2002). Building a practically useful theory of goal setting and task motivation: A 35-year odyssey. *American Psychologist, 57,* 705–717.

Long, L. D., & Cope, C. S. (1980). Curative factors in a male felony offender group. *Small Group Behavior, 11,* 389–397.

MacDevitt, J. W., & Sanislow, C. (1987). Curative factors in offenders' groups. *Small Group Behavior, 18,* 72–81.

MacKenzie, K. R. (1983). The clinical application of a group climate measure. In R. R. Dies & K. R. MacKenzie (Eds.), *Advances in group psychotherapy: Integrating research and practice* (pp. 159–170). New York: International Universities Press.

MacKenzie, K. R. (1987). Therapeutic factors in group psychotherapy: A contemporary view. *Group, 11,* 26–34.

MacKenzie, K. R. (1995). *Effective use of group therapy in managed care.* Washington, DC: American Psychiatric Press.

MacKenzie, K. R. (2001). An expectation of radical changes in the future of group psychotherapy. *International Journal of Group Psychotherapy, 51,* 175–180.

MacKenzie, K. R., & Livesley, W. J. (1983). A developmental model for brief group therapy. In R. R. Dies & K. R. MacKenzie (Eds.), *Advances in group psychotherapy: Integrating research and practice* (pp. 101–116). New York: International Universities Press.

MacLennan, B. W., & Dies, K. R. (1992). *Group counseling and psychotherapy with adolescents* (2nd ed.). New York: Columbia University Press.

MacLennan, B. W., Saul, S., & Weiner, M. B. (1988). *Group psychotherapy for the elderly.* Madison, CT: International Universities Press.

Maruish, M. E. (2002). *Psychological testing in the age of managed behavioral health care.* Mahwah, NJ: Erlbaum.

Mayerson, N. H. (1984). Preparing clients for group therapy: A critical review and theoretical formulation. *Clinical Psychology Review, 4,* 191–213.

McDermut, W., Miller, I. W., & Brown, R. A. (2001). The efficacy of group psychotherapy for depression: A meta-analysis and review of the empirical research. *Clinical Psychology: Science and Practice, 8,* 98–116.

McNary, S. W., & Dies, R. R, (1993). Co-therapist modeling in group psychotherapy: Fact or fantasy? *Group, 17,* 131–142.

McRoberts, C., Burlingame, G. M., & Hoag, M. J. (1998). Comparative efficacy of individual and group psychotherapy: A meta-analytic perspective. *Group Dynamics, 2,* 101–117.

Melnick, J., & Woods, M, (1976). Analysis of group composition research and theory for psychotherapeutic and growth-oriented groups. *Journal of Applied Behavioral Science, 12,* 493–512.

Messer, S. B. (2001). What allows therapy to be brief? Introduction to the special series. *Clinical Psychology: Science and Practice, 8,* 1–4.

Moos, R. H. (1986). *Group Environment Scale manual* (2nd ed.). Palo Alto, CA: Consulting Psychologists Press.

Moreno, K. (1994). Group treatment for eating disorders. In A. Fuhrman & G. M. Burlingame (Eds.), *Handbook of group psychotherapy* (pp. 416–457). New York: Wiley.

Najavits, L. M., Weiss, R. D., Shaw, S. R., & Dierberger, A. E. (2000). Psychotherapists' views of treatment manuals. *Professional Psychology: Research and Practice, 31,* 404–408.

Norcross, J. C., Alford, B. A., & DeMichele, J. T, (1992). The future of psychotherapy: Delphi data and concluding observations. *Psychotherapy, 29,* 150–158.

Ogles, B. M., Anderson, T., & Lunnen, K. M. (1999). The contribution of models and techniques to therapeutic efficacy: Contradictions between professional trends and Clinical research. In M. A. Hubble, B. L. Duncan, & S. D. Miller (Eds.), *The heart and soul of change* (pp. 201–225). Washington, DC: American Psychological Association.

Orlinsky, D. E., & Howard, K. I. (1986). Process and outcome in psychotherapy. In S. L. Garfield & A. E. Bergin (Eds.), *Handbook of psychotherapy and behavior change* (3rd ed., pp. 311–381). New York: Wiley.

Parloff, M. B. (1968). Analytic group psychotherapy. In J. Marmor (Ed.), *Modern psychoanalysis* (pp. 492–531). New York: Basic Books.

Parloff, M. B., & Dies, R. R. (1977). Group psychotherapy outcome research 1966–1975. *International Journal of Group Psychotherapy, 27,* 281–319.

Phares, E. J. (1991). *Introduction to personality* (3rd ed.). New York: HarperCollins.

Phipps, L. B., & Zastowny, T. R. (1988). Leadership behavior, group climate and outcome in group psychotherapy: A study of outpatient psychotherapy groups. *Group, 12,* 157–171.

Piper, W. E., & Joyce, A. S. (1996). Consideration of factors influencing the utilization of time-limited, short-term group therapy. *International Journal of Group Psychotherapy, 46,* 311–328.

Piper, W. E., Joyce, A. S., McCallum, M., Azim, H. F., & Ogrodniczuk, J. S. (2002). *Interpretive and supportive psychotherapies: Matching therapy and patient personality.* Washington, DC: Americal Psychological Association.

Riess, H., & Dockray-Miller, M. (2001). *Integrative group treatment for bulimia nervosa.* New York: Columbia University Press.

Riester, A. E., & Kraft, I. A. (Eds.). (1986). *Child group psychotherapy: Future tense.* Madison, CT: International Universities Press.

Roback, H. B., & Smith, M. (1987). Patient attrition in dynamically oriented treatment groups. *American Journal of Psychiatry, 144,* 426–431.

Rodenhauser, P. (1989). Group psychotherapy and pharmacotherapy: Psychodynamic considerations. *International Journal of Group Psychotherapy, 39,* 445–456.

Rutan, J. S. (1992). Psychodynamic group psychotherapy. *International Journal of Group Psychotherapy, 42,* 19–35.

Rutan, J. S., & Stone, W. N. (2001). *Psychodynamic group psychotherapy* (3rd ed). New York: Guilford Press.

Salvendy, J. T. (1999). Ethnocultural considerations in group psychotherapy. *International Journal of Group Psychotherapy, 49,* 429–460.

Salvendy, J. T., & Joffe, R. (1991). Antidepressants in group psychotherapy. *International Journal of Group Psychotherapy, 41,* 465–480.

Scheidlinger, S. (1987). On interpretation in group psychotherapy: The need for refinement. *International Journal of Group Psychotherapy, 37,* 339–352.

Seligman, M., & Marshak, L. E. (1990). *Group psychotherapy: Interventions with special populations.* Boston: Allyn & Bacon.

Shaffer, J., & Galinsky, M. D. (1989). *Models of group therapy* (2nd ed.). Engelwood Cliffs, NJ: Prentice-Hall.

Silbergeld, S., Koenig, G. R., Manderscheid, R. W., Meeker, B. F., & Hornung, C. A. (1975). Assessment of environment-therapy systems: The Group Atmosphere Scale. *Journal of Consulting and Clinical Psychology, 43,* 460–469.

Smith, M. L., Glass, G. V., & Miller, T. I. (1980). *The benefits of psychotherapy.* Baltimore: Johns Hopkins University Press.

Solomon, S. D. (1982). Individual versus group therapy: Current status in the treament of alcoholism. *Advances in Alcohol and Substance Abuse, 2,* 69–86.

Steenbarger, B. N., & Budman, S. H. (1996). Group psychotherapy and managed behavioral health care: Current trends and future challenges. *International Journal of Group Psychotherapy, 46,* 297–309.

Stern, M. J. (1993). Group therapy with medically ill patients. In A. Alonso & H. I. Swiller (Eds.), *Group therapy in clinical practice* (pp. 185–199). Washington, DC: American Psychiatric Press.

Stone, W. N., Rodenhauser, P., & Markert, R. J. (1991). Combining group psychotherapy and pharmacotherapy: A survey. *International Journal of Group Psychotherapy, 41,* 449–464.

Subich, L. M., & Coursol, D. H. (1985). Counseling expectations of clients and nonclients for group and individual treatment modes. *Journal of Counseling Psychology, 32,* 245–251.

Taylor, N. T., Burlingame, G. M., Kristensen, K. B., Fuhriman, A., Johansen, J., & Dahl, D. (2001). A survey of mental health care provider's and managed care organization attitudes toward, familiarity with, and use of group interventions. *International Journal of Group Psychotherapy, 51,* 243–263.

Tinsley, H. E. A., Bowman, S. L., & Ray, S. B. (1988). Manipulation of expectancies about counseling and psychotherapy: Review and analysis of expectancy manipulation strategies and results. *Journal of Counseling Psychology, 33,* 99–108.

Toseland, R. W., & Siporin, M. (1986). When to recommend group treatment: A review of the clinical and research literature. *International Journal of Group Psychotherapy, 36,* 171–201.

Tschuschke, V., & Dies, R. R. (1994). Intensive analysis of therapeutic factors and outcome in long-term inpatient groups. *International Journal of Group Psychotherapy, 44,* 185–208.

Unger, R. (1989). Selection and composition

criteria in group psychotherapy. *Journal for Specialists in Group Work, 14,* 151–157.

Vakoch, D. A., & Strupp, H. H. (2000). The evolution of psychotherapy training: Reflections on manual-based learning and future alternatives. *Journal of Clinical Psychology, 56,* 309–318.

Velasquez, M. M., Maurer, G. G., Crouch, C., & DiClemente, C. C. (2001). *Group treatment for substance abuse: A stages-of-change therapy manual.* New York: Guilford Press.

Vinogradov, S., & Yalom, I. D. (1989). *A concise guide to group psychotherapy.* Washington, DC: American Psychiatric Press.

Waltman, D. E., & Zimpfer, D. G. (1988). Composition, structure, and duration of treatment: Interacting variables in counseling groups. *Small Group Behavior, 19,* 171–184.

Wetzler, S. (Ed.). (1989). *Measuring mental illness: Psychometric assessment for clinicians.* Washington, DC: American Psychiatric Press.

White, J. R., & Freeman, A. S. (Eds.). (2000). *Cognitive-behavioral group therapy.* Washington, DC: American Psychological Association.

Wong, N. (1983). Combined individual and group psychotherapy. In H. I. Kaplan & B. J. Sadock (Eds.), *Comprehensive group psychotherapy* (3rd ed., pp. 374–401). Baltimore: Williams & Wilkins.

Woods, M., & Melnick, J. (1979). A review of group therapy selection criteria. *Small Group Behavior, 10,* 155–174.

Yalom, I. D. (1995). *The theory and practice of group psychotherapy* (4th ed.). New York: Basic Books.

Author Index

Aaltonen, J., 296
Abelsohn, D., 438
Abelson, R. P., 6
Abidin, R. R., 411
Abraham, K., 33
Abramowitz, J. S., 195
Abramson, L., 228, 235
Ackerman, N., 401, 413, 416, 417, 431, 464
Adams-Webber, J., 286
Addis, M. E., 182, 205, 527
Adessky, R. S., 208
Adler, A., 226
Agresta, J., 199
Ahn, H., 543, 544
Ahola, T., 360, 374, 379
Ainsworth, M. D. S., 94
Alakare, B., 296
Alarcon, R. D., 195
Alcaine, O., 203
Alexander, F., 81, 358
Alexander, J. F., 338, 414, 438, 441, 442, 445
Alexander, P. C., 303
Alford, B. A., 526
Allen, D. M., 324, 326
Alloy, L., 228, 235
Allport, G. W., 275
Alomohamed, S., 320
Alonso, A., 539
Alsup, R., 151
Altman, N., 71, 73, 86, 92
Anastopoulos, A. D., 438
Andersen, S. M., 94
Anderson, A., 283
Anderson, C. M., 448

Anderson, C. W., 16, 17
Anderson, H. D., 446, 448
Anderson, K., 228
Anderson, T., 543
Anderson, W., 110, 118
Andrews, J. D. W., 324, 326
Andrews, S., 322
Angel, E., 177
Angus, L. E., 288, 302, 303
Antony, M. M., 183, 191, 193, 194, 195, 196, 204, 205, 213, 525
Apfelbaum, B., 501
Aponte, H. J., 414, 416, 434, 435, 438
Appelbaum, S. A., 351
Appignanesi, R., 275
Arciero, G., 289
Ariel, S., 403
Arieti, S., 226
Arizmendi, T. G., 535
Arkowitz, H., 262, 319, 337, 344
Armstrong, E., 389
Arnkoff, D., 344, 345
Aron, L., 70, 71, 72, 87, 102
Asay, T. P., 543, 544
Asher, S., 465
Atkinson, D. R., 525
Atwood, B., 71, 73
Atwood, G. E., 71, 161
Atwood, J. D., 448
Auerbach, A., 249
Auerbach, J. S., 95
Austad, C. S., 351, 352, 354, 387
Austin, G., 224
Azim, H. F. A., 94, 524

Babcock, J. C., 465
Bacal, H. A., 384
Bach, S., 36
Bachrach, H., 56
Bader, E., 474
Bagnini, C., 469, 470, 474, 475, 476
Bahrey, F., 533
Bailey, S., 228
Baker, K. D., 302
Baldwin, L. M., 406, 411
Baldwin, M., 406, 424, 425
Bales, R. F., 404
Balfour, H. G., 384
Balint, E., 358
Balint, M., 358
Ballinger, B., 151
Bandler, R., 373
Bandura, A., 116, 120, 184, 186, 200, 227, 489
Bankart, C. P., 142
Banmen, J., 484, 485
Bannister, D., 286, 296, 302
Barber, J. P., 94, 240, 362
Barber, S. P., 36
Barkley, R. A., 438, 441
Barlow, D. H., 189, 190, 192, 193, 194, 195, 196, 202, 204, 205, 214, 215, 238, 452, 525
Barnhardt, T. M., 94
Barrett, M. S., 136
Barrett, W. H., 151
Barrett-Lennard, G. T., 108, 112
Barry, W. A., 474
Barten, H. H., 355, 358
Bartholomew, K., 94

Basch, M. F., 351
Basescu, S., 43
Bates, A., 239
Bateson, G., 286, 376, 401, 409, 428, 431
Baucom, D. H., 402, 452, 465, 490, 492, 503
Beach, S. R., 402
Beardslee, W. R., 451
Beavers, W. R., 408, 409, 412
Beavin, J. H., 359
Beck, A. T., 191, 224, 227, 230, 231, 233, 234, 235, 237, 238, 242, 243, 252, 254, 262, 276, 318, 358
Beck, J., 245, 262
Becker, E., 151
Becker, R. E., 199, 213, 536
Becvar, D. S., 439
Becvar, R. J., 439
Bednar, R. L., 517, 518
Bedrosian, R., 237
Beebe, B., 71, 74, 75
Beels, C. C., 468, 476
Behar, E., 203
Behrends, R. S., 95
Behrens, B. C., 468
Beidel, D. C., 211
Beier, E. G., 318
Bell, N., 131
Bellack, A. S., 182, 199, 215
Bellak, L., 358
Benefield, R. G., 208
Benjamin, J., 71, 72, 74, 75, 78, 101
Bennett, M. J., 361
Bennun, I., 434
Berchick, R., 238
Berg, I. K., 378, 379, 380, 383, 386, 447, 497
Bergan, J., 203
Berger, P. L., 445
Bergin, A. E., 1, 5, 12, 493
Bergman, J. S., 388
Berman, E. B., 494
Berman, J. S., 136, 302
Berman, J., 236, 251
Berman, W. H., 387
Berne, E., 358, 367, 368, 369, 383, 390
Bernheim, H., 26
Bernstein, D. A., 200, 201, 202
Bertagnolli, A., 237
Bertrando, P., 431

Best, K. M., 111
Beutler, L. E., 14, 262, 320, 327, 339, 344, 535, 544
Bevilacqua, L. J., 507
Bibring, E., 358
Binder, J. L., 116, 363, 388
Binswanger, L., 150, 169
Bion, W. R., 71, 88
Birchler, G., 494
Birchwood, M., 239
Bishop, S., 237, 238, 406, 411
Blackburn, I., 237, 238
Blatt, S. J., 54, 95
Blau, J. S., 196
Blechner, M. J., 85, 102
Blehar, M., 94
Bloch, S., 538
Bloom, B., 465
Bloom, B. L., 350, 351, 352, 353, 361, 383, 384, 390
Blowers, C., 238
Bodin, A. M., 378, 481
Boggs, S. R., 441
Bohart, A. C., 111, 119, 122, 133, 136, 142, 143, 144, 153, 170, 171, 175, 295, 299, 323, 324, 326, 334, 336
Boisvert, C., 133
Bollas, C., 76
Bongar, B., 5
Bonney, W. C., 539
Boocock, A., 239
Borduin, C. M., 402, 408
Borkovec, T. D., 200, 201, 203, 214, 238
Boscolo, L., 374, 403, 414, 431
Boss, M., 150, 169
Bostrom, A., 237
Boszormenyi-Nagy, I., 401, 416, 420, 421, 424, 470
Botella, L., 272
Bouman, T. K., 197
Bourque, P., 200
Bowen, M., 468, 470, 471, 472, 485
Bower, G., 254
Bowlby, J., 75, 94, 226, 468, 487
Bowman, S. L., 524
Box, S., 420
Boyd-Franklin, N., 403, 434
Bozarth, J. D., 122, 127, 136
Brabender, V., 545
Bracke, P., 168

Bradbury, T. N., 402, 464
Brandsma, J., 374
Bratton, S. C., 133, 135
Bray, J. H., 403, 452, 503, 545
Brehm, J., 354
Breismeister, J. M., 440
Brenner, C., 27, 32, 45, 63
Brestan, E. V., 441
Breuer, J., 18, 26, 27, 38, 39, 357
Breunlin, D. C., 402, 403, 452
Bricker, D., 256
Bridges, S. K., 287, 288
Briggs, R., 86
Bright, J. I., 302
Bright, P., 337
Brink, D. C., 144
Broderick, C. B., 463, 467, 471
Brodley, B. T., 107, 119
Brodsky, G. A., 440
Bromberg, P., 71, 72, 73
Bronfenbrenner, U., 442
Bronner, E., 286
Brooks, G., 403
Brooks, N., 238
Brown, G., 191, 243
Brown, L. S., 280, 290
Brown, R. A., 519
Brown, S., 525
Brown, T. A., 205, 210, 238
Bruening, P., 390
Bruner, J., 224
Bruynzeel, M., 195
Bry, B. H., 403, 434
Buber, M., 151, 152, 155, 156, 162, 168, 299
Budenz, D., 237
Budman, S. H., 351, 352, 353, 354, 356, 361, 373, 388, 389, 391, 469, 543
Bugental, J. F. T., 151, 152, 153, 155, 156, 157, 158, 159, 164, 166, 168, 169, 176
Bulik, C. M., 197
Bumberry, W. M., 406
Burg, J., 388
Burlingame, G. M., 388, 518, 519, 538, 544, 545
Burman, B., 465
Burns, D., 237, 245, 248, 249
Burns, J. A., 445
Burr-Harris, A. W., 408
Butcher, J. N., 351, 352, 353, 526
Butler, G., 238, 239

Butler, S. F., 362, 388, 389
Butollo, W., 338
Byers, S., 233
Byng-Hall, J., 416

Caballo, V. E., 215
Cade, B., 356
Cain, D. J., 144, 176
Callaghan, G. M., 208
Calzada, E. J., 438
Campbell, D., 431, 433
Campbell, F., 236
Campisi, T., 197
Camus, A., 151
Cantor, N., 109
Cantwell, D. P., 409
Carkhuff, R., 240
Carlson, J., 361, 391
Carlson, R., 328
Carmin, C., 238
Carr, A. C., 36, 434, 465
Carter, B., 403
Carter, E., 405
Carter, F. A., 197
Carter, R. T., 337, 338
Caspi, A., 109
Cassidy, J., 487
Castonguay, L. G., 208, 214
Catherall, D. R., 469
Cavell, T. A., 410
Cecchin, G., 374, 403, 414, 431
Celano, M. P., 403, 406, 416
Celantana, M., 279
Cerny, J. A., 205
Chadwick, P., 239
Chalkley, A. J., 238
Chamberlain, P., 409
Chambless, D. L., 14, 135, 143,
    192, 208, 239, 337, 338, 409
Chapman, A. L., 489
Charcot, J. M., 26
Cheselka, O., 42
Chiari, G., 272
Chisholm-Stockard, S., 136
Chomsky, N., 224
Christensen, A., 200, 202, 203,
    465, 468, 489, 490, 492,
    503
Christie, J., 238
Churchill, S., 150
Cirillo, S., 403
Clabby, J. F., 199
Clark, D. A., 239

Clark, D. C., 230, 234, 235, 238
Clark, D. M., 204, 238, 239
Clarke, J. C., 200, 212
Clarkin, J. F., 360, 388
Cleveland, J. D., 539
Cloitre, M., 215
Clore, G., 253
Clum, G. A., 207, 208
Cobb, J. A., 411
Cobb, J., 238
Coche, E., 526
Coche, J., 526
Cochran, B. N., 202
Coffin, W., 402
Cohen, L. R., 215
Colapinto, J., 434, 435, 437, 438
Cole, S. W., 94
Coleman, V. D., 525
Collins, A., 253
Comas-Díaz, L., 113
Combrinck-Graham, L., 406
Combs, G., 501
Conger, R. D., 412
Connell, G. M., 426
Connell, L. C., 426
Cook, P. F., 277
Coonerty, S., 338
Cooper, A. M., 39, 40, 94
Cooper, M., 177
Cooper, Z., 240
Cope, C. S., 539
Copley, B., 420
Corcoran, K., 523, 525
Corsini, R. J., 5
Costello, E., 238
Cotton, P., 243
Cottraux, J., 210
Coursol, D. H., 524
Cox, B. J., 207
Coyne, J. C., 409, 430
Cozzi, J. J., 402
Crago, M., 535
Craig-Bray, L., 277
Craske, M. G., 189, 190, 194, 196,
    202, 204, 205, 209, 238
Criswell, E., 175
Crits-Christoph, P., 36, 38, 45, 94,
    236, 240, 363, 519
Crits-Cristoph, P., 362
Crocket, K., 294, 312
Cromwell, R. L., 286
Crouch, C., 519
Crutchley, E., 431

Cuerdon, B. A., 383
Cullington, A., 238
Cummings, N. A., 337, 358, 361,
    383, 388
Cunningham, P. B., 402, 445
Curry, J., 228, 236
Curtis, R., 73, 81, 87, 92
Cushman, P., 167

Dahlen, E., 239
Daiuto, A. D., 402, 452, 503
Dana, R. H., 525
Daniel, S. S., 402, 403, 448, 452,
    453
Dasberg, H., 360, 388
Dattilio, F. M., 507
Davanloo, H., 359, 362, 363, 383
Davidovitz, D., 544
Davidson, J., 239, 245, 262
Davies, J. M., 71, 72, 73, 90, 102
Davis, M., 213, 236
Davison, G., 228
Davison, G. C., 215
Davison, K. P., 539
Day, J., 409
DeCarvalho, R., 170
Deffenbacher, J., 239
Dehle, C., 489
De Jong, P., 378, 380
de Jonghe, F., 11
Dekker, J., 11
DeLeon, P. H., 358
DeMichele, J. T., 526
Dempsey, D. J., 286, 302
Denniston, J. C., 196
Denton, W., 402, 465, 487, 488,
    489
DeRubeis, R. J., 236, 237, 519
de Shazer, S., 350, 355, 356, 359,
    360, 371, 373, 378, 379, 380,
    383, 386, 391, 446, 447, 448,
    497
Devins, G. M., 212
Diamond, G. S., 402
Dickerson, M., 196
Dickerson, S. S., 539
Dickerson, V. C., 499
Dickey, M., 402
Dicks, H. V., 467, 468, 474
DiClemente, C. C., 327, 339, 360,
    519
Diekstra, R., 228
Dierberger, A. E., 544

Dies, K. R., 521, 524, 525, 526,
    529, 531, 532, 533, 539
Dies, R. R., 515, 516, 517, 518,
    520, 521, 522, 523, 524, 525,
    526, 527, 528, 529, 530, 531,
    532, 533, 535, 536, 537, 538,
    539, 543, 544, 545
DiLollo, A., 294
Dimen, M., 71, 74
Dimidjian, S., 205
Dishion, T. J., 409
Dixon, A. E., 465
Doane, J. A., 445
Dobson, K. S., 227, 236, 262
Dockray-Miller, M., 536
Doherty, W. J., 448, 464
Doidge, N., 53, 54
Dolan, Y. M., 379
Dollard, J., 19, 20, 318
Donovan, J. M., 470, 508
Dougher, M. J., 202
Dowd, E. T., 331
Downie, F., 191
Dozois, D., 227
Drake, R., 243
Draper, R., 431
Dreelin, E. D., 406
Drescher, J., 74
Drewry, S., 390
Drost, L., 195
Druck, A., 64
Dryden, W., 239
DuBois, D., 236
Duncan, B. L., 136, 142, 326, 328,
    333, 336, 359, 479, 498
Dupuy, P., 168
Durand, V. M., 199
Dweck, C. S., 112, 120
D'Zurilla, T. J., 200

Eagle, M., 41, 43, 49, 53
Ecker, B., 289, 290, 291, 300, 311
Edelman, R. E., 192
Edelstien, M. G., 356
Efran, J. S., 277, 289, 301
Ehlers, C. L., 205
Ehrenberg, D., 90
Eifert, G. H., 216
Eisenberg, N., 410
Eisengart, S., 448
Elder, G. H., 109
Eldridge, K., 200
Elias, M. J., 199

Elkin, I., 236
Elkins, D. N., 175
Ellenberger, H., 177
Elliott, R., 18, 107, 109, 115, 135,
    136, 137, 144, 170, 171, 290,
    303, 323, 370
Ellis, A., 227, 228, 358, 522
Ellman, S., 63
Elster, J., 243
Emery, G., 224, 262, 318
Emmelkamp, P. M. G., 183, 195
Engels, G., 228
Epictetus, 225
Epp, L. R., 151, 155, 169
Epstein, L., 81
Epstein, N., 240, 243, 254, 406,
    411, 414, 438, 465, 490,
    492
Epstein, R., 110
Epston, D., 280, 293, 294, 296,
    297, 301, 302, 312, 357, 371,
    385, 446, 499
Epston, P., 3
Erbaugh, J., 242
Erickson, B. A., 371
Erickson, K. K., 373
Erickson, M. H., 358, 372, 374,
    376
Erickson, R. C., 519
Erikson, E. H., 29
Eron, J. B., 281, 290
Estrada, A. U., 402, 452
Eunson, K., 237
Evans, M., 237
Evans, S. A., 388, 389
Everstine, D. S., 373
Everstine, L., 373
Eyberg, S. M., 438, 441, 445
Eysenck, H. J., 184, 185

Fabes, R. A., 410
Faidley, A. J., 279, 298, 299
Fairbairn, W. R. D., 25, 70, 71, 72,
    73, 94, 473
Fairburn, C. G., 240
Falloon, I. R. H., 439, 440, 448,
    451
Fanger, M. T., 352, 379
Fanning, P., 213
Farber, B. A., 144
Farber, B. L., 136
Farber, E. W., 412
Farrell, D., 367

Farrelly, F., 374
Fauber, R. L., 301
Faulkner, R. A., 402
Fay, A., 351
Fay, L. F., 471
Feather, B. W., 318
Federn, P., 54
Feixas, G., 286, 302
Feldman, L. B., 402, 403, 494
Fennell, M., 238
Fensterheim, H., 333
Ferber, A., 468, 476
Ferebee, I., 200
Ferenczi, S., 357, 358
Fergus, K. D., 207
Fincham, F. D., 402, 464
Fink, C. M., 207, 211
Fink, P. J., 526
Finkelhor, D., 411
First, M. B., 182, 183, 184, 191,
    193, 205, 212, 214
Firth-Cozens, J., 339
Fisch, R., 356, 359, 374, 378, 383,
    391, 428, 481, 482, 484
Fischer, A. R., 525
Fischer, C. T., 153, 154
Fischer, J., 523, 525
Fishman, H. C., 436, 438, 476
Fiske, S., 231, 232
Fitzpatrick, M., 338
Fivush, R., 274
Flannagan, C., 256
Flavell, J., 231
Fleming, B., 245
Fletcher, K. E., 438
Foa, E. B., 195, 196, 197, 199, 209,
    232, 239, 248
Fodor, J., 226
Fogarty, T. F., 471
Fogel, A., 297
Follette, V. M., 202, 303
Follette, W. C., 208
Follette, W. T., 383
Fonagy, P., 56, 57, 74, 95
Ford, R. Q., 54
Forgatch, M. S., 440, 441
Fosha, D., 328
Fosshage, J., 75, 81, 82, 86
Foucault, M., 275
Fowler, D., 239
Fraenkel, P., 3, 15, 463, 464, 467,
    469, 473, 485, 489, 490, 493,
    503, 506, 508

Framo, J. L., 413, 416, 417, 467, 474
Frances, A., 239, 360, 388
Frank, E., 205
Frank, J. B., 5
Frank, J. D., 5, 320
Frank, K. A., 75, 87, 92, 324, 331, 332, 333, 334
Frankel, J., 86
Frankel, L., 438
Frankl, V. E., 151, 168, 226
Franklin, A. J., 338
Franklin, M. E., 197, 199
Fransella, F., 273, 286, 302
Frawley, M. G., 71, 73, 102
Freedheim, D. K., 5, 357
Freedman, J. H., 501
Freeman, A. S., 536, 545
Freeman, A., 233, 243, 245, 248, 252, 256, 262
Freeman, J., 294
French, T. M., 81, 358
Freud, A., 31, 41, 47
Freud, S., 11, 18, 28, 30, 31, 36, 38, 39, 40, 41, 42, 49, 53, 69, 70, 74, 76, 85, 93, 94, 275, 353, 354, 357, 362, 364, 371, 383, 387
Frie, R., 177
Fried, D., 94
Friedman, M., 151, 152, 155, 156, 157, 162, 168
Friedman, S., 352, 356, 361, 373, 379, 391
Fristad, M. A., 451
Fritzler, B. K., 207
Fromm, E., 70, 71, 75, 76, 85
Fromm-Reichmann, F., 54, 70, 76, 81, 87
Fuchs, C., 228
Fuhriman, A., 388, 518, 538, 545
Fukuyama, M., 286
Furman, B., 360, 374, 379
Furmark, T. L. G., 200

Gaelick-Buys, L., 199
Galatzer-Levy, R., 56
Gale, J. E., 402
Galinsky, M. D., 515, 516, 517
Galvin, J., 155
Gans, J. S., 526
Garety, P., 239
Garfield, S. L., 1, 5, 12, 351, 529

Garfield, S., 245
Garmazy, N., 111
Garnefski, N., 228
Garratt, C., 275
Garske, J. P., 5
Gartner, R., 86
Gavazzi, S. M., 451
Gedo, J., 36
Geiss, S. K., 465
Gelder, M., 238
Geldschlager, H., 286
Gelfand, L., 237
Gelles, R. J., 438
Gendlin, E. T., 107, 109, 114, 117, 120, 123, 127, 128, 132, 133, 136, 144, 170, 289, 295
Gensler, D., 86
Gergen, K. J., 276, 386, 445
Gershoff, E. T., 410
Gerson, M.-J., 86, 326, 338
Ghent, E., 71, 83
Giannetti, V. J., 361, 463
Gibbon, M., 191
Gigerenzer, G., 226
Gil, E., 426
Gilbert, M., 494
Gill, M. M., 30, 36, 39, 40, 41, 63, 70, 82, 91, 358, 501
Gillett, R., 280
Gilligan, S. G., 359, 361, 362, 379, 391
Gilmore, J., 230, 231, 232
Gingerich, S., 199
Gingerich, W. J., 360, 448
Ginsberg, B. G., 406
Giordano, F., 168
Giordano, J., 416
Giorgi, A., 150
Gislon, M., 338
Glass, C., 344, 345
Glass, G. V., 17, 383, 519
Glassman, N. S., 94
Glen, A. I., 238
Glynn, S., 438
Gold, J., 319, 321, 323, 324, 325, 326, 330, 331, 333, 335, 336, 338, 340, 345
Goldberg, A., 36
Goldfried, M. R., 170, 200, 208, 215, 227, 319, 336
Goldiamond, I., 209
Goldman, A., 503
Goldman, E. M., 302

Goldman, R., 363
Goldner, V., 74, 469
Goldstein, A., 337
Goldstein, A. P., 215
Goldstein, M. J., 206, 215, 409, 445, 448
Gonzo, M., 431
Goodman, G., 108, 123
Goodman, P., 358
Goodnow, J., 224
Goolishian, H. A., 415, 446
Gordon, D., 374
Gordon, J. R., 203
Gordon, T., 108
Gorman, J. M., 12, 19, 193, 205
Gotlib, I. H., 230, 235, 409
Gottman, J. M., 411, 465, 490
Gottschalk, L. A., 288
Gould, R. A., 207
Goulding, M. M., 356, 360, 369, 371
Goulding, R. L., 356, 360, 368, 369
Gournay, K., 239
Graap, K., 195
Grace, C., 338
Grawe, K., 170
Gray, P., 42, 53, 63
Gray, S. H., 420
Green, L., 190
Green, M., 90
Greenberg, H., 76
Greenberg, J. R., 82
Greenberg, J., 42, 71, 75
Greenberg, L. S., 107, 109, 115, 118, 119, 124, 125, 133, 135, 136, 142, 144, 170, 231, 290, 295, 303, 311, 323, 324, 332, 336, 340, 468, 485, 487, 488, 503
Greenberg, R., 238
Greenberger, D., 248
Greenburg, L. S., 370
Greene, A. F., 525
Greene, B. L., 467
Greenson, R. R., 39, 41, 44, 46, 50, 59, 60
Greist, J. H., 286
Grencavage, L. M., 14
Grinder, J., 373
Grondin, J., 149
Gross, J., 197
Grunebaum, J., 420

Guerin, P. J., Jr., 471
Guerney, B. G., 108, 401, 441
Guerney, L., 441
Guevremont, D. C., 438
Guidano, V. F., 227, 252, 262, 289, 324
Gunther, L. M., 196
Guntrip, H., 473
Gurman, A. S., 2, 3, 10, 15, 286, 326, 338, 351, 352, 353, 354, 391, 402, 403, 412, 424, 463, 464, 466, 467, 469, 473, 481, 485, 489, 490, 493, 494, 495, 496, 503, 506, 508, 544
Gustafson, J. P., 357, 360, 361, 363, 544

Haaga, D., 228, 234, 235, 237
Haddock, G., 239, 240
Hadley, S. W., 127
Haley, J., 356, 359, 371, 372, 374, 376, 377, 383, 390, 391, 405, 428, 442, 468, 476, 477, 479, 481
Haley-Banez, L., 525
Halford, W. K., 468, 490, 508
Hall, C. S., 520
Hamby, S. L., 411
Hammen, C., 230
Hampson, B. B., 408, 409, 412
Han, H., 215
Hanna, F. J., 168, 171
Hansen, N. D., 525
Hardke, L., 288
Hardy, K. V., 15, 469, 507
Harper, R., 228
Harrington, R., 236
Harris, A., 70, 71, 74
Harrison, R., 254
Hart, J., 207
Harter, S. L., 278, 303
Hartlage, S., 228
Hartman, S., 403
Hartmann, H., 31, 33
Haruki, Y., 142
Hatgis, C., 182
Havens, R. A., 372
Haw, J., 196
Hawk, L. W., 192
Hawton, K., 200
Hayes, A., 337
Hayes, S. C., 8, 15, 187, 202, 203, 209

Haynes, S. N., 215
Hazan, C., 94
Hazlett-Stevens, H., 200
Healey, B. J., 338
Heath, E. S., 384
Heavey, C. L., 503
Hecker, J. E., 207
Hedges, M., 15
Heffere, R. W., 410
Heidegger, M., 150
Heimberg, R. G., 192, 199, 213, 238, 239, 536
Heitler, S., 338
Hellcamp, D., 338
Helmeke, K. B., 403
Hembree, E., 232, 239
Hendricks, M. N., 123, 135, 137
Henggeler, S. W., 402, 408, 438, 439, 442, 443, 444, 445
Henry, W. P., 388
Hepworth, J., 448
Herbener, E. S., 109
Hermans, H. J. M., 276, 286, 287, 312
Hermans-Jansen, E., 287
Herschell, A. D., 438, 441
Hersen, M., 182, 192, 215
Hertel, R. K., 474
Hexum, A. L., 374
Hibbert, G., 238
Hill, C. E., 136
Hiller, T., 379, 380
Hillman, J., 167
Hinkle, D., 281, 286
Hirsch, I., 70, 71, 78, 82
Hirsch, S. I., 409
Hoag, M. J., 519
Hodes, M., 409
Hodges, L. F., 195
Hodgson, A. B., 339
Hodgson, R., 197
Hoffman, I. Z., 71, 79, 82, 83
Hoffman, L., 284, 403, 445
Hoffman, P. D., 409
Hofmann, S. G., 238
Hofstee, W. K. B., 6
Hogarty, G. E., 415, 448
Holdstock, T. L., 112, 119
Holland, P., 409
Hollon, S. D., 11, 135, 143, 236, 237
Holmes, D. S., 94
Holmes, S. E., 532

Holt, R. R., 29
Holzman, L., 289, 301, 302
Honig, A., 451
Hoogduin, C. A. L., 208
Hooley, J. M., 402, 409, 451
Hope, D. A., 239
Horney, K., 70, 71, 74
Hornung, C. A., 524
Horowitz, L. M., 94
Horowitz, M. J., 231, 363
Hovarth, A. O., 170
Howard, K. I., 519, 528
Hoyt, M. F., 351, 352, 353, 354, 355, 356, 357, 358, 359, 360, 361, 365, 367, 368, 369, 370, 371, 373, 374, 376, 379, 380, 381, 383, 384, 385, 386, 387, 388, 389, 390, 391, 469, 498
Hubble, M. A., 328, 359, 498
Hudson, P., 379
Huey, S. J., 445
Hulley, L., 289, 290, 291, 300, 311
Husserl, E., 150

Imber-Black, E., 405
Ingram, R. E., 16, 232, 234, 235
Iwamasa, G. Y., 211

Jackson, D. D., 358, 359, 376, 401, 428, 463, 468
Jackson, D. N., 95
Jacobson, E., 35, 200, 201
Jacobson, G., 384
Jacobson, N. S., 200, 202, 205, 206, 465, 468, 469, 489, 490, 492, 494, 503, 508
Jaffe, J., 75
James, S. E., 406, 416
James, W., 150, 152
Jameson, J. S., 196
Janet, P., 26
Jarrett, R., 237
Jaycox, L. H., 199
Jensen, J. P., 493
Jerremalm, A., 183
Joffe, R., 526
Johnson, B., 465
Johnson, I. H., 525
Johnson, L. D., 358
Johnson, S., 452
Johnson, S. M., 124, 133, 416, 417, 465, 468, 485, 487, 488
Johnson, Z., 134

Jome, L. M., 525
Jones, M. C., 184
Jones, R., 240
Jordan, C., 449
Jordan, P. L., 402
Josephson, A. M., 441
Jouriles, E. N., 503
Joyce, A. S., 76, 94, 518, 519, 524
Joyce, P. R., 197
Jung, C. G., 150
Juster, H. R., 239

Kadis, L. B., 368
Kahn, J., 409
Kaiser, H., 360, 383, 384
Kaley, H., 53
Kanas, N., 519, 522
Kanfer, F. H., 199, 215
Kantor, D., 424
Karoly, P., 16, 17, 198
Kaslow, F. W., 402, 403, 407, 416
Kaslow, N. J., 403, 406, 416
Kassel, J., 235
Katon, W., 236
Kaul, T. J., 517
Kautto, J. G., 471
Kazak, A. E., 403
Kazdin, A. E., 200, 430, 444
Keefler, J., 448
Keenan, M., 238
Kegan, R., 231
Kehrer, C. A., 202
Keijsers, G. P. J., 208
Keim, J., 428, 477, 479, 494
Keisler, D. J., 523
Keith, D. V., 424, 425, 426, 427
Kelley, H. H., 489
Kelly, G. A., 3, 224, 227, 274, 276,
    279, 280, 281, 286, 289, 290,
    292, 295, 298, 300
Kempen, H. J. G., 312
Kempler, W., 424
Kerig, P., 410, 411
Kernberg, O. F., 31, 35, 36, 54, 275
Kierkegaard, S., 149, 159
Kiesler, D. J., 469
Kihlstrom, J. F., 94, 230
Kingdon, D. G., 239
Kingreen, D., 286
Kirk, J., 200
Kirsch, I., 11
Kitayama, S., 55
Kivlighan, D. M., 528, 532, 535

Klapp, B., 286
Klein, M. H., 136, 286
Klein, M., 70, 88, 473
Klein, R. H., 519, 523
Klerman, G. L., 200, 337, 339
Klimes, I., 238
Klock, K., 402
Klosko, J. S., 205
Kniskern, D. P., 402, 463
Knox, S., 136
Koenen, K. C., 215
Koenig, G. R., 524
Koenigsberg, H. W., 36
Kohlenberg, B. S., 209
Kohlenberg, R. J., 133, 209
Kohut, H., 25, 31, 52, 71, 89, 275
Kolden, G. G., 136
Kolod, S., 92
Kool, S., 11
Kopelowicz, A., 403
Koshikawa, F., 142
Koss, M. P., 351, 352, 353, 526
Kovacs, M., 231, 232, 237, 252
Kozak, M. J., 197, 209, 239
Kraft, I. A., 539
Krasner, L., 184, 215
Krasnow, A. D., 527
Kreider, J. W., 359
Kris, E., 31
Kroenke, K., 239
Kuch, K., 207
Kuehlwein, K., 379
Kuipers, E., 239
Kupfer, D. J., 205
Kurtines, W. M., 438

L'Abate, L., 414, 438, 449
Lachmann, F. M., 75, 82, 86
Ladouceur, R., 200
Laing, R. D., 151, 155, 168, 177
Lam, K. N., 211
Lambert, M. J., 543, 544
Lambert, M., 236
Lammers, M. W., 208
Lane, J. S., 136
Lang, P. J., 207
Langs, R. J., 49
Lankton, C., 372, 374
Lankton, S. R., 372, 373, 374,
    390
Lappin, J., 477, 479, 494
Laszloffy, T. A., 15, 469, 507
LaTaillade, J. J., 492

Latham, G. P., 529
Lather, P., 276
Latimer, P., 196
Lawlis, F., 518
Lawrence, E., 200
Lawrence, W. G., 85
Layden, M., 233, 256
Lazarus, A. A., 12, 184, 227, 320,
    322, 325, 327, 329, 345, 351,
    355, 358, 383
Lazarus, R., 230, 231
le Grange, D., 409
Leahy, R. L., 241, 251
Lebow, J. L., 2, 344, 345, 402, 416,
    452, 465, 493, 503
LeBow, M., 301
Lee, T., 445
Leeuw, I., 196
Leff, J., 409, 503
Leggett, E. L., 112, 120
LeGrange, D., 240
Lehr, W., 424
Leitenberg, H., 197
Leitner, L. M., 170, 279, 290, 296,
    298, 299
Lerner, B., 133
Lerner, M., 151
Lester, D., 243
Leszcz, M., 522
Leung, A. W., 192
Levant, R. F., 108, 111, 133, 403,
    449, 452
Levenson, E. A., 71, 82, 85
Levenson, H., 328, 362, 363, 388,
    389, 544
Leventhal, H., 230, 231
Levine, J., 237
Levitt, H., 288, 303
Levy, K., 95
Lewandowski, A. M., 278, 281
Lewellen, A., 449
Lewicki, P., 113
Lewin, K. K., 358
Liberman, R. P., 199, 403, 438
Lichtenberg, J. D., 75, 82, 86
Liddle, H. A., 2, 335, 338, 403,
    445, 452
Lieberman, M. A., 536, 538
Lief, H., 494
Lietaer, G., 108, 113, 115, 128,
    133, 144, 303
Lindahl, I.-L., 183
Lindahl, K., 410, 411

Lindholm, B. W., 411
Lindsley, O. R., 184
Lindzey, G., 520
Linehan, H., 339, 344
Linehan, M. M., 202
Liotti, G., 227, 252, 262, 324
Lipsey, M. W., 17
Lipsius, S. H., 526
Livesley, W. J., 95, 530, 533
Lobovits, D., 294
Locke, E. A., 529
Loewenstein, R. M., 31
Lolas, F., 288
London, P., 7
Long, L. D., 539
Loosen, P., 236
Lorenzini, R., 296
Losee, M. C., 207
Loundy, M. R., 403
Lovell, K., 239
Lovibond, P. F., 212
Lovibond, S. H., 212
Low, J., 323
Low, S. M., 403
Luborsky, L., 17, 38, 44, 45, 94, 302, 363
Luckman, T., 445
Lukens, M. D., 289
Lukens, R. J., 289
Lund, T. W., 281, 290
Lunnen, K. M., 543
Lusterman, D.-D., 403, 452, 453
Lustman, P. J., 237
Lyddon, W. J., 272
Lynn, S. J., 5
Lyons, A., 151, 175
Lyons-Ruth, K., 52

Mabe, P. A., 441
Macalpine, I., 39
MacDevitt, J. W., 539
MacKenzie, K. R., 338, 516, 524, 530, 533, 538, 543
MacKune-Karrer, B., 402, 452
MacLennan, B. W., 539
Madanes, C., 359, 414, 430, 476, 481
Madigan, S. P., 302, 371
Magagna, J., 420
Magee, R. D., 403
Magnavita, J. J., 328, 402
Mahler, M., 35
Mahoney, M. J., 131, 224, 226,

227, 262, 273, 276, 277, 289, 301, 312
Mahrer, A. R., 159
Main, M., 94
Malan, D. H., 36, 356, 358, 359, 362, 363, 364, 383, 384
Manderscheid, R. W., 524
Mangrum, L. F., 402, 410
Mann, J., 251, 351, 359, 363
Manning, W. H., 294
Manus, G. I., 467
Marcel, G., 151
Marcotte, D., 331, 333, 339
Margolin, G., 465, 468
Margraf, J., 184, 215
Mari, M. T., 302
Markert, R. J., 526
Markman, H. J., 402, 403, 411, 464, 492, 508
Markowitz, J. C., 11, 200, 236
Marks, I., 183, 184, 196, 204, 239
Markus, H. R., 55, 232
Marlatt, G. A., 203
Marmor, J., 318
Marris, P., 95
Marsh, D. T., 402, 403, 452
Marshak, L. E., 539
Martell, C. R., 205
Martin, J., 295
Maruish, M. E., 523
Mascolo, M. F., 277, 297, 302
Massman, P., 251
Masten, A. S., 111
Matano, R., 151
Mattick, R. P., 212
Maurer, G. G., 519
May, R., 149, 150, 151, 152, 153, 154, 155, 158, 159, 164, 167, 168, 169, 176, 177
Mayerson, N. H., 523, 528
Maynard, P. E., 438
McCabe, R. E., 194, 196
McCallum, M., 94, 524, 533
McCann, L., 18
McCarter, R., 337
McCarthy, B. W., 464
McCleary, L., 409
McClintic, K., 338
McCrady, B. S., 508
McCullough, L., 322, 367
McCullough-Vaillant, L., 362
McDaniel, S. H., 403, 448, 452,

453
McDermut, W., 519
McDonald, A. L., 402
McDougall, J., 76
McElwain, B., 169, 170, 171
McFall, R. M., 190
McFarlane, W. R., 416, 448, 449, 451
McGarvey, A., 235
McGoldrick, M., 403, 405
McGovern, T. V., 528
McIntosh, V. V., 197
McKay, D., 197
McKay, M., 213
McMain, S., 261
McNeel, J., 370, 371
McRoberts, C., 519
Meeker, B. F., 524
Meichenbaum, D., 227, 230, 231, 232, 247
Melamed, B. G., 207
Melancon, S. M., 209
Melby, J., 412
Melnick, J., 523, 527
Meltzoff, J., 4, 8
Mendelowitz, E., 168
Mendelson, M., 242
Mennin, D., 238
Menzies, R. G., 200
Merbaum, M., 227
Mercier, M., 237
Merleau-Ponty, M., 150, 157
Merluzzi, T., 239
Messer, S. B., 2, 3, 5, 7, 10, 12, 14, 17, 18, 20, 34, 36, 37, 64, 93, 94, 101, 171, 302, 311, 319, 320, 321, 322, 324, 333, 345, 351, 353, 362, 363, 364, 365, 367, 385, 386, 387, 494, 526
Metalsky, G., 228
Meuser, K. T., 503
Meyer, A.-E., 132
Michels, J., 136
Mikesell, R. H., 452, 453
Miklowitz, D. J., 200, 206, 402, 445, 448, 451
Miles, M. B., 536
Miller, I. J., 170
Miller, I. W., 519
Miller, N. E., 19, 318
Miller, N., 406, 447
Miller, R. R., 196
Miller, R., 251

Miller, S. D., 136, 142, 326, 328, 333, 336, 359, 360, 378, 379, 447, 498
Miller, T. I., 17, 519
Miller, W. R., 136, 142, 208
Miltenberger, R., 198
Mineka, S., 209, 210
Minuchin, P., 434
Minuchin, S., 401, 434, 436, 437, 438, 442, 476
Miranda, J., 234
Mischel, W., 185, 227
Mitchell, S. A., 25, 70, 71, 72, 74, 75, 81, 83, 94, 102
Mittelman, B., 467, 473
Mitterer, J., 286
Mock, J., 242
Moleiro, C., 320
Molina, B., 525
Moliner, J. L., 302
Molnar, C., 214
Monarch, N. D., 403
Monheit, J., 151
Monk, G., 293, 294, 301, 312
Montalvo, B., 401, 434
Montes, J. N., 302
Montuori, M., 151
Moore, D. W., 411
Moore, M. K., 303
Moore, R., 237
Moos, B. S., 411
Moos, R. H., 411, 524
Moreno, K., 519
Morgan, H., 196
Morin, C. M., 192
Morrison, K., 17, 171
Morss, J., 301, 302
Mosconi, A., 431
Mosher, L., 151, 170
Moss, D., 149
Moustakas, C., 151
Muenz, L. R., 94
Mueser, K. T., 199, 200, 402, 438, 452
Mumford, E., 383
Munoz, R. F. L. G., 211
Muran, J. C., 45, 94, 102
Murphy, G. E., 237, 245
Murray, H. A., 150

Nadelson, C. C., 474
Najavits, L. M., 215, 544
Nardone, G., 430

Nathan, P. E., 12, 19, 193
Naugle, A. E., 208
Neal, J. H., 499
Nedate, K., 142, 211
Neiderhiser, J. M., 410
Neimeyer, G. J., 277, 281, 286, 292, 302, 311
Neimeyer, R. A., 226, 236, 273, 274, 276, 277, 281, 283, 286, 287, 288, 289, 292, 294, 297, 300, 301, 302, 303, 311, 312
Neisser, U., 6, 110, 274
Nelson, R. O., 187
Nemeroff, C. J., 198
Nerin, W. F., 486
Newell, A., 224
Newman, C., 233, 319
Newman, F., 289
Newman, M. G., 201, 214
Neziroglu, F., 197
Nezu, A. M., 200
Nichols, M. P., 434, 438, 467, 474, 476, 485, 500, 506
Nichols, W. C., 494
Nietzsche, F., 149, 150
Norcross, J. C., 2, 12, 14, 15, 19, 142, 193, 319, 345, 360, 526
Noshirvani, H., 239
Notarius, C. I., 411
Nudelman, S., 197
Nuechterlein, K., 409
Nurse, A. R., 402, 410
Nutt, R., 403
Nuzzo, M. L., 272

O'Brien, W. O., 215
O'Donohue, W., 184, 215
Ogden, T., 73
Ogles, B. M., 236, 388, 543
Ogrodniczuk, J. S., 524
O'Hanlon, W. H., 356, 359, 372, 374, 379, 391, 446
O'Hara, M. M., 112, 113, 134, 151, 168, 170, 176
O'Leary, K. D., 465
Ollendick, T. H., 14
Olson, D. H., 406, 408
Orange, D. M., 71
Oremland, J., 42
Organista, K. C., 211
Orlinsky, D. E., 170, 519, 528
Ornstein, P. H., 358
Orsillo, S. M., 191, 203

Ortony, A., 253
Öst, L.-G., 183, 200
Owens, D., 409

Padesky, C. A., 248
Pantone, P., 86
Paolino, T. J., 494, 508
Papero, D., 471, 472
Papouchis, N., 338
Papp, P., 403, 414, 431
Parad, H. J., 358
Parker, I., 294, 303
Parkes, C. M., 95
Parks, B. K., 170
Parloff, M. B., 517, 526
Parsons, T., 404
Passman, V., 338
Patterson, C., 406
Patterson, G. R., 409, 411, 440, 441
Patterson, J., 498
Paul, B., 474
Paul, N., 474, 476
Paul, S., 378, 388
Payne, L. L., 196
Pearce, J. K., 416
Pearson, P. T., 474
Peen, J., 11
Peet, B., 375
Peller, J. E., 379, 388
Pelzer, K., 338
Penn, P., 403
Pennebaker, J. W., 539
Pepitone-Arreola-Rockwell, F., 525
Pepper, C. M., 430
Perez Foster, R., 92
Perloff, J., 237
Perls, F. S., 358
Perret, J.-F., 131
Perret-Clermont, A.-N., 131
Persons, J., 237, 242, 245, 262
Peterson, C., 228
Peveler, R. C., 240
Phares, E. J., 521
Phelps, P. A., 352, 359
Phillips, A., 76
Phillips, J., 161
Philpot, C. L., 403, 452
Phipps, L. B., 524
Piasecki, J., 237
Pierson, J. F., 151, 168, 169, 176
Pine, F., 25

Pinsker, H., 367
Pinsof, W. M., 326, 333, 338, 402, 452, 465, 469, 470, 493, 494, 508
Piper, W. E., 94, 518, 519, 524, 533
Plaud, J. J., 216
Portnoy, D., 157
Prata, G., 374, 403, 414, 431
Pretzer, J., 245
Price, R., 379
Prochaska, J. O., 12, 15, 142, 325, 327, 339, 360
Procter, H. G., 284, 289
Prout, M., 196
Prouty, A. M., 403
Prouty, G. F., 133
Pugh, C., 438
Puhakka, K., 168
Pulver, S., 62
Purdon, C., 239
Purser, R., 151, 175

Qaiser, M., 81, 92
Quille, T., 338
Quitkin, F., 237

Rachman, S. J., 184, 185, 210
Racker, H., 71, 83, 88
Raffle, C., 196
Rait, D., 464, 470, 493
Rampage, C., 16, 507
Randall, D. A., 539
Rank, O., 150, 164, 357, 358
Rankin, H., 197
Rankin, L. A., 465
Rapaport, D., 30
Rapee, R. M., 239
Raskin, J. D., 278, 281, 312
Raskin, N. J., 108, 126
Raskin, P. M., 144
Rasmussen, A., 363
Raue, P. J., 208
Ray, D., 133, 135
Ray, P., 176
Ray, R. S., 411
Ray, S. B., 524
Ray, W. A., 428
Razin, A. M., 2
Ready, D., 195
Rehm, L., 227, 228, 247
Reich, W., 33
Reinecke, M., 228, 235, 236, 241, 243, 262

Reiss, D., 410
Reiss, D. J., 448
Renfrey, G. S., 211
Rennie, D. L., 109, 136, 171, 290, 326, 336
Resick, P. A., 239
Rhodes, J. W., 318
Rice, D., 151
Rice, D. G., 464
Rice, J. K., 464
Rice, L. N., 107, 109, 117, 125, 144, 170, 290, 323
Richeport-Haley, M., 372, 377
Riess, H., 536
Riester, A. E., 539
Riley, S., 239
Roback, H. B., 523, 537
Roberto, L. G., 424, 425, 426
Roberto-Forman, L., 470, 472, 473
Roberts, A., 144
Roberts, J., 235, 405
Robinson, L. A., 236, 302
Robson, P., 238
Rocchi, M. T., 296
Rodenhauser, P., 526
Rodriguez, B., 344, 345
Roemer, L., 191, 203
Rogers, C. R., 107, 108, 109, 111, 112, 115, 116, 117, 119, 121, 123, 126, 127, 128, 134, 135, 136, 142, 144, 151, 275
Rogers, G., 235
Rohrbaugh, M. J., 481, 482, 483, 498
Rollnick, S., 142
Romanelli, R., 320
Romano, P., 203
Rombauts, J., 108, 144
Roodman, A. A., 208
Rosen, H., 231, 379
Rosen, J. C., 197
Rosen, S., 374
Rosenbaum Asarnow, J., 409
Rosenbaum, R., 122, 383, 385
Rosenfarb, I., 409
Rosenfeld, H. A., 54
Rosenthal, R., 367
Rosenzweig, S., 332
Rosman, B., 401
Rossi, E., 374, 376
Rossi, S., 374
Roth, G., 175

Rothbaum, B. O., 195, 239
Rounsaville, B., 337
Rourke, M. T., 403
Rowan, J., 150
Rowan, T., 359
Rowe, C., 338
Rowe, M. K., 196
Rowland, M. D., 402, 445
Rubio, E., 287
Runyan, D., 411
Rusck, G., 390
Rush, A. J., 224, 236, 237, 262, 318
Russell, C., 406
Rutan, J. S., 518, 522, 536
Ryan, N., 236
Ryckoff, I. M., 409
Ryle, A., 323, 339

Saayman, G. S., 438
Sachs-Ericsson, N., 451
Safran, J. D., 45, 94, 102, 230, 231, 241, 251, 261, 262, 331, 332, 333, 334, 336, 339, 345
Sager, C. J., 467, 473
Saleebey, D., 301
Salkovskis, P. M., 195, 215, 238, 239
Salovey, P., 231, 232
Salvendy, J. T., 525, 526
Sampson, H., 42, 363
Sandell, R., 57, 93
Sanders, M. R., 468
Sanderson, W. C., 10, 193
Sandler, A. M., 75
Sandler, J., 64, 75
Sanford, M., 409
Sanislow, C., 539
Sano, N., 196
Santa-Barbara, J., 411
Santisteban, D. A., 403, 430, 452
Sapirstein, G., 11
Sartre, J.-P., 151
Sassaroli, S., 296
Satir, V., 401, 406, 424, 425, 428, 463, 468, 484, 485, 486
Saul, S., 539
Savard, J., 192
Sawyer, J., 236
Sayama, M., 361, 388
Schaap, C. P. D. R., 208
Schaefer, C. E., 440
Schafer, R., 43, 47, 49
Scharff, D. E., 416, 474

Scharff, J. S., 416, 417, 420, 470, 474, 475, 476
Scheidlinger, S., 536
Schermer, V. L., 519
Schewe, P. A., 402
Schindler, D., 468
Schlesinger, G., 49
Schlesinger, H., 383
Schlesinger, S., 240
Schmidt, N. B., 201
Schneider, K. J., 18, 149, 150, 152, 153, 154, 155, 158, 159, 164, 165, 166, 168, 169, 170, 171, 175, 176
Schneider, W. J., 494
Schnicke, M. K., 239
Schoenwald, S. K., 402, 445
Schrader, S. S., 463, 467, 471
Schrodt, G., 238, 244
Schroeder, M. L., 95
Schulberg, H., 236
Schumer, F., 401
Schwartz, M. S., 202
Schwartz, R. C., 402, 403, 452, 467, 474, 500, 506
Searles, H., 54, 71, 76, 91
Sears, R. R., 318
Sechehaye, M. A., 54
Seeman, J., 144, 176
Segal, L., 356, 391, 430, 481, 484
Segal, Z., 203, 230, 234, 241, 251, 261, 262, 332, 334, 336
Segraves, R. T., 469, 494
Seiden, D. Y., 211
Seifer, M., 448
Seikkula, J., 296
Seligman, M., 170, 227, 228, 539
Selton, R., 226
Selvini, M., 403
Selvini-Palazzoli, M., 403, 431, 433
Selzer, M. A., 36
Serlin, I. A., 159
Serrano, A. C., 402
Sewell, K. W., 286
Sexton, T. L., 338, 438, 441
Shaffer, J., 515, 516, 517
Shafran, R., 240
Shapiro, D., 251, 339
Sharp, J., 151, 168
Shaver, P. R., 94, 487
Shaw, B. F., 224, 230, 262, 318
Shaw, D. A., 411

Shaw, S. R., 544
Shea, M., 236
Shear, M. K., 205
Shectman, F., 387
Shelton, R., 236, 237
Shiang, J., 351
Shlien, J. M., 108, 111, 115, 129, 133, 144
Shmulker, D., 494
Shoebridge, P., 236
Shoham, V., 402, 452, 481, 482, 483, 498, 503
Short, D., 359
Shostrom, E. L., 121
Shotter, J., 297
Sifneos, P. E., 358, 359, 362, 363, 364, 383
Silbergeld, S., 524
Silliman, B., 402
Silverstein, O., 403, 431
Simmons, D. S., 464
Simms, S., 403
Simon, G., 236
Simon, K., 243, 245, 262
Simoneau, T. L., 451
Simons, A. D., 237, 245
Simpson, L., 434
Siporin, M., 519
Skinner, B. F., 184, 186
Skinner, H. A., 411, 439
Skolnick, N. J., 71
Skolnikoff, A., 56
Skynner, A. C. R., 471, 474
Slade, P., 239
Small, L., 358
Smilansky, E. M., 420
Smith, D., 142
Smith, M. C., 525
Smith, M. L., 17, 519
Smith, M., 523, 537
Snyder, C. R., 16
Snyder, D. K., 402, 410, 468, 494
Sobel, R., 401
Sokol, L., 238
Soldano, K. W., 451
Sollod, R. N., 338
Solomon, A., 234, 235
Solomon, H. C., 184
Solomon, M., 474
Sonis, W. A., 402
Sorgato, R., 431
Sorrentino, A. M., 403
Soulios, C., 207

Spark, G., 420, 421
Speed, J., 388
Spence, D. P., 18
Spence, D., 300
Spence, S., 236
Sperry, L., 256, 361, 391, 403
Spiegel, D. A., 238
Spillman, A., 17, 94
Spinelli, E., 150, 169
Spinks, S., 494
Spitzer, R. L., 191
Spotnitz, H., 81
Sprenkle, D., 406
Stanley, S. M., 402, 464, 492
Stanton, M. D., 477, 479, 494
Stayner, D. A., 95
Steenbarger, B. N., 543
Steer, R. A., 191, 242, 243
Steinhauer, P. D., 411
Steketee, G. S., 239, 248, 409
Sterba, R., 45
Sterling, M., 152, 153, 162, 163
Stern, D. B., 73
Stern, D. N., 74, 75, 114
Stern, M. J., 539
Stern, R., 183, 196
Sterner, U., 183
Stewart, B., 237
Stewart, J., 237
Stickle, T. R., 402, 452, 503
Stockton, L., 283
Stockwell, T., 197
Stoller, R., 74
Stolorow, R. D., 71, 73, 161, 169
Stone, W. N., 518, 526
Storm, C. L., 403
Straus, M. A., 411
Street, L., 196
Stricker, G., 317, 319, 321, 322, 324, 325, 330, 331, 333, 335, 336, 337, 340, 344, 345, 493
Strosahl, K. D., 202, 203
Strupp, H. H., 116, 127, 351, 363, 388, 544
Stuart, G. L., 214
Stuart, R. B., 468, 489
Stunkard, A. J., 172
Subich, L. M., 524
Suddath, R., 451
Sullivan, H. S., 70, 71, 72, 73, 74, 76, 79, 80, 81, 91, 94, 383
Sullivan, P. F., 197
Summerfeldt, L. J., 191

Sweeney, P., 228
Swiller, H. I., 539
Swindle, R., 239
Swinson, R. P., 183, 191, 193, 195, 196, 204, 207, 213
Szalita, A., 91
Szapocznik, J., 430, 438

Tallman, K., 111, 119, 136, 142, 170, 171, 295, 299, 323, 336
Talmon, M., 351, 379, 383, 384, 385
Tanaka-Matsumi, J., 211
Tang, T., 237
Tarrier, N., 195, 239, 240
Tassinari, R., 205
Tataryn, D. J., 94
Tauber, E. S., 90
Tausch, R., 136
Taylor, E. T., 149
Taylor, N. T., 526
Taylor, S., 231, 232, 239
Taylor, T., 402
Teasdale, J. D., 203, 228
Telch, M. J., 205, 238
Teleska, P. A., 516, 523, 528, 537
Terhune, W. S., 184
Thase, M. E., 11, 236
Their, P., 286
Thibaut, J. W., 489
Thomas, C., 209, 210
Thomas, J. C., 214
Thomas, M. B., 400, 401, 445
Thompson, C., 70, 74, 81
Thompson, M. G., 151
Thrasher, S., 239
Ticho, E. A., 47, 361
Tillich, P., 151, 154
Tinsley, H. E. A., 524, 528
Tirelli, M., 431
Tishby, O., 17, 94
Toarmino, D., 8, 15
Tobin, D., 338
Todaro, J., 197
Todd, T. C., 403, 477, 479, 494
Tokins, M., 262
Tolman, E., 226
Tomas, M., 431
Tomm, K., 371
Tompkins, M., 245
Tompson, M., 409
Toms, M., 119
Tonigan, J. S., 208

Torres, J. S., 525
Toseland, R. W., 519
Touliatos, J., 411
Toyokawa, T., 211
Treat, S. R., 494
Treat, T. A., 214
Trexler, L., 243
Trierweiler, S. J., 344
Trower, P., 239
Truax, C., 240
Tsai, M., 133, 209
Tschuschke, V., 539
Turk, C., 238
Turk, D., 231, 232
Turkington, D., 240
Turner, M. K., 441
Turner, R. M., 196
Turner, S. M., 211

Ullmann, L. P., 184
Ulrich, D. N., 420, 470
Unger, R., 523

Vakoch, D. A., 544
Vallis, T., 230
van Aalst, G., 11
Van Balen, R., 108, 111, 144
VandenBos, G. R., 358
van der Mast, C. A. P. G., 195
Vandiver, V., 449
Vara, L. S., 197
Vasco, A. B., 301
Vaughn, C., 409
Veale, D., 239
Velasquez, M. M., 519
Ventura, M., 167
Vetere, A., 437
Vincent, N., 301
Viney, L. L., 288, 302
Vinogradov, S., 523
Visher, E. B., 406
Visher, J. S., 406
Visser, S., 197
von Bertalanffy, L., 404
Vontress, C. E., 151, 155, 169

Wachtel, E. F., 86
Wachtel, P. L., 10, 43, 64, 86, 92, 318, 321, 323, 324, 325, 326, 332, 338, 340, 345
Wadden, T. A., 172
Wade, W. A., 182, 214
Wadlington, W., 168

Waelder, R., 31
Wahl, K., 239
Wakefield, J., 43
Waldron, S., 56
Wall, S., 94
Wallerstein, R. S., 25, 56, 57, 64
Walley, L., 238
Walsh, F., 406
Walsh, R. A., 169, 170, 171
Walsh, S. R., 402
Walter, J. L., 379, 388
Walters, M., 403, 416
Waltman, D. E., 527
Wamboldt, F. S., 410
Wamboldt, M. Z., 410
Wampold, B. E., 12, 14, 17, 101, 136, 143, 156, 170, 171, 302, 320, 543, 544
Ward, C., 242
Ward, D. M., 445
Warner, R., 451
Warren, C. S., 7, 36, 37, 93, 351, 353, 362, 363, 364, 365, 367, 385, 386, 387
Warren, R., 214
Warshaw, S. C., 71
Waters, E., 94
Watson, J. C., 133, 136, 150, 153, 171
Watzlawick, P., 359, 375, 378, 386, 390, 428, 432, 481, 482
Weakland, J. H., 355, 356, 359, 376, 378, 391, 428, 481, 482, 484
Weber, C., 286
Webster-Stratton, C. H., 402, 438, 441
Wedding, D., 5
Weeks, G. R., 374, 469, 494
Weinberger, J., 14, 332, 336
Weiner, M. B., 539
Weiner-Davis, M., 356, 360, 379, 391, 415, 446, 497
Weinshel, E. M., 46
Weinstein, S. E., 449
Weiss, J., 42, 363
Weiss, R. D., 544
Weiss, R. L., 494
Weissman, M. M., 200, 337
Weissman, S., 243
Wells, A., 239
Wells, R. A., 351, 352, 359, 361, 463

Welwood, J., 160
Wertz, F. J., 150, 170
Wessels, H., 183
Westen, D., 17, 77, 94, 102, 323, 363
Wetzel, R. D., 237
Wetzler, S., 525
Wexler, D. A., 109, 117, 125
Wheeler, J. G., 202, 203
Wheelis, A., 151
Whisman, M. A., 235, 465
Whitaker, C. A., 406, 424, 425, 426, 427
White, J., 238
White, J. R., 536, 545
White, M., 3, 280, 293, 294, 296, 297, 301, 302, 357, 359, 371, 385, 415, 446, 448, 499
White, S., 465
Whiting, R. A., 405
Whittaker, J., 236
Whorf, B., 224
Wickwire, K., 207
Wile, D. B., 501, 502, 503
Wilk, J., 379
Willi, J., 474
Williams, A., 494
Williams, J. B. W., 191
Williams, J. M. G., 203

Williams, K. E., 208
Williams, R. A., 419, 430
Wills, R. M., 494
Wilson, D. B., 17
Wilson, G. T., 182, 193
Wilson, J., 239
Wilson, K. G., 202
Winnicott, D. W., 25, 48, 71, 72, 73, 89, 101, 473
Winokur, M., 3, 5, 333, 360, 388
Winslade, J., 293, 294, 301, 312
Winston, A., 94
Winter, D. A., 301, 303, 312
Witenberg, E., 87
Wolfe, B. E., 170, 337, 345
Wolitzky, D. L., 34, 41, 43, 49, 53
Wolpe, J., 183, 184, 201, 358
Wolstein, B., 78, 88
Wong, N., 526
Woo, S., 409
Wood, J. K., 112
Wood, K. A., 403
Woods, M., 523, 527
Woods, S. W., 205
Woody, S. R., 193, 208
Woolfolk, R. L., 7, 10
Worrall-Davies, A., 409
Wright, F., 238
Wright, J. H., 208

Wright, J., 238, 244
Wynne, L. C., 401, 409, 508

Yalom, I. D., 150, 151, 152, 155, 156, 159, 161, 162, 169, 176, 177, 517, 520, 521, 523, 527, 528, 531, 532, 533, 535, 536, 538, 545
Yapko, M. D., 352, 356, 359, 383
Yartz, A. R., 192
Yingling, L. C., 402
Yontef, G., 107, 125
Young, J., 233, 237, 256
Young, M., 248

Zapparoli, G., 338
Zarate, R., 403
Zastowny, T. R., 524
Zeig, J. K., 357, 359, 361, 362, 372, 373, 376, 391
Zetzel, E. R., 39, 44
Ziegler, P., 379, 380, 382, 390
Zimmerman, J. L., 499
Zimpfer, D. G., 527
Zimring, F. M., 111, 126, 136
Zinbarg, R. E., 210
Zois, C., 365
Zumaya, M., 287, 288

Subject Index

Page numbers followed by an *f* indicate figure, *t* indicate table

ABC model, 228. *See also* Cognitive therapy
Acceptance-based treatment, 202–203. *See also* Behavior therapy
Adolescents, integrative approaches and, 338. *See also* Family therapy
Agape, 92
Agency
  description, 112–113, 155
  questions, 380, 499
  See also Personal–agentic level
Aggression
  borderline personality and, 35
  case illustration, 95–100
  relational approaches to, 74–75
Aggressive drives, 25, 28–29. *See also* Psychoanalysis
Agoraphobia
  description, 254
  integrative approaches and, 338–339
  panic control treatment for, 203–205
  See also Exposure treatment; Phobias
Americal relational theory, 25. *See also* Psychoanalysis
Anal stage of development, 29
Analytic neutrality
  change and, 53
  description, 47–49

See also Stance of the therapist
Anger
  case illustration, 95–100
  in marital therapy, 487
Anxiety
  acceptance-based treatments and, 203
  behavior therapy and, 183
  borderline personality and, 35
  case illustration, 211–214*t*
  cognitive therapy and, 238–240, 247–248, 252, 253–255
  description, 81
  development of self-system and, 72–73
  drive pressure and, 29
  exposure treatment and, 194–197*t*
  integrative approaches and, 337
  learning history and, 186
  panic control treatment for, 203–205
  psychoanalytical theory and, 30, 31–32
  relational approaches to, 80–81, 94
  relaxation training and, 201
  resistance and, 40–41
Applicability of treatment
  behavioral approaches, 210–211, 493
  cognitive–behavioral family therapy, 445

cognitive therapy, 252–257
description, 14–16
existential–humanistic psychotherapies, 169
experiential–humanistic approaches to marital therapy, 486–487, 488–489
experiential symbolic family therapy, 427–428
group psychotherapies, 539
integrative approaches, 336–338, 497
intergenerational–contextual family therapy, 424
object relations family therapy, 420
person-centered psychotherapy, 133–135
postmodern approaches, 300–302, 499, 501, 502–503
psychoanalysis, 53–55
psychoeducational approach to family therapy, 451
relational approaches, 92–93
structural and strategic approaches, 430, 438, 481, 484
systemic family therapy, 433–434
transgenerational approaches to marital therapy, 473
Arousal, in relational therapy, 81

Assessment
  behavior therapy and, 187–192,
    190f
  brief therapy and, 355
  case illustration, 257–258
  cognitive therapy and, 241–243
  description, 7–9
  existential–humanistic
    psychotherapies and,
    153–154
  family therapy and, 410–412,
    436, 442
  group psychotherapies and,
    523–525
  integrative approaches to,
    325–327
  person-centered approach to,
    118–119
  of personality, 7
  postmodern approaches to,
    280–288, 282f, 285f
  in psychoanalysis, 33–36
  relational approaches to, 77
Assimilative integration
  description, 12–13, 321–322
  trends and, 345
  See also Integrative approaches
Attachment
  marital therapy and, 487
  relational approaches and, 75
  research support for, 94–95
  understanding, 417
Attention
  refocusing, 247–248
  research support and, 94
  See also Presence
Attributional bias, in a marriage,
    466–467
Automatic thoughts
  anxiety and, 254
  case illustration, 259
  challenging, 246
  description, 230
Autonomy
  anxiety and, 254–255
  differentiation and, 471
  within the family, 407
  person-centered approach to,
    112
  relational approaches to, 79–80
  a sense of agency in, 112–113
Avoidance
  depression and, 205–206

phobias and, 194
  relational approaches to, 81
Avoidant personality, 94

Beck Anxiety Inventory, 243. See
    also Self-report
    questionnaires
Beck Depression Inventory (BDI-
    II), 191, 242–243. See also
    Self-report questionnaires
Behavior
  cognitive theory of, 6–7
  personality and, 185–186
  psychoanalytical theory and,
    30–31
  See also Behavior therapy;
    Cognitive–behavioral
    therapy
Behavior modification
  description, 184
  via parent training, 441
Behavior therapy
  applicability and ethical
    considerations of,
    210–211
  assessment and, 187–192, 190f
  case illustration, 211–214t
  change and, 209–210
  cognitive therapy and, 248
  description, 182–184, 192–193
  examples of, 203–207
  historical background, 184–185
  marital therapy and, 468,
    489–493
  personality and, 6, 185–187
  practice of, 193–203, 197t
  psychological health and, 187
  therapeutic relationship and,
    207–209
  trends and, 214–215
  See also Cognitive therapy
Behavioral approach test (BAT),
    189. See also Assessment
Behaviorism, 150
Benevolent neutrality
  change and, 53
  description, 47–49
  See also Stance of the therapist
Biofeedback, 202
Biogenetic systems
  description, 277
  diagnoses and, 278–279
Biological predisposition, 44

Bipolar disorder
  behavior therapy and, 206–207
  family functioning and, 409
Bisexuality, relational approaches
    to, 74, 101
Borderline personality
  dialectical behavior therapy and,
    202
  integrative approaches and,
    337–338, 339
  person-centered approach to,
    132–133
  psychoanalytical theory and, 33,
    35–36, 54
Boundaries
  enactment and, 480
  family functioning and, 408,
    434–435
  in a marriage, 478
  in relational approaches, 86–87
  of the self, 112
Bow-tie interview
  case illustration, 307f–308
  description, 284–286, 285f
  See also Assessment
Bowen family systems therapy,
    470–473. See also Marital
    therapy
Brief therapy
  case illustration, 366–367,
    369–371, 374–376,
    381–383, 385
  description, 350–352, 352–354,
    353t, 385–387, 389
  Ericksonian, 371–383
  future of, 387–389
  group psychotherapies and,
    526–527
  historical background,
    357–360
  managed health care and, 10
  marital therapy and, 481–484,
    495–497
  models of, 361–362
  psychodynamic
    psychotherapies, 362–367
  reasons for, 354–357
  redecision therapy and
    transactional analysis,
    367–371
  single-session therapy, 383–385
  structure of, 360–361f
  See also Multimodal therapy

Case illustration
  behavior therapy, 211–214*t*
  brief therapy, 366–367,
    369–371, 374–376,
    381–383, 385
  cognitive therapy, 257–261
  description, 17–18
  existential–humanistic
    psychotherapies, 171–175
  group psychotherapies,
    539–543
  integrative approaches, 340–344
  marital therapy, 503–506
  person-centered psychotherapy,
    137–142
  postmodern approaches,
    282f–283, 284–285f,
    291–292, 293–294,
    303–310, 305f, 307f
  psychoanalysis, 57–62
  relational approaches, 95–100
Castration anxiety, relational
    approaches to, 74
Catastrophizing
  challenging, 246
  description, 234
  See also Cognitive distortions
Categorizing maladaptive
    behavior, 7
Catharsis, 115
Cathexis, 29
Challenge, a sense of agency and,
    112–113
Change
  existential–humanistic
    psychotherapies and, 152
  strategic family therapy and,
    428–429
  transcendence and, 171
  transtheoretical therapy, 325
Change mechanisms
  in behavior therapy, 209–210
  description, 13–14
  in existential–humanistic
    psychotherapies, 168–169
  in group treatments, 534*t*,
    538–539
  in integrative approaches,
    335–336, 496–497
  in marital therapy, 475–476,
    486, 488, 493
  in person-centered therapy,
    131–133

  in postmodern approaches,
    299–300, 499, 502
  in psychoanalysis, 51–53
  in relational approaches,
    90–92
  See also Curative factors;
    Responsibility of change
Children
  integrative approaches and,
    338
  person-centered approach to,
    133
  of troubled marriages, 465
  See also Family therapy
Choosing a technique
  description, 9, 12
  psychoanalysis and, 55
Clarification
  case illustration, 60
  description, 41
  See also Interpretations
Classical conditioning
  description, 184
  learning history and, 186
Client-centered therapy. *See*
    Person-centered
    psychotherapy
Clinical interview
  in behavior therapy, 190–191
  in psychoanalysis, 33–36
  See also Assessment
Cognitive–behavioral analytic
    systems psychotherapy
  depression and, 337
  diagnoses and, 327
  practice of, 328
  research support for, 340
  See also Integrative approaches
Cognitive–behavioral therapy
  applicability of, 445
  family therapy and, 414*t*,
    438–445
  historical background, 318
  personality and, 186
  research support for, 135,
    236–238
  See also Behavior therapy;
    Cognitive therapy
Cognitive distortions
  case illustration, 258–259
  description, 233–234
  labeling, 248
  in a marriage, 466

Cognitive specificity hypothesis,
    252–253
Cognitive theory
  change and, 210
  of personality, 6–7
  See also Behavior therapy
Cognitive therapy
  applicability of, 252–257
  assumptions of, 229–230
  case illustration, 257–261
  for depression, 234–235,
    236–238
  description, 224–225, 230–234,
    238–240
  historical background, 225–229
  practice of, 240–252
  research support for, 339
Cognitive triad, 230–231
Collaboration
  in cognitive therapy, 240–241,
    242
  goal setting and, 328
  in integrative approaches,
    333–334
  in postmodern approaches, 300
  See also Therapeutic relationship
Collaborative couple therapy,
    501–503. *See also* Marital
    therapy
Commitment
  consolidation of, 167
  description, 155
Common-factors approach to
    integration
  description, 320
  personality and, 322
  See also Integrative approaches
Communication
  attending to, 290, 295–296
  double bind, 401, 429–430,
    432–433
  within the family, 407
  family functioning and, 408
  feedback loops, 404
  in a marriage, 466
  negotiation coaching, 480
  person-centered approach to,
    113–115
  skills training in, 199–200, 207,
    490, 491–493
  strategic family therapy's focus
    on, 428–430
  symptoms as, 76, 79

Comparisons of psychotherapies
    a framework for, 3–4
    value structure of, 7
Compromise formations, 31
Concordant countertransference,
    88–89. *See also*
    Countertransference
Concurrent countertransference
    case illustration, 99
    description, 88–89
    See also Countertransference
Conditioning, 184
Conflicts, relational assessment of,
    77
Conflictual relationship themes
    description, 38
    relational approaches to, 75
    research support for, 93–94
Confrontation
    case illustration, 59–60
    description, 41
    in person-centered therapy, 129
    with resistance, 165–166
    See also Interpretations
Congruence
    description, 113
    marital therapy and, 486
    in person-centered therapy, 128
    research support for, 136
    See also Incongruence
Connection, lack of, 73
Consciousness
    countertransference and, 88
    realms of, 73
    See also Unconscious
Constructivism
    assessment and, 280–288, 282f
    brief therapy and, 385–387
    cognitive therapy and, 226
    contribution to relational
        approaches, 72
    family therapy and, 415t
    historical background, 274
    marital therapy and, 481–484
    See also Postmodern approaches
Continuing education, in brief
    therapy, 388–389
Coping questions
    description, 380
    in marital therapy, 498–499
Coping styles, 77
Cormorbidity, behavior therapy
    and, 210

Corporatization of mental health,
    10. *See also* Managed
    health care
Countertransference
    analytic neutrality and, 48
    brief therapy and, 354, 363
    case illustration, 60, 95–100
    change and, 51–53
    as a curative factor, 91–92
    description, 49–51
    family therapy and, 418, 423
    historical background, 27
    integrative approaches and, 332,
        334
    marital therapy and, 475
    mutual enactment and, 82–85
    person-centered therapy and,
        129–131
    relational approaches and,
        87–90
    trends and, 63
    working alliance and, 44–45
Couple therapy
    behavioral approaches to,
        202–203, 489–493
    bow-tie interviews and,
        284–286, 285f
    case illustration, 381–383,
        503–506
    description, 463–467, 469–470
    ethical considerations, 15
    evolution of psychotherapy and,
        3
    experiential and humanistic
        approaches to, 484–489
    historical background, 467–469
    integrative approaches to,
        493–497
    postmodern approaches to,
        497–503
    research support for, 503
    structural and strategic
        approaches to, 476–484
    systems-oriented approaches to,
        5
    transgenerational approaches to,
        470–476
    trends and, 506–507
    See also Family therapy
Creativity, 111
Criticisms of psychotherapy,
    167–168
Cruelty, 74

Cultural factors
    applicability of treatment and,
        14
    assessment and, 8, 326
    behavior therapy and, 211
    Bowen family systems therapy
        and, 473
    cognitive therapy and, 225
    countertransference and, 130
    description, 15–16
    diagnoses and, 187
    existential–humanistic
        psychotherapies and, 169
    family therapy and, 403, 438
    in goal setting, 9
    group psychotherapies and, 525
    integrative approaches and, 338
    person-centered approach to,
        113, 134
    postmodern approaches to, 280,
        300–301, 310–311
    psychoanalysis and, 54–55
    relational approaches and, 77,
        92
    relationship to psychotherapy,
        10
    See also Multiculturalism
Curative factors
    in behavior therapy, 209–210
    cognitive–behavioral family
        therapy, 444–445
    description, 13–14
    in existential–humanistic
        psychotherapies, 168–169
    in experiential symbolic family
        therapy, 427
    in group treatments, 538–539
    in integrative approaches,
        335–336
    in intergenerational–contextual
        family therapy, 423–424
    in object relations family
        therapy, 419–420
    in person-centered therapy,
        131–133
    in postmodern approaches,
        299–300, 448
    in psychoanalysis, 51–53
    in psychoeducational
        approaches to family
        therapy, 451
    in relational approaches, 90–92
    in strategic family therapy, 430

in structural family therapy, 437–438
in systemic family therapy, 433
See also Change mechanisms
Current trends
in behavior therapy, 214–215
description, 18–20
in existential–humanistic psychotherapies, 175–176
in group treatments, 543–545
in integrative approaches, 344–345
in marital therapy, 506–507
in person-centered therapy, 142–144
in postmodern approaches, 310–311
in psychoanalysis, 62–64
in relational approaches, 100–101

Death, existential–humanistic psychotherapies and, 152
Defense analysis
description, 42
relational approaches to, 81–82
See also Interpretations
Defense styles, relational assessment of, 77
Definition of psychotherapy, 1, 4–5, 8
Dependency
anxiety and, 254–255
cognitive therapy and, 256
evolution of, 109
Depression
Beck Depression Inventory (BDI-II), 191
behavior therapy and, 205–206
cognitive therapy and, 234–235, 236–238, 244, 252
family functioning and, 409
integrative approaches and, 337, 339–340
learned helplessness model of, 228
mindfulness-based treatments and, 203
psychotherapy vs. medication, 11
relational approaches and, 94
schemata and, 232

social skills training and, 199–200
Depth oriented brief therapy
description, 290–292
resistance and, 295
See also Postmodern approaches
Desire, relational approaches to, 75
Destiny, existential–humanistic psychotherapies and, 151–153
Determination, multiple, 30–31
Development of the family, 405–406. *See also* Family
Development, psychological
brief therapy and, 354–355
dialogical approach to, 152–153
person-centered approach to, 115–116
personality and, 6–7
psychoanalytical theory and, 27–28, 29
relational approaches to, 72, 75, 84
Diagnosis
behavior therapy and, 187, 188
brief therapy and, 355
in cognitive therapy, 243–244
description, 7
existential–humanistic psychotherapies and, 154
family functioning and, 401, 407
group psychotherapies and, 523–524
integrative approaches and, 325
person-centered approach to, 118–119
postmodern approaches to, 278, 301, 311
psychoanalysis and, 34–35
relational approaches to, 77, 98
role of in assessment process, 8–9
semistructured interviews and, 191
See also DSM
Dialectical behavior therapy
borderline personality and, 337–338
description, 202
research support for, 339
See also Behavior therapy

Dialog. *See also* Assessment
Dialog, assessment via, 8
Dialogical approach, 152–153
Diaries in assessment, 189–190f.
See also Assessment
Dichotomous thinking, 233. *See also* Cognitive distortions
Differentiation, 471
Directives, in marital therapy, 479
Discovery-oriented therapies, 143
Disease model, relational approaches and, 76, 98
Disengagement, in a marriage, 478. *See also* Marital therapy
Disorders, 7
Dissociation
description, 81
relational approaches to, 73–74
research support for, 94
Distortions in thinking. *See* Cognitive distortions
Double bind communication
description, 401
in family therapy, 429–430, 432–433
See also Communication
Dream analysis, relational approaches to, 85
Drive–defense model, 32
DSM
assessment and, 191
behavior therapy and, 187, 188
brief therapy and, 355
description, 7
family functioning and, 407
integrative approaches and, 327
psychoanalysis and, 34–35
relational approaches and, 76
relational functioning scale in, 402
role of in assessment process, 8–9
See also Diagnosis
Dyadic–relational systems
bow-tie interviews and, 284
description, 277
psychological health and, 279–280
See also Relationship
Dynamic unconscious, 73. *See also* Unconscious
Dysthmia, 337. *See also* Depression

Eclecticism, technical
  description, 320
  in marital therapy, 493–494
  personality and, 322
  trends and, 344–345
  See also Integrative approaches
Ego, in working alliances, 45–45
Ego instincts, 28–29
Ego psychology, 25, 31. *See also*
  Psychoanalysis
Embodied meditation, 159. *See*
  also guiding
Emotional processing, 209–210
Emotional reasoning, 233. *See also*
  Cognitive distortions
Emotionally focused therapy
  applicability of, 133
  marital therapy and, 468,
    487–489
Emotions
  bipolar disorder and, 206
  countertransference and, 88–90
  infantile, 74
  person-centered approach to,
    114–115, 118
  research support for, 137
Empathy
  aggression and, 74
  compared to joining, 479
  countertransference and, 89–90
  description, 49
  to foster a working alliance, 45
  in person-centered therapy, 122,
    127–128, 133
  in postmodern approaches, 298t
  in relational approaches, 81–82
  research support for, 136, 170,
    208
  See also Communication;
    Listening skills
Empirically supported
    relationships (ESR)
  description, 12
  trends and, 19
Empirically supported treatments
    (EST)
  description, 12, 13
  person-centered psychotherapy
    and, 143–144
  trends and, 19
Empty-chair technique
  case illustration, 140–141, 370
  description, 124

research support for, 170
  See also Gestalt therapy; Role
    playing
Enactment
  in existential–humanistic
    psychotherapy, 159–160
  in marital therapy, 479–480
Encounter
  activation of presence via,
    161–163
  with resistance, 163–167
Endurance questions, 380
Enmeshment, in a marriage, 478
Environment
  assessment and, 326
  change and, 209
  multisystemic therapy and, 443
  personality and, 186
  that reinforces behavior,
    182–183, 197–199
Epigenesis, 277
Ericksonian therapies
  brief therapy and, 371–383
  strategic family therapy,
    428–430
Ethical considerations
  behavior therapy, 211
  description, 14–16
  existential–humanistic
    psychotherapies, 169
  group psychotherapies, 539
  integrative approaches, 336–338
  person-centered psychotherapy,
    133–135
  postmodern approaches,
    300–302
  psychoanalysis, 55
  relational approaches, 92–93
Evocative unfolding, 139–140. *See*
  also Gestalt therapy
Evolution of psychotherapy, 2–3
Exceptions questions
  description, 380
  family therapy and, 447–448
  in marital therapy, 498
Existential–humanistic
    psychotherapies
  applicability and ethical
    considerations of, 169
  assessment and, 153–154
  case illustration, 171–175
  change and, 168–169
  description, 151–153

historical background, 149–151
  practice of, 154–168
  research support for, 169–171
  trends and, 175–176
Experience
  enactment and, 159–160
  encouraging in the moment,
    85–86
  existential–humanistic
    psychotherapies and,
    151–153
  incongruency and, 116–117
  learning history and, 186
  organizing principles shaping,
    73
  person-centered approach to,
    113–114, 120
  relational approaches to, 76–77,
    81, 84
  of the self, 115
  See also Constructivism
Experienced split, 125
Experiential processing, 170
Experiential reflection, 151–153
Experiential symbolic family
    therapy, 424–428. *See also*
    Family therapy
Experiential therapy
  applicability and ethical
    considerations of, 133–135
  assessment and, 118–119
  family therapy and, 413t,
    424–428
  marital therapy and, 484–489
  practice of, 119–126
  research support for, 135–137
  trends and, 142–144
  See also Marital therapy
Exploratory psychotherapy
  integrative approaches and,
    321
  vs. psychoanalysis, 36
Exposure treatment
  change and, 209–210
  in cognitive therapy, 249
  description, 183, 194–197t
  in integrative approaches, 337
  with posttraumatic stress
    disorder, 239
  See also Behavior therapy;
    Phobias
Expressed emotion
  bipolar disorder and, 206

Expressed emotion *(continued)*
family functioning and,
409–410
Expressive psychotherapy
vs. psychoanalysis, 36
research support for, 93–94

False self accommodation, 80
Family
description, 403–405
development of, 405–406
functioning of, 402–403,
406–410, 434–435
See also Family therapy
Family therapy
assessment and, 410–412
bipolar disorder and, 206–207
cognitive–behavioral therapy
and, 438–445
description, 451–452
ethical considerations, 15
evolution of psychotherapy and,
3
experiential and humanistic,
424–428
historical background,
400–403
integrative approaches and, 338
intergenerational–contextual,
420–424
models of, 412, 413t–415t, 416
postmodern approaches to, 289,
445–448
psychoanalytical theory and,
416–420
psychoeducation and, 448–451
relationship to marital therapy,
464
strategic, 428–430
structural, 434–438
systemic, 430–434
systems-oriented approaches to,
5
See also Family; Marital therapy
Fear
exposure treatment and,
194–197t
modeling and, 200
Feedback
in group treatments, 535
loops, 404
nonverbal, 164–165
in strategic family therapy, 429

See also Communication;
Feedback loops
Feedback loops, 404. *See also*
Communication; Feedback
Feelings, person-centered
approach to, 114. *See also*
Emotions
Feminist therapy
description, 15–16
marital therapy and, 469, 507
See also Postmodern approaches
Five-factor model of personality,
6. *See also* Personality
theory
Fixation, 29–30
Fixed role therapy, 274, 292–293.
See also Postmodern
approaches
Flexibility
within the family, 407
in person-centered therapy, 129
Focusing-oriented psychotherapy
applicability of, 133
change and, 132
goal setting and, 121–122
techniques and strategies of,
122–123
See also Person-centered
psychotherapy
Free association
in psychoanalysis, 37
in relational therapy, 80–81
resistance and, 40–41
Freedom. *See*
Existential–humanistic
psychotherapies. *See also*
Presence
Frustration, aggression and, 74
Functional analysis
applicability of, 210
depression and, 206
description, 187–188
in marital therapy, 490–491, 495
See also Assessment
Functional family therapy
applicability of, 445
description, 441–442
See also Family therapy
Functioning
of the family, 406–410
person-centered approach to,
116
Fusion, 471

Future orientation
description, 111
in Ericksonian therapies, 373
Future trends
in behavior therapy, 214–215
in brief therapy, 387–389
description, 18–20
in existential–humanistic
psychotherapies, 175–176
in group treatments, 543–545
in integrative approaches,
344–345
in marital therapy, 506–507
in person-centered therapy,
142–144
in postmodern approaches,
310–311
in psychoanalysis, 62–64
in relational approaches,
100–101

Generalized anxiety disorder
cognitive therapy and, 238
description, 254
See also Anxiety
Genital stage of development, 29
Genograms, 472–473. *See also*
Bowen family systems
therapy
Genuineness
description, 128–129
research support for, 136, 170,
208
Geriatric patients, integrative
approaches and, 338
Gestalt therapy
change and, 132
confrontation and, 120
disappearance of, 3
empty-chair technique, 124,
140–141, 170, 370
integrative approaches and, 338
personality and, 110
research support for, 135
techniques and strategies of,
123–124
view of dysfunction, 118
See also Person-centered
psychotherapy
Goal-oriented treatment, 10
Goal setting
in behavioral approaches to
martial therapy, 490–491

Goal setting *(continued)*
  in brief therapy, 356
  in cognitive–behavioral family
      therapy, 440
  description, 9
  in experiential–humanistic
      approaches to marital
      therapy, 486, 487–488
  in group treatments, 528–529
  integrative approaches to,
      328–329, 496
  in intergenerational–contextual
      family therapy, 421
  in object relations family
      therapy, 417–418
  person-centered approach to,
      121–122
  postmodern approaches to,
      289–290, 446, 498, 500,
      502
  in psychoanalysis, 37–38
  in psychoeducational
      approaches to family
      therapy, 449
  in relational approaches, 78–79
  in structural and strategic
      approaches, 428–429, 436,
      478, 483
  in systemic family therapy,
      431–432
  in transgenerational approaches
      to marital therapy, 472, 475
Gratification, in psychoanalysis,
      48–49
Group treatment
  applicability and ethical
      considerations of, 539
  assessment and, 523–525
  case illustration, 213, 539–543
  change and, 538–539
  historical background, 515–519
  personality and, 519–522
  postmodern approaches to, 289
  practice of, 525–536, 529*f,* 534*t*
  therapist self-disclosure within,
      537–538
  trends and, 543–545
  See also Psychoeducation
Growth
  dialogical approach to, 152–153
  family therapy and, 424–428
  person-centered psychotherapy
      and, 119–120, 143

  potential for, 111, 113
  See also Self-actualization
Guiding
  in cognitive therapy, 246–247
  in existential–humanistic
      psychotherapy, 157–159

Health, psychological. *See*
      Psychological health
Heterosexuality, relational
      approaches to, 74, 101
Historical perspective
  behavior therapy, 184–185
  brief therapy, 357–360
  cognitive therapy, 225–229
  description, 4–5
  evolution of psychotherapy, 2–3
  existential–humanistic
      psychotherapies, 149–151
  family therapy, 400–403,
      430–431
  group psychotherapies,
      515–519
  integrative approaches, 317–322
  marital therapy, 467–469
  medicalization of psychotherapy
      and, 10–11
  person-centered psychotherapy,
      107–109
  postmodern approaches,
      272–275
  psychoanalysis, 24–25, 26–27,
      62–63
  relational approaches, 69–72
Holding environment
  description, 48–49
  in family therapy, 418
  in marital therapy, 474–475
  presence as, 168
  See also Psychoanalysis
Homework
  in brief therapy, 361*f*
  in cognitive therapy, 249–250
  in family therapy, 422, 425
  in integrative approaches, 330
  in marital therapy, 470, 480
  in postmodern approaches,
      294–295
Homosexuality, 74
Homosexuality, relational
      approaches to, 101
Hopelessness scale, 243. *See also*
      Self-report questionnaires

Human development
  brief therapy and, 354–355
  dialogical approach to,
      152–153
  person-centered approach to,
      115–116
  personality and, 6–7
  psychoanalytical theory and,
      27–28, 29
  relational approaches to, 72, 75,
      84
Humanism
  family therapy and, 413*t,*
      424–428
  marital therapy and, 484–489
  See also Existential–humanistic
      psychotherapies; Marital
      therapy; Postmodern
      approaches
Hypnosis, evolution of
      psychoanalysis and, 26

I–thou relationship
  case illustration, 173
  as a change mechanism, 169
  in existential–humanistic
      psychotherapy, 162–163
  See also Therapeutic
      relationship
Imagery, cognitive therapy and,
      248
Incongruence, 116–117. *See also*
      Congruence
Individualism, 112. *See also*
      Autonomy
Infantile neurosis, 39–40
Information processing
  brief therapy and, 363
  person-centered approach to,
      117–118
Insight
  case illustration, 61
  change and, 51–53
  description, 13
  in family therapy, 423
  in marital therapy, 468–469
  person-centered approach to,
      132
  relational approaches to, 91
Insight-oriented marital therapy,
      468–469. *See also* Marital
      therapy
Instinctual drives, 28–29

Instructing, in
    existential–humanistic
    psychotherapy, 158–159
Integrative approaches
    applicability and ethical
        considerations of, 336–338
    assessment and, 325–327
    case illustration, 340–344
    change and, 335–336
    description, 2
    historical background, 317–322
    marital therapy and, 470,
        493–497
    personality and, 322–323
    practice of, 327–332
    psychological health and,
        323–325
    research support for, 338–340
    therapeutic relationship and
        stance and, 332–335
    trends and, 19–20, 214, 344–345
Integrative behavioral couples
    therapy, 202–203. See also
    Behavior therapy
Intentionality, consolidation of,
    167
Interactions
    interpretations as, 42–43
    mutual enactment and, 82–85
    person-centered approach to,
        112
    psychopathology and, 118
    relational approaches to, 75, 77
Intergenerational–contextual
    family therapy, 413t,
    420–424. See also Family
    therapy
Internalized working model, 75
Interpersonal approach, 69–71
Interpersonal skills
    activation of presence via,
        161–163
    description, 13
    group psychotherapies and, 532
    relational approaches and, 94
Interpretations
    case illustration, 59–62
    change and, 51–53
    description, 13, 41–43
    empathy and, 49
    in existential–humanistic
        psychotherapy, 168–169
    in person-centered therapy, 122

relational approaches to, 85
    trends and, 63
Interview, clinical. See Clinical
    interview
Intimacy, need for, 74
Intrapsychic conflict, 29
Intuitive knowledge, 113–114
Inventories, as assessment, 8
Isolation, 152

Jamming, 483–484
Joining
    description, 479
    in relational approaches, 81–82

Knowledge
    postmodernism and, 5
    of the self, 113–114

Laddering
    case illustration, 304–305f
    description, 281–284, 282f
    See also Assessment
Learned helplessness, 228
Learning
    emphasized in group treatment,
        520
    orientation to the future and,
        111
    personality and, 186
    potential for, 110–111
Libidinal drives, 25, 28–29. See also
    Psychoanalysis
Listening skills
    in existential–humanistic
        psychotherapy, 157–159
    in family therapy, 448
    to foster a working alliance, 45
    in relational approaches, 81
    See also Empathy
Loss
    brief therapy and, 354
    of possibilities, 92
Lust, need for, 74

Managed health care
    brief therapy and, 359–360,
        387–388
    description, 10
    diagnoses and, 278
    psychoanalysis and, 54
    standardized treatment and,
        193

Marital therapy
    behavioral approaches to,
        202–203, 489–493
    bow-tie interviews and,
        284–286, 285f
    case illustration, 381–383,
        503–506
    description, 463–467, 469–470
    ethical considerations, 15
    evolution of psychotherapy and,
        3
    experiential and humanistic
        approaches to, 484–489
    historical background, 467–469
    integrative approaches to,
        493–497
    postmodern approaches to,
        497–503
    research support for, 503
    structural and strategic
        approaches to, 476–484
    systems-oriented approaches to,
        5
    transgenerational approaches to,
        470–476
    trends and, 506–507
    See also Family therapy
Masochistic tendencies, 74
Meaning, consolidation of, 167
Meaninglessness,
        existential–humanistic
        psychotherapies and, 152
Medicalization of psychotherapy,
        10–11. See also Managed
        health care
Medication
    cognitive therapy and, 244–245
    description, 9
    family therapy and, 207, 403,
        412, 416
    integrative approaches and,
        332
    medicalization of psychotherapy
        and, 11
    postmodern approaches to,
        278–279, 296
    psychoanalysis and, 44
    relational approaches and, 76, 93
Memory
    case illustration, 61
    research support and, 94
    wishes and, 28
Metapsychology, 30

Mind reading, 233. *See also* Cognitive distortions

Mindfulness-based treatment, 202–203. *See also* Behavior therapy

Miracle question
case illustration, 381
description, 380
family therapy and, 447–448
in marital therapy, 498

Modeling, 200

Motivation, relational approaches to, 75

Motivational interviewing, 142–143

Mourning of lost possibilities, 92

Multiculturalism
behavior therapy and, 211
Bowen family systems therapy and, 473
cognitive therapy and, 225
description, 15–16
diagnoses and, 187
existential–humanistic psychotherapies and, 169
family therapy and, 403, 438
group psychotherapies and, 525
integrative approaches and, 338
marital therapy and, 469, 507
person-centered approach and, 113
in postmodern approaches, 300–301, 310–311
See also Cultural factors

Multimodal therapy
assessment and, 327, 355
diagnoses and, 325
personality and, 322
See also Brief therapy; Integrative approaches

Multiple determination, 30–31

Multisystemic therapy
applicability of, 445
description, 442–444
See also Family therapy

Mutual confirmation, 162–163. *See also* Therapeutic relationship

Mutual enactment, in relational approaches, 82–85

Mutuality, 87. *See also* Therapeutic relationship

Narcissistic personality
integrative approaches and, 337–338
psychoanalytical theory and, 33, 54

Narrative couple therapy, 499–501. *See also* Marital therapy

Narrative Process Coding System, 288. *See also* Assessment

Narrative therapy, 293–294. *See also* Postmodern approaches

Needs, relational approaches to, 75

Negotiation coaching, 480

Neutrality
change and, 53
description, 47–49
See also Stance of the therapist

Noncompliance. *See* Resistance

Nondirective therapy. *See* Person-centered psychotherapy

Object relations theory
borderline personality and, 35–36
countertransference and, 89–90
description, 25
family therapy and, 416–420
historical background, 70–71
marital therapy and, 473–476
relationship and, 52
trends and, 63
See also Psychoanalysis

Observational assessment
description, 8, 189
using in family therapy, 410–412
See also Assessment

Obsessive–compulsive personality
case illustration, 61–62
change and, 210
description, 254
exposure treatment and, 194–197t
integrative approaches and, 337
relational approaches and, 94
relaxation training and, 201
response prevention treatment for, 197
Yale–Brown Obsessive–Compulsive Scale (Y-BOCS), 191

Oedipal conflict
description, 29
relational approaches to, 75

Operant conditioning
description, 184
personality and, 186
treatment practices and, 197–199

Oral stage of development, 29

Orientation towards the future, 111

Outcome measures, 188–189

Overgeneralization, 234. *See also* Cognitive distortions

Panic attacks, record of, 190f

Panic control treatment (PCT), 203–205

Panic disorder
cognitive therapy and, 238
description, 254
exposure treatment and, 194–197t
integrative approaches and, 337
panic control treatment for, 203–205
relaxation training and, 201

Parent training
applicability of, 445
description, 440–441
See also Family therapy

Parenting, relational approaches to, 75

Pathological compromise formations, 31

Pathology
behavior therapy and, 187
description, 6–7
existential–humanistic psychotherapies and, 151–153
family functioning and, 408–410
group psychotherapies and, 522–523
integrative approaches to, 323–325
person-centered approach to, 116–118
postmodern approaches to, 278–280
psychoanalysis and, 31–33, 54
relational approaches to, 76–77

Patterns of experiences
  assessment and, 153–154
  description, 151
Pause, therapeutic, 158
Penis envy, relational approaches
      to, 74
Perfomative social therapy, 176. *See
      also* Existential–humanistic
      psychotherapies
Person-centered psychotherapy
  applicability and ethical
      considerations of, 133–135
  assessment and, 118–119
  case illustration, 137–142
  curative factors, 131–133
  description, 107
  historical background, 107–109
  personality and, 109–116
  practice of, 119–126
  psychological health and,
      116–118
  research support for, 135–137
  therapeutic relationship and
      stance and, 127–131
  trends and, 142–144
Personal–agentic level
  bow-tie interviews and, 284
  description, 277
  laddering assessment and,
      281–284, 282*f*
  psychological health and, 279
  See also Agency; Personality
Personality
  behavior therapy and, 185–187
  brief therapy and, 355
  existential–humanistic
      psychotherapies and,
      151–153
  group treatment approaches to,
      519–522
  integrative approaches to,
      322–323
  person-centered approach to,
      109–116
  postmodern approaches to,
      275–278
  psychoanalytical theory of,
      27–31
  relational approaches to, 72–75
  research support and, 94
  See also Psychoanalysis
Personality pathology
  cognitive therapy and, 255–257

psychoanalytical theory and,
      33
Personality theory
  concept of, 5
  description, 6–7
Personalization, 233–234. *See also*
      Cognitive distortions
Phallic stage of development, 29.
      See also Development,
      psychological
Pharmacotherapy. *See* Medication
Phobias
  agoraphobia, 203–205, 254,
      338–339
  behavior therapy and, 183
  description, 254
  exposure treatment and,
      194–197*t*
  modeling and, 200
  psychoeducation and, 193–194
  relational approaches and, 93
  See also Exposure treatment
Planned short-term therapy. See
      Brief therapy
Play therapy, in family therapy, 426
Pleasure principle, 28, 30
Positive connotation, 432. *See also*
      Reframing
Positive regard, unconditional
  description, 127–128
  research support for, 170, 208
Postmodern approaches
  applicability and ethical
      considerations of, 300–302
  assessment and, 280–288, 282*f*,
      285*f*
  brief therapy and, 385–387
  change and, 299–300
  contribution to relational
      approaches, 72
  description, 272
  evolution of psychotherapy and,
      3
  family therapy and, 415*t*,
      445–448
  historical background, 5,
      272–275
  to marital therapy, 497–503
  personality and, 275–278
  practice of, 288–297
  psychological health and,
      278–280
  research support for, 302–303

therapeutic relationship and,
      297–299, 298*t*
  trends and, 310–311
Posttraumatic stress disorder
  cognitive therapy and, 239
  exposure treatment and, 195
  relaxation training and, 201
  See also Trauma
Practice of psychotherapy
  behavioral approaches, 193–203,
      197*t*, 490, 491–493
  cognitive–behavioral family
      therapy, 440–444
  cognitive therapy, 240–252
  description, 19
  existential–humanistic
      psychotherapies, 154–168
  experiential–humanistic
      approaches to marital
      therapy, 486, 487, 488
  experiential symbolic family
      therapy, 425–427
  group psychotherapies,
      525–536, 529*f*, 534*t*
  integrative approaches, 327–332
  integrative approaches to
      marital therapy, 495–496
  intergenerational–contextual
      family therapy, 421–422
  object relations family therapy,
      418–419
  person-centered psychotherapy,
      119–126
  postmodern approaches,
      288–297, 446–448,
      498–499, 500–501,
      501–502
  psychoanalysis, 36–47
  psychoeducational approaches
      to family therapy, 449–450
  relational approaches, 77–87
  structural and strategic
      approaches, 429–430,
      436–437, 478–480,
      482–484
  systemic family therapy,
      432–433
  transgenerational approaches to
      marital therapy, 472–473,
      475
Preflective unconscious, 73. *See
      also* Unconscious
Prescriptive therapy, 339

Presence
    assessment and, 153–154
    as a change mechanism,
        168–169
    cultivation of, 155–157
    as a goal, 157–161
    interpersonal activation of,
        161–163
Primary-process thinking, 28
Problem-focused treatment, 10
Problem–solution loop, marital
    therapy and, 483
Problem-solving training
    description, 200
    in marital therapy, 491–493
    skills training and, 207
Problematic reaction point, 125
Process–experiential
    psychotherapy
    applicability of, 133
    change and, 132
    diagnoses and, 119
    goal setting and, 121–122
    research support for, 135, 340
    techniques and strategies of,
        124–125
    See also Person-centered
        psychotherapy
Progressive relaxation training,
    200–202. See also
    Relaxation
Psychic determinism, 30
Psychic energy, 28–29
Psychic structures, 27–28
Psychoanalysis
    applicability of, 53–55
    assessment process in, 33–36
    brief therapy and, 362–367
    case illustration, 57–62
    curative factors, 51–53
    description, 24–26, 150
    ethical considerations, 55
    family therapy and, 413t,
        416–420
    group psychotherapies and, 517
    historical background, 26–27,
        69–71
    personality and, 6, 27–31
    psychological health and, 31–33
    research support for, 55–57
    therapeutic stance and, 47–51
    therapy practice, 36–47
    trends and, 62–64

Psychoanalytically oriented
    psychotherapy, 36. See also
    Psychoanalysis
Psychoeducation
    case illustration, 213
    description, 193–194
    family therapy and, 207, 415t,
        448–451
    in panic control treatment, 204
    social skills training and, 199
    See also Behavior therapy;
        Group treatment
Psychological development
    brief therapy and, 354–355
    dialogical approach to, 152–153
    person-centered approach to,
        115–116
    personality and, 6–7
    psychoanalytical theory and,
        27–28, 29
    relational approaches to, 72, 75,
        84
Psychological health
    behavior therapy and, 187
    description, 6–7
    existential–humanistic
        psychotherapies and,
        151–153
    group psychotherapies and,
        522–523
    integrative approaches to,
        323–325
    person-centered approach to,
        116–118
    postmodern approaches to,
        278–280
    psychoanalysis and, 31–33
    relational approaches and,
        76–77
Psychophysiological assessment,
    191–192. See also
    Assessment
Psychosexual development, stages
    of, 29
Punishment
    behavior therapy and, 197–199
    personality and, 186

Rational–emotive behavior
    therapy
    description, 228
    family therapy and, 439
    See also Cognitive therapy

Reactance, brief therapy and, 354
Reactivity, 190
Realities
    family therapy and, 445–446
    multiple, 113
    visions of, 386–387
Reality principle, 28
Reappearance hypothesis, 110
Redecision therapy, brief therapy
    and, 367–371
Referral for testing, from
    psychoanalysis, 33
Referral to different type of
    therapy
    description, 14
    from person-centered
        psychotherapy, 134
    from postmodern approaches,
        278–279
    from psychoanalysis, 34, 55
    from relational approaches, 78,
        92–93
Reflection
    compared to interpretation, 122
    in relational approaches, 81–82
Reframing
    in brief therapy, 378
    description, 390n
    in existential–humanistic
        psychotherapy, 158–159
    in family therapy, 429, 432
    in marital therapy, 480
Regression
    description, 29–30
    relational approaches and, 92
Regressive transference neurosis,
    39. See also Transference
Reinforcement
    behavior therapy and, 197–199
    personality and, 186
Relapse
    in brief therapy, 361f
    cognitive therapy and, 237–238,
        250
Relational approaches
    applicability and ethical
        considerations of, 92–93
    assessment and, 77
    brief therapy and, 363–365
    case illustration, 95–100
    curative factors, 90–92
    historical background, 69–72
    practice of, 77–87

psychological health and, 76–77
research support for, 93–95
therapeutic relationship and
stance, 87–90
trends and, 100–101
Relationship
brief therapy and, 355
change and, 51–53
conflictual themes in, 38
functioning of, 402, 465–467
group psychotherapies and, 521,
532, 535
skills training and, 199–200
See also Family; Family therapy;
Marital therapy;
Therapeutic relationship
Relaxation training
behavior therapy and, 200–202
cognitive therapy and, 249
integrative approaches and, 330
systematic desensitization and,
183
Repertory grid technique, 286.
See also Assessment
Repression
historical background, 27
relational approaches to, 74
research support for, 94
Research support
for behavior therapy, 183
of case illustration usage, 18
for cognitive therapy, 234–235,
236–238
description, 16–17
for existential–humanistic
psychotherapies, 169–171
for group psychotherapies,
518–519
for integrative approaches,
338–340, 344
for marital therapy, 503
for person-centered
psychotherapy, 135–137
for postmodern approaches,
302–303
for psychoanalysis, 55–57
for relational approaches, 93–95
for single-session therapy,
383–385
therapeutic relationship, 207
Resistance
cognitive therapy, 251–252
description, 40–41

encounter with, 163–167
family therapy, 418, 422, 425, 429
focus on, 36
integrative approaches to,
331–332
interpretations of, 41–43
in person-centered therapy, 126
postmodern approaches to, 295
relational approaches to, 81–82
working through, 46
Response prevention, 197. See also
Behavior therapy
Responsibility
in cognitive therapy, 241
existential–humanistic
psychotherapies and,
151–153, 162–163, 169
Responsibility of change
description, 12
in family therapy, 427
See also Change mechanisms
Restructuring
description, 479–480
in marital therapy, 488
Revisitation, 165
Rituals in the family, 405,
432–433
Role of the therapist
in behavioral approaches to
martial therapy, 493
in brief therapy, 355–356
in experiential–humanistic
approaches to marital
therapy, 486, 488
in group treatments, 535–536
in integrative approaches to
marital therapy, 496–497
in postmodern approaches to
marital therapy, 501, 502
self-disclosure in group
treatment and, 537–538
in structural and strategic
approaches to marital
therapy, 480–481
in transgenerational approaches
to marital therapy,
475–476
Role playing
case illustration, 370
in cognitive therapy, 249
empty-chair technique, 124,
140–141, 170, 370
social skills training and, 199

Roles of family members,
405–405
Satir model of marital therapy,
485–487. See also Family
therapy; Marital therapy
Scaling questions
case illustration, 381
description, 380–381
in family therapy, 447–448
in marital therapy, 498
Schemas, personality and, 6–7
Schemata
activated during termination,
251
brief therapy and, 363
description, 230, 231–233
identifying via transference, 241
in personality disordered
patients, 256
Schizophrenia
existential–humanistic
psychotherapies and, 170
family functioning and, 409
family therapy and, 401,
448–451
integrative approaches and, 338
person-centered approach to,
117, 133
psychoanalysis and, 54
relational approaches to, 76, 91
Science of psychotherapy, 19
Sculpting, 486. See also Satir model
of marital therapy
Secondary-process thinking, 28
Security, need for, 74
Seduction theory, 32
Selective abstraction, 234. See also
Cognitive distortions
Self
postmodern approaches,
275–278
as a process, 115
See also Personality
Self-actualization
marital therapy and, 486
potential for, 111
relational approaches to, 79–80
See also Growth
Self-attunement, 488
Self-confrontation method,
286–287. See also
Assessment

Self-disclosure
　　description, 12
Self-disclosure *(continued)*
　　in existential–humanistic
　　　　psychotherapy, 161
　　in group treatments, 537–538
　　in person-centered therapy,
　　　　128
　　in relational approaches, 90
　　research support for, 136
　　during termination, 126
Self-efficacy, person-centered
　　　　approach to, 131–132
Self-esteem
　　marital therapy and, 485, 486
　　relational approaches to, 72, 94
Self-fulfilling prophecies, 324
Self-help treatment, 207–208
Self psychology
　　borderline personality and,
　　　　35–36
　　countertransference and, 89–90
　　description, 25, 31
　　historical background, 71–72
　　relationship and, 52
　　trends and, 63
　　See also Psychoanalysis
Self-report questionnaires
　　in cognitive therapy, 242–243
　　description, 8, 191
　　using in family therapy,
　　　　410–411
　　See also Assessment
Self-system, relational approaches
　　　　to, 72–73
Selves-in-context, 112
Semistructured interview,
　　　　190–191. *See also* Clinical
　　　　interview
Sexual drives. See Libidinal
　　　　drives
Sexual holonic mapping, 287–288.
　　　　See also Assessment
Sexuality
　　postmodern approaches to,
　　　　287–288
　　relational approaches to, 74
"Should" statements, 234. *See also*
　　　　Cognitive distortions
Single-session therapy, 383–385.
　　　　See also Brief therapy
Skeleton key question
　　description, 380

in marital therapy, 498
Skills training
　　in cognitive therapy, 249
　　communication, 199–200, 207,
　　　　490, 491–493
　　in marital therapy, 468,
　　　　489–490, 491–493
　　relaxation, 183, 200–202, 249,
　　　　330
Social anxiety
　　case illustration, 211–214t
　　cognitive therapy and, 239
Social class
　　behavior therapy and, 211
　　psychoanalysis and, 53–54
Social–linguistic systems
　　description, 277
　　psychological health and, 280
Social phobia, exposure treatment
　　　　and, 194–197t
Social skills training
　　in cognitive therapy, 249
　　description, 199–200
Solution-focused therapy
　　brief therapy and, 378–383,
　　　　380t
　　family therapy and, 447–448
　　marital therapy and, 497–499
Specialization in psychotherapy,
　　　　19–20
Splitting, borderline personality
　　　　and, 35–36
Stages of psychosexual
　　　　development, 29
Stance of the therapist
　　behavior therapy, 207–209
　　description, 11–13
　　existential–humanistic
　　　　psychotherapy, 155–168
　　experiential symbolic family
　　　　therapy, 427
　　group psychotherapies,
　　　　536–537
　　integrative approaches,
　　　　332–335, 496–497
　　intergenerational–contextual
　　　　family therapy, 422–423
　　marital therapy, 472, 475–476,
　　　　480–481, 486, 488
　　object relations family therapy,
　　　　419
　　person-centered therapy,
　　　　127–131

postmodern approaches,
　　　　297–299, 298t, 448, 499,
　　　　502
　　psychoanalysis, 47–51
　　psychoeducational approaches
　　　　to family therapy, 450–451
　　relational approaches, 82, 87–90
　　strategic family therapy, 430
　　structural family therapy, 437
　　systemic family therapy, 433
Standardized treatment, 192–193
Stimulus generalization, 186
Strategic therapy
　　brief therapy and, 376–378
　　family therapy and, 414t,
　　　　428–430
　　marital therapy and, 476–484
Strengths, relational approaches
　　　　and, 76
Stress, escalating, 437
Structural family therapy
　　description, 414t, 434–438
　　marital therapy and, 476–484
　　See also Family therapy
Structure of therapy
　　behavioral approaches, 193–203,
　　　　197t, 490, 491–493
　　cognitive–behavioral family
　　　　therapy, 440–444
　　cognitive therapy, 240–252
　　description, 19
　　existential–humanistic
　　　　psychotherapies, 154–168
　　experiential symbolic family
　　　　therapy, 425–427
　　group psychotherapies,
　　　　525–536, 529f, 534t
　　integrative approaches,
　　　　327–332, 495–496
　　intergenerational–contextual
　　　　family therapy, 421–422
　　object relations family therapy,
　　　　418–419
　　person-centered psychotherapy,
　　　　119–126
　　postmodern approaches,
　　　　288–297, 446–448,
　　　　498–499, 500–501,
　　　　501–502
　　psychoanalysis, 36–47
　　psychoeducational approaches
　　　　to family therapy, 449–450
　　relational approaches, 77–87

strategic family therapy, 429–430

structural and strategic approaches to marital therapy, 478–480, 482–484

structural family therapy, 436–437

systemic family therapy, 432–433

transgenerational approaches to marital therapy, 472–473, 475

Structured Clinical Interview for DSM-IV (SCID-IV), 191. *See also* Assessment; Clinical interview; DSM

Structured interview
as assessment, 8
in behavior therapy, 190–191
See also Clinical interview

Substance abuse
behavior therapy and, 203
integrative approaches and, 338
relational approaches and, 93

Suggestions in treatment, 36–37

Supportive psychotherapy
vs. psychoanalysis, 36
research support for, 93–94

Symptoms
of anxiety, 255
assessment of in behavior therapy, 188–192, 190*f*
brief therapy and, 355
Ericksonian therapies and, 371–372
marital therapy and, 477, 480
psychoanalytical theory and, 27, 31–33, 34–35
relational approaches to, 76, 78–79, 98

Systematic desensitization, 183. *See also* Behavior therapy

Systematic treatment selection, 327

Systemic approaches. *See* Family therapy; Marital therapy

Systemic family therapy, 414*t*, 430–434

Technical eclecticism
description, 320
in marital therapy, 493–494
personality and, 322

trends and, 344–345
See also Integrative approaches

Technical neutrality. *See* Analytic neutrality

Tenderness, need for, 74

Termination
from brief therapy, 354, 361*f*
case illustration, 100
from cognitive therapy, 250–251
description, 9, 13
from family therapy, 418–419, 427, 430
from group treatment, 532
from integrative approaches, 332
from marital therapy, 475, 484
from person-centered therapy, 126
from postmodern approaches, 296–297
from psychoanalysis, 46–47
from relational approaches, 87

Theoretical integration, 320–321. *See also* Integrative approaches

Therapeutic eclecticism, 128–129

Therapeutic pause, 158

Therapeutic relationship
assessment of, 77
in behavior therapy, 207–209
in brief therapy, 363
change and, 51–53
with children, 133
in cognitive therapy, 240–241, 241–242
description, 11–13
in existential–humanistic psychotherapy, 162–163
in family therapy, 418, 423–424, 427, 448, 450–451
in group psychotherapies, 536–537, 544
in integrative approaches, 318, 332–335, 336
in marital therapy, 470
mutual enactment and, 82–85
in person-centered therapy, 122, 127–131
in postmodern approaches, 297–299, 298*t*
in psychoanalysis, 47–51
in relational approaches, 70, 80, 87–90

working alliance aspect of, 44–46

Therapeutic stance
behavior therapy, 207–209
description, 11–13
existential–humanistic psychotherapy, 155–168
experiential symbolic family therapy, 427
group psychotherapies, 536–537
integrative approaches, 332–335, 496–497
intergenerational–contextual family therapy, 422–423
marital therapy and, 472, 475–476, 480–481, 486, 488
object relations family therapy, 419
person-centered therapy, 127–131
postmodern approaches, 297–299, 298*t*, 448, 499, 502
psychoanalysis, 47–51
psychoeducational approaches to family therapy, 450–451
relational approaches, 82, 87–90
strategic family therapy, 430
structural family therapy, 437
systemic family therapy, 433

Therapist role
in assessment, 8
in brief therapy, 377
description, 12
in person-centered therapy, 121, 132
in postmodern approaches to marital therapy, 499
in termination, 87

Therapist training, in brief therapy, 388–389

Therapy, 9–11. *See also* Practice of psychotherapy

Time-limited therapy, 10. *See also* Brief therapy; Managed health care

Training of therapists in brief therapy, 388–389

Trait theory, 6, 185. *See also* Personality theory

Transactional analysis
brief therapy and, 367–371

Transactional analysis *(continued)*
  disappearance of, 3
Transcendence, change and, 171
Transference
  analytic neutrality and, 48
  case illustration, 59–61, 95–100,
    342–343
  change and, 51–53
  in cognitive therapy, 241
  countertransference and, 49–50
  as a curative factor, 91–92
  description, 39–40
  in family therapy, 418, 423
  focus on, 36
  historical background, 26–27
  interpretations of, 41–43
  in marital therapy, 470, 475
  mutual enactment and, 82–85
  in person-centered therapy,
    129–131
  in postmodern approaches,
    298–299
  research support for, 94
  resistance and, 40–41
  trends and, 63
  working alliance and, 44–45
  during working through phase
    of treatment, 46
Transference cure, 80
Transgenerational approaches,
    470–476
Transtheoretical therapy
  assessment and, 327

diagnoses and, 325
research support for, 339
See also Integrative approaches
Trauma
  conditioning and, 184
  dissociation and, 73
  posttraumatic stress disorder as a
    result of, 195, 201, 239
  relational approaches to, 77, 93
Treatment. *See* Practice of
    psychotherapy
Treatment planning
  assessment and, 188
  in cognitive therapy, 241–242,
    243–244
Trends
  description, 18–20
  in existential–humanistic
    psychotherapies, 175–176
  in group treatments, 543–545
  in integrative approaches,
    344–345
  in marital therapy, 506–507
  in person-centered therapy,
    142–144
  in postmodern approaches,
    310–311
  in psychoanalysis, 62–64
  in relational approaches,
    100–101
Triangulation, 435
Two-person psychology. *See*
    Relational approaches

Unbalancing interventions, 480
Unconditional positive regard
  description, 127–128
  research support for, 170, 208
Unconscious
  description, 30
  experience and, 73
  See also Consciousness
Unfinished business, 125
Unstructured interview, 190–191.
    See also Assessment;
    Clinical interview
Unvalidated unconscious, 73. *See
    also* Unconscious

Vivification of resistance, 164–165.
    See also Resistance

Wishes
  description, 28, 30
  intrapsychic conflict and, 29
Working alliance, 44–46. *See also*
    Therapeutic relationship
Working through phase of
    treatment, 46, 61. *See also*
    Psychoanalysis

Yale–Brown
    Obsessive–Compulsive
    Scale (Y-BOCS), 191. *See
    also* Clinical interview